Community Health Care Nursing

Principles for Practice

Community Health Care Nursing

Principles for Practice

Edited by

Sheila Twinn PhD, BA(Hons), PGCEA, RHV, RGN, RSCN

Senior Lecturer, Department of Nursing, Faculty of Medicine, The Chinese University of Hong Kong; Formerly Lecturer, Department of Nursing Studies, King's College, University of London, UK

Barbara Roberts MSc, BA, RGN, RSCN, QN, RNT, CHNTCert

Nursing Education and Research Consultant; Formerly Professional Adviser in District Nursing, English National Board for Nursing, Midwifery and Health Visiting, London, UK

Sarah Andrews MSc, RGN, DN, CPT, PGCEA

Co-Director of Nursing, Camden and Islington Community Health Services NHS Trust, and Director of Nursing First; Formerly Director of The Queen's Nursing Institute, London, UK

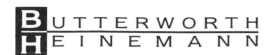

BUTTERWORTH HEINEMANN

Butterworth-Heinemann
Linacre House, Jordan Hill, Oxford OX2 8DP
A division of Reed Educational and Professional Publishing Ltd

℞ A member of the Reed Elsevier plc group

OXFORD   BOSTON   JOHANNESBURG
MELBOURNE   NEW   DELHI   SINGAPORE

First published 1996

© Reed Educational and Professional Publishing Ltd 1996

British Library Cataloguing in Publication Data
A catalogue record for this book is available from the British Library

ISBN 0 7506 1590 7

Typeset by Keytec Typesetting Ltd, Bridport, Dorset
Printed and bound in Great Britain by Clays Ltd, St. Ives plc

Contents

Contributors

John Atkinson BA, RGN, NDNCert, DipEd, DNT
Research Assistant

Cynthia Atwell RGN, OHNCert, CertEd(FE)
Principal Occupational Health Nursing Adviser, Railways Occupational
Health Ltd

Ann Bergen BA, MSc, RGN, DipN, DNCert, CertEd, DNT
Lecturer, Department of Nursing Studies, King's College, London

Jennifer Billings MSc, BSc(Hons), RGN, PGDipHV, DipN
Research Assistant

Annabel Broome BA, MSc, ABPsS, CPsychol
Chartered Psychologist, Annabel Broome Associates, Weymouth, Dorset

**Sarah Cowley BA, PhD, PGDipEd, RGN, RCNT, DipN, RHV, FWT,
HVT**
Senior Lecturer, Department of Nursing Studies, King's College, London

June Crown MA, MB, BChir, MSc, FRCP, FEPHM
Director, SE Institute of Public Health, Kent

Sue Davies MSc, BSc, RGN, HV
Lecturer, Postgraduate Research Centre, Sheffield North Trent College
of Nursing and Midwifery, Sheffield

Liz Day RGN, NDN, HV, PGCEA, BA, MA(Gerontol)
Senior Lecturer

Faye Doris MEd, RN, RM, ADM, PGCEA
Senior Midwife, Lecturer Practitioner, RD and E Hospitals, Exeter

John Dreghorn BA, RGN, DipPS, DipDN
Scottish Office, Home and Health, Department of Nursing Glasgow
Caledonia University, Glasgow, UK

Virginia Dunn BSc, MSc, Dip Christian Studies
Fellow and Macmillan Clinical Lecturer in Palliative Nursing, National
Institute for Nursing, Radcliffe Infirmary, Oxford

Dorothy Ferguson BA(Hons), MPH, RGN, SCM, RHV, OHNC, HVT
Lecturer, Department of Health and Nursing Studies, Glasgow Caledonia
University, Glasgow

Sarah Forester BSc, RGN, HVcert
Professional Officer (Education), Health Visitors Association, London

Kate Harmond MA, BA(Hons), SRN, RMN, SCM
Regional Nurse Adviser, Public Health Department, NHS Executive, South Thames, London

Sally Kendall PhD, BSc(Hons), RGN, RHV
Reader in Nursing, Buckinghamshire College, High Wycombe

Denise Knight RGN, RHV, BSc(Hons), MSc(Nursing), MSc(Psych), PGDE, RNT
Scheme Tutor(BSc Hons), Specialist Nursing Practice (Community)

Kate Lock BSc(Hons), RGN, DipDN
District Nursing Sister, Exeter

Ann Mackenzie MA, PhD, RGN, DN, RNT, DipEd
Professor of Nursing, Chinese University of Hong Kong

Alison Norman DMS, RGN, RM, RHV
Executive Director of Nursing and Clinical Director of Primary Care, Combined Health Centre, Stoke-on-Trent

Fedelmia O'Gorman BA(Hons), RGN, RHV
Health Visitor, Ormeau Road Health Centre, Belfast

Mary Pearce RGN, ONC, School Nurse Cert
School Health Nurse, Didcot Health Centre, Didcot

Liz Porter BA, PGCEA, RGN, RM, HV, CPT
Lecturer in Health Studies, Department of Sociology and Social Policy, University of Southampton

Sheila Roy
Director, Newchurch & Co Ltd, London

Kate Saffin MPhil, RN, RHV, CPT
Health Services Research Officer, Unit of Health Care Epidemiology, University of Oxford. Formerly: Professional Head of School Nursing, Oxford Community NHS Trust

David Sines BSc(Hons), PhD, RMN, RNMH, RNT, PGCTHE, FRCN
Professor of Community Health Nursing, Faculty of Social and Health Sciences, University of Ulster at Jordanstown, Northern Ireland

Verena Tschudin BSc(Hons), MA, RN, RM, DipCouns
Senior Lecturer, University of East London

Michael Weir BSc(Hons), MB, ChB, MFPHM
Director of the Crosthwaite Trust

Carole Whittaker RN, RM, RHV
Assistant Director of the Crosthwaite Trust

Lesley Whyte MPhil, BA, RGN, DNCert
Lecturer/Practitioner, Glasgow Caledonian University, Glasgow

Angela Williams BSc, RGN, DipDN
ICRF Research Sister, Churchill Hospital, Oxford

Preface

To edit a book in an area as complex as community health care nursing has been an exciting challenge. When the work started NHS reforms were in their infancy. As the text is published we are witnessing the dawn of a primary care led NHS with primary health care nursing set to become the pivotal specialism within nursing. Our intention is to provide practitioners and students with the opportunity of considering and exploring principles that not only inform current practice but also the future development of practice. In order to achieve this we have included contributions from authors from a range of disciplines and practice settings who have drawn on research based practice and professional expertise to discuss and debate principles underpinning care. In adopting this approach we have not attempted, nor indeed considered it appropriate to discuss the practice of individual professional groups within community health care nursing. However authors have drawn extensively on published material to illustrate principles for practice. Where possible examples from more than one professional group have been used, although in some cases this has not been feasible. In this situation it is anticipated that readers will draw on this material to apply the principles to their specific area of practice.

The pace of change in primary health care is unprecedented and editing a book at this time on a topic such as community health care nursing has not been an easy task for two main reasons; firstly the nature of change and secondly the diversity of practice. The changes not only relate to health care legislation but also to changes within the nursing profession. These seemingly continual changes have required us to constantly review the content of the book, as well as creating anxiety that there will inevitably be more changes before the book is available to readers. The contribution of nurses to commissioning and purchasing of services provides an example. The diversity of practice in community health care nursing provided our second major challenge in selecting a framework from which to organize the chapters within the book. Attempting to address principles for practice within practice settings ranging from public health nursing in the community to caring for acutely sick people in their own homes and the eight sub-specialities of the community practitioner (UKCC, 1994) demonstrates the challenge. However, although we believe that each discipline within community health care nursing has an individual and particular contribution to make to patient and client care there are principles for practice that are common within these different professional groups and it is these which have been developed within this text.

Another debate related to the term used to describe nurses practising at a specialist level in the community. Two policy documents *New World, New Opportunities* (NHSME, 1993) and *Report on Propos-*

als for the Future of Community Education and Practice (UKCC, 1991) used very different terms to describe the same practitioners in the community. The UKCC (1994) further added to the debate by introducing the term specialist practitioner and referring to specialist community nursing education and practice. After much discussion the decision was taken to use the term community health care nurse rather than either primary health care nurse or specialist community nurse. We believe this term sets community nursing firmly in the context of primary health care, while maintaining some consistency with the policy of the professional regulatory body.

A criticism of edited books, particularly with a large number of contributors, is that it creates a 'Smorgasbord' effect for readers. Although acknowledging this criticism, we believe this effect can be beneficial to readers, especially those studying at degree level, as it provides a range of different perspectives and views which should encourage practitioners to debate and challenge some current practices in the delivery of care. We have tried not to alter the authors' individual styles but have provided an introduction to each part of the book giving an overview of the major issues for discussion. We have cross referenced chapters where relevant and we hope readers will agree that the range of authors provides a stimulating resource text in which they can delve to explore practice issues in which they have a particular interest.

It is inevitable that there is repetition between chapters relating to the implementation of key health reforms, notably the *The NHS and Community Care Act* (1990) and *The Health of the Nation; a strategy for health in England* (1992) as well as the parallel strategies in Scotland, Wales and Northern Ireland which have become core objectives of the NHS. We are aware that the text largely relates to community health care nursing in the United Kingdom. However we hope that readers in other countries can gain from the principles underlying practice in various settings.

We make no apology for not focusing separate chapters on issues such as gender, culture or sexual orientation. We believe these issues to be fundamental to the delivery of high quality care, and as a consequence consider these issues should be integrated in the discussions informing principles for practice throughout the book. In addition we recognise that there are other topics such as clinical supervision that have not been addressed specifically. Although partly a consequence of the pace of change, it is also because we believe the significance of topics such as these require more consideration than can be given in a book considering principles for practice. Topics such as clinical supervision will therefore make up a series of texts for practitioners that will expand on issues contained in this book.

Finally we anticipate that practitioners and students alike will find this text useful in developing their practice to meet the changing demands of health care provision.

Sheila Twinn
Barbara Roberts
Sarah Andrews

1

Introduction–nursing for community health: changing professional issues

Sheila Twinn

● Introduction

Nursing, and nursing in the community in particular, has had to adapt to major changes which have arisen not only from government policy and the changing needs of society but also from within the profession itself. Policy changes involving major reorganizations of health and social services, with the consequent changes in nursing practice, have occurred on a continuous basis for nearly two decades. The more recent demand for value for money within the health service has also contributed to the demands made on practitioners (Audit Commission, 1992). Society and the health needs of individuals and communities in society continue to change in response to changing patterns of morbidity and mortality, demographic trends and increasing levels of stress. This has required practitioners to rethink the focus of their practice as well as the strategies used for patient and client care. Changes within the profession itself, such as a new strategy for nurse education, skill mix and the demand for outcome measures, require practitioners to reassess their professional expertise.

In addition, a range of policy documents has been produced which have particular relevance for nurses practising in the community. Documents such as *New World, New Opportunities* (NHSME, 1993a) identify specific contributions to the development of primary health care nursing (the term used to describe nurses with a post-registration qualification working in the community) in both policy formation and direct patient and client care. Other documents, such as that from the professional regulatory body, the United Kingdom Central Council for Nursing, Midwifery and Health Visiting (UKCC, 1991; UKCC, 1994), describe proposals for nurses practising in the community using the term community health care nursing. It is important to observe the difference in title used by these two significant documents to describe qualified practitioners in the community, which perhaps is indicative of some of the changes and issues currently facing practitioners. In this book the title community health care nursing has been chosen to describe the eight groups of specialist practitioners working in the community (UKCC, 1994). A similar debate occurs about the definition of community (McMurray, 1994). Here it has been defined as any place where people live and work in their ordinary lives and where interaction takes place between individuals, groups and communities; a definition which is reflected in later chapters of this book.

The aim of this chapter is therefore threefold: to explore the implications of the changing professional issues for community health care nursing, drawing on the development of the profession from both a historical and professional perspective, the changing emphasis in health care and issues fundamental to high-quality patient and client care. It is anticipated that using this approach will provide readers with a framework from which to consider not only the current context of community health care nursing but also future developments in practice.

● **Development of community health care nursing**

Historical context

In considering the historical factors influencing the development of nursing in the community, it is neither possible nor appropriate to include specific details of the different professional disciplines. It is obviously more appropriate for readers with an interest in a particular discipline to explore other sources of literature, particularly since most of the literature on the historical development of community health care nursing considers specific disciplines such as district nursing rather than the more generic concept of nursing in the community. However, there are some factors which are common to the development of different disciplines practising in the community. The first of these factors relates to the origin of the profession. This issue in itself raises an interesting debate for community health care nursing, since within district nursing and health visiting Florence Nightingale identified a common historical association between the two professional groups. Baly (1989), in her description of the role Nightingale played in the development of public health nursing, demonstrates the link between this activity and caring for sick people at home. A particularly important aspect was her recognition of the need to train nurses to care for people in their own homes, which led to communication with William Rathbone about the future direction of district nursing. Although Nightingale was not directly responsible for establishing either service, her influence is undeniable. In addition, many authors describe her as the first nursing theorist (George, 1990). This association also provides evidence of the deep historical roots of health visiting and district nursing. However, this association did not continue, with professional friction and misconceptions of each other's role developing between them.

The development of community psychiatric nurses (CPN) and community mental handicap nurses (CMHN) has little association with Florence Nightingale. Indeed, Thompson (1990) states that the 'Nightingale legacy has left the mental handicap nurse marginal to the main profession' and argues for the continuation of the association between CMHN and social services particularly in relation to the preparation of practitioners. Community psychiatric nursing developed directly from a hospital-based service and therefore it could be argued has a different philosophical base for care. The recent development of the practice nurse is again removed from the traditional development of health visiting and district nursing. Indeed, Stilwell (1991) suggests that the rapid growth of the number of practice nurses directly relates to government policies, in particular the introduction of the General Practitioner contract in 1990. This relatively new development in community health care nursing has met with mixed reactions from the more traditional practitioners and has added a further dimension to the context in which practitioners work in the community. Although this brief discussion is not able to consider all the different disciplines identified in community health care nursing, it demonstrates some major differences in the origins of these professional disciplines, which in part can be described in philosophical terms, and perhaps contributes to the difficulties experienced by practitioners in developing a common identity.

The difficulty in achieving a common identity can also be traced to the development of policies in health care, with perhaps once more the major division occurring between health visiting and district nursing and other practitioners in the community. The development of the Primary Health Care Team (PHCT) provides an illustration of this phenomenon. Government publications, such as circular CNO(77)8 (DHSS, 1977), set out the team members of PHCT, specifically identifying district nurses and health visitors as members of that team. However, there was no provision for CPNs or CMHNs to join PHCTs, reinforcing the isolation of these two groups in the community. Although the Harding Report (1981) highlighted some of the problems of community health care nurses working in PHCTs, particularly in urban areas where practitioners were once more taking responsibility for a geographical population, government policy continued to support the concept of the PHCT – a commitment which has continued and grown.

The Cumberlege Report continued the division of community practitioners by suggesting that 'CPN and mental handicap nurses should not be core members (of the PHCT), but should nevertheless work closely with the NNS (Neighbourhood Nursing Service) with a view to eventually becoming integrated' (DHSS, 1986). More recently, the GP contract, although providing enormous opportunity for practitioners to market community health care nursing, has highlighted the difficulty of practitioners such as CMHNs in providing a service that GPs wish to purchase on a continuing basis (Naughton, 1993b). It is interesting that when exploring policy issues in the context of the historical development of community health care nursing, the influence of organizational factors becomes evident.

Although government policy has obviously influenced the development of nursing in the community, other factors have played a significant role. These factors not only include issues directly relating to practitioners, such as preparation and management, but also the professional context of community health care nursing. Indeed, an understanding of these issues is essential if the current context of practice is to be understood by practitioners in order to benefit patient and client care.

Professional context

Despite the changing emphasis from secondary to primary health care, and an increasing number of policy documents raising the profile of practitioners in the community, Roy (1991) argues that community health care nurses continue to seek reassurance of the significance of their contribution to the health care of individuals and communities. In part this phenomenon may be attributed to factors such as the division that has developed among the different disciplines of community health care nurses and the lack of a cohesive identity among practitioners. Indeed, until the publication in 1991 of the UKCC report on the proposals for the future of community education and practice, there had been little attempt even to identify those practitioners included within the concept of community health care nursing.

This phenomenon is more clearly demonstrated in a brief review of the literature. Kratz (1982), in her paper on excellence in community health care nursing, confines her discussion to health visitors, district nurses, midwives and community psychiatric nurses. In a publication providing a comprehensive review of research and developments in community nursing, the authors state they have confined their definition to those 'most closely involved in the day to day work of providing primary care', describing these as health visitors, district nurses, health authority treatment room nurses and practice employed nurses (Baker *et al.*, 1987). In the author's view this definition highlights two observations; first the fact that at the time of publication of this review health visitors demonstrated a reluctance at being included within the definition of nursing, and secondly, the almost interchangeable use of the term treatment room nurse and practice nurse for practitioners who had quite different professional responsibilities.

It is interesting that the Cumberlege Report, the first major policy document reviewing the role of nurses practising in the community, continued to differentiate among those practitioners included within the term 'community nursing' (DHSS, 1986). Indeed, an explicit definition is given of the term community nursing, stating it is used to discuss 'the services provided generally by health visitors, district nurses, school nurses and their support staff of registered and enrolled nurses' (DHSS, 1986). The definition goes on to state that where the work of practitioners such as CPN is described, the specific name of the practitioner will be used. However, a similar report undertaken for the Welsh Office adopted a different approach of using client groups with whom nurses practise to identify professional groups in the community (Welsh Office, 1987). Although Butterworth (1988) highlighted the need for community health care nurses to present a strong collective identity, it is interesting that he also differentiated, at the time of this publication, between community health care nurses and health visitors.

The most recent review of community health care nursing in England, although using the term 'primary health care nurse', provides a much more extensive definition by including within this term all those practitioners 'working outside hospital who have been fully prepared through training and education for the clinical responsibilities needed to deliver primary health care in the community' (NHSME, 1993b).

It is evidence such as this which illustrates not only the opportunity for confusion of role experienced by many practitioners, but also the complexity of relationships among the different professionals. It can be argued that this confusion has contributed to the need to seek continued reassurance of their contribution to health care. In addition, organizational factors, including the preparation and management of practitioners, contribute to the context in which community health care nurses currently practise, which has implications for the development of practice of patient and client care.

● **Preparation and management of community health care nursing**

The inconsistency in the professional preparation of practitioners in the community provides a useful illustration of the implications of organizational factors to the current context of community health care nursing. This is particularly so since the inconsistency is related equally to both the professional and academic components of courses. Undoubtedly this anomaly has been emphasized by the phenomenon which requires health visitors to obtain an additional statutory registrable qualification, whereas the preparation for school nurses is still not mandatory. Although this illustration is particularly relevant because of the similarities in practice of these two groups of practitioners, a similar situation has existed with practice nurses. The requirement by the UKCC (UKCC, 1994) for common standards of preparation overcomes the problems of inconsistency in professional preparation; however, the continuing anomaly of a statutory qualification for one professional group remains, creating feelings of elitism and resentment among practitioners. Although the introduction of shared learning among students on post-registration courses has begun to address these issues, discrepancies remain contributing to negative effects on teamwork and hindering a common professional identity.

The management structure of nurses working in the community remains a complex issue, which is neither appropriate nor possible to address in detail in this book. However, there are some issues which are particularly relevant to the development of community health care nursing which will be explored in general terms, to provide an understanding of the contextual setting for the current situation experienced by many practitioners. The first and most significant of these issues is the recurrent reorganization of the National Health Service (NHS).

Although the changing structure of the NHS is considered in depth in Chapter 2, in the context of current practice, it is perhaps relevant to consider here the major influences on community health care nursing. The reorganization of the NHS in 1974 provides an important starting point, since it was then that district nurses, health visitors and school nurses were removed from their roots in the Local Authority structure to become part of the NHS. Some authors suggest this move provided a major stimulus for practitioners in seeking reassurance for the continuation of their existence, particularly as their practice and contribution to health care was compared with that of the acute sector (Robinson, 1985). Although it is possible to argue that until the implementation of the NHS and Community Care Act 1990 further reorganizations had little effect on field staff, the continued reorganizations have contributed to the difficulty of developing a cohesive team, particularly since some districts lost their discrete community units (Baker *et al.*, 1987).

The influence of the personnel responsible for managing community health care nurses is also a significant factor in its development. Although previous reorganizations had provided for management of practitioners by community health care nurses, organizational units were frequently quite distinct. This is illustrated by the situation where health visitors were organized and managed as a distinct district-wide service and district nursing was managed as another quite separate unit. An important recommendation of the Cumberlege Report (DHSS, 1986) was that each Neighbourhood Nursing Team should be headed by a manager chosen for his/her management skills and leadership qualities. The fact that the professional discipline was less significant than the managerial skills of the individual, stimulated a major debate among practitioners. Clay (1986) highlighted the issue of so much professional energy being invested in the debate of whether a health visitor could manage district nurses rather than on the more significant practice issues which were raised in the report. Although this illustration relates to only two of the disciplines within community health care nursing, it provides another example of the issues which have hindered the development of a cohesive approach to patient and client care.

● Organization of the Profession and Professional Practice

In considering the implications of organizational factors on the development of a profession or professional group, two issues require addressing: first the organization of the profession, and secondly, the organization of practice. The organization of the profession has influenced the development of community health care nursing in several different ways. The first and perhaps most significant relates to the size of the workforce within each discipline. The Audit Commission (1992) demonstrated that over half of the community health expenditure funded nursing activity. However, if this nursing activity is broken down into professional groups, 24% of the expenditure resources district nursing whereas only 4% is used to resource community psychiatric nursing. Although these figures may reflect the size of the workforce, it raises questions about the extent to which this allocation necessarily reflects the health needs of the population. Indeed, it could be argued that with the workforce of practice nurses doubling between 1988 and 1990, questions should be asked as to whether resources are being used to the best effect in patient and client care. Without systematic observation of the service it is impossible to answer this type of question. In addition, questions such as these contribute to the rivalry and mistrust which, although decreasing, continues to exist between some practitioners.

The organization of this workforce is also an important issue within the development of community health care nursing and one that has become more complex following the implementation of the NHS and Community Care Act 1990. The Roy Report (NHSME, 1990) attempted to address this issue by suggesting five different models for organizing and managing nursing practice in the community. The implementation of the NHS and Community Care Act 1990, however, overtook these recommendations by establishing community trusts and GP fund-holding practices. Although the implications of these structures are discussed in detail in Chapters 2 and 10, respectively, the significance and complexity of these changes in ensuring the effective use of resources must be acknowledged.

The professional organizations responsible for community health care nursing have also contributed to its development. For some organizations, such as the Health Visitors Association, this involved active participation of the organization and its members, to maintain the distinct professional identity of health visiting. More recently, the organization has developed a different philosophy, acknowledging that health visiting is part of nursing, and has considered expanding the terms of reference to allow other community nurses to join the organization. The merger of this organization with another major trade union has facilitated this process, particularly since the Community Psychiatric Nursing Association (CPNA) has merged with the same trade union, and developments such as this facilitate professional unity over health issues in the community. Indeed, it could be argued that a weakness in the development of community health care nursing has been the apparent striving among organizations for membership rather than for the cohesive development of practitioners.

The final organizational issue influencing the development of community health care nursing relates to the statutory bodies responsible for professional education and the regulation of the profession. In 1983, the statutory bodies responsible for the education of different nursing disciplines in the community were incorporated into the National Boards for Nursing, Midwifery and Health Visiting for England, Scotland, Wales and Northern Ireland. This provided the opportunity to develop a more cohesive approach to community health care nursing. However, the National Boards responded to this opportunity in different ways, with some time elapsing before the elected membership of the English Board used the opportunity to implement shared preparation for practice and establish a Primary Health Care Committee. It is perhaps important to acknowledge that these changes were at times difficult to achieve and implement, partly because of the different opinions and perceived lack of cohesion among members of the board. A similar situation occurred within the United Kingdom Central Council for Nursing, Midwifery and Health Visiting, where the range of opinions of elected members has contributed at times to the lack of cohesiveness among practitioners, making the process of change complex.

The organization of practice raises some similar issues. One method of organizing practice is the concept of the PHCT, and some of the issues involved in practising in this way have previously been discussed. However, the work of the PHCT has been influenced by different approaches to the organization of community health care nursing. Where neighbourhood nursing teams provided the organizing focus for practice, although clear advantages for practice were demonstrated, identification of practice priorities, particularly with General Practitioners and practice nurses, created some difficulties in developing a cohesive approach to community health care. The introduction of a market economy in health care, and within that context the implementation of GP Fund Holders, has had major implications for the organization of practice. Naughton (1993a) argues that this approach to care makes increasing demands on the services of community health care nurses. She goes on to argue that GPs, in promoting the concept of the nurse practitioner, are increasingly supporting staff to attend appropriate courses. Developments such as these have both short- and long-term implications for community health care nursing. The change in legislation also introduced the concept of quality assurance and cost effectiveness to community health care nursing, both of which have significant implications for the organization of care. This has required both practitioners and managers to focus on the outcomes of practice, which has raised questions about whether the organization of practice is always appropriate to the health needs of the population. Developments such as these provide major challenges to the organization of practice among community health care nurses.

Finally, the individual practitioner's interpretation of practice continues to have implications for the organization of practice, both in terms of the development of community health care nursing and the quality of care offered to patients and clients. This issue is addressed in Chapter 3, but also has implications for the professionalization of community health care nursing.

● **Professionalization of community health care nursing**

The professionalization of community health care nursing remains a tortuous process not only because of general questions such as the extent to which nursing can be described as a profession, but also the more complex question of the different professions involved in community health care nursing. Although once again it is inappropriate in a book such as this to explore this issue in depth, it is appropriate to consider in general terms some of those factors which have influenced this process. Prior to discussing these factors it is important briefly to state the context in which the term professionalization is being used, particularly since there is no attempt to use the term in its true sociological sense. Indeed, even using the criteria, such as specialized knowledge and skills, providing a service to society, a lifetime career commitment, control over practice and a code of ethics, identified by authors such as Oermann (1991) in their debate about the professionalization of nursing, highlights the complexity of the question.

Therefore, for the purpose of this discussion a much more pragmatic interpretation of the term has been chosen. This interpretation is similar to that described in the strategy for nursing 'Vision for the Future' (NHSME, 1993b), which cites issues such as quality of care, professional development and professional and clinical leadership. It is therefore for this reason that three general issues to explore have been highlighted: the scope of professional practice, the changing professional role of practitioners, and the implications of changing policies for those roles. It is these factors which in the author's view have particularly contributed to tribalism, a phenomenon which has hindered the cohesive development of community nursing (Gordon, 1991).

In the position statement on the scope of professional practice (UKCC, 1992), professional practice was not only defined in terms of knowledge, skills, responsibility and accountability, but as a dynamic activity which must respond sensitively to the changing needs of individual patients and clients. Implicit within this definition is the changing structure of professional practice, highlighting the need for practitioners to recognize the scope of practice and in turn the implications for practice. In order to help practitioners acknowledge this changing role within the scope of professional practice, the UKCC identified the following six principles to ensure high quality care:

- that each aspect of practice is directed towards meeting the needs and serving the interests of patients and clients
- always endeavour to achieve, maintain and develop knowledge, skill and competence to respond to those needs and interests
- honestly acknowledge any limits of personal knowledge and skill and take the necessary steps to remedy any relevant deficits
- ensure that any enlargement or adjustment of the scope of professional practice be achieved without compromising or fragmenting existing aspects of care
- recognize and honour the direct or indirectly personal accountability borne for all aspects of professional practice
- avoid any inappropriate delegation to others which compromises the interests of patients and clients (UKCC, 1992).

Although readers will be familiar with these principles, it is perhaps helpful to illustrate the implications for the development of practice in the community by using one principle within one professional group.

The third principle described above requires practitioners to 'honestly acknowledge limits of personal knowledge and skill and take the necessary steps to remedy any relevant deficits' (UKCC, 1992). Using this principle as an illustration within health visiting, two particular issues are raised: the need for practitioners to develop skills in groupwork to meet changing health needs, and to collaborate with community psychiatric nurses to meet the needs of women with postnatal depression (Mac-Intosh, 1993). Where practitioners have failed to recognize limits in their expertise to meet the scope of professional practice, there are implications for quality of care, both in terms of responding to individual need as well as hindering the development of teamwork in practice. Unless practitioners are willing to recognize the principles underlying the scope of professional practice, the development of professionalism is likely to be compromised.

Implicitly linked to the scope of professional practice is the changing professional role of practitioners. The extent to which practitioners are prepared to adapt their role to meet new health needs also influences both patient care and the effectiveness of teamwork. Again an example from health visiting provides an illustration of the implications of this phenomenon in the process of professionalization. In a study of the interpretation of professional practice in health visiting, Twinn (1991) describes the development of four paradigms of practice which have particular implications for the changing role of practitioners.

The paradigms of practice, illustrated in Figure 1.1, demonstrate the different approaches practitioners may adopt for practice. The directive individual approach provides a traditional interpretation of practice, with the emphasis placed in maternal and child health. Where practitioners have adopted this approach as the predominant focus of practice, it limits their ability to respond to the changing health needs of a practice population. In contrast, the directive collective approach, while allowing a public health focus in practice, may limit practitioners to working in only traditional public health arenas rather than those appropriate to the needs of individuals and the communities in that practice setting (Ashton, 1990). A similar critique is equally applicable to the two remaining approaches to practice. Although these paradigms are not mutually exclusive, with practitioners frequently using more than one approach in their practice, the illustration highlights the need for practitioners to develop an underpinning framework for practice, informing both practice and professional judgement – a process which applies equally to other disciplines.

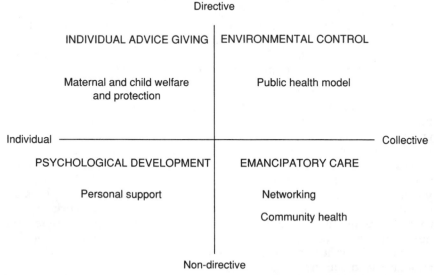

Figure 1.1 Roles and paradigms in health visiting (From Twinn, 1991, by permission)

The implications of a framework for practice are discussed in more detail in Chapter 7. However, where practitioners have developed a framework to underpin practice it not only allows them to articulate their practice but more significantly identify practice in terms of patient and client outcomes. This approach is particularly important following the implementation of the purchaser–provider model in health care. Indeed, the development of a framework to underpin practice allows practitioners not only to adapt their practice to meet changing health needs, but also to respond to the demands of changing policies in practice without fearing that these policies will lessen their professional contribution to health care. It is in ways such as this that changing professional roles have contributed to the professionalization of community nursing.

Changing policies have been equally influential in changing professional roles which in turn has influenced the professionalization of community health care nursing. Although the implications of these policies are considered in greater depth later in this chapter, there are particular policies which have significant implications for the professional role of community health care nurses. The implementation of a market economy in health care provides just one example. The policies resulting from the NHS and Community Care Act 1990 have far-reaching implications for community health care nursing which are outlined in later chapters in this book, but in terms of professionalization the introduction of skill mix plays a major role. Although the literature demonstrates the contentious nature of skill mix (Gibbs *et al.*, 1991), skill mix has been implemented to a greater or lesser extent in community health care nursing (Laurent, 1992; Cowley, 1993). Despite the research published by Lightfoot and Baldwin (1992), suggesting that disciplines within community health care nursing have different perceptions of the value of skill mix, there is little doubt within the current professional climate that skill mix provides an important challenge to the professional expertise of practitioners in the community – a challenge that must be addressed from the perspective of the quality of patient and client care.

The implementation of Project 2000 has obviously contributed to the skill mix debate, since this group of practitioners, although not holding a post-registration qualification in community health care nursing, have been prepared to practice equally in an institution or community setting. Indeed Project 2000 nurses provide care which complements that provided by highly qualified community practitioners, without necessarily compromising the philosophy that better qualified nurses provide better quality of care (Centre for Health Economics, 1992). Undoubtedly the introduction of Project 2000 has provided practitioners with the opportunity to reconsider their professional practice in the light of the need to provide high-quality but cost-effective care. It is issues such as this, which although challenging, need to be considered if practitioners are to continue the development of community health care nursing to meet future needs and challenges.

It is clear therefore that there is a range of issues which have influenced and will continue to influence the professional development of community health care nursing. Although some of these issues appear stimulating and exciting to practitioners, others will be less so, perhaps to the extent of appearing threatening. However, whether practitioners agree or disagree with the changes it is important that practitioners understand the issues involved in the changes, so that debate, supported by appropriate evidence, can take place to further professional development. It is obvious that this debate will need to occur within the changing emphasis in health care currently facing practitioners in the community.

● **Changing emphasis in health care: the implications for community health care nurses**

The brief discussion about the implementation of skill mix highlights the implications of policy changes for practitioners. However, the implementation of skill mix is only one of the major policy changes which have taken place over recent years, many of which are significant for community health care nurses; in particular in the changing emphasis of health care. Although once again these changes are discussed in detail in later chapters in the book, it is important to consider in general terms the implications of these major changes for community health care nursing. Despite the definition of a major policy document differing among practitioners and different disciplines, there are specific policies which have influenced the emphasis in health care and it is these which are considered in the following discussion.

Perhaps the most significant in terms of health care has been the change in emphasis from institution to community care. Within this context there has also been a shift in emphasis from secondary to primary care. Although these policy changes have implications for practitioners, the change in community care introduced in April 1993 perhaps has the greatest significance for practice. Some practitioners will view this opportunity positively, as described in Chapter 30 in the discussion on case management, whereas others have concerns as to the extent to which this change in policy erodes the contribution of health care to vulnerable members of the community. Another very significant change is the shift away from acute health care to health promotion. Although this change in emphasis was first demonstrated in 1986 in the consultative document produced by the Conservative Government (Secretary of State for Social Services, 1986), the implementation of the General Practitioner Contract in 1990 particularly highlighted the implications for community health care nursing (Turner, 1990). In addition, policy changes have influenced not only lifestyles of individuals and communities, but also perceptions of dependency levels and episodes of care. Although these issues are explored in detail in later chapters in the book, some are particularly significant to the development of community health care nursing and the perceptions practitioners have of one other's contribution to patient care. The most fundamental of these issues in the author's view is that of the implementation of community care.

Readers will be familiar with the requirement for Local Authorities to 'become responsible in collaboration with medical, nursing and other interests for assessing individual need, designing care arrangements and securing their arrangements within available resources' (DoH, 1989).

In addition, some practitioners will have considerable experience in the implementation of the Act, particularly in the assessment of health need. Indeed, a major concern about the implementation of the Act related to the fundamental conflict created for authorities in identifying need, then having a statutory responsibility to meet that need in a climate of diminishing resources and no ring-fencing of funds.

The Act also raised questions about the relationship between social and health care. Jackson (1993) describes different projects which have been established around the country in an attempt to overcome the problems of roles and relationships among social service and health care staff. The importance of an integrated assessment and referral system is clearly highlighted in providing high-quality care, particularly since it is often difficult to make a clear distinction between the different needs of patients and their carers. However, there is also the question of the extent to which the service provided meets needs as determined by the patient or client, which is particularly significant when considering the narrow grey line between social and health care. It is issues such as these which raise questions about the working relationship between practitioners and their colleagues in social services, in particular partnership in care.

Indeed, the relationship between social services and health care highlights the need for interprofessional collaboration if patient needs are to be met. Jackson (1993) highlights the significance of a clear distinction between needs assessment and case management to prevent the formation of a resource-led rather than a needs-led service – an approach which requires skilled interprofessional collaboration. Although this issue is discussed in depth in Chapter 30, it is important to note here that intercollaborative work between health care and social services practitioners has frequently failed to provide high-quality care (Audit Commission, 1992).

Evidence such as this highlights the significance of this policy change in the development of community health care nursing. It demands effective teamwork, not only among other disciplines within nursing in the community, but also among other professionals and voluntary groups. It requires practitioners to recognize gaps in service provision and respond to those service gaps using strategies based on the purchaser–provider philosophy. It requires practitioners clearly to articulate their practice, and in particular practice outcomes, so that other health care workers can be used where appropriate. This highlights the importance of skill mix in this approach to care. Finally, it requires practitioners clearly to acknowledge their particular expertise and make appropriate referrals to other practitioners.

The publication of the *Health of the Nation* (DoH, 1992) is a culmination of several documents demonstrating a change of emphasis in government policy from a sickness service to a health service. The White Paper argues that the overall goal of the government is to improve the health of the nation by adding years to life and life to years. It goes on to argue that this will be achieved through public policies, healthy surroundings, healthy lifestyles and high-quality health services. It states that it recognizes these are not new goals but those identified in the World

Health Organisation publication *Health For All in the Year 2000* (WHO 1978, 1985). However, what is new is the commitment to health promotion and disease prevention as well as treatment, care and rehabilitation. Indeed, the White Paper claims a commitment to improving and maintaining health rather than merely health care.

In order to achieve this the White Paper highlights five areas as key areas. These key areas were selected using the following criteria:

- the area should be a major cause of premature death or avoidable ill health
- effective interventions should be possible, offering significant scope for improvement in health
- it should be possible to set objectives and targets and monitor progress towards them.

Using these criteria the key targets were identified as coronary heart disease and strokes, cancers, mental illness, HIV/AIDs and sexual health and accidents. In each of these key areas targets for action were identified; to reduce the death rate from breast cancer in the population invited for screening by at least 25% by the year 2000 provides an example of one such target. It is interesting that the targets generally relate to very specific epidemiological data rather than issues in social policy which caused considerable criticism of the document. Indeed, despite the government's stated commitment to health and health promotion, the total lack of any mention of poverty raises questions about the extent of this commitment in reality. Despite this serious omission, the publication of a document demonstrating a major commitment to health promotion and disease prevention, with particular reference to mental health, has implications for nurses working in the community, which are discussed in detail in Chapter 3. However, the direct link between the targets and health data has particular relevance to the development of community health care nursing as practice responds to identified health needs.

Indeed, the response to identified health need illustrates further the changing emphasis in health care which has resulted not only from the introduction of GP Contracts, including screening programmes for people over 75, but also from the emphasis on health need identified from epidemiological data. Recent (1993) figures from the HMSO's *Population Trends* illustrated a decrease in the infant mortality rate to 7.4 per 1000 live births, but an increasing suicide rate among men. Evidence such as this provides a stimulus for practitioners to reconsider workloads and ensure that practice is needs-led rather than by rituals and traditions. In addition, this changing emphasis provides the opportunity for practitioners within community health care nursing to focus more on health promotion, particularly in primary prevention, than they have done previously. In order to achieve this it is necessary for practitioners to recognize the contribution made by the different disciplines in the community and to work collaboratively to achieve high-quality care, a process which will require many practitioners to develop their skills in teamwork.

However, it is not only changing health policies that have led to a change in emphasis in health care, but also changes in social structure and in turn the lifestyle of individuals and communities. The growing population of elderly people, with the increasing demands on their carers, presents a shift in practice profiles. The increasing number of people who are HIV positive highlights the continuing need for health promotion and health education, particularly since little success has been achieved to date in the treatment of AIDs. The growing incidence of poverty and homelessness also makes increasing demands on community health care nurses and the quality of care they can offer to people living in adverse social situations.

This changing social structure has coincided with an increasing incidence of stress-related illness. Although this increase relates to both physical and mental health problems, mental health issues particularly highlight altered trends in health needs. The consequences of mental ill health is demonstrated in certified sickness levels, increasing levels of substance and alcohol abuse and increasing suicide rates, particularly among young men. This evidence highlights not only the need for practitioners in the community to reassess priorities in health care and the identification of health need, but also the growing demand for practitioners with expertise in mental health to collaborate and liaise with other practitioners.

Within this changing social structure homelessness has emerged as a major challenge to health care. This is demonstrated not only by the number of people sleeping on the streets or in hostels, but also by the number of families currently dependent on bed and breakfast accommodation for their home. The challenge for practitioners in meeting needs presented by this group of people is considerable, partly created by the difficulties frequently experienced by people who are homeless in registering with a GP and partly because the traditional service provision, for a variety of reasons, is inappropriate. Health schemes such as those run in hostels for the homeless illustrate how health needs can be met (Pollock, 1993). Although the implications for community health care nursing are discussed in detail in Chapter 17, for many practitioners this is a very different approach to practice, highlighting not only the need to reconsider practice in the context of the health needs of different populations, but also in the development of practice.

Indeed, the changing lifestyle of many individuals and communities has significant implications for developments in practice. The most obvious is the need for practitioners to base their practice on identified health needs of the practice population, involving the use of epidemiological data and practice profiling. Although this intervention is discussed in detail in Chapter 23, it is important to acknowledge the importance of practitioners working closely with colleagues within the field of public health. In using this approach to practice it also allows practitioners to meet the requirements of Commissioning Agents which is essential to the development of community health care nursing. It also highlights the need for practitioners to develop and implement innovative approaches to practice, moving on from traditional areas which for some practice populations are no longer appropriate – a process which some practitioners may find both demanding and challenging.

Another significant issue influencing the emphasis in care is the changing definition of episodes of care and dependency levels of clients and patients. Although the complexity of identifying appropriate dependency measures in community health care nursing has been identified (Durand, 1989; Hays, 1992), there is clear evidence to suggest that patient dependency levels are increasing. This not only relates to factors such as increasing numbers of frail elderly living in the community, but also to the introduction of schemes such as Hospital at Home (Young, 1991). Although for many practitioners, particularly those with a major responsibility for health promotion, it is inappropriate to describe care in terms of dependency levels, the increasing complexity of health promotion is equally apparent. Indeed, developing effective strategies in health promotion to meet the health needs outlined earlier involves high levels of skill and collaboration. In addition, the increasing demand for practitioners to measure the impact of nursing interventions adds to the complexity of the situation, particularly since it is an area of practice in which developments have been relatively slow (Barriball and Mackenzie, 1992).

Throughout this discussion of the changing emphasis in health care, the implications for practice have been repeatedly highlighted. It is this type of evidence which demands that practitioners reconsider their practice to ensure it meets changing health needs. In order to achieve this outcome, practitioners will need to use research findings to underpin new directions in practice. Although it is evident that practice must adapt to current health needs, there are fundamental practice issues which have not changed and are essential to the process of providing high-quality care. Since these fundamental issues, such as the values and beliefs of practitioners, underpin the different concepts and practice interventions explored in the book, it is important to consider these issues in relation to the current context of community health care nursing.

● **Fundamental issues in practice**

Although the earlier discussion emphasizes the changing practice of community health care nursing, there are practice issues which are fundamental to providing high-quality care. The most significant of these factors must relate to the values and beliefs of the practitioner. It is the values and beliefs of practitioners which influence their approach to patient and client care, an issue which is discussed in more depth in Chapter 7. However, a major factor influencing these values and beliefs relates to the ethical principles of the practitioner. Although the issue is explored in detail in Chapter 9, the ethics underpinning practice provide a fundamental issue in the development of current and future practice in community health care nursing. Implicitly related to the ethics of the practitioner is his/her respect for individuals and client groups, particularly those people to whom discriminatory practice is evident. This not only includes people from ethnic minority groups, but also the elderly or people with different sexual orientations. However, fundamental to these issues is the knowledge and understanding of the practitioner, highlighting the essential role of research and the implementation of research findings in practice. Although these fundamental practice issues are not unique to community health care nursing, there are factors which are significant to practitioners specifically working in community settings and therefore frequently working in relative professional isolation.

The first of these arises within the ethical dimension of practice. Tschudin (1992) suggests that caring is a basis for ethical issues in nursing. Although caring is itself a complex concept to define, with definitions varying with different contexts and professions, there are specific issues which arise in nursing in the community. Perhaps the most significant of these are the different dimensions of caring with which the practitioner is involved. Caring not only involves the patient or client but equally the carers of that person. Although nurses working in an institutional setting might quite rightly argue that their caring also extends to the family of the patient, it is a very different situation when the carer is providing the majority of the care, with the practitioner supporting and complementing that care. It raises questions about how practitioners work with both the carer and the person. This is particularly relevant when the person and the carer have different needs which may even be conflicting, a situation which is not unusual when working with vulnerable groups such as people with learning difficulties, children and the elderly. This may influence the development of the caring relationship with both the individual and their carer, and the implications for practice are discussed further in Chapter 13.

The relationship with the carer, however, is not the only factor highlighting the uniqueness of caring in community health care nursing. The setting in which that caring is carried out is also significant and may challenge the values and beliefs of practitioners. Obviously, with practitioners working in people's homes and other community settings they are exposed to an enormous range of situations, some of which may be either challenging or even threatening. The practitioner needs to adapt to these different settings, offering respect and care to patients and clients, a process which requires skill and expertise from the practitioner.

The different settings in which the practitioner works implicitly requires involvement with many different client groups, demonstrating the breadth of the definition of community. Among these groups are people from ethnic minorities, many of whom continue to receive an inferior quality of service. This situation may result from either practice or service provision. The need for the improvement of services to meet the needs of specific ethnic groups has been argued. The study undertaken by Cameron et al. (1988) demonstrated that black clients received proportionally less resources than white clients. Both of these situations provide illustrations of the discriminatory practices which continue to influence the quality of care offered to some patients and clients.

However, these practices are not restricted to people from ethnic minority groups. Research studies demonstrate that elderly people also experience reduced quality of care both in terms of practice and service provision. It is perhaps important to also acknowledge that these practices are also associated with gender and sexual orientation. Cameron et al. (1988) demonstrated that elderly female carers received less resources than elderly male carers. Discriminatory practices towards people with different sexual orientations has been particularly significant since the rapid increase in HIV infection. Although it is now acknowledged that heterosexual, rather than homosexual, transmission is now a major source of communicating the HIV virus, research suggests that attitudes of practitioners in the community remain negative to working with people with AIDs (Bond et al., 1990). Indeed, any discriminatory practice obviously influences the quality of care, demonstrating the fundamental role of the values and beliefs of practitioners to practice.

An important factor contributing to discriminatory practice relates to the knowledge of practitioners, which in turn influences their values and beliefs. The use of research plays an important role in informing both knowledge and understanding, and the significance of research in the development of practice has been highlighted in the report published by the Department of Health on research and development in nursing (DoH, 1993). In community health care nursing the significance of research and the implementation of research findings are equally important, but again there are some factors which relate specifically to practitioners in the community; in particular the scarcity of published research, support for practitioners undertaking research, the utilization of research findings in practice and finally the need to develop excellence in practice through the expansion of Nursing Development Units (NDUs).

The relative paucity of published research in community health care nursing obviously makes it difficult for practitioners to access material to use in the development of practice. In part, this absence of research highlights the difficulties practitioners experience in attracting funds for community projects. Both the changing emphasis in health care and the *Report of the Taskforce on the Strategy for Research in Nursing, Midwifery and Health Visiting* (DoH, 1993) are welcomed as a method of overcoming this issue. However, many practitioners need support in developing their research skills. This support not only relates to appropriate expertise and skills, but also support in terms of management – a situation which has become more complex following the implementation of the purchaser–provider philosophy in health care. However, where research does exist, practitioners also need support in its implementation and the relatively small number of NDUs in the community may have contributed to this situation. Where NDUs have been established they provide the opportunity for practitioners to develop expertise in practice which obviously has implications for the quality of care. Indeed, the importance of research to the quality of practice is demonstrated in the following chapters by the continuous attempt to use research to illustrate the foundations of practice and issues within practice.

● **Conclusion**

This review of developments in community health care nursing illustrates not only the continuing change facing practitioners, but also the significance of fundamental practice issues to high-quality care. It is unlikely that this situation will change, since both society and health needs will continue to change as we move towards the twenty-first century. So if community health care nursing is considered within this context, it demonstrates that for practice to continue to develop practitioners will need to strive towards four aims:

- responding to continuing changes in practice
- developing proactive changes in practice
- adapting and developing practice
- offering high-quality care within existing resources.

Developing a proactive approach to practice is particularly significant in moving practice forward and facing the challenges of continuing change. However, the research literature in managing change clearly illustrates the needs of individual practitioners involved in the process, particularly the need for support. Butterworth and Faugier (1992) argue that support should be in the form of clinical supervision, and government policy demonstrates the requirement for clinical supervision for practitioners (NHSME, 1993a). In community health care nursing, where practitioners have less opportunity for prolonged contact with an appropriate supervisor, peer support plays an important role. Because of the working methods of practitioners in the community, peer support may come from different disciplines, particularly where PHCTs have been well established. It is issues such as this which highlight once more the importance of continuing education and professional development.

It is anticipated that the following chapters will provide both practitioners and students with one method of continuing their professional development. However, since the book has been developed to meet the needs of the range of practitioners working in the community, issues have been explored from general principles as a foundation for practice. In approaching topics in this way, the discussion, research and analysis can be drawn on by a range of practitioners, contributing to the development of excellence in practice.

References

Ashton, J. (1990) The health of towns and cities. *Health Visitor*, **63**(12), 413–415

Audit Commission (1992) *Homeward Bound: A New Course for Community Health*, HMSO, London

Baker, G., Bevan, J.M., McDonald, L. and Wall, B. (1987) *Community Nursing Research and Recent Developments*, Croom Helm, London

Baly, M.E. (1989) Florence Nightingale and the development of Public Health. *Humane Medicine*, **5**(Autumn), 37–45

Barriball, K.L. and Mackenzie, A. (1992) The demand for measuring the impact of nursing interventions: a community perspective. *Journal of Clinical Nursing*, **1**, 207–212

Bond, S., Rhodes, T., Philips, P., Setters, T., Foy, C. and Bond, J. (1990) HIV infection and AIDS in England: the experience, knowledge and intentions of community nursing staff. *Journal of Advanced Nursing*, **15**, 249–255

Butterworth, T. (1988) Breaking the boundaries, *Nursing Times*, **84**(47), 36–39

Butterworth, T. and Faugier, J. (1992) *Clinical Supervision and Mentorship and Nursing*, Chapman and Hall, London

Cameron, E., Badger, F. and Evers, H. (1989) Old, needy and black. *Nursing Times*, **84**(2), 38–40.

Centre for Health Economics (1992) *Skill Mix and the Effectiveness of Nursing Care*, University of York, York

Clay, T. (1986) *Community Nursing after Cumberlege*, Conference Paper 3 June, Solihull

Cowley, S. (1993) Skill mix for whom? *Health Visitor*, **66**(3), 166–168, 171

DHSS (1977) *Nursing in Primary Health Care*, HMSO, London

DHSS (1986) *Neighbourhood Nursing – A Focus for Care*, HMSO, London

DoH (1989) *Caring for People: Community Care in the Next Decade and Beyond*, HMSO, London

DoH (1992) *The Health of the Nation: A Strategy for Health in England*, HMSO, London

DoH (1993) *Report of the Taskforce on the Strategy for Research in Nursing, Midwifery and Health Visiting*, Department of Health, London

Durand, I. (1989) Nurse/patient dependency in community nursing. *Nursing Times*, **85**(26), 55–57

George, J. (ed.) (1990) *Nursing Theories*, 3rd edn, Prentice-Hall Englewood Cliffs, N.J.

Gibbs, I., McCaughlan, D. and Griffiths, M. (1991) Skill mix in nursing: a selective review of the literature. *Journal of Advanced Nursing*, **16**, 242–249

Gordon, P. (1991) *The Responsibilities of Nursing Service Providers and Practitioners for Patients in the Community*, A consensus conference on nursing in the community, South East Thames Regional Health Authority, Bexhill

Harding Report (1981) *The Primary Health Care Team*, Report of Joint Working Group of the Standing Medical Advisory Committee and the Standing Nursing and Midwifery Advisory Committee, HMSO, Amersham

Hays, B.J. (1992) Nursing care requirement and resource consumption in home health care. *Nursing Research*, **41**(3), 138–143.

Jackson, C. (1993) Your role or mine? *Health Visitor*, **66**(4), 124–126

Kratz, C.R. (1982) Community nursing – prescription for excellence? *Nursing Times*, 21 April, 676–682

Laurent C. (1992) Mixed feelings. *Nursing Times*, **88**(30), 57–58

Lightfoot, J. and Baldwin, S. (1992) *Nursing by Numbers?* Setting staffing levels for district nursing and health visiting services, SPRU University of York, York

MacIntosh, J. (1993) Postpartum depression: women's help-seeking behaviour and perception of cause. *Journal of Advanced Nursing*, **18**, 178–184

McMurray, A. (1994) *Community Health Nursing*, 2nd edn, Churchill Livingstone, Melbourne

Naughton, B. (1993a) Funds of opportunity. *Nursing Times*, **89**(17), 63

Naughton, B. (1993b) The marketing imperative. *Nursing Times*, **89**(19), 52–54

NHSME (1990) *Nursing in the Community*, NHS Management Executive, London

NHSME (1993a) *New World, New Opportunities: Nursing in Primary Health Care*, Department of Health, London

NHSME (1993b) *A Vision for the Future*, Department of Health, London

Oermann, M.H. (1991) *Professional Nursing Practice: A Conceptual Approach*, Lippincott, New York

Pollock, L. (1993) Positively Parker Street. *Nursing Times*, **89**(17), 18–19

Robinson, J. (1985) Health visiting and health. In *Political Issues in Nursing*, vol. 1 (ed. R. White), Wiley, Chichester

Roy, S. (1991) The future of community nursing. *Primary Health Care Management*, **1**(7), 4–5

Secretary of State for Social Services (1986) *Primary Health Care: An Agenda for Discussion*, HMSO, London

Stilwell, B. (1991) The rise of the practice nurse. *Nursing Times*, **87**(24), 26–28

Thompson, T. (1990) Targets for Action – Practice. In *An Action Plan* (ed. J. Brown), SPSW Publishing, York

Tschudin, V. (1992) *Ethics in Nursing*, 2nd edn, Butterworth-Heinemann, Oxford

Turner, J. (1990) The new G.P. contract: a case for concern? *Nursing Times*, **86**(20), 27–28

Twinn, S. (1991) Conflicting paradigms of health visiting: a continuing debate for professional practice. *Journal of Advanced Nursing*, **16**, 966–973

UKCC (1991) *Report on Proposals for the Future of Community Education and Practice*, UKCC, London

UKCC (1992) *The Scope of Professional Practice*, UKCC, London

UKCC (1994) Programmes of Education Leading to the Qualification of Specialist Practitioner, Registrar's letter 20/1994, UKCC, London

Welsh Office (1987) *Nursing in the Community*, Report of the Review of Community Nursing in Wales, Welsh Office Information Division, Cardiff

WHO (1978) *Health For All in the Year 2000*, World Health Organisation, Geneva

WHO (1985) *Targets for Health for All*, World Health Organisation, Regional Office for Europe, Copenhagen

Young, L. (1991) Hospital at home. *Primary Health Care*, May, 26–27

Part I

Changes in health care

In common with health care systems throughout the world, the National Health Service (NHS) in the UK is undergoing significant changes as the twentieth century draws to a close. This part of the book examines these changes and explores their implications for nursing practice in the community.

This changing pattern in health is reflected in health care provision, with an increasing emphasis on primary rather than secondary health care. In the 1970s the World Health Organisation (WHO) initiated the *Health For All in the Year 2000* project (WHO, 1978), which has been adopted by member states throughout the world. In the UK the publication of the document *The Health of the Nation* (DoH, 1992) demonstrated the commitment to health promotion and disease prevention rather than medical treatment. Chapter 2 focuses on the changing emphasis in health care and the structural changes occurring within the NHS, introducing the concept of purchaser and provider in health care provision. The tension competition creates in a managed health care system may allow for increased quality, efficiency and effectiveness, but may also result in further fragmentation of a system that is already complex. Chapter 3 describes the 'Health for All' movement developed by the WHO and introduces the principles of the 'Health of the Nation' document. The authors go on to use the 'Healthy Cities' project to discuss the relationship between primary health care and public health, and explore the responsibilities of the nurse as an advocate and citizen. The shift from secondary to primary health care is considered in detail in Chapter 4. The author of this chapter highlights some of the factors contributing to and influenced by this shift, such as the growing polarization of wealth, shifts in patterns of economic activity and the increasing awareness of the health service consumer and the importance of the public voice in health planning and development. For nurses working in the community, the need to respond to consumer needs and requirements may radically alter the way in which the service has been traditionally provided, requiring more flexible and rapidly responsive practitioners.

The changing focus in health care is developed in Chapter 5, in which the authors explore a new vision for health care. This thought-provoking chapter provides practitioners not only with the opportunity of reconsidering the philosophy underpinning health care, but also approaches to practice. Indeed, the authors' proposed paradigm for health care presents practitioners with a major challenge as the provision of patient and client care moves towards the twenty-first century. The challenge is continued, although in a different context, in the final chapter of this part. Here the author explores the health care needs of people with disability and handicaps, stressing in particular the need for individuals to strive for independence. This goal has considerable implications for community health care nurses in facilitating clients in achieving maximum health and social gain.

While this part of the book focuses on the changes in health care systems, the editors are aware that change continues and uncertainties remain in the provision of patient and client care. However, this changing world highlights the importance of community health care nurses developing their role and maximizing opportunities as professional boundaries blur and the need for flexibility of skill transfer and sharing information increases.

References

DoH (1992) *The Health of the Nation: A Strategy for Health in England*, HMSO, London

WHO (1978) *Health for All in the Year 2000*, World Health Organisation, Geneva

2

The changing organization of health care: setting the scene

Kate Lock

● **Introduction**

Community health care nursing in the 1990s is evolving within a health service which is changing rapidly. The changes have implications for both the structure and the content of community health care nursing. In order to meet this challenge it is necessary to understand the way that health care in the UK is organized and how it has responded to the reforms placed upon it, especially the NHS and Community Care Act 1990 which was implemented in April 1993. This chapter attempts to explain these changes and put them into the context of health care. The reforms imply a shift in thinking about both health and social service support. These are discussed, with the implications for community health care nursing considered.

● **Historical developments**

Review of UK health service changes until 1989

The health service was created as a result of the recognition of the need for welfare provision between the two World Wars. The Beveridge Report (Beveridge, 1942) outlined the basis for a health system which was comprehensive, accessible to all, and free at the point of need, paid for through national insurance and income tax contributions. The National Health Service, one of the first in the world, was established on 5 July 1948.

The NHS has continued to expand since 1948. It now employs over a million workers (OPCS, 1992). In 1974 and 1982 significant reorganizations of the structure of the NHS were completed. The first reforms attempted to unify the management system, creating a three-tier system of Regional Health Authorities, Area Health Authorities and District Health Authorities. Family Practitioner Committees co-ordinated the care offered by General Practitioners who were self-employed medical contractors within the NHS. The structure emphasized consensus management between disciplines as a way of improving and unifying management. The reorganization of 1982 disbanded the Area Health Authorities, the functions of which were shared between District and Region, enabling the District Health Authorities, as smaller units, to achieve more localized decision-making.

These reorganizations were, in part, financially led. The NHS was perceived to be consuming increasingly more public money, and changing the management structure was seen as the key to controlling costs. However, as costs and demands for health care continued to rise and coincided with a worsening economic climate of the country, the need to reorganize the service once again was recognized.

Consumer expectations

The NHS remains one of the most popular national institutions. Every government has declared absolute support for the concept. However, people's expectations of the NHS have changed significantly over the years. At the formation of the health service, health professionals considered they knew better than patients as to what constituted good health care and no patient or client voice was built into the structure of the NHS. The growth of patient care groups, often people with specific health needs, led to the creation of the Community Health Councils (CHCs) in 1974, which acted to counter concern over public accountability in a bureaucratic and paternalistic health service (Klein and Lewis, 1976).

In the 1980s several reports were published showing the increasing dissatisfaction with the delivery of care in the NHS. The British Social Attitudes Survey undertaken in the 1980s showed that of those interviewed, 87% identified the need to improve waiting list times for surgery, and 73% wanted improvement in staffing levels of nurses and doctors in hospital. In addition, while the majority of the public were content with the NHS as a whole, an increasing number were dissatisfied with the experience of outpatient clinics and that of being an in-patient (Bosanquet, 1988).

In the late 1980s the government responded to this expression of public dissatisfaction by promoting 'consumerism' within the NHS. This replaced the more collectivist ideals of the Community Health Councils with the notion that the NHS should respond to individuals as consumers through the introduction of a market ethos throughout the management and structure of the organization (Mahon *et al.*, 1994).

Economic imperatives

Up to, and including, the 1982 reorganization, governments believed that given the right management structure, cash limits would be respected and the cost of the NHS would be contained. When this did not happen in practice, as savings in one area were spent in others, the government began to impose cost-limiting policies more directly. When this in turn had limited effect, a major change of organization within the

NHS was decided upon. This was promoted in part by the belief that if a system rewarded good practice and freed up local management to make more local financial decisions, poor practice would wither and money would be saved. This thinking ran through many government initiatives at the time, including those in education and the welfare system.

The Black Report (Black, 1980) related patterns of illness to socio-economic status, showing that poorer members of society had the greater health need and the lowest life expectancy. The health service has not always planned services to meet the greatest needs. Indeed as Hart (1971) identified, the reverse is true, with the health requirements of the poorest section of society such as those who are unemployed, who are homeless and those with long-term physical and mental health needs receiving the least attention. To ensure that equality of health provision remains a realistic goal, the organization of the NHS must have these people's health needs at its centre.

● **The new order**

Working for patients

In January 1989 the government published the White Paper 'Working for Patients' which was to radically alter the organization of health care in the NHS. The NHS and Community Care Act enshrining these changes in law was passed in 1990. The changes made by this Act have been the most far-reaching experienced by the NHS since its inception in 1948.

The NHS was perceived by the government as being dogged by bureaucracy which was highly inefficient. In addition it perceived wastage of public money, which, according to the prevailing thought, should be redirected, as far as possible, into the private sector (Butler, 1994). However, in reality, the NHS was, by international comparison, one of the most cost-efficient health systems, providing extremely high quality care to individuals both in their own homes and hospital (Scheiber and Poullier, 1989). It provided universal health care coverage, the majority of which was delivered free at the point of need. Low costs were attributed in part to low administrative costs because in the UK there is no system of direct payment by users.

However, there were indeed significant problems with its organiza-tion. The management system pre-1985 was structured to favour the independence and power of professional groups above those of managers employed to direct resources and balance the books. The medical team in particular were free within the NHS to exercise their clinical judgement independent of managerial constraints (Harrison and Wistow, 1993). The system of general management introduced following the Griffiths Report in 1983 began to address some of these issues. It aimed to prioritize health input within financial constraints and to produce performance indicators relating to the work of health professionals and improve information systems. While these may have saved some money, research has shown that these savings were not significant (Butler, 1992).

These ideas were further developed in the White Paper *Working for Patients* (DoH, 1989). Six essential features of the reforms emerged:

- there should be a consolidation of managerial control in line with government directives
- funding of health should reflect the size and dependence of the population as a whole rather than care and treatment provided for specific individuals in hospitals
- capital assets would be charged for in similar ways to private capital to give equity between public and private competition
- systems to define the costs of the services would be created
- systems of medical and health audit would be introduced at all levels
- the clinical freedom of medical practitioners would be subject to the constraints of financial planners.

The internal market competition in the NHS

In the commercial world, the notion of competition within a market economy is easily understood, but within health care the validity of the concept of competition is less clear. In business, competition relies on the identification of the cost of each 'product', or element of service which may be an operation or the provision of medical diagnosis, as well as assessment of the quality of each aspect of service. This offers the purchaser of services a choice from which provider to buy services based on the cost-effectiveness and quality of the provision.

Working for Patients introduced a new form of health care organization with separation within the NHS between those people that purchase health care and those that provide it. This split would then create an NHS market, and the possibility of competition within health care provided in Britain (see also Chapter 8). The majority of the providers of both hospital and community health services have chosen to take on trust status under the terms of the 1990 Act. They set their own standards of care, closely directed by central government, and, from 1995, will be able to offer their own terms and conditions of employment. Trusts have strict financial constraints placed upon them by central government through the office of the NHS Executive, and must break even each year within the financial limits placed on them. The trusts have gradually evolved over the past five years so that by the end of 1992, 95% of all provider units had trust status (Bartlett and Le Grand, 1994). Health care may also be provided by independent and voluntary agencies as contracted by purchasers.

The purchasers, as defined in the Act, are the District Health Authorities (DHAs), the Family Health Services Authorities (FHSAs) employing GPs, and GP fund holders. From 1996, DHAs and FHSAs will merge to form new Health Commissions. These purchasers are responsible for identifying the health needs of the local community and the services required to meet these needs. In order to make these decisions they have directed providers to collate information about the quality and cost of services they offer. In addition, they should ascertain from the community what health care it requires by undertaking surveys and questionnaires. On the basis of this information, providers then decide which services to buy and from where to purchase them. Purchasers then place contracts to buy health services from providers, ensuring continuation of existing services or commissioning new or altered services according to local need.

The majority of contracts placed by purchasers have so far been block contracts, which means that a purchaser is buying a service without stipulating how much service or how many patients should be treated. However, increasingly, under government guidance, they are placing contracts on cost and volume and contracts on cost per case. These contracts clearly define how many patients and/or service episodes will be bought (Appleby *et al.*, 1994) and include standards for achievement related to quality of service and clinical effectiveness.

Alongside this process, there has been a scaling down of the size of the previously powerful Regional Health Authorities (RHAs). In October 1993, the government released plans initially to merge the existing 14 RHAs in England into eight, with their abolition planned for April 1996 (see detail in Chapter 8).

Quality in health services

Quality management has been important in the commercial world for the past 15 years, and terms such as Total Quality Management (TQM) have come to represent a more efficient and often more humane way of running systems which in turn contribute to a more consistent product or service with respect for the contribution of all employees. This understanding of quality emerged slowly in the health service. The Griffiths Report (Griffiths, 1983) recognized the need to tighten the management of the NHS and clarify the lines of accountability. General managers were appointed, and given both managerial and budgetary control over their units. These were often, but not necessarily, health professionals, and, often for the first time, were systematically given extra training in both people and budgetary management (Thompson, 1993).

In addition, all parts of the health delivery system are required to produce regular data on the quality of care and patient satisfaction with the services provided. To encourage this, responsibility for the audit of the NHS was transferred to the Audit Commission, which now makes regular reviews of the NHS. Some of the first information to be released from the Audit Commission related to the number of days patients stayed in hospital. Later, waiting times for operations were released, then the accuracy of appointment times and the choice of menu of hospital food. More recently, the system of quality assurance has become more sophisticated, with an increasing number of aspects of health service, including primary health and community care provision, being evaluated. In fact, in the summer of 1994 league tables of trusts and hospitals were compiled and published (DoH, 1994).

Nurses have also implemented quality assurance programmes initially through standard setting and the use of programs such as Monitor. Standards describe the minimum level of care delivered which would be considered acceptable for a particular task or situation. Once this standard has been established and is familiar to the team, audit can be used to measure how closely practice matches the standard. Standards have been effectively used in such fields as pressure area care, using quantifiable measures such as the Norton and Waterlow scores (Waterlow, 1985). The report *A Vision for the Future* (NHSME, 1993) urges nurses actively to audit their work, and the review of this report published in April 1994 (NHSME, 1994) stated that 79% of the sample of nursing units had auditing systems in place. More sophisticated methods of audit are being used to test the quality of wards or nursing units. In a study by Redfern *et al*. (1992) it was found that three of the most commonly used systems – Monitor, Senior Monitor and Qualpacs – have good cross-reliability, with closely matching scores for the different aspects of care measured. However, critics of these systems argue that information of this sort often does not measure outcomes of care, which are essential if the value and effectiveness of health care is truly assessed.

Outcomes of care

In order to decide how well the health service functions, and therefore how to focus resources, purchasers require outcomes of health care intervention to be measured. However, producing reliable and accurate information on the outcomes of health care is extremely difficult. For example, although comprehensive mortality statistics are available, the cause of death does not reliably reflect the condition of the patient related to care and treatment given and so extrapolating from these is difficult. Other researchers have tried to evaluate the improvement in quality of life experienced, referred to as Quality Adjusted Life Years (QALYs) (Torrance, 1986). QALYs give a measure of the predicted improvement a certain procedure could give a patient, which should help in decision-making about the services offered in a contract. However, they have proved subjective and difficult to use in practice. Indeed, Hopkins and Maxwell (1990) commented that 'QALYs are more like research tools than indicators to audit outcomes'. Essentially, they represent an attempt to systematize moral decision-making, making objective a subjective process. The QALYs debate has resulted in more questions being created than answered (Gray, 1993). In addition, these measures are more appropriate for the assessment of medical care than nursing practice. Measurement of outcomes of care are a challenge to both practitioners and researchers, although the advent of benchmarking and the development of predictive care pathways will aid this process. The fragmentation of provider units may reduce the capacity to produce accurate information about long-term outcomes of health intervention, making it difficult to gather data from several different services which provide elements of care to individual patients.

Unit cost analysis

If a true picture of the effectiveness of health care interventions is to be achieved, quality assurance and clinical audit must be matched to financial information. The NHS has historically allocated budgets for whole hospital departments, but must now determine the costs of a typical total hip replacement, a normal birth or a 'package' of community care. This requires the development of systems devoted to cost analysis and this process is still in the early stages of development. Community nursing is in a similar situation, with reliable data on unit costs scarce and uneven between areas (Appleby *et al.*, 1994).

Purchaser choices

As information on both quality and cost becomes available, it should be possible for purchasers to decide which providers give the best quality and most cost-effective services. For example, some GP fund holders have opted to pay for a mental health counsellor on site whose costs can be offset against outpatient appointments which the GPs considered ineffective and for which there were often long waiting lists (Glennerster *et al.*, 1994). Another example is provided by Plymouth and Torbay Health Trust which introduced specialized dermatological consultation into GP practices, on the basis that this is both a cheaper and more acceptable service to the patient (Manning and Dunning, 1994).

It is too early to produce information which shows significant improvements in efficiency through creative contracting by purchasers. While fund holders are moving towards a cost-per-case basis of contracting, District and Family Health Services Authorities are still largely arranging block contracts. Furthermore, activity increases of trusts seen since the reforms started have not proved to show increased efficiency, but rather are considered by some to be a reflection of the considerable finance which fuelled the reforms (Bartlett and Le Grand, 1994).

The Community Care Act

The second major change in the environment of the delivery of health care was the long awaited implementation of the Community Care Act in 1993. Although this was part of the NHS and Community Care Act passed in 1990, progress on the community aspect has been delayed. However, given the radical nature of the changes implied, some authors argue that the long preparation time eased implementation (Harrison, 1993).

For the past 30 years, government policy and health professional thinking have both favoured the close of long-stay care beds managed in the NHS, and their replacement with community services. Thus beds for the frail elderly, disabled and those with chronic mental health problems have been closed in large numbers since the early 1960s. For example, in-patient beds for those with mental health problems reached their peak in 1954. In 1972 there were 100 000 in-patient beds in this sector; by 1985, it had dropped to 65 000 (Hunter, 1993). The care for these people was shifted to the community. In reality this has often meant support by members of the person's family, very often their mothers and wives, who have been given little support (Green, 1988; Carers' National Association 1993). The reduction in bed numbers has not been accompanied by a comparable increase in community health or social services, and many disabled people have 'fallen through the net' of community provision (Hunter, 1993). It was in this context that the Community Care Act was introduced.

The Community Care section of the Act does for the social services what the other part of the Act did for health. Indeed, the Act had two equally important driving imperatives. The first was that people should stay in their own homes for as long as possible and the resources needed to keep them there should be made available, if necessary from the money which previously paid for people to be kept in residential or nursing homes or hospital beds. The second imperative was the extension of the free market into the welfare system, creating purchasers and providers, as in the health sector, and the introduction of the notion of competition with the aim of driving down cost and improving quality. The Act was mainly concerned with the social needs of people with physical and mental health problems and those with learning disabilities.

This new system allows a much greater degree of flexibility in the provision of services. Service provision should be needs led, rather than service led. That is, the assessment should reveal, for example, what is needed by a person to stay at home rather than assessing whether they need home help, meals on wheels or other services. This has led to some very creative thinking in developing planned intervention. For example, if a person needs to eat in the evening, the social services might pay a public house to provide that meal. It has led to the provision of Health Care Assistants (HCAs) out of normal hours, at weekends, evenings and overnight. Service providers are now attempting to diversify to meet new demand, providing home care overnight and during unsociable hours (Dobson, 1994a).

The demand for home care services has fast outstripped supply, and Local Authorities have been unable to meet the need using HCAs employed by social services departments. This has led to a flourishing of private and voluntary agencies providing HCAs and other kinds of social input (Dobson, 1994b). So far it seems that, while they are expanding, they are not all yet flexible enough to adequately meet the needs of disabled people (Social Policy Research Unit/York Health Economic Consortium, 1993).

The development of information systems about the quality of services has been slow, as in health care. Social services departments were required to accredit all residential and nursing homes in the first year of operation of community care, and those homes that failed to meet expectations are not used, at least as first choice, by social services. Accreditation of home care services has taken longer, but in due course all providers of domiciliary care will need to meet stringent requirements.

Home owners and managers of home care agencies have complained that the accreditation system does not truly reflect the quality of their services (Langan and Taylor, 1994), but it is recognized that some measurement of quality is important and that it takes time and experience to implement new schemes such as accreditation. So far, community care can be seen undoubtedly to have allowed some very frail people to remain in their own homes longer, receiving the services they need. It is anticipated that the reduction of use of residential homes, and to a lesser extent, nursing homes, will free a considerable block of money to provide care in people's own homes. An inevitable result of this will be that some residential and nursing homes may be put out of business (King's Fund Centre/Nuffield Institute, 1994).

Implications for community health care nursing

The Community Care Act clearly draws a distinction between the care given by HCAs, as being social care, and that provided by nurses as health care. Although this may appear obvious, the clarification of these terms has led to some considerable changes in working practices. It has long been recognized that much care given by district nurses was more appropriately defined as social care, and should be given by staff under social services management.

Redefining health and social care has led to many districts referring much of the routine care they provided to social services, leaving practitioners more time for assessment and the treatment of health problems and health promotion (White, 1994). The role of the community health care assistant (nursing auxiliary) has come sharply into focus and some health trusts are reluctant to continue to pay for the social care they have been providing. Some differing models have emerged, but trends suggest social services will increasingly assume responsibility for parts of mental health budgets in the future, and there is evidence to suggest the success of multidisciplinary community-based mental health resource teams (Audit Commission, 1994). In addition, as community health care nurses become familiar with care management, they have taken on this function with patients with whom they are very closely involved and who have high-dependency health needs. Close co-operation and good communication channels are necessary for this cross-working to function efficiently (Rogers, 1994).

● The emphasis on primary health care

Shifting responsibilities for acute care

Primary health care has been boosted by two important changes in hospital treatment: the increase in day-case surgery and the early discharge of patients into the community.

In a continued effort to reduce the cost and improve the efficiency of hospital beds, day surgery has become increasingly popular. It is in part a response to better surgical techniques, including keyhole surgery, as well as the recognition of the harm an extended stay in hospital may result in for a patient. Surgery, such as cataract removal, varicose vein surgery and dilatation and curettage, previously involving several days in hospital, is now carried out as a day case or with an overnight stay (Morgan, 1992). Whereas, in 1981, 12.7% of all surgery was included within the category of day cases, by 1991/92, 20.6% was done on a day-case basis (HMSO, 1993). This obviously reduces the cost of such a procedure to the hospital, since a day-case unit is as much as 30% cheaper to run than an average theatre unit (NHSME, 1991). Day surgery is also popular with consumers (Audit Commisson, 1992).

Coupled with the increasing use of day surgery is the trend of early discharge of patients. There are several reasons for this, the first of which is the recognition that, as with day cases, people recover at least as well, if not better, in their own home than in hospital. Secondly, those attempting to reduce the cost of health care have argued that it is cheaper for people to recover at home rather than in hospital. Finally, with a clarification of health and social care, as soon as a person's needs become predominantly social, through care management, they are able to move to living either at home or in residential accommodation suitable to their needs. The average patient stay in acute beds for all ages has fallen from 12.5 days in 1981 to 8.8 in 1990/91 (DoH, 1993a).

As bed occupancy has fallen over the past five years, and throughput increased (Perrin, 1992), the government has congratulated itself on treating more people with the same amount of resources. However, there has been much debate as to the real quality of this change. Although waiting lists remain high, numbers of people waiting have decreased slightly, but it is unclear from the statistics exactly what this means for particular patients (Frankle and West, 1993). In addition, Frankle and West (1993) point out that day cases are inexplicably absent from all waiting lists statistics in Britain.

As patients are discharged earlier from hospital, there has been debate as to whether this has increased readmission rates. Indeed, government statistics do not report the readmission of patients. However, in the mental health field, UK and USA studies do not show an increased level of readmission following a shorter but more intensive in-patient stay.

Preventive work

Recent changes have recognized the importance of financing preventive health care, and in line with the WHO/UNICEF Alma Ata declaration for 'Health For All by the Year 2000' (1978), the government published its *Health of the Nation: A Strategy for Health in England* White Paper (DoH, 1992), which defined target areas for health promotion, which are coronary heart disease, cancer, mental illness, accidents and HIV/AIDS and sexual health. The health strategy focuses on individual behaviour and sets to discourage smoking, reduce the fat content of diet, reduce the incidence of suicide and increase the use of condoms both to reduce the spread of HIV and unwanted, mostly teenage, pregnancy.

Many health authorities have welcomed these initiatives and health promotion departments have taken on an increased role as a result. However those targets, such as reducing by half the rate of conception among the under-16s by the year 2000, avoid the larger issue of the influence of other factors on health which are often related to socio-economic circumstances rather than individual behaviour. As the Black Report (Black, 1980) so sharply illustrated, socio-economic conditions have by far the greatest effect on a person's health, and more recent researchers have underlined this by stating that 'the most effective way of improving health is to make incomes more equal' by raising the standard of living of the poorest in society (Quick and Wilkinson, 1991).

There is resistance to legislate changes such as banning tobacco advertising, or lifting the restriction on giving contraceptive advice to teenagers under 16 without the consent of their parents, both of which could contribute towards meeting the targets set out in 'Health of the Nation'. Although some more forward-looking health promotion departments have seized the opportunity given by these health promotion targets to extend the remit of their work to take in issues of poverty, poor housing and access to appropriate advice as part of their health promotion work, many have criticised the 'Health of the Nation' targets for failing to tackle the socio-economic problems which underlie ill health (Caraker, 1994).

In conjunction with the 'Health of the Nation' targets, GPs have been given financial incentives to run health promotion clinics and collect data on health behaviour such as smoking and uptake of cervical smears. Although scepticism has been voiced as to whether these clinics actually improve health behaviour or morbidity rates (Cassidy, 1994), their existence must be considered to be contributing to an improvement in the health of the nation. Indeed, despite difficulties such as those identified above, the renewed emphasis on health promotion must be welcomed as a step forward in creating a health rather than a sickness service.

Consumer expectations

The recipient of health care is now increasingly being described in government literature as a consumer of the health care services. This language is accompanied by an attitude which tries to put the needs of the client before the needs of the institutions which serve the client. The Griffiths reports (Griffiths, 1983, 1988) advocated this approach. It was also central to the *Working for Patients* White Paper (DoH, 1989), emphasizing the need for patients to be given both information and choice about health care services.

This move led to information being made available to users of health services at every level so that patients know what they can expect from the service. This information also gives them a minimum standard by which to judge the care they receive. In addition, it has been made easier for patients to change their GP. Once a patient is in consultation with the health professional, they are encouraged to take an active part in their care, be involved in care planning and be given choices of treatment, with the necessary information needed to make that choice. Most importantly, DHAs, FHSAs and hospitals are required to make clear and effective the process of complaints so that grievances can be quickly addressed by the individuals concerned and the institutions.

Criticisms of the consumerist ideal

There is no doubt that the move for consumers to have more information and control over their care is beneficial for both patients and health professionals. However, the implementation has so far ignored some crucial factors. There is an inherent inequality between health professionals and patients, as there is between most professionals and their clients. While information can and should be given to patients, the practitioner has the advantage of a professional education and training. This can lead to the professional holding both the majority of the information and the power in relation to a patient's health which has implications for the philosophy of partnerships in health care.

The emphasis on the responsibility of the patient to obtain the health care they need, rather than the system to provide it, inevitably favours those patients with a strong voice. These tend to be educated patients and clients skilled in the use of the services – generally those from the higher socio-economic groups in the community. Conversely, those disenfranchised or with less self-esteem are bound to lose out in obtaining the health care they need in this new phase of consumerism. Ironically, as has been seen above, there is no doubt that those disenfranchised are those with the greatest health needs and therefore with most to lose.

The present drive to improve the consumer's experience of health care focuses almost entirely on the individual, ignoring the potential of groups such as Community Health Councils (CHCs) and pressure groups to represent the views of the public and challenge the service (Winkler, 1989). However, public accountability within the NHS has been reduced as a result of recent reforms. CHCs now have limited statutory powers, and while they must be consulted, there is little responsibility on the services to respond to their concerns. In addition, the latest reforms have meant that CHCs have not only lost their right to attend Trust board meetings, but also have fewer members of the public on these boards, than for predecessor health authorities with more members appointed directly from region or government (Searle, 1993).

Economic imperatives

As the country emerges from the economic recession of the late 1980s, the majority of employees in the NHS understand that there are no longer unlimited resources with which to fund the health service. The difficult choice as to where best to target the limited resource available is a key debate and there are some factors which must direct that debate, over which central government and managers of the service have little control.

Population

The population of the UK is not rising significantly, but, like all developed countries, the proportion of the population over 65 is increasing. In 1988, 8.9 million of the population was over 65; 15.6% of the total population. By 2011, that figure will rise to 9.7 million; 16.2% of the population. In addition, the proportion of the elderly who are over 80 years old will rise from 22% of all elderly people in 1988 to 27% in 2011. This change is coupled with a demographic fall in the numbers of middle-aged people, the group who are both carers and wage earners supporting the elderly (Wells, 1992). This situation has left the nation with the structural problem of large numbers of dependent elderly people and fewer middle-aged people to support them.

Technology

Research in health care funded by both industry, charities and government bodies such as the Medical Research Council have continued to improve the diagnosis and treatment of many diseases and illnesses. Indeed, there remains the belief that technology can give the ultimate answer to illness. However, as documents such as 'Health of the Nation' (DoH, 1992) have demonstrated, it has now been recognized that government-led initiatives to improve the health status of the population must go beyond an ever increasing spiral of expenditure on drugs and technology. Health status ultimately depends as much on people's social and economic situation, education and lifestyles as the ability of technology to cure them once they have become sick (Wyke, 1994).

Nevertheless, the advances made in health science have had a great impact on health care structures. New drugs have been developed which not only avoid intrusive surgery but also improve the control of disease, such as the new generation of chemotherapeutic agents. Diagnostic techniques have dramatically improved. Imaging the fibreoptics technology has allowed professionals to identify health problems and sometimes treat an individual without the need for surgery.

Resource allocation

Government attempts to decide where scarce resources must be spent have always been heavily criticized by different sections of the health professions. In the 1970s, in response to the obvious inequity of distribution of resources, the government of the day created the Resource Allocation Working Party for England. This organization had the responsibility for developing formulae for resource allocation based on the need for health care using mortality figures. Areas of need were allowed to grow more rapidly and those that were over-resourced were limited in their growth. Although this was successful in reducing inequalities between areas, it only limited growth, rather than actually reducing the size of over-resourced areas.

Present financial arrangements have taken this process further, based on the philosophy that money should follow patients, and that purchasers, having collected information on the health needs of their communities, should buy services at a competitive rate to meet those needs. It was anticipated that within this system uneconomic or unnecessary services would wither, while those giving appropriate value for money services should expand.

Funding for purchasers is now based on population figures for each area, adjusted for mortality and age-profile. This new system referred to as Weighted Capitation Formulae (WCF) aims to buy health gain, rewarding health authorities for improving their health statistics. In practice, the WCF has channelled funds away from deprived areas, where statistics show poor health, and moved them into more prosperous areas such as the south-east of the country. Thus some of the poorest areas of Birmingham and Manchester face the threat of substantial cuts (Jacobson, 1990; Appleby, 1992), while the area of Greater London was also identified as being heavily over-resourced. The government planned that secondary care provision in London should lose substantially to other areas of the country. The response from organizations following the realization of the magnitude of cuts suggested prompted the government to commission a special enquiry, which resulted in the Tomlinson Report (Tomlinson, 1992). This, and the subsequent Department of Health report, suggested that London's health budget should concentrate on primary health care while merging and closing some of the large teaching hospitals (DoH, 1993b). WCF is now under review, as difficulties in the system have become clearer.

Within each DHA, considerable discussion has taken place as to how to use the allocation of money, since purchasers are now required to collect information on local needs and the views of the local population. Basing decisions that take account of local views is a complex process. An example of this kind of consultation has been provided by Oregon in the USA, which, in effect, balloted the local population as to which illnesses should be treated. The results of these ballots were used to make up priorities for health spending (Fox and Howard, 1993). However, later reports suggest that the list compiled has still not been put into operation, despite years of discussions. In addition, under this system certain conditions would be given few or no resources, such as AIDS-related diseases, and others such as tuberculosis and appendicitis would be given a very high priority. Whether UK health authorities would be inclined to use such a model is open to question, but some commentators have suggested that such consultation with the public is inevitably non-egalitarian since participation is unequal and the publics views are less well informed (Hunter, 1993).

However, some DHAs have identified significant areas of deprivation and channelled funds accordingly. This is illustrated by one district where 70% of the development budget was directed towards primary health care following a needs survey (Whitehead, 1994). National directives through documents such as the 'Patient's Charter' and the 'Health of the Nation', place imperatives on DHAs in the allocation of funds, but generally they have far more freedom than previously in placing contracts and spending money in the way they choose.

● Nursing changes

Nursing has always been subject to change. Registration legislation and the formation of the General Nursing Council in 1919 ensured consistency of education and practice across the country (Baly, 1980). More recently there has been an increasing emphasis on professionalizing nursing practice. The use of independent nursing research to inform practice and the increasing specialization of nurses, with their advancing skill, has further strengthened this process (Hopps, 1994). The early 1960s saw the start of degree courses for nurses, and it became more common for nurses to take on university education as part of their career structure. The implementation of 'Project 2000' (UKCC, 1986) removed nurse education from hospital control and limited the use of student nurses in service provision. New emphasis is being placed on appropriate academic education linked to professional practice for all nurses. Health care assistants also receive training, generally through the National Vocational Qualification scheme.

Much debate has ensued as to the status of the Health Care Assistants. The Royal College of Nursing has so far rejected attempts to admit them as members on the grounds that only professionally educated personnel can be said to carry out nursing. The debate avoids the central issue, which is that of grade mix and skill mix which in effect may reduce the quality of nursing input. Carr-Hill *et al*. (1992) have observed, 'the quality of care was better the higher the grade (and skill) of the nurses who provided it'. In addition the King's Fund Report on the NHS reforms comments: 'There has been surprisingly little attempt to conduct a proper evaluation of the cost effectiveness of skill mix changes . . . [and] little attention has been paid to evaluating the broader impact on costs and quality . . . of care provided' (Robinson and Le Grand, 1994).

Implications for community health care nurses

The changes in the NHS raise many questions for the community health care nurse, and the UK Chief Nurses' Report (DoH, 1994) attempts to answer some of these questions for all branches of nursing and midwifery as the twenty-first century approaches. The report acknowledges the shift of care from hospital to community and the increasing importance of teamwork with other professionals. In addition, the report predicts that nursing will need to be more concerned with the efficiency and effectiveness of the care provided. Finally, the Chief Nurses foresee that in order for nursing to take up the challenges of the massive changes occurring in the health service as well as the profession, there will need to be substantial investment in the existing staff. This will need to include investment in training, innovation and research in practice, as well as much closer co-ordination between all levels of staff and policy-makers if the potential of the profession is to be realized (DoH, 1994).

This is to be welcomed in the context of community health care nursing. For many years this branch of the profession has been seen as the poor cousins of those who are hospital based. With increasing numbers of people who would have traditionally been nursed in hospital now being cared for at home, all disciplines within community health care nursing will become more important. Indeed, with the clarification of differences between health and social input by the Community Care Act, practitioners must now take up the challenge of their health care remit, especially their role in health promotion with all members of the community. Alongside this role, community health care nurses will be able to exercise and develop increasing skills as more acutely ill people are nursed at home. As this trend is extended, the boundaries between practitioners in the community will need to become increasingly flexible.

● **Conclusion**

The Chief Nurses' Report (1994) observed the change of direction for community health care nurses and recognized that the change may not always be appreciated by the public. It is therefore the responsibility of community nurses to consult and inform the public as changes are made. Although nurses have always striven to assert their role as advocates of both individuals and their carers, with the increasing responsibility for health care being placed on the individual receiving care, the need for intelligent, informed advocates for individuals and their families has never been stronger. Community health care nurses are ideally placed to take up this role.

GPs and purchasers will increasingly define the specific services they wish to purchase from the community health care nursing service. Practitioners must be involved in the process and welcome audit as a way of demonstrating their worth. Audit must move away from the simple collection of figures to include more qualitative assessments of the effectiveness and quality of community health care nursing. It is neither appropriate nor desirable to have this process determined by purchasers or managers in the provider sector whose main agenda is financial saving.

The opportunities for community health care nursing to take on a major role in the care of frail and sick people and the promotion of health among the well has never rested more upon the ability of practitioners to be flexible, confident and competent in defining the needs of individuals and their families and structuring their work to meet those needs.

References

Appleby, J. (1992) NHS distribution of funds unfair. *British Medical Journal*, **304**, 70

Appleby, J. *et al*. (1994) Monitoring managed competition. In *Evaluating the NHS Reforms* (eds R. Robinson and J. Le Grand), King's Fund Institute, London

Audit Commission (1992) *Homeward Bound: A New Course for Community Health*, HMSO, London

Audit Commission (1994) *Finding a Place: A Review of Mental Health Services for Adults*, HMSO, London

Baly, M. (1980) *Nursing and Social Change*, Heinemann, London

Bartlett, W. and Le Grand, J. (1994) The performance of trusts. In *Evaluating the NHS Reforms* (eds R. Robinson and J. Le Grand), King's Fund Institute, London

Beveridge, W. (1942) *Social Insurance and Allied Services* (the Beveridge Report), CMD 6404, HMSO, London

Black, D. (1980) *Inequalities in Health: Report of a Research Working Group*, DHSS, London

Bosanquet, N. (1988) An ailing state of national health. In *British Social*

Attitudes, the 5th Report (eds R. Jowel, S. Witherspoon and L. Brook), Gower, Aldershot

Butler, J. (1992) *Patients, Policies and Politics*, Open University Press, Birmingham

Butler, J. (1994) Origins and early development. In *Evaluating the NHS Reforms* (eds R. Robinson and J. Le Grand), King's Fund Institute, London

Caraker, M. (1994) Health Promotion – time for an audit. *Nursing Standard*, **8**(20), 32–5

Carers' National Association (1993) *Speak Up, Speak Out*, quoted in Spurgeon, P. (1993) *The New Face of the NHS*, Longman, London

Carr-Hill, R. *et al*. (1992) *Skill Mix and the Effectiveness of Nursing Care*, Centre for Health Economics, University of York

Cassidy, J. (1994) Nurse-led screening is a waste of time. *Nursing Times*, **90**(5), 6

Chief Nurses' Report (1994) *The Challenges for Nursing and Midwifery in the 21st Century*, Chief Nurses of England, Scotland, Wales and Northern Ireland/ Department of Health, London

DoH (1989) *Working for Patients*, HMSO, London

DoH (1990) The NHS and Community Care Act, HMSO, London

DoH (1992) *The Health of the Nation: A Strategy for Health in England*, HMSO, London

DoH (1993a) *Statistical Bulletin 1993/2*, quoted in Harrison, A. (ed.) (1993) *Health Care UK, 1992/3*, King's Fund Institute, London

DoH (1993b) *Making London Better*, HMSO, London

DoH (1994) *League Tables of Health Trusts in the UK*, Department of Health, London

Dobson, R. (1994a) Valley of care. *Community Care*, **1031**, 10

Dobson, R. (1994b) Big Business. *Community Care*, **1031**, 16–17

Fox, D. and Howard, L. (1993) Rationing care in Oregon. *Health Affairs*, Summer

Frankle, S. and West, R. (1993) *Rationing and Rationality in the NHS*, Macmillan, London

Glennerster, H. *et al*. (1994) GP fundholding: wild card or winning hand? In *Evaluating the NHS Reforms* (eds R. Robinson and J. Le Grand), King's Fund Institute, London

Gray, A. (1993) Rationing and choice. In *Dilemmas in Health Care* (eds B. Davey and J. Popay), Open University Press, Buckingham

Green, H. (1988) *Informal Carers* (OPCS Social Survey Division, Series GH5, No. 15, Supplement, A), HMSO, London

Griffiths, R. (1983) *NHS Management Enquiry*, DHSS, London

Griffiths, R. (1988) Does the public serve? The consumer decision. *Public Administration*, **66**, 195–204

Harrison, A. (ed). (1993) *Health Care UK, 1992/3*, King's Fund Institute, London

Harrison, S. and Wistow, G. (1993) Managing health care: balancing interests and influence. In *Dilemmas in Health Care* (eds B. Davey and J. Popay), Open University Press, Birmingham

Hart, J.T. (1971) The inverse care law. *Lancet*, **i**, 405–412

HMSO (1993) *Health and Personal Social Services Statistics for England*, HMSO, London

Hopkins, A. and Maxwell, R. (1990) Contracts and quality of care. *British Medical Journal*, **300**, 919–922

Hopps, L. (1994) The development of research in nursing in the UK. *Journal of Clinical Nursing*, **3**, 199–204

Hunter, D. (1992) The move to community care with special reference to mental illness. In *In the Best of Health?* (eds E. Beck *et al*.) Chapman and Hall, London

Hunter, D. (1993) *Rationing Dilemmas in Health Care*, NAHAT, London

Jacobson, B. (1990) *Health in Hackney: Annual Public Health Report for 1990*, City and Hackney Health Authority, London

King's Fund Centre/Nuffield Institute (1994) *Fit for Change? Snapshots of Community Care Reforms*, KFC/NI, London

Klein, R. and Lewis, J. (1976) *The Politics of Consumer Representation*, Centre for Policy Studies, London

Langan, J. and Taylor, M. (1994) Bending the rules. *Community Care*, **1035**, 30–31

Mahon, A., Wilkin, D. and Whitehouse, G. (1994) Choice of hospital for elective surgery referral: GPs' and patients' views. In *Evaluating the NHS Reforms* (eds R. Robinson and J. Le Grand), King's Fund Institute, London

Manning, S. and Dunning, M. (1994) Every day in every way. *Health Service Journal*, **104**(5393), 27–28

Morgan, M. (1992) Waiting lists. In *In the Best of Health?* (eds E. Beck *et al.*), Chapman and Hall, London

NHSME (1991) *Day Surgery; Making it Happen*, NHSME Value for Money Unit/HMSO, London

NHSME (1993) *A Vision for the Future*, Department of Health, London

NHSME (1994) *Testing the Vision*, A report on the progress of the first year of 'A Vision for the Future', Department of Health, London

OPCS (1992) *Social Trends 22*, HMSO, London

Perrin, J. (1992) Administrative and financial management of health care services. In *In the Best of Health?* (eds E. Beck *et al.*), Chapman and Hall, London

Quick, A. and Wilkinson, R. (1991) *Income and Health*, Socialist Health Association, p. 5

Redfern, S. *et al.* (1992) The reliability and validity of quality assessment measures in nursing. *Journal of Clinical Nursing*, **1**, 47–51

Robinson, R. and Le Grand, J. (1994) *Evaluating the NHS Reforms*, King's Fund Institute, London, p. 185

Rogers, J. (1994) Collaboration among health professionals. *Nursing Standard*, **9**(6), 25–26

Scheiber, G. and Poullier, J. (1989) International health care expenditure 1987. *Health Affairs*, **18**(3), 169–177

Searle, C. (1993) The consumer voice. In *Dilemmas in Health Care* (eds B. Davey and J. Popay), Open University Press, Buckingham

Social Policy Research Unit/York Health Economic Consortium (1993) *Caring for People Who Live at Home*, SPRU/YHEC, York, UK

Thompson, D. (1993) Developing managers for the 1990's. In *The New Face of the NHS* (ed. P. Spurgeon), Longman, London

Tomlinson, B. (1992) *Report of the Inquiry into London's Health Service – Medical, Education and Research*, HMSO, London

Torrance, G.W. (1986) Measurement of health status utilities for economic appraisal: a review. *Journal of Health Economics*, **5**, 1–30

UKCC (1986) *Project 2000: A New Preparation for Practice*, United Kingdom Central Council for Nursing, Midwifery and Health Visiting, London

Waterlow, J.A. (1985) A risk assessment card. *Nursing Times*, **89**(32), 52–53

Wells, N. (1992) Responses to changes in demography and patterns of disease. In *In the Best of Health?* (eds. E. Beck *et al.*), Chapman and Hall, London

White, D. (1994) *The District Nurse and the Community Care Act*, Unpublished MA thesis, Exeter University

Whitehead, M. (1994) Is it fair? Evaluating the equity implications of the NHS reforms. In *Evaluating the NHS Reforms* (eds R. Robinson and J. Le Grand), King's Fund Institute, London

WHO/UNICEF (1978) *'Health for All by the Year 2000'* Declaration following

Alma Ata Conference, WHO, Geneva

Winkler, F. (1989) *Post the Review: Community/Consumer Representation in the NHS with Specific Reference to Community Health Councils*, GLACHC, London

Wyke, A. (1994) The future of medicine. *The Economist*, 19 March, 3–5

3

Health for all, healthy cities

Kate Harmond and June Crown

● Introduction

This chapter outlines some of the wider issues which affect the health of communities and individuals, and gives practical examples of how the community health care nurse can play a role in health gain for the population. It analyses the principles initially endorsed by the World Health Organisation (WHO) in its 'Health for All' strategy and outlines some of the types of collaborative work which have proved successful in the 'Healthy Cities' project. The close links between health, social and economic policies and the implications, with examples, for community health care nurses are discussed.

The UK strategy for health, *The Health of the Nation* (DoH, 1992) is introduced and the key areas and targets within this strategy are explored. The development of consumer-focused care is then described, together with *The Patient's Charter* (DoH, 1991) and the elements of this that have particular application in the community (DoH, 1995).

Finally some of the most recent innovations in health care practice are highlighted, with specific emphasis on community-based developments, and these are linked with organizational changes in the NHS. Throughout this chapter, the role and responsibilities of the community health care nurse as a professional, as an advocate and as a citizen remain the focus of attention, with the promotion of health and the prevention of disease acting as common linking themes.

● Health for all

The 'Health for All' strategy was launched by the World Health Organisation in 1978 at a conference held in Alma Ata, in the former Soviet Union. There were several pressures which led to this major policy initiative. For example, in developed countries demographic changes were taking place, with rising proportions of older people in the population, making increasing demands on health services. Technical developments in medical care were encouraging people to expect 'cures', even when this was unrealistic. In addition, there was increasing emphasis on hospital-based health care, at the expense of primary and community-based care. All these trends were resulting in rapidly rising costs of health care, as measured by the percentage of Gross National Product (GNP) spent on health services, with no compensating improvements in health status in the population. Meanwhile, developing countries were still experiencing population growth, high levels of infant mortality, malnutrition and deaths from preventable diseases. Although all these problems could be addressed by primary health care services and preventive programmes such as family planning and immunization, in many places, the main health care developments were in secondary and tertiary care (see Chapter 10).

The Alma Ata conference gave the WHO the opportunity to declare its commitment to health rather than to the treatment of disease, and to emphasize for the first time the importance of primary health care. The WHO stated firmly that primary health care should be the central function and main focus of any health care system, and underlined the importance of accessibility as a guiding principle for planning services, with health care being located as close as possible to where people work and live.

The declaration went on to emphasize that primary health care should be relevant to the special needs of individuals, communities and nations, and acceptable to the society it aims to serve. It discussed the importance of effective social policies to support good health; these include education, sufficient and safe supplies of food and water and proper sanitation. The promotion of good health and the prevention of illness were given high priority, with family planning and immunization held as examples of good practice.

In 1985 the European Region of WIIO published a report on the 'Health for All' policy and targets (WHO, 1985) which concluded that significant improvements in a population's health will be achieved by the implementation of policies which include:

Equity.   There are significant differences, both between and within communities, in the health experience of advantaged and disadvantaged groups. Major improvements in health status would be achieved if the levels of the most deprived could be raised to those of the most advantaged people. It was considered that progress will be made in this area through social and economic developments (education, employment, housing) rather than through changes in health care.

Health promotion.   The development of health policy, at both national and local levels, should not concentrate on the diagnosis and treatment of disease, but should address the whole range of health interventions, with particular emphasis on health promotion. This includes health promotion focused on individual behaviour, for example smoking, abuse of drugs and alcohol, diet, and at the macro level of organizational and environmental matters, for example, air pollution and a safe water supply.

Multisectoral action.   The prerequisites for health, including factors such as a secure role in society, freedom from the fear of war, and the main determinants of health (factors in the physical, economic and social environments), can only be changed if there is co-operation across all sectors. This means that government agencies at national and local levels must work together with industry, as well as with business and professionals; their combined efforts must include concern for quality and cost-effectiveness.

Public participation. Well-informed and well-motivated citizens are important partners in the setting of priorities and the implementation of health programmes. 'Health for All' is essentially a 'bottom-up' approach which needs the facilitation of 'top-down' political commitment.

Reorientation of health services. The basic health care needs of a community should be met by accessible high-quality primary health care. This requires all health services to incorporate health promotion and disease prevention as part of their repertoire of care.

These principles aim to achieve the outcomes of:

- ensuring equity in health
- adding life to years by helping people to achieve their full physical, mental and social potential
- adding health to life by reducing disability and disease
- adding years to life by increasing life expectancy.

The 38 'Health for All' targets established by the European Office (WHO, 1985) were endorsed as policy by all the WHO European Member States, including the UK, and have subsequently been updated (WHO, 1991; WHO, 1992).

● Health of the nation

Following the publication of the 'Health for All' targets by the WHO, several governments drew up health strategies for their own countries.

In England, the Department of Health produced *The Health of the Nation: A Strategy for Health in England* (DoH, 1992). This specifically endorsed the 'Health for All' strategy and its stated aim is to secure continuing improvement in the general health of the population by 'adding years to life and life to years'. It also adopted the approach of target setting as a method of defining the direction of desired change, setting goals for the rate of change and establishing means of measuring progress. Five 'key areas' were selected for attention, on the basis that they represent a major burden of disease, and information on methods of prevention is already available. These five areas are:

- coronary heart disease and stroke
- cancer
- mental health
- HIV/AIDS and sexual health
- accidents.

Targets have been set in each of these areas, with associated action plans and timetables. The document stresses the need for 'healthy alliances' (multisectoral action) in order to achieve these targets.

The 'Health of the Nation' document has been criticized on the grounds that it focuses on issues related to individual behaviour (smoking, alcohol consumption) and avoids matters of public policy such as poverty, unemployment and the physical environment. It has also been pointed out that many of the targets are in line with current trends, such as the falling mortality from coronary heart disease, so that it is possible the targets may be achieved with minimal extra effort.

The 'Health of the Nation' document was followed by the publication of *Targeting Practice: The Contribution of Nurses, Midwives and Health Visitors* (DoH, 1993a). This document draws attention to the important role all nurses can play in achieving 'Health of the Nation' targets. Practitioners have an education role, by informing and empowering people to change behaviour and make healthy choices, as well as influencing professional practice and the delivery of health care, making it more accessible and sensitive to the needs of service users, thus improving uptake of preventive services and encouraging early reporting of symptoms. A further important role of the community health care nurse is to influence environmental change through professional advice on health hazards in either the workplace or the community in which people live. Community health care nurses are often recognized and respected in their localities and provide an important role model not only for people with whom they are in direct contact, but also for the wider community. Personal health behaviour in matters such as smoking, diet, exercise and participation in prevention programmes is therefore of particular importance as a contribution to the population's health.

Coronary heart disease and stroke

The main targets in this area are reductions in mortality from coronary heart disease and stroke. It is anticipated that these will be reached by reductions in risk factors such as smoking, diet, obesity, blood pressure and alcohol consumption. All community health care nurses can contribute to this work. For instance, behaviour can be influenced by advising on lifestyles as part of professional contact with individuals as well as in more formal screening and health promotion clinics. Such advice is effective and important at certain key times, such as in antenatal clinics and child health clinics. Community health care nurses also have increasing opportunities to advise individuals on lifestyle and rehabilitation following surgery and other hospital treatments; this is especially possible with decreasing lengths of in-patient care and the increased use of day treatments.

Cancer

Reductions in mortality from lung, breast, cervical and skin cancers are the main targets in relation to cancer. The achievement of lung cancer targets depends on reduction in risk factors, predominantly smoking, which also applies to coronary heart disease. Here again, the contribution of community health care nurses to behaviour change, through individual advice, smoking cessation clinics and other focused health promotional activities, and personal example, is of importance in the overall programme.

The main prospects of reduction in breast and cervical cancers are through screening programmes. Community health care nurses can inform women about the availability of preventive services and about the nature of the tests, reassure them about participation and counsel them about results. Where appropriate, they can also show leadership and example by themselves attending for screening. Nurses can play a major part in the provision of screening services and work with colleagues to achieve high standards of quality of care, which improve both uptake and satisfaction among women.

Reduction in skin cancer can be achieved by reducing exposure to sunlight. The main contribution of practitioners is therefore through education, particularly in child health clinics, school clinics and as part of work with community groups (see Chapter 15).

Mental health

A reduction in suicide rates, both for the general population and among severely mentally ill people, is the challenge set in the area of mental health. This is perhaps the most challenging of the five target areas, and the one where success will be most difficult to achieve. The contribution of community psychiatric nurses is clear, through their support for people with mental illness, particularly those who have been discharged from hospital care. However, other community health care nurses have important preventive roles through the provision of support, particularly during vulnerable episodes in people's lives such as the postnatal period and following bereavement. Knowledge of clients at risk of these situations enables practitioners to detect depression at an early stage and the provision of support for individuals and groups can help to reduce stress associated with key life events such as retirement, redundancy or homelessness.

HIV/AIDS and sexual health

The main aim in the area of sexual health is to reduce the incidence of HIV and other sexually transmitted diseases as well as reducing the number of unwanted pregnancies, especially among young people. Again, in this area the main contribution is through education, targeted at high-risk and vulnerable groups. Community health care nurses can participate in this by using opportunistic contact, for example in family planning clinics where the practitioners can influence the provision of services, making them more acceptable to young people. There is a key education role for community health care nurses in schools, which is discussed in Chapter 14.

Accidents

Reductions in death rates from accidents among children under 15, young people (15–24) and older people (65 and over) are set as targets to be achieved. Community health care nurses have a key role in achieving this target both through group activities, education sessions and advice to individuals. When visiting people at home, opportunities will arise to advise on the removal of hazards and if necessary to ensure that action is taken; for example, by obtaining help to secure appropriate window locks and fireguards or deal with unsafe electrical equipment.

The 'Health of the Nation' is a welcome statement of the government's commitment to improving the health of the population, and clearly identifies targets which community health care nurses must address when working with individuals and groups in the community. However, their impact will be limited unless there is complementary action at local and national levels in the development of health policy and the establishment of 'Healthy Alliances'.

● **Healthy alliances**

The 'Health for All' strategy emphasizes the importance of multisectoral action, and 'Health of the Nation' talks of 'healthy alliances'. In both cases this means that health improvement cannot be brought about by the health care sector, or any other sector, acting alone. Progress is only made by the collaborative action of statutory agencies (education, housing, health, social care), commerce and industry and voluntary bodies acting at both local and national levels. There are many examples of 'healthy alliance' projects and initiatives throughout Europe, North America and Australia (Ashton, 1992). A specific example focuses on the promotion of children's health in inner London and involves an alliance between the local authority, the District Health Authority and the Family Health Services Authority (DoH, 1993b).

● **Healthy cities**

The 'Healthy Cities' project was initiated by the WHO to bring together and support cities across Europe developing health strategies using the 'Health for All' framework. The project has now extended to cities worldwide and has become the 'Healthy Cities' movement (Tsouros, 1990). It includes the principles of health promotion set out in the Ottawa *Charter for Health Promotion* (WHO, 1986) and the principles of the *European Charter on Environment and Health* (WHO, 1989).

Participating cities are expected to:

- reduce inequalities in health status and in access to the prerequisites for health within the city
- develop healthy public policies at the local level
- create physical and social environments that support health
- strengthen community action for health
- help people develop new skills for health
- reorient health services in accordance with the health strategy and the principles of health promotion.

Many places have now adopted this approach to policy and service development even if they are not part of the 'Healthy Cities' project. Although 'Healthy Cities' work is led by local government, health agencies inevitably play a significant role in both policy and project development. The opportunities for community health care nurses to contribute to 'Healthy Cities' based approaches to health care are numerous. These initiatives rarely require extra resources, but are much more dependent on attitude, innovative ideas and multi-agency team-work. They are consistent with the priorities which most Health Authorities have declared and are underpinned by the educational philosophies established for nurses in the UK through *Project 2000* (UKCC, 1986) and for doctors through *Tomorrow's Doctors* (General Medical Council, 1993).

Inequalities in health status can be reduced by professionals focusing their work among the most vulnerable people in the community, such as homeless people, travellers, ethnic minority groups, single parents and chronically ill and disabled people. This enables the provision of flexible and easily accessible services in or near people's homes, to encourage the participation of those who have little motivation and who may lack the physical, psychological or economic resources needed to travel to formal health care facilities. Community health care nurses are important public health advocates at the local level, particularly for the vulnerable groups of the population, since their professional training and continuing development and education make them natural participants in community planning groups. Indeed, practitioners' knowledge of health and of the local population allows them to analyse problems, assess possible solutions and put forward practical proposals for implementation (see Chapter 23).

Health-promoting physical and social environments at both the micro and the macro levels need to be created. Within people's homes the community health care nurse can advise individuals on diet, hygiene and physical hazards, as well as supporting people with relationship problems, encouraging activities which reduce social isolation and offering health education, issues which can also be addressed in various group situations. All these activities contribute to the empowerment of the population which leads to strengthening of community action for health and provides citizens with knowledge about health and helps them to develop the skills allowing them to make healthy choices.

Nurses are the single largest group of health professionals, both in hospitals and in the community. They therefore have the greatest opportunities to contribute to the reorientation of health services and this can be done through either individual care or with groups giving advice on health, the prevention of disease or its recurrence, and rehabilitation. In addition, practitioners can work together to focus on policy development and improvement in the quality of care in departments or services.

●   **Health and social policy**

'Healthy Cities' and 'Healthy Alliances' are based on the need for integrated health-promoting policies across many sectors at local level in order to improve the health of the population. For many health hazards, the same arguments apply at national and international levels. Such hazards, environmental ones, do not recognize man-made boundaries. This was acknowledged in the UK at the time of publication of *Health of the Nation*, when a Cabinet-level interdepartment group was established to consider the health impact of the policies of all government departments and to co-ordinate action.

Indeed, the link between poverty and ill health has been well documented and analysed since 1980 when the Black Report highlighted the correlation between health and socio-economic status by publishing a number of health indices (Davidson and Townsend, 1982). Further work has suggested that the 'health gap' in society has grown wider, even though there is a general trend towards improvement on indicators such as perinatal mortality (Kumar, 1993; Eames *et al.*, 1993).

Housing policy also has a major impact on health. Connelly and Crown (1994) show there is no doubt that poor health can precipitate homelessness, and that homelessness, either as a street-dweller or as a homeless family statutorily accommodated in an inadequate dwelling, can impair health. They also argue that poor-quality housing with inadequate facilities affects health. Recent government policies favouring and subsidizing home ownership and reducing the stock of local authority housing and housing association accommodation, and affordable private-rented housing, have led to large increases in the number of homeless people, especially those who are poor, chronically ill or disabled or otherwise vulnerable (see Chapter 17).

Transport policy affects health and wellbeing in many ways, and policies which favour cars and other forms of road transport have direct effects on air pollution which are associated with respiratory and other diseases as well as contributing to the 'greenhouse effect'. Cheap and reliable public transport, using rail and water as well as roads, can help people with access to work and services they need, such as health care, while reducing environmental damage, stress and accidents.

Education has a crucial relationship with health, and is a key determinant of the socio-economic status of adults. It directly affects levels of knowledge about health and, more importantly, it affects employment opportunities, self-esteem, empowerment and hence many behavioural patterns (Policy Studies Institute, 1994). Traditional patterns of education such as pre-school, school and higher education now need to be complemented by continuing education to allow people to acquire new skills required by advancing technologies, so as to retain their employability and reduce the impact of rapidly changing work requirements and redundancy.

An inevitable part of population empowerment and health promotion, which has implications for social policy relating to health, is increased user involvement in service planning and provision. This change has been endorsed by government policy in a wave of initiatives to make public sector services more responsive and accountable to their consumers. *The Patient's Charter* (DoH, 1991) was published with the aim of improving the quality of health care delivery to the public, while maintaining the principles of the NHS, that services should be available to every citizen on the basis of the clinical need, regardless of ability to pay, and that the service should be funded mainly by general taxation. The Charter sets out 10 rights to NHS care, and defines nine national charter standards. Charter standards relate to quality issues, for example for privacy and acceptance of cultural beliefs, equal access to premises regardless of psychomotor or sensory disability, and the availability of information to patients' relatives. Maximum waiting times for ambulances and in-patient, outpatient and accident departments are defined, together with recommendations about the cancellation of operations. The Charter also endorses the profession's initiative in introducing the concept of the 'named nurse' who is responsible for the co-ordination of care.

Many of the Charter's high profile national initiatives have concentrated on acute hospital issues, most notably waiting lists and waiting times. It has been less widely recognized that the Charter Rights and Standards apply to all users of the NHS, including those in primary, community and non-acute settings. New additions to the Charter have specifically focused on general practitioner services and the community services provided by nurses, health visitors and midwives (DoH, 1995). Local charter standards have been developed in many of these units by staff working alongside clients in areas such as mental health, elderly care and children's services.

● Conclusion

'Health for All' is a powerful and cohesive strategy which underpins much policy development in the UK and elsewhere. Its implementation requires the extension and improvement of primary health care, as well as the development of broader based health policies. Community health care nurses can have pivotal roles in these activities and must ensure that their training, education and practice enable them to play a full part.

References

Ashton, J. (ed.) (1992) *Healthy Cities*, Open University Press, Milton Keynes
Connelly, J. and Crown, J. (eds) (1994) *Homelessness and Ill Health*, Royal College of Physicians, London
Davidson, M. and Townsend, P. (1982) *Inequalities in Health*, Penguin, London
DoH (1991) *The Patient's Charter*, HMSO, London
DoH (1992) *The Health of the Nation: A Strategy for Health in England*, HMSO, London
DoH (1993a) *Targeting Practice: The Contribution of Nurses, Midwives and Health Visitors*, HMSO, London
DoH (1993b) *The Health of the Nation: Target*, Issue 4, Department of Health, London
DoH (1995) *The Patient's Charter and You*, HMSO, London
Eames, M., Ben-Shlomo, Y. and Marmot, M.G. (1993) Social deprivation and premature mortality: regional comparison across England. *Br. Med. J.*, Oct., 1097–1102
General Medical Council (1993) *Tomorrow's Doctors: Recommendations on Undergraduate Medical Education*, GMC, London

Kumar, V. (1993) *Poverty and Inequality in the UK: The Effects on Children*, National Children's Bureau, London

Policy Studies Institute (1994) Policy Studies Institute Report, 100 Park Village East, London, UK

Tsouros, A.D. (1990) *WHO Healthy Cities Project: A Project becomes a Movement. Review of Progress 1987–1990*, World Health Organisation, Copenhagen

UKCC (1986) *Project 2000: A New Preparation for Practice*, United Kingdom Central Council for Nursing, Midwifery and Health Visiting, London

WHO (1985) *Targets for Health for All*, World Health Organisation, Regional Office for Europe, Copenhagen

WHO (1986) *Charter for Health Promotion*, no. 4, iii–v, *Health Promotion 1*, World Health Organisation, Copenhagen

WHO (1989) *European Charter on Environment and Health*, World Health Organisation, Copenhagen

WHO (1991) *Targets for Health for All: The Health Policy for Europe*, World Health Organisation, Regional Office for Europe, Copenhagen

WHO (1992) *Targets for Health for All: The Health Policy for Europe*, World Health Organisation, Regional Office for Europe, Copenhagen

4

Secondary to primary health care shift

Sheila Roy

Health care is being affected by a number of trends, all of which will impact upon the delivery of services within the NHS as a whole. That change, which is necessary in delivering community services, is becoming increasingly accepted by all leading health care policy-makers and has achieved a consensus across all the political parties. Forces such as fundamental social, demographic and technological change, as are illustrated in Figure 4.1, are creating an opportunity significantly to improve services to the ultimate users with the pressures, such as the structural reform, taking place within the NHS and the need to ensure cost-effective services providing the motivation for change.

● Forces for change

There are a number of forces for change impacting upon community services, and in particular the shift from secondary to primary care. These will fundamentally alter the provision of health care in general, and community services in particular, within a very short time-scale.

Demographic changes

The impact of changes in the demography of the UK, shown in Figure 4.2, has been well documented. A major factor in the future will be a rise of 32% in those living beyond the age of 85 before the end of the century.

At the same time, assuming that most people have children in their twenties, the pool of available carers for this age group will decline by 5%. At present, there are nearly seven people aged 60–74 to everyone aged over 85. By the end of the century the pool of carers, unpaid and often unacknowledged, will have significantly shrunk, whereas the demand for their services will have risen.

Paradoxically, at the same time there will be a growth at the other end of the age spectrum, with a rise in the number of those aged under 5

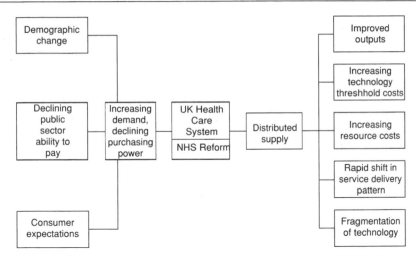

Figure 4.1   UK health care forces for change (Source: Newchurch & Co.)

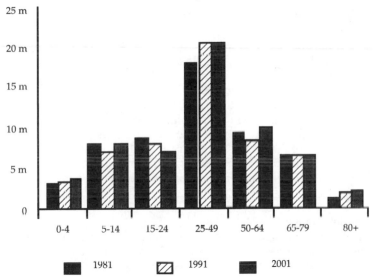

Figure 4.2   Demographic change, 1981–2001 (Source: Office of Population Censuses and Surveys Population Projections 1989 Based)

in the next 10 years of over 10%. As can be seen in Figure 4.3, these age groups account for a significant proportion of the health care spend at the present time. These trends, therefore will have a significant impact in shifting the focus of health care towards the delivery of services in the community, with a greater emphasis on health promotion and maintenance rather than treatment.

As people have started to live longer, the expectation of the quality of life during that extended period of old age has also risen. A high quality of life does not equate with traditional institutional care. This shift in attitudes has been recognized by recent government initiatives

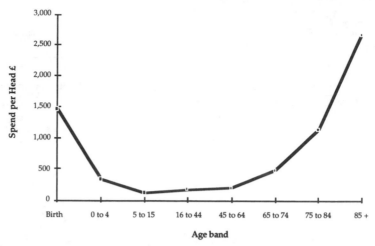

Figure 4.3 NHS health care spend by age group (Source: The government's expenditure plans 1992/93–1994/95, Department of Health and OPCS departmental report, 1993)

such as *The Health of the Nation* (DoH, 1992) and *The Patient's Charter* (DoH, 1991), both of which will lead to greater challenges to current patterns of service delivery and quality. The recent annual report from the Association of Community Health Councils for England and Wales (ACHCEW, 1993) states that 86% of community health councils (CHCs) have received an increase in complaints about the health service since April 1992. Of those CHCs which reported an increase in complaints, 58% considered the increase to be substantial and another 8% said that increases had doubled. It is interesting to note that 61% of CHCs believe that the Charter was the major cause of the increase in complaints.

Social change

Running concurrently with these demographic shifts are a number of social changes impacting upon the way we lead our lives and how we expect to interact with society. Not least among these is a general increase in levels of articulation among the public at large.

This trend has a particular impact upon community services when one considers that those currently entering pensionable age, who are traditionally high users of community services, represent the first generation of home owners, dual income earners and well pensioned to reach old age.

This growth in individual purchasing power is a general phenomenon. Real disposable income has risen inexorably in recent years, and as people have met their basic material needs, their attention has turned to other areas such as entertainment, travel and, not least, health care. This rise in purchasing power is likely to continue, and as people live longer, so their expectation of quality of life during the extended period of old age will rise, and it is likely they will be prepared to use some of their purchasing power to secure this.

Technological change

Technological change has been impressive over the past few years. Increasingly, technologically driven change has affected every aspect of how we run our lives. Critically, the way we view technology has also changed, with a general expectation that new products will work. The revolution in manufacturing techniques and quality control pioneered by the Japanese has brought about a sea-change in how we view technology. This change in attitude has an impact upon the delivery of health care. Those needing care expect to be treated, and for the treatment to be successful.

At the same time, much of the heavy investment made in information technology within the NHS has had little discernible effect on improving its efficiency. The revolution in thinking on how to harness the potential of technology seems to have largely passed the NHS by. For example, the increasing use of bar codes in a number of areas of everyday life over the past few years is only now appearing in health care.

The widespread use of drugs to control symptoms of many chronic conditions, especially mental illness, is having a dramatic effect on the need for long-term care. Improvements in dispensing technology have led to drug doses being planned much more sensitively to the needs of individual patients so that socially debilitating side-effects can be much reduced. This has a significant effect on the need for carers in the community and the skills required of professional staff.

● **Changes in practice**

Health care procedures are changing rapidly. Over the past 12 years the average length of stay in an acute hospital has fallen from 9.4 to 6.1 days, as illustrated in Figure 4.4.

As techniques become increasingly sophisticated, so the proportion of interventions carried out on a day basis or otherwise outside the traditional acute hospital setting is expected to rise substantially. Already

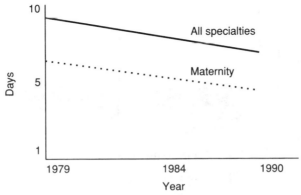

Figure 4.4 Changes in average length of stay (acute and maternity), 1979–90 (Source: Health and Personal Social Services Statistics for England, Department of Health, 1992)

the number of day cases carried out each year has doubled since 1979 to over 1.1 million. Even when a stay in hospital is required, advances in treatments have allowed average lengths of stay in acute specialities to fall by over a third in the past ten years to 6.1 days, a trend which has been mirrored in maternity care.

The reduction in the time spent by a patient in an acute setting does not necessarily reduce the amount of care and support required, but does shift the location of its delivery; for example, the increasing number of elderly people who are having cataract operations carried out as day cases. While these patients will receive their main course of treatment in an acute setting, they will still require continuing support from community services to ensure a return to full fitness. Similarly, elderly patients undergoing hip replacement operations can be discharged much earlier and rehabilitated in their home environment through well co-ordinated programmes of care across all agencies. It is partly due to the advances in technology and changed patterns of practice that there is a shift away from secondary to primary and community care and that this can be successfully achieved.

At the same time, there has been a rise of 14% in the numbers of patients treated (Figure 4.5). Over the same time, the growth in the proportion receiving acute services has risen by 38% to 5.7 million. However, the number of in-patient beds has declined from 370 000 to 270 000, with 120 000, or 45%, of those being classified as acute. New techniques such as lithotripsy high-energy shock waves to shatter kidney and gall stones, chemical treatments for gastric ulcers, CAT scanners and EMI resonators are all reducing the need for surgical intervention and long stays in hospital. Increasingly, patients are being discharged into the community at a higher level of dependency.

Changes have also occurred in the delivery of certain types of care,

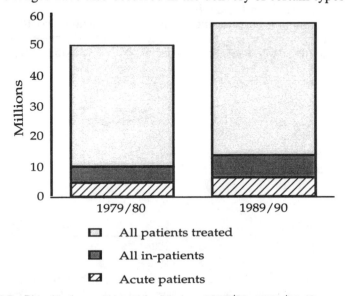

☐   All patients treated

▨   All in-patients

▨   Acute patients

Figure 4.5 Rise in the number of patients, 1979/80–1989/90 (Source: Health and Personal Social Services Statistics for England, Department of Health, 1992)

and this is particularly evident among care of the elderly. Over the past 10 years there has been a 150% increase in the number of residential care places. Much of this growth has been created by the private sector, which has increased its share of the residential care market from 37% to 60%.

Furthermore, the care of people who either have learning disabilities or are chronically mentally ill has undergone substantial change, with the numbers in residential NHS care having fallen dramatically in recent years. Over the past decade, the total number of mentally ill and people with learning disabilities in residential NHS care has fallen by over a third (Figure 4.6).

Within mental health, the drive in recent years has been to complete the process of closing institutions and freeing people from enforced dependence on rigidly controlled patterns of care. As a result, policy-makers have had to balance a number of often conflicting demands, including questions over the amount of influence they can legitimately exercise over people's lives and the provision of adequate care to ensure the safety of users and other members of society. In an effort to help resolve this, there has been an effort to devolve and share responsibility. The inclusion of the needs of these people in the 'Care in the Community' initiative is an attempt to provide care on an individually planned basis at the same time as creating a separation of roles

Structural change

The NHS reforms have radically altered the picture of the NHS. Critically, a division has been drawn between the commissioning of services and the provision of them. While they may attach different labels to the process, this division has gained a broad consensus among the political parties. This has led to an increasingly complex and fragmented pattern of care which users may find difficult to access (Figure 4.7).

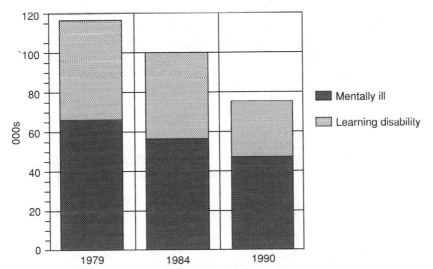

Figure 4.6 Numbers of mentally ill and people with learning disabilities in residential NHS care, 1979–90 (Source: Newchurch & Co. Estimates, 1992)

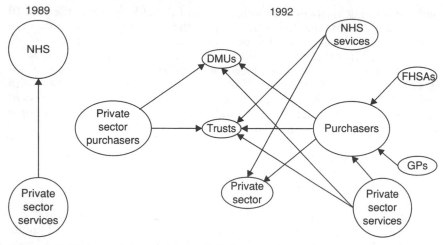

Figure 4.7   Structural change in the NHS (Source: Newchurch & Co.)

Structural change can also be seen in the increased specialization of services. Services for specific care groups, such as those with HIV/AIDS, diabetes, asthma or learning disabilities are increasingly being treated by specialist teams which include staff from both the secondary and primary sectors. This development will also have an important impact upon the way community services are delivered in the future and sets a model of good practice for an integrated approach to care across a number of agencies.

The complexity of this picture is further increased by the changes promulgated in the local authority sector. Social Services departments have been given the lead role in many areas previously seen as the preserve of the NHS, especially in the long-term care of people who are elderly, mentally ill or have learning disabilities. From 1 April 1993, the assessment of all people with special needs is now made in conjunction with Social Services. Already problems have been experienced among both users and health care professionals by the establishment of clear demarcation lines which are further fragmenting the delivery of the service, and instead of the creation of a seamless service, enormous barriers have been erected across agency boundaries.

Definition of primary and secondary care

The population's initial point of contact with the NHS is usually via the primary care portal. It is generally accepted that primary care includes:

* Family Health Services provided by General Medical Practitioners (GPs), dentists, opticians and pharmacists which are in contact with the Family Health Services Authorities (FHSAs)
* health promotion and disease prevention provided and managed by District Health Authorities (DHAs)

- community health services provided by either Trusts or Directly Managed Units (DMUs) including district nurses, health visitors, school nurses, paramedical services and others.

Primary care can also have a wider definition, which is not universally acknowledged. This definition embraces the above, but additionally includes:

- services which the patient refers themselves to without initial referral to any health care professional; for example, family planning services and chiropodists
- services which are provided in a non-primary health care setting; for example, patients seen in an accident and emergency department to obtain primary care
- outpatient and day-care services, where the GP still has clinical responsibility for the patient
- support from Local Authorities which could include housing, education and input from Social Services, which may take the form of social workers or home support.

In general, primary care has a local focus, with an emphasis on ease of accessibility.

Secondary care is typified by the local district general hospital (DGH). It is here that the patient is normally referred to from the primary care setting should they require specialist acute diagnosis and treatment. The central feature of a DGH is the ability to admit medical and surgical emergencies through an accident and emergency department. District general hospitals also provide an outpatient department, where patients are seen both before and after medical and surgical treatment, facilities to carry out operations, a maternity department, together with support services such as pharmacies, pathology and radiography.

Traditional view of the DGH as a focus of secondary care

Although the vast majority of people only ever have health care contact at primary level, much attention and finance has been focused within secondary care, and most especially within the local district general hospital. Only 15% of patients treated by the NHS are seen in a hospital, although roughly 55% of the NHS budget is allocated to hospital-based care (Figure 4.8).

The main argument that has been used to defend the secondary sector as a centre of care is the high visibility of medical interventions and clinical outcomes. Community and primary care have, by their very nature, been less visible due to the diversity of the services and the delivery of these as near as possible to the patient's own home. Increasingly this situation is changing. The rapid development of new medical technology has revolutionized the delivery of care, allowing shorter lengths of stay after surgery and more complex procedures being carried out in a variety of settings.

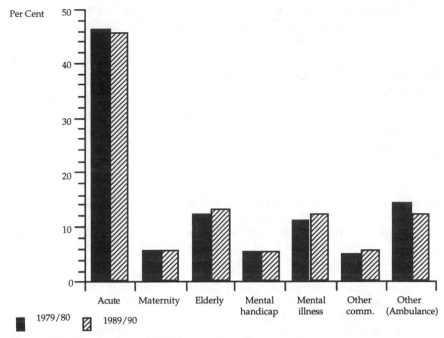

Figure 4.8 Distribution of NHS spending (Source: The government's expenditure plans 1992/93–1994/95, Department of Health and OPCS departmental report, 1993)

The culture of dependency on hospital-based care

It has been widely acknowledged that in order to increase the shift away from secondary to primary care, the traditional reliance on the local district general hospital as the focus of care must be broken. This problem is especially relevant in inner cities. Inner city residents rely on their local hospital to provide both the relevant secondary care and primary care in an appropriate location. Many visit the accident and emergency department of their local hospital in order to receive treatment that would be more appropriately carried out in a primary care setting; for example, 40% of attendees at the accident and emergency department at King's Hospital, London, fit this category. This inflow of patients creates longer delays for those who should be treated in an accident and emergency department and causes inconvenience for those who present themselves for treatment in the inappropriate setting.

In order to combat the hospital dependency problem, the idea has recently been floated to provide 24-hour GP surgeries within the district general hospital. However, this scenario still does not completely solve the problem. Patients are still presenting themselves for treatment in an inappropriate setting, when they really should be educated into seeking treatment from their local GP surgery. The reality is, however, that re-educating the public will not suffice if the services on offer within the primary care sector are substandard and not meeting the needs of the population.

Funding arrangements

Spending on health care within the UK has risen steadily, to a point where the NHS currently accounts for nearly £30 billion, or 14.4% of all government spending, compared with a figure of 12.0% in 1979. Spending has also risen in the private sector to over £5 billion. This is a significant market, and the split between commissioning or purchasing and providing services has opened up the prospect of alternative suppliers of services coming forward.

With low barriers to entry and huge demand, alternative suppliers are likely to compete for business. This competition may come from both within and outside the NHS, although in the short term, competition is more likely to come from within the health service, not only from adjacent suppliers, but also from GPs. In the longer term, competition from the private sector, or even local authority social services departments or voluntary agencies, will become critical.

The transfer of lead responsibility to local authorities for long-term care and the creation of purchasing budgets for many non-emergency services is leading to a major reduction of the purchasing power of DHAs acting in isolation. The impact on NHS Trusts and directly managed units that focus on the provision of community services will be enormous. The proactive have a vast array of potential income sources. Those relying on the benevolence of local NHS policy-makers who might wish to see a shift of service provision into the community will quickly suffer and may raise serious questions about their viability.

If the present patterns of service delivery are to continue with no change to the present internal NHS division of allocated monies shown in Figure 4.9, this would necessitate an even larger increase in funding to

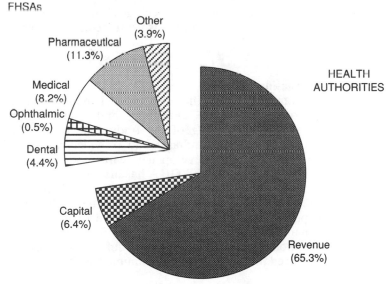

Figure 4.9 Distribution of NHS expenditure, 1991 (Source: The government's expenditure plans 1992/93–1994/95, Department of Health and OPCS departmental report, 1993)

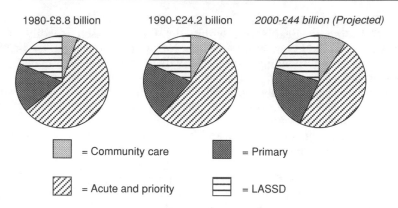

1980-£8.8 billion   1990-£24.2 billion   2000-£44 billion (Projected)

▦ = Community care   ▪ = Primary

▨ = Acute and priority   ▤ = LASSD

Figure 4.10 Expenditure on community health and care services, 1979–2000 (Source: The government's expenditure plans 1992/93–1994/95, Department of Health and OPCS departmental report with Newchurch and Co. Estimates, 1993)

meet the cost of delivery. This is one of the reasons why attention has been focused upon a shift to primary from secondary care. Projected forward at the present rate of growth and maintaining patterns of service delivery in their current form, by the year 2000 the NHS would need a budget of £44 billion, (Figure 4.10).

On the evidence of previous years, this growth would not automatically generate increased quality in the delivery of the service to the public; in fact, evidence supports the opposite. Where funding has been continuously reduced, increased throughput, lowered waiting lists and different patterns of service delivery have emerged. Alongside the emergence of GP fundholding, increased patient choice, value for money initiatives and the introduction of capital charges, there is a growing momentum for change and a shift of emphasis from secondary to primary care.

Changing purchasing strategies

As the internal market within the NHS takes shape and stabilizes, district health authorities are now examining and evaluating their purchasing strategies. The uncoupling of the traditional hospital/DHA relationship has meant that both purchaser and provider can examine patterns of care and subsequently develop new care models. The pre-reform entanglement of the hospital and DHA has meant that inappropriate care patterns have evolved, with a heavy reliance on patient referrals to a secondary care setting. The DHA, now purchasing health care on behalf of its local population, can now respond more easily to techno-logical and social change. Existing purchasing patterns are already being challenged and new models are evolving, with a definite emphasis on a shift to care being centred in a primary and community setting.

The influence of the FHSA on primary care

Both FHSAs and GPs have realized that in order to improve the provision and quality of health care, they must enter into a closer partnership. Added to this partnership is the increasing involvement and co-operation with the DHA. Some FHSAs and DHAs are already entering into joint commissioning partnerships, with the still legally separate DHA and FHSA now calling themselves purchasing commissions. This welcome integration should also lead to a greater integration of primary and secondary care services.

The Patient's Charter

From April 1993, *The Patient's Charter* came into effect in the primary care setting. GPs and other primary health care professionals are drawing up quality standards for their own surgery or health centre. Standards should cover the following areas:

- improving the quality of information given to patients about local community health services
- improving the complaints, suggestions and comments procedures on local health care issues
- improving the transfer of patients' records from one surgery to another.

In addition, GPs and primary health care teams are drawing up and setting quality standards for their own practices and health centres. For example, some practices and health centres are improving the way in which they give results of tests, the organization of health promotion clinics, and improving facilities for the disabled. FHSAs are also liaising with local medical committees, individual GPs and primary health care professionals to set local voluntary standards. Examples of local standards include:

- how long a patient waits before getting an appointment with their GP
- how long a patient can be expected to wait to see a GP or nurse
- how quickly a patient can reach a GP or nurse in an emergency.

Patterns of service

A constant problem for health authorities is the tension between the demands for a centralized large district hospital that offers a comprehensive range of services and also for a decentralized provision of health care offered in the local community. The increase in technological change is allowing a gradual compromise between these two patterns of care. Procedures which used to require hospital admission, often involving a subsequent post-procedural stay, can now be carried out on a day-case or outpatient basis. Some episodes can even be carried out totally in a community setting, often in a GP's surgery.

Changing patterns of access

The traditional feature of secondary care acute services is that access is usually controlled by a GP, referring the patient for treatment in a secondary care setting. This pattern has remained rigid in the past, but there are signs that there is a shift away from this pattern. The changing ideas and practices that the recent reforms have introduced into the NHS have meant that new patterns of health care are emerging.

● **A window of opportunity**

While the changes described above are real, they can be viewed as an opportunity as much as a threat to community services. It is recognized by all leading health care policy-makers that the weighting of health care expenditure towards the acute sector cannot continue. Although the share of spending devoted to acute services has declined slightly in the past 10 years, this shift has been small. To ensure the necessary diversion of resources, community services will need to make a strong case to health care purchasers.

An ageing, more affluent population, with high expectations of quality services, is an attractive market for private sector suppliers. The speed with which the private sector has managed to gain a majority share of the market for residential care serves to illustrate how quickly previously accepted ways of doing things can change.

The shift from secondary to primary care

These forces are creating a momentum which is inevitable. Changes in funding, increasingly articulate populations, the growth of GP fundholding and the drive to establish programmes of value for money are all determining the need for change, as is illustrated in Figure 4.11. If nurses, midwives and health visitors are to meet this challenge, they must ensure that they are proactively responding rather than resisting the changes about them. There has never been such a time for nurses and other health care professionals working within the community environment to drive and take control of the changes which surround them.

Community nursing embraces the wide range of services provided by district nurses, health visitors, GP-based practice nurses, school nurses, community psychiatric nurses, mental handicap nurses, community midwives and specialist nurses such as family planning, Macmillan, stoma and continence nurses. These services range from the direct nursing of sick, convalescent or very ill patients to the wide spectrum of health promotion and disease prevention activities provided to the community as a whole, families and particular care groups such as children, elderly and disabled people, and those with mental health problems and learning difficulties.

At this critical time, nurses must see themselves within the context of health care delivery by a range of health care professionals, and the services which are delivered should be jointly agreed across a whole spectrum of disciplines. The measurements of quality existing at the moment in the community is invalid. Figure 4.12 illustrates this point by showing a number of contacts by a variety of health care professional groups. It is immediately apparent that this comparison of contacts across

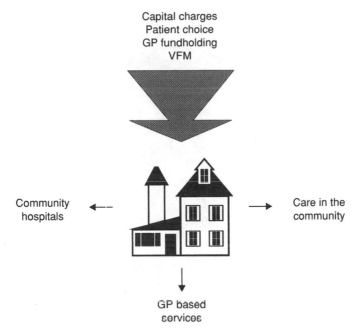

Figure 4.11 Pressures creating the shift of resources to primary care (Source: Newchurch & Co., 1993)

disciplines is inappropriate and has no meaning. Why then does this continue to be the predominant measure for community services? Nurses, midwives and health visitors should ask themselves continuously:

- **Who will buy my service in the future?**
- **How much will they buy?**
- **Based on what?**

Development of outcomes

The existing measures of community services are invalid, as has been demonstrated. Nurses, health visitors and midwives, as well as other health care professionals, must take the initiative and develop measures which are a true reflection of the input of value of their service. The risks associated with not taking this step are enormous, with continuing judgements being made on the basis of cost only, with no determining factor of quality. If health care professionals are to ensure optimum delivery of services to the user, they must take responsibility for this area.

Skill mix

Over the years, significant attention has been focused on skill mix. Manpower is the most significant cost in the provision of care. Throughout the NHS, it is estimated that manpower accounts for 76% of the cost base, of which 31% is accounted for by nurses, midwives and health visitors, which amounts to £5.2 billion. It is no surprise that attention is

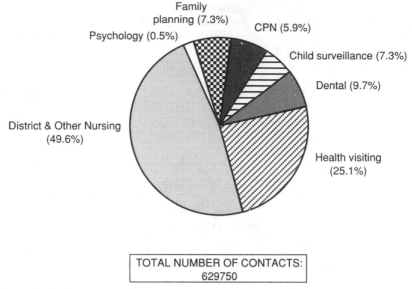

TOTAL NUMBER OF CONTACTS:
629750

Figure 4.12 Illustration of the breakdown of a number of contacts by professional group (Source: Newchurch & Co., 1993)

consistently focused on this group, and attempts made to reduce costs while maintaining high-quality services. A 1% saving on nursing across the board constitutes £52 million, and in any hard-strapped provider unit, a proportionate amount is significant to their survival and ability to survive. Still there is an enormous variation across the country in the numbers of staff to population, and the grade mix utilized.

Invariably there is no account taken of other disciplines and the skills and contribution that they have to offer, or the interface or overlaps which occur between them. The contracting processes which are now in place necessitate cost efficiency. Dilution of skill mix not only means a reduction in the unit cost of delivery, but can also improve the quantity and quality of the input by the use of most appropriate staff group. Figure 4.13 shows a typical picture of grade mix across three professional groups: district nursing, health visiting and school nursing.

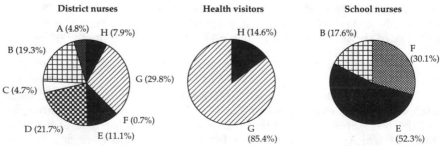

Figure 4.13 Typical picture of staff by grade by professional group (Source: Newchurch & Co., 1993)

As can be seen, the grade mix in district nursing and school nursing has been partly adjusted, but not so within health visiting. Many health visitors maintain that it is impossible for a dilution of grades to take place without de-skilling the professional group. This attitude is invalid when used at the same time as health visitors are complaining on the one hand of excessive clerical work and on the other of being unable fulfil their role with families rather than small segments of populations. Health visiting is a valued and valuable professional group, but the invisible nature of the role that they perform means that they are not perceived by everyone to be of value. This they must quickly address.

Both district nurses and health visitors must also review the percentage of teaching grades which generates an overhead cost on their services. At a time when the numbers of post-registration students being trained is diminishing, this cost must be reviewed. Nurses and health visitors must ensure, first, that they are training and educating appropriate numbers for the future, particularly as there is a large number of community staff approaching retirement age, and secondly, that there is a balance in the numbers of community practice teachers to oversee the educational programmes.

A further element which cannot be ignored is that of qualifying Project 2000 nurses. Since September 1992, there have been 834 nurses completing their programmes. These newly qualified nurses are now prepared to work in both the hospital and community setting and a framework within which they are able to work must be created if we are to realize the vision of 1989 when training started.

The creation and development of GP fundholding has added a further dimension to the purchasing of care. Individual practices now have the ability to buy certain services; these are:

- specified hospital services: namely, in-patient elective surgery, outpatient and diagnostic investigations – emergency admissions and medical admissions are excluded
- staff costs of the practice, excluding the GPs' salaries
- drugs prescribed and dispensed.

From April 1993, the list was extended to include:

- community services
- some mental health services.

Community services cover district nurses, health visiting, family planning and paramedical services including physiotherapy, speech and occupational therapy. Fundholders can also purchase care for people with learning difficulties and mental health services including community psychiatric nursing.

Initially, GP fundholders have been required to purchase services from NHS provider units. From April 1994, fundholders will be permitted to purchase a limited number of services, such as physiotherapy and chiropody, from providers who may be outside the NHS. In future years it seems likely that restrictions on the purchase of other services will also be relaxed. This will result in competition for the provision of community services from GP-run services and the private sector and voluntary agency services, as well as from other community units.

The threat of competition is already having a significant impact on the way community services are delivered. Many community units are seeking to lock into their local GPs by aligning their services with GP practice populations and ensuring that community nursing services are part of an integral primary health care team. Skill mix reviews are being introduced to improve productivity and to assist in reducing wait times and lowering costs.

An immediate risk in the system is, however, the allocation of funds and the calculation of budgets. Some Regions are already proposing to allocate monies on a capitation formulae. This may in no way relate to the present flows of money and may dramatically impact on the levels of service at present delivered to some populations. Figure 4.14 illustrates the major differences which exist within one District, and the variation of spend which exists.

If looked at against the map of deprivation for the same areas, it can be seen that, not surprisingly, the areas of lowest spend are the most highly deprived of the population, and the areas of highest spend correspond to more articulate populations with better provision from GP practices. Anecdotally, nurses and health visitors know that this situation exists, and has existed for a long time, and yet it is still possible consistently to find examples of this mismatch throughout any community.

It is accepted that a differential spend may be wholly appropriate dependent upon the population need based on deprivation, but is it correctly focused now? The exercise of mapping elements of the population indices against the number of staff delivering care repeatedly demonstrates that a mismatch exists between resource and need. Exam-

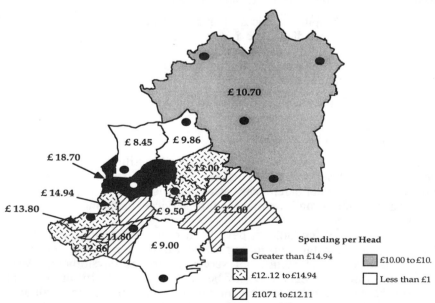

Figure 4.14 Map showing a range of spend on health care professionals for a District by electoral ward (Source: Newchurch & Co., 1993)

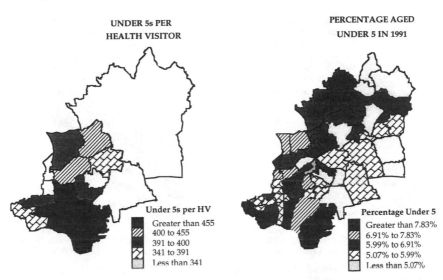

Figure 4.15 Example of mismatch between local population need and delivery: health visitors to under 5s (Source: Newchurch & Co., 1993)

ples of this are seen in the following illustrations. Figure 4.15 shows the concentration of under 5s by electoral ward within a population, compared with the density shown by shading against the number of health visitors to under 5s in the same population

Figure 4.16 illustrates a similar pattern for district nurses compared to over 65s. These particular indicators are chosen as one group most served by that particular health care professional, but other indices can be added to build up the picture of deprivation; for example, single parents, unemployment, and the elderly living alone.

It would appear that there is an underprovision in some areas where the care group is in high concentration and overprovision in areas of low concentration. As can be seen, the geographical areas may be large and the population dense in some areas, and the number of practices covered within the area may be numerous. For this reason the attachment of staff may be very appropriate for one practice population and less so for another. The problem arises in that, with the present information systems, it is difficult to obtain a more clear picture in the majority of areas, and this must be remedied as soon as possible.

The way forward

A number of opportunities have developed for community staff to create and deliver a very different pattern of services in the future. Too often they have been constrained by money and imagination. The areas on which community staff should immediately focus include: quality and outcome measures; skill mix and unit costs; multi-agency working; and

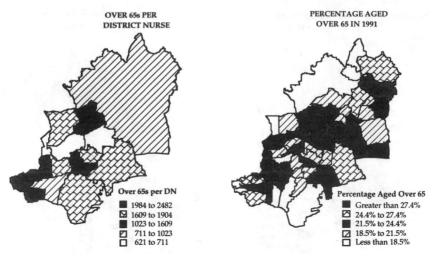

Figure 4.16 Example of mismatch between local population need and delivery: district nurses to over 65s (Source: Newchurch & Co., 1993)

education and training. The changes within society alongside the NHS reforms have created a window of opportunity which they must utilize.

References

ACHCEW (1993) Annual Report 1992/93, Association of Community Health Councils for England and Wales, London.

DoH (1991)*The Patient's Charter*, HMSO, London.

DoH (1992)*The Health of the Nation: A Strategy for Health in England*, HMSO, London.

5

A new vision for health care

Michael Weir and Carole Whittaker

A new kind of health policy is required which takes account of the many and varied factors which influence health far beyond the specific elements of the health services themselves.

(Margaret Whitehead, *The Health Divide*)

● **Introduction**

What is health status?

Several years ago one of the authors of this chapter was working in Africa attempting to introduce family planning strategies to rural communities. The evidence indicated that longer spacings between births would reduce the distressingly high death rates of young babies and of mothers in labour. However, the initiative had little appeal to the women in the villages and made limited impact on the problem. Fertility was the currency of status in a society where a woman's principal value was her ability to produce offspring. Any interference with this role would have had serious implications for her standing and personal viability. The Western scientific appreciation of the health needs of these women contrasted sharply with their own understanding. A clash of interpretations of what health actually meant had emerged.

It would be a mistake to believe that such conflicts are only to be found in developing countries, as they characterize the health debate globally. In the 'developed world', the need to be accepted by one's peers and therefore drink or smoke or abuse drugs as they do, can have more relevance than warnings about the consequences of such actions. For some, the termination of pregnancy is seen as a woman's right; for others, it is the senseless destruction of a life. Health, rather than being a fixed concept, reflects the belief system of the culture and individuals in question. Respecting the wishes of the individual while working for collective improvement is the challenge confronting health care planners.

At a national level, prevailing political, scientific and socio-economic factors determine how health is understood and how health care is provided. Again differing interpretations of the same problem are advocated by a spectrum of agencies. In the UK, the impact of poverty and unemployment on health and the influence of cigarette advertising on teenage smoking are interpreted differently by the major political parties. For better or for worse health care holds centre stage in the struggle between different political and ideological interests. To date, the size of the health budget, the volume of patients treated, the length of waiting lists and the numbers of doctors and nurses employed by the National Health Service (NHS) have been taken as the major indicators of commitment or indifference in the health debate. Unfortunately, such crude monitoring of activity and input alone gives little information about the effectiveness of attempts to cure or care. What all shades of political opinion need to give greater emphasis to is the outcome of services and the impact of expenditure on the public health.

It is easy to agree that health services should be concerned to protect, promote and restore health, that their principal goal should be to improve health status by the most effective, efficient and appropriate means available. But how does one measure health status and who determines the parameters to be employed? Is it merely a measure of the levels of illness in society or should it embrace wider indicators of individual and collective wellbeing? Such philosophical considerations and their practical implications should lie at the heart of the debate about the fate and purpose of health services. This would give greater balance in these times of unrest and uncertainty, as many powerful authorities compete to present their visions for the future of health care.

Times of change

The past decade has witnessed an unprecedented level of challenge and change to the way health care is managed and directed. To a large degree the principal motivation has been financial, as governments have sought to control expenditure through a variety of approaches. To this end the NHS has been through a succession of major reorganizations in the pursuit of improved quality and accountability. More recently, these changes in general and fiscal management have been intensified by a philosophical shift to market forces and away from the perceived limitations of a State-run bureaucracy.

Other agencies have expressed their concerns less about how the ship is run and more about the actual direction in which it is heading. The World Health Organisation's *Health for All by the Year 2000* initiative has championed preventive medicine and identified specific outcome goals which would have major implications for the planning and philosophy of care (WHO, 1985). *The Black Report* (Townsend and Davidson, 1982) and *The Health Divide* (Whitehead, 1992), in establishing a clear appreciation of the contribution of poverty and social deprivation to ill-health, have lent support to calls for direct government action to influence these factors.

Challenging the status quo

To those concerned to improve the public health, reviewing the management and direction of health care should be ongoing processes.

However, it is the contention of these authors that attempts to improve health services must be complemented by a fundamental review of the scientific and philosophical assumptions which underpin the health care model currently employed. This, we consider, is the major challenge awaiting health care professionals and one which has greater implications for the way care is provided than many, if not all, of the recent changes.

Though it is seldom made explicit in medical and nursing training, the scientific basis of practice is based upon certain assumptions of the nature of human life. It is evident that these assumptions can no longer be scientifically justified and that they are imposing major obstructions to attempts to improve the health of the nation. To a large degree modern medicine, despite its employment of high technology in diagnosis and treatment, still strictly operates within the mechanistic paradigm which developed from the ideas of René Descartes and Sir Isaac Newton three centuries ago (Capra, 1983). In the light of developments in modern physics, systems theory and the social sciences, together with evidence of stasis in attempts to improve prevention and treatment of many illnesses, a direct challenge to these assumptions is long overdue (Weir, 1991).

In this chapter the justification will be presented for complementing reviews of the management, funding and direction of health care with a review of the philosophical principles which underpin services. The definition, origins and limitations of the existing health care paradigm will be presented together with the new thinking in science which has emerged in recent times. The implications for health care of the new thinking will be outlined and an extended range of care defined. Examples will be presented of how the new range might have an improved impact in attempts to care for and cure individuals with heart disease and cancer. The applications of unconventional therapies will be discussed and the staff and service requirements of working with the new paradigm examined.

● **The existing paradigm**

There is nothing included in the concept of the body that belongs to the mind, and nothing in that of mind that belongs to the body.
(The Cartesian division)

What is a paradigm

Essentially a paradigm is the constellation of beliefs, values and techniques shared by members of a given scientific community. It reflects the prevailing world view about the nature of existence and effectively defines the ground rules by which scientific investigation should progress. Although only an approximation to reality, it determines how problems should be understood and how enquiry should proceed. The science historian Thomas Kuhn introduced the concept of a paradigm in an attempt to explain how the understanding of life and thereby scientific thinking has evolved over time (Kuhn, 1962). He proposes that scientific thought does not evolve in a smooth way but involves periodic revolutions as the old belief system becomes increasingly redundant and the search for a superior understanding is initiated.

The German physicist Fritjof Capra has argued that there is currently a shift to a new paradigm as scientists across a broad spectrum of disciplines are making discoveries which question and challenge the basic postulates of the existing scientific belief system (Capra, 1983). To understand how the existing mechanistic or reductionist paradigm emerged, and helped determine the parameters of modern health care, it will be necessary to make a brief historical review of the ideas of a number of individuals who have influenced modern-day thinking.

During the sixteenth and seventeenth centuries leading thinkers and philosophers of the Western world attempted to devise a new method of scientific enquiry free from dogma and superstition. Their observations were to challenge the cultural and religious traditions of the day. Nicolas Copernicus and Galileo Galilei, from the results of their investigations of the planets, questioned man's perceived role as the principal position in God's creation. Galileo's contention that science should restrict its investigations only to those objective properties which could be measured and quantified, further demystified the ways of understanding the cosmos. An appreciation of the universe in inanimate and mechanical terms began to replace 'the notion of an organic and living entity' (Capra, 1983).

In England, Francis Bacon also formulated clear methods of objective scientific enquiry and advocated that nature should be 'bound into service' and that the aim of science was to 'torture nature's secrets from her'. A new and very masculine philosophy of science, far different from the pursuit of wisdom and a harmonious interaction with nature, was emerging. However, it is the contributions of René Descartes and Sir Isaac Newton which are widely recognized for establishing the framework of the new world view. Both were devoutly religious men who, while accepting the existence of God the creator, sought to establish a legitimate way of scientific enquiry. Descartes is most widely known for the method of scientific enquiry he developed and the Cartesian division – his postulation of the separation of mind from body.

Descartes believed that the material universe was a machine and worked according to mechanical laws. Thus a legitimate means of scientific enquiry was to reduce a system to its components and study each in isolation from the others. His work was given greater validity by Newton's support for a mechanistic world view and the development of a system of advanced mathematics to support this thesis. The Newtonian/ Cartesian, or reductionist, or mechanistic world view are all names given to the paradigm which has developed from the work of these giants of philosophy and science. Importantly, and of particular relevance to the argument the authors now present, the belief in the certainty of scientific knowledge has been directly challenged by modern physics which has demonstrated 'that there are no absolute truths in science, that all our theories and concepts are limited and approximate' (Capra, 1983). If this is the case, then every scientific theory is potentially replaceable by a more appropriate model.

The biomedical model

Descartes, himself a physician, extended his mechanistic thinking to the study of medicine. He postulated that the body could be understood as a machine or clock and studied completely independently of the mind. The biomedical model is the resulting health care interpretation of this thinking. The advances made in biology in the nineteenth century, particularly through the work of Rudolf Virchow and Louis Pasteur, consolidated the integration of mechanistic thinking into medicine. Virchow, who formulated cell theory in its modern form, postulated that illness involved structural changes at cellular level, thus establishing cellular biology as the basis of medical science. In recent times, the identification of DNA and the appreciation of its role in essential life processes has further consolidated the pre-eminence of reductionist thinking. As a consequence of these collective insights, attempts are made to reduce problems to molecular phenomena, with the aim of finding a mechanism that is central to the problem.

Another pioneer of reductionist medicine, Louis Pasteur, studied micro-organisms and demonstrated the correlation between bacteria and disease. Claude Bernard, the great physiologist and a contemporary of Pasteur, advocated that factors other than the virulence of the pathogen were important contributors to the development and progression of infectious disease. He proposed that a more complex ecological or holistic mode of interaction of host, environment and germ was involved. However, despite Bernard's insights it was 'the germ theory' of Pasteur which won the day. Interestingly, while not minimizing the importance of Pasteur's contribution, the modern-day understanding of the spread of infectious diseases lends great support for Bernard's holistic interpretation. The major breakthrough in reducing the levels of the principal killer infections in this country was effected before the development of vaccines or effective antibiotic treatment regimens, and was related to improvements in sanitation, housing, nutrition and education (McKeown, 1976).

A result of a reductionist emphasis on the germ and the molecular process effectively moved the focus from patient to the disease. An understanding of the disease entity as something independent of the individual initiated the trend towards disempowerment of the patient, depersonalization of the health care system and specialization in medical practice. As will be demonstrated later, many of these 'disease entities', far from being independent of patients, can be directly influenced by them.

The adoption of the Cartesian division has meant that physicians ignore the mind's contribution to organic illness and those concerned with mental health have paid little attention to the body. Psychiatry has focused its efforts on the chemistry of the brain and on the dynamics of mental illness rather than mental health. Thus medication is central to attempts to combat the mental illnesses of these days. Even Freud, in the pursuit of scientific credibility for his work, specifically created his theories of the psyche within the Newtonian/Cartesian paradigm. Not surprisingly, his later ideas on the importance of Eros and Thanatos, the love and death principles, which equate well with a holistic approach, received little support from his followers (Grof, 1985).

Interestingly, although Newton and Descartes were devoutly spiritual men, the application of the reductionist approach to the mind and its comprehension as a product of the brain have been important steps in the process of despiritualizing the appreciation of human existence. In contrast to their initial stance, a system of medicine has evolved which denies the divine and mystical essence of life. Those followers of Freud who questioned the mechanical understanding of the psyche and sought to investigate the spiritual were obliged to break with their mentor and develop new schools of transpersonal psychology to explore this dimension (Jung, 1963; Assagioli, 1974, 1976). To date, their ideas have had little influence on academic psychology or the practice of mainstream health care.

Reductionist medicine
The separation of mind from body, the understanding of the physical body and human behaviour in mechanistic terms, the central importance of the surgical intervention or 'magic bullet', rather than the individual in his recovery, and the disregard of the intuitive and the spiritual lie at the heart of the Western health care model. In the next section the reasons will be presented why a continued adherence to this understanding needs to be challenged.

● **Why change?**

If health care continues unquestioningly to accept the theories of yesteryear, it will stand accused of not being scientific in its approach.

For health care personnel exhausted by a succession of reorganizations, the prospect of yet more change and upheaval is unlikely to be met with enthusiasm. In reality, the development and implementation of a new paradigm in health care would have profound implications for the entire service and the role of every health care professional. The following seven subsections represent some of the reasons why the active consideration of a different or expanded model is justified.

The pursuit of excellence and scientific purity
The concept of quality management is based upon an ongoing process of questioning and challenge. There is no reason why the basic assumptions employed in care should not receive the same scrutiny as the management and financial systems employed. The past success of Japanese industry can be related to the involvement of staff in quality initiatives and the challenging of established practice in the pursuit of excellence. Such a process allows for the continual evolution of organizations and the active participation of staff in change.

Challenging the existing belief system or paradigm would also be consistent with the philosophy of science proposed by Karl Popper (Popper, 1965). Popper believes that without the process of challenging and replacing established ideas, as well as theories and concepts, true science cannot be practised. He suggests that the absence of mechanisms for self-questioning and challenge result in dogma and atrophy and eventual redundancy of that particular system. By Popper's reasoning, if health care continues unquestioningly to accept the theories of yester-year, it will stand accused of not being scientific in its approach.

No concept of health/health status/quality of life

A consequence of applying the mechanistic approach to health care has been an emphasis on illness and molecular biology. Mechanistic medicine has no meaningful appreciation of positive health or wellness and hence no strategy to promote it. As readers will recall, the ground rules of reductionist science promoted by Virchow, Descartes and Newton specifically excluded subjective and qualitative measures. Only reproducible and objective observations are accepted as valid data. Thus quality of life and concepts such as happiness and contentment have no meaningful definition or role in services. If no appreciation of health or quality of life exists, then attempts to measure health status must be restricted to quantitative data which merely informs about the prevailing levels of illness. A deeper appreciation of wellbeing and the factors which promote and protect individual and collective health are required. This would allow for the evolution of more appropriate and effective approaches to treatment programmes, health promotion and preventive medicine.

Consumer demand

The introduction of complementary therapies into the NHS has already started, although evidence suggests that this is being done in a poorly co-ordinated and undirected way (Addington-Hall *et al.*, 1993; Weir *et al.*, 1995). Evidence suggests that individuals are seeking out alternative medicine and are effectively voting with their feet and spending power. The size of the shift is considerable. In the USA, in 1990, Americans made an estimated 425 million visits to providers of certain unconventional therapies. This number is greater than the total number of visits to primary care physicians in that year and represents an expenditure of $13.7 billion (Eisenberg *et al.*, 1993).

It is difficult to equate these figures to the UK, but they represent a clear sign of dissatisfaction with conventional care. If the NHS is to be truly responsive to market forces, and the wishes of the consumer, these trends must be noted by those who purchase care on their behalf. Some direction and guidance is required if confusion, waste and possible harm are to be avoided. It is also very important to recognize the danger of the emotional and financial abuse of individuals once they move outside areas of accountable care. Under such circumstances, patients may delay presentation when conventional care can anticipate significant benefits. For those concerned with protecting and improving the public health, it is important to make sense of these developments and explore and examine the value of the new thinking.

The limitations of current practice

The interest in alternative approaches is fuelled by dissatisfaction with conventional treatment options. There are many areas of health care where progress in improving the outcome of care has been minimal in recent times. The following quote from *The Oxford Textbook of Medicine* makes the point very succinctly (Horrobin, 1988):

> *Medicine has acquired the attitude of pure science where things are done with no clear practical end in terms of benefit to the patient. . . . With perhaps two exceptions, peptic ulcer and renal failure, there is no common disease in which it is possible to demonstrate convincingly that those receiving treatment in 1985 are much better off than those receiving the best treatment in 1960. In other common conditions there is nothing that medicine has done which has dramatically improved either the survival or the comfort of patients.*

These areas of stasis include preventive medicine, where no effective way of preventing many of the major killer cancers, heart disease or mental illness exist. Progress has been minimal in recent decades in improving the survival prospects of people with the major killer cancers or reducing inequalities in health. Indeed, inequalities in health in northern England appear to be widening in a way which cannot be explained by behaviour alone (Phillimore *et al.*, 1994). The previous Chief Medical Officer, Sir Donald Acheson, also made this same point (Acheson, 1990):

> *This conclusion is that the forty years since the introduction of the NHS have seen little progress in the reduction of inequalities in health among the various social groups. Indeed for some variables the difference has grown.*

The failure to effect improvements across such a broad spectrum of activities should lead one to question the appropriateness of the existing health care model. Health care reforms designed to provide services in a more cost-effective and user-friendly way are by themselves unlikely to address the many areas of stasis in health care practice. Existing practices should be challenged and a major examination of the scientific thinking underpinning care initiated.

Stress and health

In recent decades there has been a growing awareness of the association of psychosocial factors with organic disease (Pelletier, 1977). In the development and recurrence of cancer and heart disease, such factors have been shown to have a higher predictive value than medical parameters (Lynch, 1979; Ruberman *et al.*, 1984; Ramirez *et al.*, 1989; Morris *et al.*, 1994). Likewise programmes of psychosocial intervention have been shown to prolong the life of cancer patients (Speigal *et al.*, 1989) and start to clear atheroma from diseased coronary arteries (Ornish *et al.*, 1990).

Cannon's fight and flight mechanism (1932), Selye's General Adaption Response (1950) and developments in psychoneuroimmunology help to explain many of the interactions of mind and body. Likewise,

Sterling and Eyer's (1981) research into the biological basis of stress-induced illness and Henry's (1982, 1983) explanation of the contribution of mental states to cancer and heart disease, provide plausible descriptions of other mechanisms of interaction. The intimate relationship of mind with body helps explain how chronic states of deprivation and unhappiness are associated with disruption of essential self-regulation processes and the development of organic illness. It also opens up the possibility of positive mood states and mental attitudes being employed to enhance the individual's self-healing potential. Extensive research into biofeedback, autogenics and meditation has confirmed that mind can favourably influence physiology (Pelletier, 1977).

In the light of such 'hard' evidence to the contrary, the continued adherence to Descartes' mind–body separation in the way illness is understood and treated must be challenged.

Consciousness research

Research in many areas of progressive psychology has consistently revealed findings which cannot be explained by mechanistic science and the traditional conceptual framework of psychiatry, psychology and medicine. It raises questions about how one should respond to the insights of Jung (1963), Maslow (1962, 1969), Moody (1975, 1977), Grof (1985, 1987), Shealy and Myss (1993), and many others. Are they to be ignored and the belief maintained that consciousness is the product of the brain, or is it time to develop an expanded model of mind which includes spirituality and goes beyond the boundaries of time and space?

Jung's concepts of the collective unconscious, a common reservoir of experience and information shared by humanity, and synchronicity, the interdependence of internal mental/emotional experience and the external world, present an understanding of consciousness which interconnects the individual, the community and the environment. This is an ecological model consistent with a mystical world view and also with the principles of new thinking in science (Capra, 1975). Unfortunately, the concept of consciousness in the biomedical model is poorly developed and would have great difficulty accommodating these exciting theories. If the existing paradigm cannot accommodate new observations, should it not be challenged and revised? The limitations of an existing paradigm should not be allowed to disregard the legitimacy of new, reproducible findings.

General paradigm shift

The move away from the limitations of mechanistic science to a new world view is occurring in many areas of scientific endeavour. The following areas have particular relevance for this discussion.

The new physics

The world view emerging from modern physics can be characterised by words such as organic, holistic and ecological. The universe is no longer seen as a machine made up of a multitude of objects but has to be pictured as one indivisible whole whose parts are essentially interrelated and can be understood only as patterns of a cosmic process. . . . An increasing number of scientists are aware that mystical thought provides a consistent and relevant philosophical background to the theories of contemporary science, a conception of the world in which the scientific discoveries of men and women can be in perfect harmony with their spiritual aims and religious beliefs.

(Capra, 1983)

Systems theory
The development of general systems theory, which looks at the world in terms of relationships and integration, has challenged the exclusivity of the mechanistic model. In this approach, systems are understood as integrated wholes whose properties cannot be reduced to those of the smaller unit. It is essentially concerned with the principles of organization and explores the dynamics of relationships. It directly challenges the exclusivity and independence of any part or component of a whole and has direct implications for the growing specialization of modern medicine.

Changes in other disciplines
There is also pressure for a move towards a holistic appreciation of chemistry (Prigogine, 1980; Prigogine and Stengers, 1984), biology (Sheldrake, 1981), ecology (Lovelock, 1979) as well as psychology.

Collectively the preceding seven subsections summarize some of the reasons why the model employed in health care can be responsibly challenged. Indeed, the authors would suggest that it is irresponsible to continue providing services exclusively within such a restrictive model. If the existing paradigm or belief system cannot be challenged despite the weight of hard evidence against it, then dogma has once again won the day. Under these circumstances, the belief that science is concerned with the search for truth rather than with the defence of established thinking is clearly in question. The authors do not advocate that the reductionist model is wrong or that it should be completely disregarded. Rather its limitations should be recognized and the validity of new thinking acknowledged. An expanded understanding is required which integrates the strengths of the old with the potential of the new. In the next section some of the concepts the 'New Health Care' will need to incorporate will be proposed.

● **Requirements of the 'New Health Care' model**

Reductionism and holism, analysis and synthesis, are complementary approaches that, used in proper balance, help us obtain a deeper knowledge of life.

(Fritjof Capra, *The Turning Point*)

Discrimination

The challenge confronting health care is the development of a paradigm which retains the strengths of existing practice but expands the conceptual model to accommodate the insights gained from the new physics, behavioural medicine, systems theory and transpersonal psychology. This will be an exercise requiring careful reflection and discrimination. As it is health care professionals who will be required to implement the new thinking, they must be actively involved in its creation and refinement. In the views of these authors the 'New Health Care', should acknowledge and embrace the concepts discussed in the following subsections (Weir and Whittaker, 1995a).

The dynamics of health

The health spectrum

Wellness --- Illness

An understanding of health as a continuum is required which incorporates the spectrum of influences which lead to illness, recovery and wellness. Epidemiological evidence indicates that disharmony at the personal, social and environmental levels can be associated with the development of illness (Townsend and Davidson, 1982; Whitehead, 1992; Morris *et al.*, 1994). Lawrence Le Shan, who has pioneered psycho/spiritual care for people with cancer, identifies meaning and enthusiasm as the central promoters of wellbeing (Le Shan, 1990). Peace of mind, a loving family and a supportive community have all been recognized as protectors and promoters of health (Lynch, 1979). Therefore, it may be argued that achieving greater levels of happiness and fulfilment would have a positive impact on one's ability to stay well? If this is so, the pursuit of these qualities should be a central consideration in the development of the new model.

Wellness

The absence within the biomedical model of any practical understanding of wellness or strategies to promote it, presents a clear challenge to progress. Likewise, the interrelationship of individual, societal and ecological wellbeing is also difficult to accommodate using a reductionist model. A systems approach is required if a comprehensive appreciation of the dynamics of health is to be developed at the physical, mental, emotional and spiritual dimensions of the individual as well as at the levels of community and planet. Without this expanded understanding of the factors which generate disease or lead to wellness, the development of meaningful strategies for preventive medicine and health promotion is not possible.

Perhaps, as the modern physicists discovered, some guidance may be gained from Eastern thought (Capra, 1975). The philosophy and techniques of yoga, which constitute a comprehensive system for promoting the health of body, mind and spirit, are worthy of consideration. The concepts of enlightenment and the expansion of consciousness should also receive attention as should Jung's idea of individuation and Maslow's processes of self-realization and self-actualization. Given that the pursuit of happiness was seen to be worthy of inclusion in the American Constitution, the authors suggest that health care should be equally idealistic and follow suit.

Mind–body medicine

The separation of mind from body, like the belief that the nervous system is distinct from the immune system, is a reflection of the old paradigm and the mind set of the researchers who identified them. The new paradigm must include a revised understanding of mind, body and their interrelationships. To a degree some concessions have already been made by conventional medicine. The placebo effect is a well-established phenomenon in which the individual's anticipation of change directly influences the body's physiology, immune function and biochemistry. In its research methods, high-technology medicine has had to allow for the influence of the minds of patient and investigator on the outcome. The double blind control trial is specifically designed to determine if the agent under investigation has any therapeutic impact above and beyond the changes patients induce in themselves.

The acceptance of the legitimacy of mind–body interactions opens up a whole new area of therapeutic intervention. Mental techniques can be employed to influence the physiological and immunological basis of health and illness. Many Eastern philosophies believe that emotions and feeling are communicated to the body by the breath (prana). By working directly with the breath it is therefore possible to access and interact with many dimensions of the individual's inner world. Breathing and meditation techniques have actions which range from a calming effect to the mobilization of repressed emotional and energetic material.

A range of therapies is also available which is specifically focused on the body as opposed to the mind. These aptly named bodywork therapies endeavour to release energetic and emotional blocks, with resultant benefits for psychological and physical health. Techniques such as Rolfing and deep massage operate on the belief that feelings and thoughts are reflected in the physical organism, manifesting themselves in posture, movement and aches and pains. As the body and the psyche are so intimately related, working on either will affect the other.

Clearly, all the dimensions of mind–body interactions cannot be accommodated within the existing understanding of the human organism. As the pure scientists have found in their investigations of matter, it is necessary to view the human organism from physical and energetic standpoints.

The human energy system

In addition to an integration of the known neural, immunological, biochemical and neuroendocrine pathways, the new model should consider the human energy field or aura. Thus emotions and feelings can be relayed to the body through biochemical and energetic pathways. These phenomena may possibly be explained by concepts like meridians, the subtle bodies and the chakra system which are central to many Eastern and mystical philosophies (Gerber, 1988; Shealy and Myss, 1993; Gyatso, 1994). An energetic understanding would help provide the framework to explain approaches such as Chinese medicine and its concepts of life energy, balance and complementarity, as well as homeopathy, acupuncture and spiritual healing which are nonsensical under the biomedical model.

While not denying that some processes are clearly organic and others psychological, the authors' work leads them to propose that the concept of a *body–mind continuum* should be introduced. In some way, unresolved past experience can be encoded in the mind–body continuum and continue to impact the individual's physical and emotional wellbeing. The energetic and timeless qualities of the mind–body continuum will need to be explained by a radically different understanding of the human being (Chopra, 1989; Zohar, 1990). Indeed, the roots of many illnesses will be found at this level, influences which disrupt mind and body and lead to the various manifestations of illness. Conventional medicine's concentration on molecular and cellular chemistry must be complemented by approaches which address these dynamics if a true impact on the illnesses is to be achieved.

The lines of enquiry which require one to accommodate mind–body interactions and an energetic understanding of the human organism in the new model necessitate that a spiritual understanding of the psyche also be included.

Spirituality

The new model should include an appreciation of human spirituality. The work of the pioneers of transpersonal psychology, together with the phenomena of near death and out-of-body experiences (Moody 1975, 1977; Lorimer, 1984), strongly suggest that there is an element of the human psyche which exists independently of the brain. Likewise, deep meditation techniques (Gyatso, 1990, 1994) and Stanislav Grof's work with non-ordinary states of consciousness (Grof, 1985, 1987) provide valuable insights into the spiritual nature of the psyche. A useful model which attempts the challenging task of incorporating a spiritual dimension into the anatomy of the unconscious is presented by the creator of the therapeutic system *psychosynthesis* (Assagioli, 1976).

A belief in the spiritual dimension of existence is central to all the world's great religions and mystical traditions. Many 'primitive peoples', most notably the North American Indians, have a philosophy of life based upon the spiritual essence and interdependence of all aspects of creation. Thus the actions of the individual have implications for his family, community and the greater environment. For those wishing to explore this spiritual model of ecology, the ideas and writings of Chief Seattle remain avant-garde and inspirational. Professor James Lovelock's Gaia hypothesis, an appreciation of this planet as a living sentient entity, gives some scientific credibility to the ideas of this pioneer of planetary ecology (Lovelock, 1979).

Healing
A model which includes mind–body interactions, the human energy system and spirituality will allow for the inclusion of the concept of healing. Healing can be concerned with work on the emotional, psychological, energetic and spiritual dimensions of humans. The techniques of healing not only include kindness, reassurance, words, touch but may involve interaction on energetic or spiritual levels. In some way, certain individuals appear to be able to interact with the deeper levels of human consciousness and initiate beneficial change. By addressing and resolving obstacles within the mind–body continuum, an improved sense of wellbeing and ability to avoid and combat illness may be anticipated (Brennan, 1988). To explain this phenomenon, insights can be gained from a study of the philosophy and techniques of the Shaman and the traditional healing practices of the world's indigenous peoples (Casteneda, 1968; Harner, 1980; Halifax, 1982).

The process of healing through the resolution of long-standing hurts, or dysfunctional behaviour, and the achievement of a clearer connection with the divine is not seen as merely for those confronting illness. It is in effect the journey to enlightenment that many spiritual traditions outline, and lies at the heart of the human potential movement which developed in the USA. It is also central to the 12-step programme so successfully employed by Alcoholics Anonymous and to progressive approaches to addiction in general. Thus, healing also has an essential role to play in the creation and expression of positive health and wellness.

Transformation
The ability of individuals to connect with hidden inner resources and go through radical psychospiritual change to achieve a greater sense of peace and purpose is an important potential to be included in the new model. For patients facing a life-threatening illness the opportunity exists to confront and resolve long-standing inter- and intrapersonal difficulties which may well have been factors in the development of their *dis-ease* (Le Shan, 1990). According to Joseph Campbell, the journey into the darkness of the unconscious and the potential for spiritual rebirth is depicted in mythologies across cultures and across time. In *A Hero with a Thousand Faces* (1970) he presents these common themes from the myths of many different peoples. The concept of transformation lies at the heart of many spiritual traditions, including Christianity and Buddhism (Welch, 1982; Gyatso, 1990, 1994). It represents, one may believe, the new frontiers of true health promotion.

The role of the health care professional
The new paradigm with its different approach to illness and recovery will have many implications for the way in which professionals

work with patients. A deeper and more open connection will require a new power balance of partnership rather than the dependence-promoting, paternalistic expert and patient contact. Many of the protections of the professional role will be redundant, although the need to work within agreed professional boundaries is not questioned. For professionals who wish to work on emotional, psychological and spiritual dimensions with patients, it is incumbent upon them that they have first explored these areas within themselves. The need for careful supervision and support for staff working in this way is paramount.

● **Developing the 'New Health Care'**

The challenge for true health care is to achieve the right synthesis of mechanistic treatment with a strategy which promotes quality of life and mobilizes the self-healing potential.

How can one interpret this new paradigm and provide care which combines the strengths of the mechanistic and holistic approaches? Insights on how the challenge may be addressed can be gained from progressive thinkers within the NHS. Malcolm McIllmurray's range of hospital and community services for people with cancer in Lancaster and South Cumbria and Peter Nixon's work with heart patients at Charing Cross Hospital demonstrate that a patient-centred approach to major illness is possible (Nixon 1982, 1984; McIllmurray *et al.*, 1986). Patient and client care requires a range of interventions from the high-technology, mechanistic through to psychosocial support. Perhaps the following categorization will be helpful in defining the spectrum of care more clearly. Collectively, the interventions are concerned to address the illness, improve quality of life and support the self-healing potential. Though each dimension has a particular point of emphasis which distinguishes it from the others, the model represents a way in which conventional and progressive approaches can be employed together (Weir and Whittaker, 1995b).

An expanded model of care

Reductionist
This involves the appropriate application of the range of technical skills which have been acquired from one's professional training. These include diagnosis, surgical and medical interventions, prescribing medication and many aspects of good nursing care. The *reductionist* approach is applicable to understand the presenting complaint and plan the necessary intervention. As outlined previously, the illness is understood in terms of the identified disruptions of behaviour, biochemistry, physiology or anatomy. Appropriate steps to restore balance through a variety of interventions are then initiated. Effectively, patients are passive recipients of the health professionals' skills and only their compliance with the treatment is required. The reductionist approach has particular relevance

for medical emergencies, but for most chronic and terminal illnesses it represents only a partial solution. Although the focus of attention is on the illness and its symptoms, this should always be undertaken in a sensitive and patient-centred way. Clearly, without competence at this level the other dimensions of care can become academic.

Humanistic

The humanistic emphasis specifically recognizes the central import- ance of clients' and patients' need for psychosocial care. It includes the provision of services specifically designed to meet the human needs of individuals, address their anxieties and loneliness and provide support and information. In addition to in-patient stays and progressive ap- proaches to psychiatry, the humanistic emphasis is central to post-treat- ment care. It is at the core of community care and is a principal mode of operation of many community and general practice personnel. The contact with the patient can be in a group or individually and may involve humour, a few words of support, basic counselling or the use of a complementary therapy. The nature of the interaction will be determined by the time available and the particular needs of the individual.

For so many conditions the individual's wellbeing and prospects for the fullest recovery are dependent upon the combined provision of reductionist and humanistic care (Speigal *et al.*, 1989; Ornish *et al.*, 1990). The importance of the humanistic dimension as a modality in itself or as an adjunct to mechanistic medicine should never be underestimated in the planning of health services. A search for the more efficient use of resources through faster turnover and less in-patient care will be shown to be false economy if, in the process, the human needs of individuals are neglected. Political and managerial expediency should never be allowed to adversely affect the outcome or quality of care professionals provide. Humanism represents the middle ground between the reductionist and holistic approaches and seeks to ensure that the comprehensive needs of the individual are addressed.

Holistic

This is a more interventionist approach, with the goal of working with patients to specifically address issues which compromise quality of life and impair prospects for the fullest possible recovery. Unlike the reductionist approach, the holistic emphasis requires the active participa- tion of the patient or client. A new client/professional relationship based on greater equality and mutual respect is therefore required. The objective is to work through any identified obstructions to improve quality of life and stimulate the self-healing potential. Responsible holistic interventions represent the new frontiers of health care and offer rich potential for cure and care. Working in a holistic way takes scientific medicine beyond the limits of the Newtonian–Cartesian paradigm to embrace the new physics and the concepts outlined earlier in the previous section concerning the 'New Health Care'.

To those whose world view remains mechanistic it is likely that holism may appear incomprehensible. It is important that such prejudices do not limit its potential, as undervaluing this range of interventions would be as short-sighted as disregarding the importance of conventional care. Identifying which individuals wish to work in this deeper and more intimate way will require particular attention. It is important that the 'therapist' works at the client's pace and does not attempt inappropriate interventions. Clearly, the qualities of compassion and intuition will be important requirements for this work.

Achieving balanced care

It is important that the humanistic and holistic approaches should not be seen as subservient to reductionism. This would merely be a reproduction of the existing model and limit the true potential of the new paradigm. The reductionist, humanistic or holistic dimensions used in isolation, independently of the others, should not be regarded as offering comprehensive care. Indeed, the authors suggest that complementary medicine is in many ways the harmonious integration of these three approaches. Achieving the correct balance of the three will be an ongoing challenge for health care providers. Monitoring of outcome and patient satisfaction will help determine how the best balance may be delivered.

Clearly, a healing impact can be achieved by any part of a patient-centred service. A caring and inspiring surgeon or radiotherapist, or the support and humour of nursing or ancillary staff, can have a superior impact to any therapy used without compassion and sensitivity. Nevertheless, the introduction of complementary therapies offers a rich potential which can help redress the imbalance between the intellectual and the curative approach on the one hand and the intuitive and healing approach on the other.

Unconventional therapies

There is an enormous number of unconventional therapies which can be employed in patient care. The challenge is determining how they may be used in a complementary way to the other dimensions of care. It is important that they are used in a responsible way which acknowledges the range and degree of their potential impact. Although therapies may be directed at particular levels of the individual, the intimacy of body, mind and spirit does not exclude effects on other dimensions. To a large degree this will be determined by the skills of the therapist, the openness, receptivity and expectation of the client and the nature of their relationship. It is this complexity of the healing exchange which invalidates many of the conventional approaches to the evaluation of the outcome of holistic care.

The therapies may be employed in a supportive, humanistic way whereby the warmth and attention of the therapist is the most important factor. Touching, be that physical contact or on an emotional or spiritual level, can open powerful channels of communication and have deep therapeutic returns. As with conventional approaches the placebo effect is operative and helps explain a good proportion of reported benefits. The commitment and investment of those who seek out alternative methods and the personal attention they receive are all very influential factors in the healing equation. Benefits also flow from the social consequences of working and meeting other people on a regular basis. The development of friendships and the sense of belonging and support can have significant and lasting returns.

The effectiveness of these therapies cannot be explained totally by the placebo effect or the personal attention patients receive. An expanded appreciation of the human organism to include energetic dimensions, the mind–body relationship and the different levels of consciousness helps make sense of some of their modes of action.

Specific modes of action

Benefits may be mediated through the improved posture induced by techniques such as yoga, osteopathy or the Alexander technique. Psychological benefits can be a result of counselling or from the improved sense of personal power which flows from regular meditation. In addition to psychological benefits, the calming effects of meditation and relaxation techniques can also induce a host of beneficial physiological changes. These may be mediated by an improved sense of control and wellbeing leading to a sustained reduction in sympathetic arousal and/or a reversal of the balance or catabolic and anabolic hormones identified in stress-induced illness.

While the *relaxation response* identified by the American cardiologist Herbert Benson has many therapeutic applications (Benson, 1975), other approaches are effective through the precipitation of a cathartic reaction. Catharsis is a particularly powerful mechanism which leads to the release of repressed emotional or energetic material stored within the *body–mind continuum*. The process can be triggered by a number of approaches including deep meditation, breathing techniques and body-work therapies. With approaches of this nature, the attendance and ongoing contact with a skilled and mature therapist are essential to ensure the process is completed and not left unresolved. Clearly, such an inappropriate conclusion to the therapeutic process can be particularly harmful to the client. However, under the right conditions profound benefits for physical and psychospiritual health can result (Grof, 1987).

Certain therapies rely upon a mechanism which can be understood in reductionist thinking and are therefore appropriate subjects for conventional evaluation. For instance, physiological improvements, through the removal of waste products, toxins, heavy metal or free radicals, are claimed to result from metabolic and cleansing therapies such as chelation or colonic lavage. On the other hand, interventions such as reflexology, homeopathy and acupuncture appear to interact with the body's energy fields to improve balance and promote self-healing. In this instance new models of evaluation are necessary. Although difficult to explain, the spiritual impact of some therapeutic approaches needs to be acknowledged (Brennan, 1988; Shealy and Myss, 1993). Certainly, 'changes' on this level can be profound, deeply moving and transformative.

Distinguishing legitimate therapies from the instruments of quackery will require ongoing vigilance and the maintenance of the highest professional standards. As the therapy is an extension of the therapist, any approach used without integrity and compassion can become invalid. This is as applicable to acupuncture as it is to plastic surgery. It is for this reason, to protect the public health, that the potential of complementary areas of unconventional practice should be embraced rather than ignored by mainstream care.

● Scope for intervention

Conceptually the origins of disease should take precedence over the nature of the disease process.

(Thomas McKeown)

To a large degree the causation and development of illness are mysteries which are unlikely ever to be fully explained by any simple theory or model. In particular, childhood terminal illness is as difficult to comprehend or explain as it is to accept. However, it is timely to consider the impact that an expanded model of health care would have for current major illnesses. Ischaemic heart disease and cancer will be reviewed and the emerging paradigm compared and contrasted with the present one.

Ischaemic heart disease

The conventional approach to the prevention and treatment of heart disease is a classical example of reductionist medicine. The heart is regarded as a pump and particular attention is directed to the patency of the coronary arteries, the obstruction of which, by the build-up of atheroma, is seen as the principal cause of angina and heart attacks. If necessary these arteries can be bypassed or mechanically cleared should the need arise. Likewise, attempts to prevent heart disease also use a reductionist approach with the identification of classic risk factors, namely high blood pressure, elevated levels of cholesterol and smoking. A variety of mechanistic interventions, including medication and low fat diets, is employed to address the problems.

In terms of reducing the incidence of the illness and the resulting death rate, both approaches have largely failed. Bypass surgery, with the exception of a minority of well-defined groups, offers no survival advantages over medical treatment alone. Both treatments are purely palliative approaches, concerned not to address the disease process but to make the symptoms less unpleasant. Likewise the attack on risk factors has regularly failed, in major studies, to reduce the death rate from the condition when compared to a control group. A leader in the *British Medical Journal*, a flagship of conventional medicine, has openly challenged the legitimacy of the approach and questioned if in fact it was not harmful (Oliver, 1992)! Although epidemiological studies reveal that only a minority of heart patients have a history of risk factors (Grayboys, 1984; Marmot, 1986), their identification and eradication remain the foundation of attempts to prevent heart disease. It is a mystery why the inappropriateness of this strategy has not been digested by many workers in preventive medicine and health education. Clearly, the reticence to change reflects the strength and hold of the old paradigm.

If the mechanics of angina are examined, more intriguing facts are revealed. There is no simple correlation between the level of chest pain and the degree of coronary artery occlusion. Thus an individual with extreme symptoms can have less disease than a patient with minimal pain. In one study, factors such as anxiety and overbreathing were identified as major contributors to the presenting complaint (Bass and Wade, 1984). The physiological disruption induced by the hyperventilation of emotional distress or exhaustion can lead, by affecting the body's pH balance, to constriction of the coronary arteries, ischaemia and infarction. It is therefore not surprising that for patients recovering from heart attacks factors such as social isolation and stress were identified as the major predictors of recurrent illness (Ruberman *et al.*, 1984). Of particular significance is an American study which has demonstrated a five-fold higher mortality rate among depressed myocardial infarction survivors (Frassure-Smith *et al.*, 1993). Collectively, these insights question the exclusivity of the mechanistic approach to heart disease and indicate that an expanded model of the illness should be developed.

The holistic model

If psychosocial factors are major predictors of heart disease and recurrent heart attacks (Lynch, 1979; Ruberman *et al.*, 1984; Frassure-Smith *et al.*, 1993), then they must be addressed. For patients with established disease this can improve clinical outcome as well as quality of life. Currently, the terror and depression which heart attacks and related surgery generate frequently go unnoticed in mainstream cardiology practice. However, Peter Nixon is a consultant cardiologist who for many years has championed and implemented a holistic understanding of heart disease (Nixon, 1982, 1984). His observations of patients led him to the clear conclusion that myocardial infarction often followed a period of emotional and physical exhaustion (Freeman and Nixon, 1985a). Others have also related the condition to overwork and various kinds of social disruption (Eyer, 1980). Nixon demonstrates that a heart attack is not necessarily a consequence of atheroma, as it bears no simple relationship to the condition of the coronary arteries. He indicates that dynamic factors caused by failure of coping with the demands of life makes a major contribution to the health breakdown (Freeman and Nixon, 1985b).

Prolonged states of exhaustion induce a metabolic catabolic state characterized by increased levels of cholesterol, blood pressure and blood clotting factors. They can also lead to impaired left ventricular function. Fear and anxiety are characterized by overbreathing which as well as inducing coronary spasm can reduce the heart's threshold for arrhythmias. Thus, a normal heart can experience ischaemia and infarction through fear and exhaustion induced changes. Clearly, a low fat diet and blood pressure tablets do not address the underlying *dis-ease* and indeed may give a false sense of security. Smoking is a way of coping with the inner states of distress and reflects the underlying emotional nature of the illness. Helping individuals to stop smoking through programmes which address their physiological distress and emotional and physical addiction to nicotine is indicated.

From his extensive clinical experience in high-technology medicine and cardiac rehabilitation, Nixon has long advocated that a biopsychosocial model be employed for clinical practice (Engel, 1982). Thus, preventive and rehabilitation services must embrace a comprehensive review of the lifestyle of individuals and the coping strategies they employ. Central importance must be afforded to the patient's ability to give and receive love, and for this reason the active involvement of the partner in the rehabilitation programme is highly desirable. Healing a wounded relationship can have profound benefits for the psyche and soma of both parties.

Scientific support for Nixon's clinical insights is provided by the results of Chandra Patel's holistic approaches to preventive cardiology. Her employment of stress management, yoga and biofeedback have not only succeeded in reducing elevated risk factors, but there are also good grounds to believe that her programmes prevent the development of coronary events (Patel *et al.*, 1981, 1985). The implications of Nixon's and Patel's work for the prevention of heart disease are truly profound and represent a cheap and effective way of combating the major killer disease of our time.

Reversing the disease process

Dean Ornish has shown that the approach is equally valid for individuals with established disease. His published scientific work with patients with advanced disease of their coronary arteries is of particular note (Ornish *et al.*, 1990). As an adjunct to conventional medical care he employed a humanistic/holistic programme to address a wide spectrum of patients' psychosocial needs. At the end of the study, the coronary arteries of the 'holistic' group had less atheroma than at the start, whereas the control group's arteries had accumulated more. The assessments were performed by independent physicians without knowing if the cases were from the intervention or control groups.

This is the first scientifically documented example of an intervention leading to the reversal of heart disease. Ornish puts particular store on his low-fat dietary programme. However, the personal experience of the authors would suggest that the total intervention, which included meditation and talking about feelings, enabled the individuals to gain control of their lives and thereby reduce the levels of exhaustion and metabolic disruption which, in Nixon's model, actively promote the disease. The appropriate application of reductionist medicine to the treatment of heart disease is not challenged. However, it is evident that an expanded model of care is particularly appropriate for people with heart disease. Indeed, the denial of the humanistic and holistic dimensions to patients not only has cost and quality of life implications, but also clinical outcome consequences which would appear indefensible both ethically and economically.

Cancer

The conventional approach to cancer is also based within the Newtonian/Cartesian paradigm. The illnesses are understood in terms of cancer cells and the cellular mechanisms involved in malignant change. Attempts are then directed at the elimination of these cells by surgery, radiotherapy and chemotherapy. The Cartesian division operates and no consideration of the mind in generating the illness or as a possible way of confronting it is included in standard practice. The illnesses have been understood at the molecular biology level and the human needs of patients given much lower priority (Cancer Relief Macmillan Fund, 1992; Addington-Hall *et al.*, 1993).

Although reductionist treatment methods can report progress with the soft-tissue cancers and leukemias, the same cannot be claimed for the major killer cancers. It is difficult to demonstrate that developments in treatment have led to any significant improvement in survival prospects in these solid tumour conditions for many decades if not generations. This point was clearly presented in a recent *Lancet* editorial which stated that despite all efforts the overall mortality rate for breast cancer remains static. It pointed out that conservative surgical treatment has the same survival benefits as a radical approach and urged those advocating extreme chemotherapeutic interventions to learn these lessons of history (Lancet Editorial, 1993).

Psychosocial needs neglected

Traditionally, NHS cancer services have focused upon treatment of the illnesses and have afforded little priority to providing psychosocial support services. Given this lack of provision it is not surprising that many of the emotional and practical needs of people with cancer, and their carers, are not met (Cancer Relief Macmillan Fund, 1992). As the psychosocial needs of cancer patients are now well appreciated, this stance is no longer tenable or defensible (Fallowfield *et al.*, 1986; Hardman *et al.*, 1989). Understandably, a growing number of NHS centres are now providing such services and employ complementary therapies and counselling in their work (Addington-Hall *et al.*, 1993). In general, these services are humanistic rather than holistic and are not seen as ways of affecting prolonged survival (Weir *et al.*, 1995a,b). This is in contrast to the philosophy of the Bristol Cancer Help Centre which advocates that patients, through the mobilization of inner resources and the employment of unconventional therapies, can play a central role in their recovery (Brohn, 1986; Weir, 1993).

The holistic approach in the care of people with cancer

It would be a mistake to be overcritical of cancer care services and underestimate the enormous benefits they offer. However, in the pursuit of greater quality it would be wrong not to examine how provision could be improved by embracing an expanded model of care. The central emphasis of this initiative is a move from cancer care to the care of people with cancer. Indeed, support for such a shift is very broadly based. The recent report of the Association of Cancer Physicians (1994), which represents mainstream practitioners of reductionist cancer medicine, emphasizes the importance of the humanistic dimensions of care to complement high-technology treatment services.

In addition to specifically addressing the psychospiritual needs of individuals, a holistic approach offers a different understanding of the development and progression of cancer. It identifies an intimate and complex interaction between the patient's wellbeing and nutritional status, the body's surveillance mechanisms and the inherent tendency it is believed humans have to produce malignant cells. When the equilibrium is disturbed, the ability to identify and destroy these cells can be impaired and illness develops. In many ways, the understanding of cancer from the reductionist and holistic standpoints is a re-run of the debate between Louis Pasteur's mechanistic and Claude Bernard's ecological view of infectious disease. The holistic view requires the allocation of greater attention to the individual's internal world (feelings, emotions, nutritional status) and external environment (relationships, physical and economic situation) than is currently the case (Simonton *et al.*, 1978; Meares, 1994; Siegel, 1988; Le Shan, 1990).

Given the intimate relationship of the immune and nervous systems, the channel for the influence of mental processes upon the progression of the disease is clear. Evidently, as one moves along the health spectrum towards the illness end, genetic, constitutional or familial predisposition to disease are triggered. If this is so, then movement in the reverse direction towards wellness, through the resolution of personal problems and the experience of greater self-worth and love, could remove some of the impairment to the body's self-healing potential. However, living longer should not be the sole or even the principal criterion of the success of this approach. Living better and dying better are also essential goals of a patient-centred service (McIllmurray *et al.*, 1986; Kubler-Ross, 1987; Levine, 1988).

Prolonged survival

Scientific support for the belief that patients can influence the disease process comes from the work of Speigal *et al.* (1989). They demonstrated that psychosocial support for women with advanced breast cancer doubled their life expectancy as compared to a control group. The work of Ramirez *et al.* (1989) also supports a relationship between psychosocial support and survival prospects in women with breast cancer. Women experiencing severe life events had a risk of relapse 5.67 times greater than women facing no such difficulties. These findings are consistent with the high incidence of cancer in areas of social deprivation or in those individuals having had a recent negative life experience (Phillimore *et al.*, 1994; Morris *et al.*, 1994). Although another study (Barraclough *et al.*, 1992) failed to reproduce the findings of the Ramirez paper, the association between psychosocial factors and cancer is clearly established.

The reductionist approach to the treatment of cancer and heart disease focuses on the manifestation of disease, be that malignant cells or atheroma. Although many benefits and effective interventions have flowed from this understanding of the illnesses, it is the underlying disease processes which promote the growth of cancer cells, compromise the body's surveillance systems and coronary arteries and destabilize the myocardium which need to be challenged. If, as some propose, the malignant process is supported by despair and autosuppression of the immune system, and if the chest pain reflects the physiological and biochemical consequences of emotional distress, then these dynamics need to be addressed through an expanded model of care. Patel, Speigal and Ornish's remarkable results can be explained by the inclusion of humanistic and holistic approaches to meet patients' needs. The improved support they received, the alleviation of personal distress and the enhancement of essential self-healing processes surely lie at the heart of their success. It is interesting to reflect what the reaction to their research would have been had the same results been achieved by a drug, a piece of technology or any approach of a mechanistic nature.

At a time when even the most reactionary medical journals advocate psychosocial support the trend to shorter inpatient stays continues to gather momentum.

(Williams and Chesney, 1993)

Moves to further eliminate the caring dimension of health care through a greater emphasis on outpatient care must only be made after deep reflections on the implications of such changes. Attention must be given to ensuring that humanistic and holistic dimensions are not completely eliminated from the care equation. To include services which address the human needs of patients alongside conventional treatment modalities requires only a small shift in thinking and a few courageous individuals to champion comprehensive care (McIllmurray *et al.*, 1986; Weir *et al.*, 1995).

● **Changing the system**

As guardians of the public health it will be for general practitioners and Directors of Public Health to determine the relative benefits of the healing and treatment modalities and commission services accordingly.

Progressive thinkers of the past identified the contribution of social and environmental pollution to the health problems of the day. Evidence indicates that many of the modern-day ills have their roots in the inner distress which the pressures and uncertainties of life can help create. The consequential disruptions of psyche and soma underpin so many of the social, emotional and physical pathologies of our times. Reductionist thinking interprets and confronts these states as distinct entities rather than symptoms or reflections of a deeper *dis-ease*. A new vision of health care is urgently required which equips individuals to confront life's challenges more successfully. This must include an appreciation of wellness and the intrapersonal, community and environmental factors which promote and compromise it.

Certain groups of personnel already employ this vision in their work. Health visiting, in particular, incorporates progressive thinking about the dynamics of health and illness and in many ways can be seen as a profession of the new paradigm. The problem such progressive practitioners often encounter is having their activities monitored and understood in unsympathetic, reductionist ways, particularly in terms of patient/client outcomes. Such an interpretation of their contribution makes practitioners such as these particularly vulnerable to 'cost-cutting' exercises and their replacement by less expensive personnel. This creates frustration and a sense of non-appreciation, which can in turn lead to a loss of enthusiasm and idealism (a move down the health spectrum no less). As it is difficult to swim against the tide, some consideration of how the total system may be influenced is required.

Influencing team consciousness

Initially, energy should be put into in-service training and team building to shift the consciousness of the health care team away from the purely mechanistic towards an extended model of care. Clearly, a change in emphasis of the entire service would have a greater impact than the random introduction of a few complementary therapies. In the authors' experience, once the scientific and epidemiological justification for the changes are appreciated and the rich potential they offer for patients and clients is grasped, enormous enthusiasm and interest at all professional levels can result. Without a true appreciation of the potential of the new thinking it is likely that new skills would be seen as merely an adjunct to conventional treatment. The opportunity to truly enhance and expand the range of care would therefore be lost.

Once a supportive professional environment has been achieved, training in specific skills will be necessary for individuals wishing to work in new ways. For some practitioners, a particular challenge will be that of working in a more intimate and personal way than is usually the case in conventional care. The renegotiation of professional boundaries and the strict maintenance of ethical standards will be necessary to prevent over-involvement with the patient or client and to minimize the risk of professional burn-out. These 'therapists' would benefit from membership of a support group and should be actively involved with their own process of personal growth. As already identified, they will require good-quality, regular supervision. Such inputs should be adequately funded from the anticipated savings on medication and 'high-tech' interventions. Attentions should also be directed to assuring the right balance of work so that personnel are not continually involved with in-depth work. The monitoring of the work through the development of appropriate scales to measure progress will be necessary. Training in basic research, data collection and computer skills is therefore indicated.

Objectivity and sensitivity

As the purchasing role becomes an accepted part of health care culture it will be for fundholding General Practitioners (GPs) and Directors of Public Health (DPHs) to determine the relative benefits of the healing and treatment modalities and commission services accordingly. A mere repackaging of the old health care system, which has failed to address so many issues successfully, would waste the opportunity to make services fit the needs of the community. Interestingly, the need for a framework for purchasing which embraces humanistic values as well as previously accepted criteria of quality has already been advocated (Goodwin, 1994).

However, as hospitals now have a financial as well as an ideological investment in treatment modalities, the pressure to buy the same 'products' as before will be intense. The authors argue that employment of high-technology interventions at the expense of the humanistic and holistic dimensions will be actively promoted. Large drug companies with huge financial resources and medical schools in defence of 'scientific' medicine will champion this cause. Unless these pressures are resisted, the scope for innovation and evolution will be lost. As the guardians of the public health it is essential that DPHs and fundholding GPs act as honest and objective brokers and purchase services which truly lead to health gain. The challenge which this exercise presents cannot be underestimated.

The authors firmly advocate that the development and acceptance of a new paradigm is essential if health care is to evolve and effectively confront the individual and community challenges of the twenty-first century. A paradigm shift according to Kuhn is a time of conceptual chaos as the zeal of the reformers is met by the misgivings and vested interests of the status quo. If at all times the goal is demonstrably to improve the outcome of care, rather than wave a particular flag in support of an established or a new procedure, it is likely that one's endeavours will be the most successful. An exciting journey awaits those practitioners who decide to tread this path of discovery. The authors wish good fortune to all those who choose to do so.

References

Acheson, D. (1990) Quoted in Townsend, P., Davidson, N. and Whitehead, M. (1933) *Inequalities in Health*, Penguin Books, London

Addington-Hall, J.M., Weir, M.W., Zollman, C. and McIllmurray, M.B. (1993) A national survey of support services for people with cancer. *British Medical Journal*, **306**, 1649

Assagioli, R. (1974) *The Act of Will*, Turnstone Press, London

Assagioli, R. (1976) *Psychosynthesis*, Penguin Books, New York

Association of Cancer Physicians (1994) *Review of the Pattern of Cancer Services in England and Wales*, ACP, London

Barraclough J., Pinder P., Cruddas M., Osmond, C., Taylor, I. and Perry, M. (1992) Life events and breast cancer prognosis. *British Medical Journal*, **304**, 1078–1081

Bass, C. and Wade, C. (1984) Chest pain with normal coronary arteries: a comparative study of psychiatric and social morbidity. *Psychological Medicine*, **14**, 51–61

Benson, H. (1975) *The Relaxation Response*, First Avon Books, New York

Brennan, B.A. (1988) *Hands of Light: A Guide to Healing Through the Human Energy Field*, Bantam Books, London

Brohn, P. (1986) *Gentle Giants*, Century Hutchinson, London

Campbell, J. (1970) *A Hero with a Thousand Faces*, World Publishing, Princeton, NJ

Cancer Relief Macmillan Fund (1992) *The Social Impact of Cancer*, Mori Research Study

Cannon, W.B. (1932) *The Wisdom of the Body*, Norton, New York

Capra, F. (1975) *The Tao of Physics*, Shambhala Publ., Berkeley, CA

Capra, F. (1983) *The Turning Point*, Flamengo, London

Castenada, C. (1968) *Teachings of Don Juan: A Yaqui Way of Knowledge*, University of California Press, Berkeley, CA

Chopra, D. (1989) *Quantum Healing*, Bantam Books, London

Eisenberg, D.M., Kessler, R.C., Foster, C., Norlock, F.E., Calkins, D.R. and Delbanco, T.L. (1993) Unconventional medicine in the United States. *New England Journal of Medicine*, **328**, 246–252

Engel, G.L. (1982) Biopsychosocial model and medical education. *New England Journal of Medicine*, **306**, 802–805

Eyer, J. (1980) Social causes of coronary heart disease. *Psychotherapy and Psychosomatics*, **34**, 75–87

Fallowfield, L., Baum, M. and Maguire, G.P. (1986) Effects of breast conservation on psychological morbidity associated with diagnosis and treatment of early breast cancer. *British Medical Journal*, **293**, 1331–1334

Frassure-Smith, N., Lesperance, F. and Talajic, M. (1993) Depression following myocardial infarction: impact on six month survival. *Journal of the American Medical Association*, **270**, 1819–1825

Freeman, L.J. and Nixon, P.G.F. (1985a) Chest pain and the hyperventilation syndrome – some aetiological considerations. *Postgraduate Medical Journal*, **61**, 957–961

Freeman, L.J. and Nixon, P.G.F. (1985b) Dynamic causes of angina pectoris. *American Heart Journal*, **110**, 1087–1092

Gerber, R. (1988) *Vibrational Medicine: New Choices for Healing Ourselves*, Bear and Co., Santa Fe, USA

Goodwin, S. (1994) Purchasing effective care for parents and young children. *Health Visitor Journal*, **67**, 127–129

Grayboys, T.B. (1984) Stress and the aching heart. *New England Journal of Medicine*, **311**(9), 594–595

Grof, S. (1985) *Beyond the Brain*, State University of New York Press, New York

Grof, S. (1987) *The Adventure of Self-Discovery*, State University of New York Press, New York

Gyatso, G.K. (1990) *Joyful Path of Good Fortune*, Tharpa Publications, London

Gyatso, G.K. (1994) *Tantric Grounds and Paths*, Tharpa Publications, London

Halifax, J. (1982) *Shaman: The Wounded Healer*, Thames and Hudson, London

Hardman, A., Maguire, P. and Crowther, D. (1989) The recognition of psychiatric morbidity on a medical oncology ward. *Journal of Psychosomatic Research*, **33**, 235–239

Harner, M. (1980) *The Way of the Shaman: A Guide to Power and Healing*, Harper and Row, New York

Henry, J.P. (1982) The relation of social to biological processes in disease. *Social Science and Medicine*, **16**, 369–380

Henry, J.P. (1983) Coronary heart disease and arousal of the adrenal cortical axis. In *Bio-behavioral Bases of Coronary Heart Disease* (eds T.M. Dembroski, T.H. Schmidt and G. Blumchen), Karger, Basel

Horrobin, D.F. (1988) Scientific medicine, success or failure? In *The Oxford Textbook of Medicine*, Section 2, Vol. 1, Oxford University Press, Oxford

Jung, C.G. (1963) *Memories, Dreams, Reflections*, Routledge and Kegan Paul, London

Kubler-Ross, E. (1987) *Aids: The Ultimate Challenge*, Macmillan, New York

Kuhn, T.S. (1962) *The Structure of Scientific Revolutions*, University of Chicago Press, Chicago

Lancet Editorial (1993) Breast cancer: have we lost our way? *Lancet*, **341**, 343–344

Le Shan, L. (1990) *Cancer as a Turning Point*, Gateway Books

Levine, S. (1988) *Who Dies*? Gateway Books, Bath

Lorimer, D. (1984) *Survival*, Routlege and Kegan Paul, London

Lovelock, J. (1979) *Gaia: A New Look at Life on Earth*, Oxford University Press, London

Lynch, J.J. (1979) *The Broken Heart: The Medical Consequences of Loneliness*, Basic Books, (ISBN 0-465-00771-6)

McIllmurray, M.B., Gorst, D.W. and Holdcroft, P.E. (1986) A comprehensive service for patients with cancer in a district general hospital. *British Medical Journal*, **292**, 669–671

McKeown, T. (1976) *The Role of Medicine: Mirage or Nemesis*, Nuffield Provincial Hospital Trust, London

Marmot, M.G. (1986) Does stress cause heart attacks? *Postgraduate Medical Journal*, **62**, 683–686

Maslow, A. (1962) *Toward a Psychology of Being*, Van Nostrand, Princeton, NJ

Maslow, A. (1969) A theory of metamotivation: the biological rooting of the value of life. In *Readings in Humanistic Psychology* (eds A.J. Sutich and M.A. Vich) Free Press, New York

Meares, A. (1994) *The Wealth Within*, Hill of Content Publishers, Australia

Moody, R. (1975) *Life after Life*, Mockingbird Books, New York

Moody, R. (1977) *Reflections of Life after Life*, Mockingbird Books, New York

Morris, J.K., Cook, D.G. and Shaper, A.G. (1994) Loss of employment and mortality. *British Medical Journal*, **308**, 1135–1139

Nixon, P.G.F. (1982) Stress and the cardiovascular system. *Practitioner*, **226**, 1589–1598

Nixon, P.G.F. (1984) Stress, lifestyle and cardiovascular disease. A cardiological odyssey. *British Journal of Holistic Medicine*, **1**, 20–29

Oliver, M.F. (1992) Doubts about preventing coronary heart disease. *British Medical Journal*, **304**, 393–394

Ornish, D., Brown, S.E., Scherwitz, W. *et al.* (1990) Can life style changes reverse coronary heart disease? *Lancet*, **336**, 129–133

Patel, C., Marmot, M. and Terry, D.J. (1981) Controlled trial of biofeedback-aided behavioural methods in reducing mild hypertension. *British Medical Journal*, **282**, 2005–2008

Patel, C., Marmot, M., Terry, D.J., Carruthers, M., Hunt, B. and Patel, M. (1985) Trial of relaxation in reducing coronary risk; four year follow-up. *British Medical Journal*, **290**, 1103–1106

Pelletier, K.R. (1977) *Mind as Healer, Mind as Slayer*, Dell Publishing, New York

Phillimore, P., Beattie, A. and Townsend, P. (1994) Widening inequality in health in northern England (1981–91). *British Medical Journal*, **308**, 1125–1128

Popper, K.R. (1965) *The Logic of Scientific Discovery*, Hutchinson, London

Prigogine, I. (1980) *From Being to Becoming: Time and Complexity in the Physical Sciences*, W.H. Freeman, San Francisco

Prigogine, I. and Stengers, I. (1984) *Order out of Chaos: Man's Dialogue with Nature*, Bantam Books, New York

Ramirez, A., Craig, T.J., Watson, J.P. and Fentimen, I.S. (1989) Stress and relapse in breast cancer. *British Medical Journal*, **298**, 291–293

Ruberman, W., Weinblatt, E., Goldberg, J.D. and Chaudhary, B.S. (1984) Psychosocial influence on mortality after myocardial infarction. *New England Journal of Medicine*, **311**, 552–559

Selye, H. (1950) *The Physiology and Pathology of Exposure to Stress*, Acta, Montreal

Shealy, C.N. and Myss, C.M. (1993) *The Creation of Health*, Stillpoint Publishing, Stillpoint, New Hampshire

Sheldrake, R. (1981) *A New Science of Life: The Hypothesis of Formative Causation*, Tarcher, Los Angeles

Siegel, B. (1988) *Love, Medicine and Miracles*, Harper and Row, London

Simonton, O.C., Mathews-Simonton, S. and Crighton, J. (1978) *Getting Well Again*, Tarcher, Los Angeles

Speigal, D., Bloom, J.R., Kraemer, H.C. and Gottheil, E. (1989) Effects of psychosocial treatment on survival of patients with metatastic breast cancer. *Lancet*, **298**, 291–293

Sterling, P. and Eyer, J. (1981) Biological basis of stress related mortality. *Social Science and Medicine*, **15E**, 3–42

Townsend, P. and Davidson, N. (1982) *The Black Report*, Penguin Books, London

Weir, M.W. (1991) Towards an holistic understanding of health and illness. *Health Visitor*, **64**, 77–79

Weir, M.W. (1993) Bristol Cancer Help Centre: Success and setbacks but the journey continues. *Journal of Complementary Therapies in Medicine*, **1**, 42–45

Weir, M.W. and Whittaker, C.H. (1995a) New Frontiers in Healthcare: Making sense of holistic medicine. In preparation

Weir, M.W. and Whittaker, C.H. (1995b) Providing Comprehensive Care: Requirements of the new healthcare model. In preparation

Weir, M.W., Zollman, C. and Addington-Hall, J. (1995) Developing psychosocial services for people with cancer: a review of six centres. *Journal of Cancer Care*, **4**, 3–10

Welch, J. (1982) *Spiritual Pilgrims*, Paulist Press, New York

Whitehead, M. (1992) *The Health Divide*, Penguin Books, London

WHO (1985) *Targets for Health for All: Targets in Support of the European Regional Strategy for Health for All by the Year 2000*, World Health Organisation, Copenhagen

Williams, R.M. and Chesney, M.A. (1993) Psychosocial factors and prognosis in established coronary heart disease. *Journal of the American Medical Association*, **270**, 1860–1861

Zohar, D. (1990) *The Quantum Self*, Bloomsbury Publishing, London

6

Images of disability and handicap

David Sines

● **Introduction**

This chapter considers the needs of people with disabilities and handicaps within the context of a paradigm that suggests that they should be encouraged to strive for independence above all other goals. In assisting others to achieve this aim, community health care nurses may find themselves central players with their clients in fostering interdependence and reciprocity to maximize opportunities for health and social gain.

Whilst disability was not afforded specific status within the five key areas of the *The Health of the Nation* (DoH, 1992), the health needs of people with a range of disabilities are considered to be the subject of a number of tangential DoH initiatives.

In recognition of the centrality of the needs of this group, the following elements of service change and development have been adapted from the 'Health of the Nation':

* increased attention to prevent the incidence and prevalence of disability
* under-reporting (recognition) due to stigma
* the need to enhance the recognition of actual needs of people at community and primary health care levels
* a requirement to raise awareness to social, emotional and psychological needs associated with longer term disablement for both individuals and their carers
* social policy changes that have accelerated care in the community initiatives (and an associated reduction in dependence on the long-stay or hospital sector)
* changes in working patterns which encourage shared learning and inter-professional teamwork
* recognition of the primacy of consumerism and self-reliance
* provision of comprehensive and systematic approaches to care delivery, continuing care and rehabilitation.

These issues will form the focus of this chapter, which commences with an analysis of the status and position of people with disabilities and handicaps in society – and the way in which public services and professional have chosen to respond to them.

● Definitions

The majority of people are unable to distinguish, through the use of everyday language, between terms used to describe forms of disability. For many, images are produced which are associated with wheelchairs or white sticks. According to the Open University (1990) there are three components to disability: the impairment, the permanence of the impairment and a significant difficulty in behaving functionally. As the authors suggest, this approach involves subjective judgements about the individual and their personal attributes:

The meaning of disability has, therefore, to go beyond the simple use of words. We have suggested that the deeper meaning of disability involves subtle judgements which take us beyond everyday spontaneous associations with a particular word. There are many words associated with disability and the situations of disabled people, some positive, most negative, but all relevant to the overall picture of what disability means in our society. (p. 15)

Definitions are therefore subjective and may provide an inappropriate means of describing people who have handicaps, impairments or disabilities. The use of such terms is also commonly associated with medical interpretations and diagnoses. However, in the final analysis people should be regarded as people first and the nature and extent of their disabilities should be described in ways which serve to empower the individual concerned to maximize independence and the potential for self-determination. In so doing it is important to regard disability as the outcome of a number of related interactions between different bodily and/or emotional impairments and the way in which opportunities are provided in the person's physical and social world. This approach provides for positive imagery and action on the part of people with disabilities and their support staff.

● Images of disability and handicap

Historically, people with disabilities have been regarded as inferior or as second-class citizens (Miller and Gwynne, 1974; Zola, 1985). Others, such as Goffman (1961), consider the actual needs of disabled persons to have been neglected by society on the basis of chosen neglect and marginalization, often misinformed by ideas that such conditions are irreversible and impossible to treat. These mythical misconceptions must be challenged if health and social care professionals are to meet their needs with any sense of conviction.

One such misconception relates to the relationship of disability and social class. The Office of Population of Censuses and Surveys (OPCS, 1988) have identified that there are $6\frac{1}{4}$ million people with disabilities in the UK. Of these, some 31% are employed compared to 69% of the general population. Disability and unemployment are therefore closely linked in some people's minds. People with disabilities may be looked upon as 'unemployable', thus reducing their status and image in society and, in turn, their social class position.

The locus for care provision is another determinant of how people regard disability. In the past, many people with disabilities were cared for in long-stay hospitals and according to Ryan and Thomas (1980) the hospital social structure serves to reinforce the dependence and incapacity of people. In such circumstances, Ryan and Thomas consider that it becomes easy to objectify people, and nurses and social workers may encourage staff to regard their clients as objects rather than people. The authors suggest that the main reasons for this process are:

- the absence of any equality or similarity between people
- the absence of the possibility that people can be anything other than prescribed by their social roles or definitions
- the absence of the acknowledgement of subjectivity, of people's own consciousness of themselves.

In a famous study by Menzies (1970), the problems facing nursing staff in under-resourced and understaffed hospitals were explained in terms of the anxiety they experience as a result of their work. In order to cope with some of the more depressing and less rewarding aspects of their job, some may bring defensive techniques into their work in an effort to disguise and assist them in externalizing work pressures. Menzies interpreted these defence mechanisms as being socially structured and developing over time following reinforcement by managers and staff:

A social defence system develops over time as the result of collusive interaction and agreement, often unconscious, between members of the organization as to what form it should take. The socially structured defence mechanisms then tend to become an aspect of external reality with which old and new members of the institution must come to terms. (p. 51)

The following are examples of some of the social defence mechanisms identified by Menzies (1970) which are still applicable today. She suggests that the following mechanisms assist staff in the accomplishment and achievement of their tasks under difficult and personally threatening conditions:

- splitting up the nurse–client relationship (distancing)
- depersonalization, categorization and denial of the significance of the individual
- detachment and denial of personal feelings
- the attempt to eliminate the need to make decisions by ritual task-performance
- reducing the weight of responsibility in decision-making by checks and counterchecks by senior staff
- collusive social redistribution of responsibility and irresponsibility
- purposeful obscurity in the formal distribution of responsibility

- reduction of the impact of responsibility by delegation to superiors
- avoidance of change.

Individuals vary in the extent to which they use these mechanisms, and the personal agendas they develop to cope with their work will be influenced by their past experiences and learning behaviours. Some of these behaviours will undoubtedly result in a detachment from the primary purpose of the nurse's role which is to provide an individually-based service to each client.

In some cases defence mechanisms may work to the positive disadvantage of the client and may cause them to become the subject of ridicule and distraction. Stockwell (1972) indicated the significance of joking behaviour in long-term care and noted that in some cases such jokes may become personalized and while introducing humour into very tense situations may cause personal embarrassment and humiliation for the person concerned. The extent to which nursing staff engage in such practices is unknown, although conformity to the social customs of the organization is understandable if one considers the pressures exerted by established staff and their allegiance to the social systems operating within health and social service agencies.

According to Matza (1964), the concept of deviant behaviour is very simple and uncomplicated and is explained in terms of straying from a path or standard. In many cases, standards are not easily defined and within the human care services there may be several, and potentially conflicting, subcultures and rules in operation. This plurality may present different rewards to different groups of staff and may result in differences of opinion. The lack of respite from caring routines may lead staff to neutralize their behaviours and to drift towards a pattern of practice which may be associated with lower standards of care. A theory of neutralization and drift was developed by Sykes and Matza (1957) and provides a helpful starting point in the understanding of the ways in which staff rationalize their behaviours. Sykes and Matza suggest that a typology of rationalizations exist consisting of five techniques of neutralization.

One other major problem confronting people with disabilities is that some may not possess the necessary skills to articulate their needs or to present their own grievances. The denial of certain basic rights to people with disabilities may also be significant for clients who rely on the integrity of their staff or 'carers' to represent their interests and to protect them from harm or exploitation. It is as a result of the acknowledgement of the needs of people with disabilities that the UK is now witnessing the development of client advocacy movements. Such schemes aim to provide an independent source of support and representation for dependent people (see Chapter 28).

Clearly the way in which care and support is provided for clients with disabilities is set to change. Professionals will be expected to adapt their behaviour and care practices to provide valued and service responses to their clients' needs and demands. The changes involved in this major cultural shift are typical of many that are currently confronting staff in both health and social care agencies. Such a process of change and its management may be described as a cycle. Adams *et al* (1976), in their analysis of staff response to change in human services in this country, pose one model for change characterized by seven stages:

First stage: *Immobilization* – a sense of shock, being overwhelmed and unable to make plans or to organize.

Second stage: *Minimization* – with a reluctance to acknowledge the change, characterized by a temporary retreat from reality and a denial that anything different is happening.

Third stage: *Depression* – when an awareness of the change dawns, there may be sporadic outbursts of anger and a sense of frustration at not knowing how to change.

Fourth stage: *Letting go* – when there is some optimism and confidence and no longer a constant reference to the way things used to be done.

Fifth stage: *Testing* – when new behaviours are tried out.

Sixth stage: *Searching for meaning* – recognized by a gradual shift towards understanding with positive talking, but with a need to step back and reflect on the meaning of the change and an acceptance that change is there to stay.

Seventh stage: *Internalization* – the new behaviour is automatic and feels comfortable; the old way is mentioned less often and then only in sentimental terms.

Other change processes are described in Chapter 29.

Nurses have already demonstrated their commitment to enact the basic values that underpin the philosophy of caring for people in the community. The NHS and Community Care Act 1990 provides the legislative framework for these changes and nurses with their clients are involved in translating the values that underpin good-quality care into action. This requires creativity, innovation, commitment and a rejection of the values of the outdated hospital culture which have been described earlier in this section.

● **A new conceptual approach to disability**

Conceptually and morally, the way in which society perceives the status of people with disabilities will determine the extent to which individuals are afforded basic human rights. In the community, opportunities to create integrated service responses have facilitated a transfer of empowerment to people with disabilities. Professional staff will be expected to respond to the expressed needs of their clients and to reduce the role distance between nurses and the people with whom they work. This is different from the traditional hierarchical communication system of the institutionalized side of health care provision. In their place, service users will demand access to planning systems, to their own case files and to participate in the review and evaluation of their service, thus reducing the status of professsionals as guardians of their future and welfare.

The move towards client-centred care clearly influences the power base of professionals. Although in theory the degree of control that staff have over their clients is reduced in the community, staff will be confronted with a potential conflict of interest, as they need to adapt to this new approach while retaining their interest in the advancement of their professional careers.

One other way in which all staff are changing is through the sharing of their skills and learning opportunities so that their clients develop to the maximum level of ability. As such, the rigid divisions that previously existed between different professions are becoming blurred, as inter-professional teamwork requires all staff to unite on an equal basis to meet the needs of their clients. Professional skills must therefore become transparent if they are to be judged as effective; in their turn, clients will expect their support staff to account in terms of measured outcomes and productivity in responding to their actual needs.

The philosophical approach of the 1990s is that of normalization or social role valorization which replaces the deviancy theories outlined previously. The new approach is based on the acknowledgement of the importance of self-image and on the image imposed upon an individual by the way in which others view that person. For people with disabilities, the theorists regard the group to be devalued by society and denied the full range of opportunities afforded to other citizens. Their world is therefore restricted and the people themselves may be prevented from fulfilling active and valued social roles. In turn, they will often be patronised by others, uninvited to participate in important life decisions that affect them, segregated from the mainstream of community life and deprived of access to local amenities in their neighbourhoods.

The negative labels that are often attributed to disability, such as *spastic*, *loony* or *invalid*, all serve to reinforce the image that society affords some of its members. Furthermore, deprived of the opportunity to participate in their community, they may also be denied the chance to prove that they are able to make an active and valuable contribution to family and community life.

Wolfensberger (1972) suggests that these ideas are morally repugnant and unjustified in modern society and suggests that all professionals must (by engaging in a process of self-reflection) examine their own values and their premise for caring. He suggests that all people have strengths, needs, abilities and wants, and when these are examined together the full potential of people can be appreciated. Outside institutions, he argues that people will regain their dignity and respect and with appropriate support will advance in their acquisition of living and social skills and competences.

In order to achieve the balance between support and autonomy, nurses will be challenged to work in partnership with their clients who from time to time may need assistance to develop the personal capacity to make decisions for themselves, particularly during periods when their autonomy may be impaired (see also Chapter 24 for a discussion on partnership).

In order for this shift in conceptual thinking to take place, it will be necessary to ensure that the barriers that exist to prevent meaningful integration are removed. Dependence on the long-stay hospital sector is one way of achieving this goal, but far more importantly will be a major change in the attitudes of carers and professionals as they strive to empower people with disabilities to assume responsibility for their own lives. However, this will require both appropriate support and the basis of informed choice.

In this new paradigm, professionals will have to accept that they do not always know best and calculated risks will become a regular feature of each person's care plan. The normalization model therefore challenges all persons involved in the care and lives of people with disabilities to engage in a model of care delivery that values clients as equal citizens. The resultant service will be judged on its ability to empower clients and upon the extent to which it provides a service that respects people's rights and dignity, builds on their wishes, further skills and competences and offers opportunities for people with disabilities to:

- integrate and participate in the lives of their local communities
- develop and sustain meaningful relationships of their choice
- engage in decision-making (on the basis of informed choice and calculated risk assessment)
- share in all aspects of the case management process (see Chapter 30)
- receive an adequate income in recognition of their ability to contribute to the local economy.

● Removing the barriers

The importance of involving people with disabilities in all aspects of community life has been emphasized. The practical aspects of translating this approach into action will now be considered.

In the first instance, nursing staff should adopt an approach to working with people with disabilities that empowers them to engage in all aspects of their care. The principle of equal opportunities underpins this concept and starts with a basic re-examination of the nurse's own values and attitudes towards disability. Acknowledgement of moral principles, such as client rights to enjoy the same range of access and opportunity in the community, is a prerequisite.

The following are examples of positive action and skills that nurses should be encouraged to acquire and engage in:

- proficiency in alternative communication systems for those people who are unable to use conventional systems (e.g. deaf–blind persons)
- advocacy skills that serve to empower clients
- political awareness and community action skills to identify and promote positive discrimination and access in the locality
- the design and development of networks of self-help and voluntary action groups

- co-ordination of local services to provide a single point of access for clients to services
- evaluation of local resources and policies to ensure that people with disabilities are provided with equal opportunities.

While these values and principles are essential, it is of equal importance to ensure that local policies are formulated in partnership with clients themselves. The principle of shared action planning (Brechin and Swain, 1987) requires that consumers are adequately prepared to participate in community life and in decision-making. Consider, for example, a person who has been in residential care for some years. Providing that person with a choice about discharge to live in the community must be accompanied with an assessment of the person's present level of communication and comprehension. After so long within an institution, personal decision-making abilities may have been reduced and it may be necessary to introduce new ideas over a period of time. This requires tact, sensitivity and patience.

A short illustration might further identify the key issues:

John had a physical disability and had lived in a long-stay hospital for several years. He had a speech impediment in the form of a stammer which was noticeably pronounced when he was anxious. He was considered for discharge to a new facility in the community. Prior to his discharge he met with his primary nurse who assisted him in prioritizing his strengths, needs, abilities and apprehensions. These were recorded for John, who had difficulty holding a pen, and were prepared for John to present to a case conference when his plan would be agreed. On the day in question, the chairperson (of unspecified professional status) was late and on arrival hurried the proceedings. He decided that it would be preferable to take evidence from the primary nurse rather than to invite John into the room in order to speed up the activity. The nurse insisted that John be invited in and this was reluctantly agreed. On entering the room he was told by the Chair that he had three minutes to present his case. Needless to say, John *became* anxious, his stammer increased resulting in him becoming almost incoherent. Eventually he was asked to leave and his written list of needs was considered in his absence.

This true story serves to demonstrate the importance of preparing both professionals and clients to share together in decision-making meetings. Careful preparation is essential and professional dominance has no place in this equation.

Skill enhancement for the client in the following areas is necessary:

- social skills
- self-help skills
- literacy
- listening

- assertiveness
- counselling
- communication
- self-awareness.

The Disabled Persons (Services, Consultation and Representation) Act 1986, in the UK, provides the framework within which such consultation should be placed. Social service authorities are required to produce evidence in their community care plans to communicate how they intend to empower people with disabilities. Community nurses also have a particular role to play in ensuring that their clients have their needs heard and responded to.

Some examples of how this might be achieved are:

- production of information leaflets about local services and opportunities
- self-advocacy forums
- consumer councils and groups
- involvement of consumers as members of local inspection teams
- membership and participation of people with disabilities in primary health care management teams.

This section calls for a new approach to people with disabilities and requires nursing staff to:

- examine their beliefs, attitudes and values towards concepts related to disability
- reflect on how informal and formal interactions with people occur and to re-examine the ground rules that govern the interactions
- promote equal opportunities for people in all aspects of community and public life
- acquire new skills aimed at empowering clients
- review the language they use to describe people with disabilities.

An examination of personal and professional values and beliefs is therefore a prerequisite for the adaptation and advancement of positive nursing practice. The next section provides a specific challenge to practitioners and illustrates both moral and ethical principles associated with human rights.

● Personal relationships and sexual identity

Issues relating to citizenship and empowerment are closely associated with civil rights. Equity and social justice arise in multiple health perspectives and become all the more important as choices are extended. One such example that spans personal, professional and moral agendas is the right to be sexual.

The need to be loved and to share love is acknowledged as a basic human right. However, for some people with disabilities the opportunities to form, develop and maintain personal relationships may be denied. These difficulties may commence in childhood and may be associated by the belief that people with disabilities are 'eternal children' and thus, by inference, are unable to function as sexually mature persons. In reality, there is little doubt that people with disabilities are as equally capable of enjoying fulfilled sex lives as other members of the general population. However, in so doing there must come the associated risks of rejection, loss, denial and, on occasions, infection.

Other influences that militate against the sexual needs of people with disabilities are those stemming from society's view of able-bodied men and women. The women's role is to be attractive and to bear children, whereas the man's sexual prowess is related to his 'macho' image and physical ability. Naturally these may not translate easily to the situation of a person with a disability, thus further rendering them to a lower status.

Nurses should be aware of these issues and seek to enable people with disabilities to:

- develop a positive self-image
- form personal friendships
- explore their own sexual identity without fear of invasion of personal privacy, judgement, criticism or prejudice
- receive information, guidance and counselling
- respect their spiritual and emotional needs
- access practical advice, education and materials to enable them to experience a full range of expressed needs.

● Responding to care needs

People with disabilities and their carers access a range of co-ordinated services. Community nurses have a significant role to play in the delivery of community care. A survey by the Royal College of Physicians (1986) found, in a review of Health Authorities in England, that there were major concerns about the level of domiciliary and respite care provided to people with disabilities. Even when services were provided, consumers were often dissatisfied with the poor choice provided for them. Another survey reported similar results (OPCS, 1988), and at least 10% of respondents stated that they required additional support from community nurses. In the same survey, 17% stated that they did not receive continence aids. The OPCS survey also found that 2.1% of people aged between 16 and 19 years have some form of disability. In at least 40% of these the underlying cause was cerebral palsy which provides a useful illustration of the key needs of people with disabilities. A wide range of needs might include: respite care provision; personal nursing care; provision of home aid and adaptations; health screening; continence advice; counselling.

People and their carers appear to rate respite care as a major need (RCN/Spastics Society, 1993). In a survey conducted by these bodies, the main interest in this facility was the provision of a flexible service that could respond to a range of needs for:

- home-based care to relieve carers for shopping trips or to attend family functions

- phased care that provided regular breaks every few weeks on a rotational basis (sometimes for holiday relief)
- informal care with volunteers in the neighbourhood
- irregular care in hostels, or in community facilities, whenever the need arose (sometimes in response to a family crisis or when care became 'just too much to manage').

None of the people surveyed wanted care in hospital settings, but rated support at home for their daily needs as their main priority, with the condition that it was provided at times directed to their individual lifestyles.

Sadly most respondents received very few services regularly and on occasions some people learnt to call for help 'only in the event of an emergency'. One other issue was the problem of confusion of whom to call upon among the many people in the community who were apparently responsible for the diverse and diffuse care functions. The concept of a single gatekeeper would appeal.

This factor has been the foundation of the community care reforms in the UK, and the emergence of the case management process has been a direct result of this (see Chapter 30). The appointment of a named person or care manager to co-ordinate all aspects of care, or in some cases enabling the client to become their own care manager, would appear to be one way of overcoming the confusion and frustration expressed by so many people with disabilities. Community nurses may be well placed to fulfil this function, with their knowledge of individual needs and of the resources of the local community.

The value of community nursing care for carers is also clearly expressed by carers. Their role extends across the age span and transcends many client groups and needs. The flexible nature of nursing provision also reduces the need for a proliferation of professionals to visit families for differentiated care provision. Their role may include the provision of:

- family counselling to enable the acceptance of the emergence of 'disability' in the family
- practical advice and assistance with aspects of daily living, including advice on the management of continence, mobility, self-help and social skills
- the delivery of therapeutic skills and care such as pain control or the 'management' of behavioural problems with some people with mental health needs or learning disabilities.

For many carers the reality of providing long-term care at home may result in personal isolation and economic deprivation. The study by the RCN and the Spastics Society referred to above, confirmed some of these needs and noted that many carers were dissatisfied with the services they received at home. Examples of difficulties were expressed as:

- the absence of respite care services
- inappropriate provision of equipment and in some cases the lack of any provision at all
- low levels of income to pay for the additional services needed

- inadequate provision by speech therapy, occupational therapy and physiotherapy services.

Consequently the gaps in service provision may be perceived by individual carers in different ways. For some, the lack of simple advice on continence or personal hygiene may have been a major problem, and for others, the lack of day and respite care services may have encouraged them to seek long-term care solutions for their problems outside the family home.

The value of practical support cannot be underestimated for many people and for their carers. Sadly the reality appears to be that limited choice persists among the services that community nurses are able to offer their clients and consequently many needs continue to go unmet. Difficulties in inter-agency collaboration compound these problems and the failure to involve service users, their informal carers and their community nurses in planning care delivery may be of particular concern.

The solutions are far from simple, but may include some of the following:

- the provision of responsive care management services to clients and their carers
- evidence of real shared care with consumers and their carers
- collaborative inter-professional teamwork in both the planning and delivery of services to clients
- more choice and flexibility in service design and accessibility for clients
- adequate finances to ensure that consumers are financially independent from the indignity of dependence on statutory service providers.

A requirement of health and social services is to listen to the views of consumers and to deliver responsive services in accordance with a series of core values. The core values identified in Table 6.1 may be used by consumers and their carers to evaluate the effectiveness and acceptability of services. However, to these should be added other values which relate to:

- the right to be informed
- the right to be consulted
- the right to be free from exploitation and excessive threat
- the right to redress and representation.

Table 6.1 Core values to evaluate effectiveness of services

Appropriateness	Services should meet needs of individuals and the population as a whole
Equity	There should be no organizational, social or geographical barriers to services and there should be a fair share of the services available to the population in accordance with need
Accessibility	As far as possible, services should be available locally
Acceptability	Services should satisfy the reasonable expectations of the population
Efficiency	Services should use resources to best effect
Effectiveness	Services should achieve the intended benefit

Adapted from the Strategic Plan for Health and Personal Social Services (Northern Ireland), 1992–97.

In conclusion to this section, carers have many needs and in many cases they possess the personal capacity to meet these needs themselves. However, the everyday demands of caring for 24-hour periods, often without respite, may take their toll, and it is the responsibility of all community nurses to assess and respond to the needs of all people with disabilities within the context of their families. To do otherwise would be to ignore the individual needs of the millions of informal carers. Further discussion on the role and responsibility of carers appears in Chapter 13.

● **Completing the circle**

Valuing people with disabilities has been a central theme in this chapter. Images of deviance no longer have a place in encouraging able-bodied and able-minded members of society to categorize people who do not accord with their perception of what constitutes the ordinary person in the street.

In their place has emerged a new approach to understanding all members of society as individuals with their own talents, strengths and needs. Community care policy has, to some extent, enabled this major shift in perception. Local neighbourhoods are beginning to demonstrate their ability and willingness to live and work alongside people with disabilities. As they do so, apparent differences may diminish and similarities may emerge to reduce the perceptual gap between disability and ability.

The key to achieving change to this degree or magnitude must be the creation of a set of cultural values to underpin the philosophy of equality. Donnison (1991) suggests that as individuals move towards the development of a united society they realize just how divided they really are. He states that a new poverty is evident that has the effect of marginalizing more groups than ever before from the mainstream activities of the society, and deepens these divisions, 'between those in the core and on the margin of the labour force'.

Implementing care in the community obviously requires a major conceptual change among community health care nurses and others, not least a requirement for them to empower people with disabilities to make their own decisions and to speak for themselves. Access to paid employment, integrated leisure facilities and opportunities to fully contribute to the life of their local communities will be required to announce that people with disabilities have achieved equal citizenship.

Thus the move to community care may be accompanied by a range of ethical, moral and political dilemmas which continue to test the professional and personal capacities of those people who aim to improve the quality of care and life for people with disabilities. As society aims to produce a more self-sufficient approach among its members, it must address the need to continue in its quest to remove the perceptual and physical barriers that restrict life opportunities for its more vulnerable members.

The task now facing community health care nurses is how best to ensure that people with disabilities are empowered and supported to respond to this challenge and to inform the debates that continue to be held on their behalf.

Maintaining the status quo is not an acceptable alternative to encouraging self-reliance and creating the social conditions that will enable all members of society to achieve their full potential with dignity, self-respect and a sense of personal fulfilment.

● **Conclusion**

This chapter has considered issues relating to the nature and presentation of disability for community nursing practitioners. During the next decade many of these issues will feature on the public and professional agenda and will continue to challenge the extent to which professionals are willing to empower people with disabilities to acquire additional rights in their quest to achieve an equitable status in society.

For the nursing profession, a major adjustment will be required in the attitudinal status afforded by its members to people with a range of disabilities. In this respect nurses will be confronted with complex decisions relating to risk-taking, empowerment and advocacy. Ethical issues underpin these abstract concepts which will soon become part of every nurse's everyday frame of reference.

The extent to which people with disabilities will be empowered to take control over their lives will be dependent upon the will of society and government policy. Extensive change is required in all aspects of public sector provision, and despite government support the UK has so far failed to legislate in favour of a policy of positive discrimination for people with disabilities.

The nursing profession has indicated its support for the empowerment of all clients and this must include those persons who have disabilities. The ultimate challange will be the extent to which nurses can influence the public and professional agenda to ensure that change is realized so that people with actual or presumed impaired autonomy are empowered to direct their own lives with equal citizenship.

References
43 & 44 Eliz. II., C.19. *The National Health Service and Community Care Act 1990*
35 & 36 Eliz. II., C.33. *The Disabled Persons (Services, Consultation and Representation) Act 1986*
Adams, J.D, Hayes, J. and Hopkins, B. (1976) *Transition: Understanding and Managing Personal Change*, Martin Robertson, London
Brechin, A. and Swain, A. (1987) *Changing Relationships – Shared Action Planning for People with a Mental Handicap,* London, Harper and Row
DoH (1992) *The Health of the Nation* (White Paper), London, HMSO
Donnison, D. (1991) Squeezed and broken on the brink, Thesis 19 April, quoted in Compton, A. and Ashwin, M. (1992) *Community Care for Health Professionals*, Butterworth-Heinemann, London
Goffman, E. (1961) *Asylums: Essays on the Social Situation of Mental Patients and Other Inmates*, Anchor Books/Doubleday, Washington

Matza, D. (1964) *Delinquency and Drift*, Wiley, New York

Menzies, I.E.P. (1970) *The Function of Social Systems as a Defence Against Anxiety. A Report of a Study on the Nursing Service of a General Hospital*, Tavistock Institute, London

Miller, E.J. and Gwynne, G.V. (1974) *A Life Apart*, Tavistock Press, London

OPCS (1988) *The Prevalence of Disability Amongst Adults*, OPCS Surveys of Disability in Great Britain, Report 1, HMSO, London

Open University (1990) *Disability – Changing Practice, Home Study Text*, K665X, Milton Keynes, Open University

RCN/Spastics Society (1993) *Day in and Day Out – A Survey of the Views of Respite Care*, RCN and the Spastics Society, London

Royal College of Physicians (1986) *Physical Disability in 1986 and Beyond*, RCP, London

Ryan, J. and Thomas, F. (1980) *The Politics of Mental Handicap*, Penguin Books, London

Stockwell, F. (1972) *The Unpopular Patient*, Royal College of Nursing, London

Sykes, G.M and Matza, D. (1957) Techniques of neutralisation: a theory of delinquency. *American Sociological Review*, **6**, 667–670

Wolfensberger, W. (1972) *The Principle of Normalisation in Human Services*, National Institute on Mental Retardation, Toronto

Zola, I.K. (1985) Depictions of disability – metaphor, messages, and medium in the media: a research and political agenda. *Social Science Journal*, **24**, 12–18

Part II

Frameworks for practice

The eight subspecialities of community nurses identified by the UKCC (1994) demonstrate not only the range of professional experience and clinical expertise of practitioners in the community, but also the variety of settings in which they practice. For example, practice nurses work predominantly in General Practitioners' premises, whereas others such as district nurses spend most of their time working in people's homes. Other community health care nurses work in community centres, schools and the workplace. Although these practitioners have some skills and knowledge in common, they also contribute different specialist and complementary expertise to the care of patients and clients.

However, there are some factors which influence all practitioners working in the community and which have a particular significance for the frameworks underpinning the care offered to patients and clients. This part of the book attempts to address four of these essential elements. Chapter 7 considers the influence of the individual practitioner's philosophy of care, as well as the structural organization in which that practitioner works. In Chapter 8 the structural organization is analysed in more depth and the implications of the contract culture for practice are discussed. The significance of ethics and values in determining a framework for practice is explored in Chapter 9. Chapter 10 considers the contribution of the different levels of prevention and care. It is possible to argue that other issues are equally influential in the development of frameworks for practice. However, in the editors' opinion the elements chosen are particularly significant in the context of clinical practice and current health care provision.

Since current legislation plays a major role in the provision of care, it is easy to understand the rationale for the selection of issues such as organizational structure. However, other factors have fundamental implications for practice. Indeed, the philosophical underpinning of practice and a firm understanding of nursing knowledge and models informing practice will also influence the quality of care given. The community health care nurse needs to develop a flexible approach in meeting the specific needs of patients and clients which may require operating at different levels of care and prevention.

The varied backgrounds of the authors are reflected in the individual styles of the chapters in this part. This approach offers readers the opportunity to assess different perspectives on some of the issues and questions that need to be considered in developing frameworks for practice. Although at times these issues may be complex and perhaps even raise conflicting ideas, it is hoped that readers will have the opportunity to think about the particular issues that are relevant to their own practice. This should provide the stimulus to take a fresh look at current practice and if appropriate develop new, or different, frameworks for practice.

Reference

UKCC (1994) Registrar's Letter CMc/MJW/PG/2/boc. UKCC, London

7

Philosophies, structures and traditions: implications for a framework for practice

Sheila Twinn

● Introduction

As community health care nurses continue to debate the development and contribution of practice to health care in a context of continuing change, an important issue for practitioners to consider is the framework underpinning their practice. This framework will not only play a significant role in determining the interpretation of practice, but also strategies for the implementation of patient and client care. Although a range of issues are relevant to the development of a framework for practice, the author suggests three issues are particularly influential. The first of these issues is the philosophy of care informing practice. The philosophy of care adopted by practitioners may be influenced by their understanding of the different theories underpinning practice or may be an explicit attempt by practitioners to develop a model for care. The second issue relates to the organizational factors influencing practice, and may be a consequence of the structure in which the practitioner works or a consequence of the working patterns practised within that community setting. The third and final issue to be considered in this chapter is that of the traditions of practice. In Chapter 1, the significance of the historical development of nursing in the community to current practice is highlighted. This process also contributes to the development of traditions in practice which has implications for the framework guiding patient and client care. Although there is a degree of interdependence between these three issues, each plays a significant role in determining the framework for practice adopted by the practitioner.

● Philosophy of care

The key targets identified in the publication *A Vision for the Future* (NHSME, 1993a) identify the essential role played by the philosophy of practice underpinning the care practitioners offer to patients and clients. However, the philosophy underpinning care will be influenced by a range of factors, some of which will result from the theoretical basis underpinning practice. Others will result from more pragmatic influences such as the introduction of the contract culture within the National Health Service (NHS) and the need for practitioners to respond to the demands of purchasers and providers. Although practitioners might feel the pragmatic approach to the philosophy of care is more realistic in the current context of health care, the theoretical basis of practice is also important since it provides the foundations from which practice can be developed to maintain high-quality care.

A theoretical foundation for nursing in the community

However, the theoretical basis of nursing in the community is not easily defined. Indeed, Chalmers and Kristjanson (1989) argue that although the theoretical basis directing practice is of primary importance in any applied discipline, the profession lacks conceptual clarity as to what determines nursing at a community level. In part, this lack of clarity is attributed to the difficulty of defining community and a discussion of some of these definitions is provided in Chapters 1 and 31. Another important factor influencing the lack of clarity in nursing in the community is the range of practice disciplines carried out in that context. Although this topic is discussed in some detail in Chapter 1, it is important to acknowledge once more the debate about the domains of practice, particularly since authors such as Geis (1991) highlight the fact that practice cannot be considered synonymous merely because home health nursing and community health nursing occur in the community.

Although the discussion by Geis refers to practice in the USA, a similar scenario is presented in the UK, with the domain of practice also ranging from public health nursing to nursing acutely sick people at home. It is possible to argue that it is inappropriate to search for a theoretical basis common to these different domains of practice; however, nursing theorists such as Orem (1991) and Roy (1970) have attempted to develop nursing models which provide a theoretical underpinning for practice in a range of clinical settings. Indeed, Hartweg (1991) describes the range of settings in which Orem's model, drawing on a theory of self-care deficit, has been developed in practice. The settings include critical care units, hospices, college student health programmes and a high rise senior centre, ranging therefore from critical care nursing to health promotion. Equally, the work of Roy, drawing on systems theory and the concept of adaptation, has been used in settings providing in-patient care as well as community and administration settings, giving a further theoretical basis for practice. (Andrews and Roy, 1986). Interestingly, both these authors have drawn on well-developed and tested theories from other disciplines, which perhaps highlights the lack of theoretical developments in nursing.

Nolan and Grant (1994) suggest that this lack of theoretical development may be a result of nursing having its roots in practice, therefore creating an uneasy relationship with theory. The limited number of empirical studies available which demonstrate the contribution of theory to practice perhaps supports this view. However, other authors such as Ingram (1991) and Vaughan (1992) argue that theory provides a useful contribution to the development of practice. Indeed, where the significance of a theoretical basis to the foundation of practice has been recognized, practitioners have been able to use this to develop practice. An example is provided by the work of Schröck and her contribution in developing the principles of health visiting (CETHV, 1993). Schrock's work, carried out nearly 20 years ago, used philosophical debates about the concept of health in an attempt to define a foundation for practice. Although some criticism has been suggested in attempting to ground practice in a concept as complex as health (Robinson, 1985), more recent work suggests that these principles continue to provide an important basis for practice (Twinn and Cowley, 1992). Nevertheless, anecdotal evidence once more questions the extent to which these principles have been demonstrated in practice-based research. However, it is neither possible nor appropriate to provide discussion of sufficient depth relating to the theoretical development of nursing in this chapter, and readers are therefore referred to texts such as Smith (1994), Marriner-Tomey (1994) and Chinn and Kramer (1991) to pursue this debate further.

The application of theory in practice

Despite the controversy of the contribution of theory to the development of nursing, practitioners have drawn on models of nursing in an attempt to inform and develop their practice in community health care nursing. One example is provided by practitioners in community psychiatric nursing using the model developed by Neuman to inform practice (Davies, 1989). Neuman's model, developed particularly for nursing in a community setting, is grounded in systems theory and the response of the client system to stressors at levels, which she refers to as interpersonal, intrapersonal or extrapersonal (Neuman, 1989). The model goes on to describe the use of nursing intervention at a primary, secondary or tertiary level to help clients obtain what Neuman describes as reconstitution in their health status. Because of the focus of this model on the 'client as a system' in interaction with the environment, practitioners in the community have considered it particularly appropriate to practice. Clark (1986) provides a further example of the contribution of this model to health visiting practice.

Other practitioners have developed this model to include the concept of community-as-client (Anderson et al., 1986). These authors argue that the development of this model is an attempt to 'put into practice the definition of public health nursing as a synthesis of public health and nursing'. This model, representing the community as eight subsystems and the response of these subsystems to stressors, attempts to provide a framework from which community nursing diagnosis gives direction to the goals and interventions of nursing practice. This approach to practice provides practitioners with another framework from which to assess the health needs of the community – a process which is discussed in detail in Chapter 23.

Other frameworks, although less well developed, also contribute to the philosophy of practice. Twinn (1991) describes a conceptual framework for health visiting practice which has evolved from two ideologies: the principles of health visiting and reflective practice. The framework illustrated in Figure 7.1 identifies the client as the central core of the structure, with the health status, health needs and health behaviour of the client integral to the central component of the framework. The fundamental role of the concepts of the client–practitioner relationship, promotion, prevention, choice and advocacy in developing effective practice strategies to identify and meet the health needs of clients, is demonstrated by the central and integrating location of these concepts in the framework. However, the author argues that the process of reflective practice is essential to the development of effective strategies since this enables practitioners to manage practice phenomena described as complexity, uncertainty, instability, uniqueness and value conflict (Schön, 1987). Indeed, it is the synthesis of practitioners' understanding of these phenomena in determining professional judgements which Schon de-

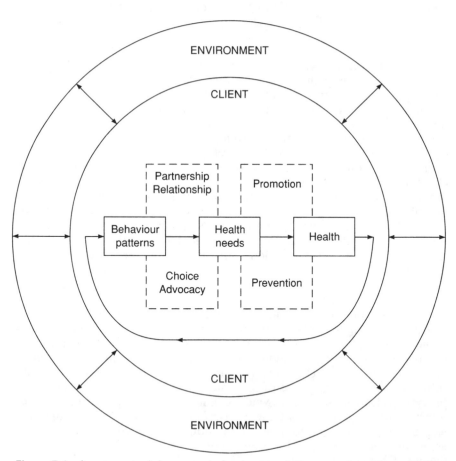

Figure 7.1 A conceptual framework for health visiting practice (From Twinn, 1991, by permission)

scribes as intuitive knowing-in-practice. The fundamental role of this process in the context of the conceptual framework and subsequent professional judgements, is represented by the dotted lines in Figure 7.1. Although the framework still requires considerable development, the author suggests this approach to practice lessens the emphasis on a task-orientated, client specific approach to that of the values and beliefs underpinning practice, so that practitioners can effectively work with clients to identify health need and adapt health behaviour as appropriate.

Mackenzie (1989) describes a framework for practice developed for district nursing which identifies 12 key activities of practice. Although some activities, such as participating in research and compiling a neighbourhood profile, are not specific to this discipline, others provide more specific activities expected of the practitioner within that particular practice environment. This framework, developed by a working party of the organization then known as the District Nursing Association, provides an illustration of the role played by professional organizations in developing a framework for practice.

● Organizational determinants

The framework for practice will not only be influenced by the practitioner's philosophy of care, but also by organizational determinants. These determinants can be divided into two major domains: first, that described as structural, and secondly, patterns of working within that structural setting. The structural setting of the practitioner will be influenced at both a macro and micro level. The macro level includes central government bodies such as the National Health Service Executive (NHSE) and professional organizations. The micro level refers to the individual practice setting of the practitioner, which for many practitioners will be within a Primary Health Care Team (PHCT). For those practitioners working within a large Trust, it is more difficult to consider this setting only at a micro level, since these structures also have significant organizational responsibilities influencing a wide range and number of staff. The other domain within this organizational determinant is the pattern of working adopted by the practitioner. In part this will be influenced by the structural setting of that practitioner, but there is evidence to suggest that within the same structural setting practitioners work independently of each other (Hutchinson and Gordon, 1992), consequently adopting different work patterns. Although the relationship between these two settings demonstrates once more the interdependent nature of factors determining the framework of practice, there are issues which are specific to each category.

The influence of the structural domain

The influence of the structural domain on the framework for practice is demonstrated at a macro level not only by legislation but also by policy documents produced by central government. The NHS and Community Care Act 1990 provides an example of legislation which created major challenges for practitioners, particularly as it requires practitioners to reassess the provision of care by the introduction of concepts such as the contract culture, a needs-based system of health care and the effectiveness and quality of care. Although these concepts have major implications for practice, evidence suggests an initial reluctance on the part of practitioners to acknowledge the significance of this legislation to the delivery of care (Rowe, 1993). The shift in emphasis by central government from secondary to primary health care, demonstrated in the policy initiative *The Health of the Nation* (DoH, 1992), once more requires practitioners to demonstrate their effectiveness in meeting the key targets determined in the document. Although this provides an exciting opportunity for nurses working in primary health care, it has implications for the framework for practice adopted by practitioners.

Government policy documents have also influenced the framework informing practice. *Neighbourhood Nursing: A Focus for Care* (DHSS, 1986) highlighted the importance of teamwork in practice as well as the need for practitioners to get out of 'their rut' by reconsidering the method of delivery of care. It was also in this document that the contribution of practice nurses to patient and client care was highlighted, which raised issues about the framework for practice for many practitioners. More recent documents, in particular, *New World, New Opportunities* (NHSME, 1993b) have continued this debate. This document, with the emphasis on auditing of practice, research and once again teamwork as key targets in developing community health care nursing to meet the demands of patient and client care, provides a clear agenda in developing frameworks for practice. In addition, the NHSE commissioning of research such as that of the *Health Visitor Marketing Project* (NHSE, 1994a) demonstrates the influence of central government to this process.

Finally, an important influence to consider is that of quasi-government organizations such as the statutory bodies: the United Kingdom Central Council for Nursing, Midwifery and Health Visiting (UKCC) and the National Boards for England, Scotland, Wales and Northern Ireland. The UKCC, with its responsibility for the regulation of the profession by controlling professional registrations and monitoring standards of practice, contributes to the development of frameworks for practice. Policy documents such as *The Future of Professional Practice—the Council's Standards for Education and Practice following Registration* (UKCC, 1994) provide an example. Indeed this document, by defining the specific learning outcomes required by practitioners entering specialist community nursing education, obviously plays a significant role in determining the framework for professional practice. The National Boards, in validating courses and monitoring the standards of those courses, provide an additional educational influence.

Those professional organizations with a dual responsibility of representing the trade union and professional rights of their members also contribute to the development of professional practice. Both the Health Visitors Association (HVA) and the Royal College of Nursing (RCN) provide examples of this type of organization. Indeed, the influence of the HVA in developing the framework for practice in health visiting can be seen in the publication of documents such as that on health profiling (Twinn *et al.*, 1990) and caring for families and children with HIV/AIDS (Gorna, 1994). The former publication, produced by one of the professional committees of the HVA, provided practitioners with a framework for profiling the health needs of practice populations prior to the implementation of legislation. More recently, publications such as *Action for Health* (HVA, 1994a) provide guidelines for practitioners to promote high-quality and effective primary health care nursing services. The trade union activities include, in particular, pay bargaining and grading of staff, both of which have implications for the delivery of care. Organizations such as the Community and District Nursing Association (CDNA), although not a trade union, provide similar important influences on practice by the production of publications such as *Key Issues in District Nursing* (Mackenzie, 1989).

At a micro level the organizational determinants influencing practice are created by the practice setting of the practitioner, which for many practitioners will be working in a PHCT possibly based in a General Practitioner's premises. The framework for practice will not only be influenced by effective teamwork and health promotion strategies, but also the contract culture now controlling this setting. The implications of this process for practitioners and the development of practice is discussed in detail in Chapter 8. For those practitioners whose practice setting remains within the NHS Trusts, the business contracts of the Trust will influence the framework for practice. However, this setting may also have implications for the framework at a macro level, as previously discussed.

Patterns of working

The pattern of working for community health care nurses, the second domain identified within organizational determinants, will not only be influenced by organizational factors but also by the traditions of practice, once again demonstrating the interdependent nature of the factors influencing the development of frameworks for practice. However, there are issues which are less dependent on the traditions of practice, in particular the development of primary health care and specialist roles. Although community health care nurses have worked in PHCTs since the 1960s, the more recent developments of programmes such as *Health for All by the Year 2000* (WHO, 1985) and the 'Health of the Nation' strategy have contributed to the development of nursing in the primary health care setting. Indeed, Scruby and McKay (1991) suggest that working patterns of community health care nurses will be influenced by the philosophy of 'Health for All' which requires practitioners to participate in fostering public participation, co-ordinating healthy public policy and strengthening community health services. However, for this approach to care to work effectively, interdisciplinary work is essential and evidence suggests the limited success of many PHCTs in working together as a team without some assistance in the process (Spratley, 1989). Indeed, the commitment of practitioners to teamwork will contribute to the framework for practice adopted by the practitioner.

The development of specialist roles in community health care nursing also has implications for patterns of working, which in turn may influence the framework for practice. The contribution of specialist practitioners to care is discussed in detail in Chapter 25; however, Charlton and Macaulay (1993) suggest that the introduction of specialist roles may lessen the expertise of general nurses working in the community, which may have implications for the framework of practice. The development of specialist roles and new patterns of working will also be influenced by the extent to which the practitioner is confined by the traditions of practice.

The tradition of practice

The tradition of practice is the final factor for consideration in the development of a framework for practice. It is possible to argue that tradition provides a negative influence to the framework guiding practice, since it may prevent practitioners from adapting practice to meet the changing demands of patients and client. However, the recent refocus of public health in health visiting demonstrates the positive contribution that tradition can also make to practice. Although this example perhaps raises the additional question of what is understood by the term tradition in the context of practice, there are two issues which appear particularly influential to the traditions of practice and will therefore be discussed in this chapter. The first of these is the development of the profession and the second is that which has been described as the rituals of practice. Indeed, the influence of the rituals of nursing practice in the acute setting is well documented by authors such as Walsh and Ford (1989), who provide examples of the implications of rituals in practice for patient care. Although evidence of the effect of rituals of practice in community health care nursing is less well described, there are implications for patient and client care and the development of practice in particular. However, it is perhaps important first to consider the influences of the development of the profession on the framework for practice, since this may contribute to the practice of ritualistic care.

Development of the professions

Although Chapter 1 attempts to set current practice within the historical development of community health care nursing, there are other issues in the development of the profession which have implications for frameworks informing practice, in particular the relationship between different disciplines in community health care nursing, the profile of the workforce and the educational roots of practitioners. Geis (1991) suggests that the emphasis in public health nursing on the continuous nature of care, wellness, health promotion and primary prevention differs considerably to that which she describes as home health nursing, with the emphasis of practice on illness-oriented care, episodic in nature and focusing on people who have either sought care for themselves or been referred by other health care professionals. These differences she claims raise issues about the preparation of practitioners, design of continuing education and research interests. Although this is an American interpretation of the relationship between community practitioners, similar differences exist in the UK. The publication of the document on the future of professional practice (UKCC, 1994) attempts to overcome these differences in perceptions of subspecialties by introducing a core component to the educational preparation of practitioners. However, anecdotal evidence suggests that differences remain in the perception of the contribution of different practitioners, with the consequent implications for the framework determining the practice offered to clients and patients.

The profile of the workforce raises further issues, particularly in health visiting, where data suggests a considerable proportion of the workforce will be reaching retirement age in the next decade (HVA, 1994b). A profile such as this raises questions as to the extent to which pracitioners adopt new approaches to care or whether they remain locked into more traditional methods. In turn, these questions raise the issue of the extent to which traditions of practice influence the philosophy of care, particularly since the introduction of the contract culture has major implications in developing a framework for practice which meets the new challenges in health care. In addition, the educational route of the practitioner may be influential in adopting a particular framework for practice. The validation process undertaken by the National Boards for programmes of community health care nursing demonstrates the range of approaches used in the preparation of practitioners.

Focus of practice

Although the educational preparation of practitioners highlights the possible interdependent nature of the development of the profession and rituals in practice, there are other independent examples of the rituals of practice which require consideration in the development of a framework for practice. The first of these is that of a focus on a specific age group which again is particularly illustrated in district nursing and health visiting. In health visiting, many practitioners have focused on the care of children under 5 which has influenced the framework for practice and prevented practitioners from adopting a needs-based approach to practice. Indeed, Hayes (1990) argues that her study demonstrated that health visitors would like to become more involved in health promotion activities but considered their current workload with children under 5 prevented them from developing this area of practice. Evidence such as this raises the additional question as to the extent to which the focus of practice is research based – a question which is particularly important to consider since the contract culture requires practitioners to focus practice on the identified health needs of practice populations.

In addition, the rituals of practice have led practitioners to focus on particular elements of practice. Health visiting provides a further example, with the focus on child health surveillance despite the lack of research evidence to support this practice (Hall, 1991). In district nursing, generally practitioners have continued to focus their practice on un-scheduled visits creating difficulties for both patients and their carers. Ellis (1995) demonstrates not only the feasibility of using timed visits, but also the appreciation of both patients and carers to the introduction of this scheme. Studies such as this highlight the important contribution of research findings in the development of a framework for practice.

Research-based practice

Research-based practice is essential if the framework is to be developed from an informed knowledge base rather than the rituals and traditions of practice. The present debate in the profession about skill mix provides an example, with practitioners highlighting their concern about the introduction of the process. Cowley (1993), in identifying the need to differentiate between grade and skill mix in the implementation of this approach to practice, goes on to discuss the importance of skill mix reviews being led by professionals to maintain high-quality patient and client care. This approach is supported by other literature which suggests that skill mix can lead to improved services by allowing community practitioners to focus their practice on those activities they are best qualified to carry out (HVA, 1994a). These issues all highlight the need for empirical research to be undertaken to examine the effects of skill mix on patient and client care, so that the framework informing practice is appropriately developed, rather than informed by rituals and tradition of practice. It is interesting that this principle was raised by the World Health Organization 20 years ago, when it identified the need for change in attitudes on the part of many health workers to the development of a community approach to practice (WHO, 1974). It is issues such as this which highlight the significance of the framework adopted for practice. However, these issues, particularly those identified within the traditions and rituals of practice, raise questions as to the opportunities provided for practitioners to develop their framework for practice from an informed research knowledge base – an approach to care which is particularly important in the current climate of the quest for excellence in practice.

● **Developing a framework for practice: contributing factors**

The development of an informed research-based framework for practice is fundamental to the provision of high-quality care and excellence in practice. However, to achieve this aim practitioners need support and opportunity in reviewing and assessing their clinical practice. The significant role that clinical supervision can play in this process has gradually been acknowledged in nursing. Butterworth and Faugier (1992) identify the contribution of this approach in developing practice, and in the field of psychiatric nursing clinical supervision has been undertaken for some time (Baker, 1992). More recently, government policy documents have also reflected the importance of this initiative with target five in the 'Vision for the Future', identifying the need for all practitioners to have access to clinical supervision (NHSME, 1993a). The review of the progress of the implementation of the targets demonstrated that 96% of units surveyed by the DoH in England had held discussions with nursing staff as to how they might develop their practice (NHSE, 1994b).

Although Bishop (1994) suggests that definitions of clinical supervision are relatively complex, she acknowledges the important role of clinical supervision in developing nursing expertise and suggests it should consist of clear expectations, criteria for quality and feedback which should involve participants, patients and management. She goes on to state there is no one correct model for clinical supervision, since local need determines the choice of approach. She suggests a model for clinical supervision which includes key ingredients such as clear feedback mechanisms, confidence in the supervisor, skilled listening and the ability to network with experts and collaborate (Bishop, 1994). These key ingredients not only highlight the demands on those responsible for clinical supervision but also the need for preparation to carry out this role. Organizations such as the HVA are currently involved in developing directives for their members involved in clinical supervision (Swain, 1995), demonstrating once more the contribution of organizations in developing a framework for practice.

However, the development of excellence in practice is a complex topic, as suggested in the recent survey of optimum practice in nursing, midwifery and health visiting (Butterworth, 1993). This research identified 18 key characteristics and 77 sub-items of optimum practice, all of which have implications in developing frameworks for practice. The report also highlights the role that Nursing Development Units (NDUs) have played in facilitating the development of excellence in practice. Although the initial development of these units has been focused in secondary care settings with little development in the community (Naish and Twinn, 1992), the greater emphasis on primary health care has led to NDUs being established in the community. The Strelley Nursing Development Unit provides an illustration of the way in which practitioners can use this resource to develop their clinical practice (Boyd *et al.*, 1993).

● **Conclusion**

With developments such as those described in this chapter occurring within nursing in the community, it provides opportunities for practitioners to reassess the framework underpinning their practice. In reassessing the framework, practitioners need to consider whether it is determined by the principles underpinning high-quality care and research-based knowledge, rather than the traditions of practice. In addition, it is important for practitioners to reconsider their individual philosophy of care, since this may have implications for the framework determining practice. The influence of organizational determinants in the framework, although equally important, is more difficult to address. It not only requires practitioners to remain politically active so that any compromise in the quality of care is minimized, but also that practitioners continue their professional development so that they can contribute positively to the process of change.

References

Anderson, E., McFarlane, J. and Hilton, A. (1986) Community-as-client: a model for practice. *Nursing Outlook*, **34**(5), 220–224

Andrews, H.A. and Roy, C. (1986) *Essentials of the Roy Adaptation Model*, Appleton-Century-Crofts, Norwalk, Conn.

Baker, P. (1992) Psychiatric nursing. In *Clinical Supervision and Mentorship in Nursing* (eds T. Butterworth and J. Faugier), Chapman and Hall, London

Bishop, V. (1994) Clinical supervision for an accountable profession *Nursing Times*, **90**(39), 35–37

Boyd, M., Brummell, K., Billingham, K. and Perkins, E. (1993) *The Public Health Post at Strelley: An Interim Report*, Nottingham Community Health NHS Trust, Nottingham

Butterworth, T. (1993) *A Delphi Survey of Optimum Practice in Nursing, Midwifery and Health Visiting*, University of Manchester, Manchester

Butterworth, T. and Faugier, J. (eds) (1992) *Clinical Supervision and Mentorship in Nursing*, Chapman and Hall, London

CETHV (1993) *An Investigation into the Principles of Health Visiting*, English National Board for Nursing, Midwifery and Health Visiting, London

Chalmers, K. and Kristjanson, L. (1989) The theoretical basis for nursing at the community level: a comparison of three models. *Journal of Advanced Nursing* **14**, 569–574

Charlton, T. and Macaulay, M. (1993) Good communication heralds successful integration: evaluation the roles of community specialists and general nurses. *Professional Nurse*, **8**(9), 600–602

Chinn, P.L. and Kramer, M.C. (1991) *Theory and Nursing*, 3rd edn, Mosby Year Book, St Louis

Clark, J. (1986) A model for health visiting. In *Models for Nursing* (eds B. Kershaw and J. Salvage), John Wiley, Chichester

Cowley, S. (1993) Skill mix: value for whom? *Health Visitor*, **66**(5), 166–168, 171

Davies, P. (1989) In Wales: use of the Neuman's systems model by community psychiatric nurses. In *The Neuman Systems Model*, 2nd edn (ed. B. Neuman), Appleton and Lange, Norwalk, Conn.

DHSS (1986) *Neighbourhood Nursing: A Focus for Care*, HMSO, London

DoH (1992) *The Health of the Nation*, HMSO, London

Ellis, J. (1995) Testing the feasibility of timed district nurses' visits. *Nursing Times*, **91**(3), 40–41

Geis, M.J. (1991) Differences in technology among subspecialities in community health nursing. *Journal of Community Health Nursing*, **8**(3), 163–170

Gorna, R. (1994) *Positive Practice*, Health Visitor's Association, London

Hall, D.M.B. (1991) *Health for All Children*, 2nd edn, Oxford University Press

Hartweg, D.L. (1991) *Dorothea Orem: Self-care Deficit Theory*, Sage Publications, Newbury Park

Hayes, E. (1990) Health visitors and health promotion. *Health Visitor*, **63**(10), 342–343

Hutchinson, A. and Gordon, S. (1992) Primary care teamwork – making it a reality. *Journal of Interprofessional Care*, **6**(1), 31–42

HVA (1994a) *Action for Health*, Health Visitors' Association, London

HVA (1994b) *A Cause for Concern: An Analysis of Staffing Levels and Training Plans in Health Visiting and School Nursing*, Health Visitors' Association, London

Ingram, R. (1991) Why does nursing need theory? *Journal of Advanced Nursing*, **16**, 350–353

Mackenzie, A. (1989) *Key Issues in District Nursing*, Paper One, District Nursing Association, London

Marriner-Tomey, A. (1994) *Nursing Theorists and their Work*, 3rd edn, Mosby Year Book, St Louis

Naish, J. and Twinn, S. (1992) Excellence in the community. *Nursing Times*, **88**(23), 45–47

Neuman, B. (1989) *The Neuman's Systems Model*, 2nd edn, Appleton and Lange, Norwalk, Conn

NHSE (1994a) *Health Visitor Marketing Project*, Project Report, Department of Health, London

NHSE (1994b) *Testing the Vision*, Department of Health, London

NHSME (1993a) *A Vision for the Future*, Department of Health, London

NHSME (1993b) *New World, New Opportunities*, Department of Health, London

Nolan, M and Grant, G. (1994) Mid-range theory building and the nursing theory gap: a respite care case study. In *Models, Theories and Concepts* (ed. P. Smith), Blackwell, Oxford

Orem, D. (1991) *Nursing Concepts of Practice*, 4th edn, Mosby Year Book, St. Louis

Robinson, J. (1985) Health visiting and health. In *Political Issues in Nursing*, Vol. 1 (ed. R. White), John Wiley, Chichester

Rowe, J. (1993) Contract culture. *Health Visitor*, **66**(10), 356

Roy, C. (1970) A conceptual framework for nursing. *Nursing Outlook*, **18**(3), 43–45

Schön, D. (1987) *Educating the Reflective Practitioner*, Jossey-Bass, San Francisco

Scruby, L.S. and McKay, M. (1991) Strengthening communities: changing roles for community health nurses. *Health Promotion International*, **6**(4), 263–269

Smith, J. (1994) *Models, Theories and Concepts*, Blackwell Scientific Publications, Oxford

Spratley, J. (1989) *Disease Prevention and Health Promotion in Primary Health Care*, Health Education Authority, London

Swain, G. (1995) *Clinical Supervision: The Principles and Process*, Health Visitors' Association, London

Twinn, S. (1991) Conflicting paradigms of health visiting: a continuing debate for professional practice. *Journal of Advanced Nursing*, **16**, 966–973

Twinn, S. and Cowley, S. (1992) *The Principles of Health Visiting: A Re-examination*, UKSC and HVA, London

Twinn, S. Dauncey, J. and Carnell, J. (1990) *The Process of Health Profiling*, Health Visitors' Association, London

UKCC (1994) *The Future of Professional Practice – The Council's Standards for Education and Practice following Registration*, United Kingdom Central Council for Nursing, Midwifery and Health Visiting, London

Vaughan, B. (1992) The nature of nursing knowledge. In *Knowledge for Nursing Practice* (eds K. Robinson and B. Vaughan), Butterworth-Heinemann, Oxford

Walsh, M. and Ford, P. (1989) *Nursing Rituals, Research and Rational Actions*, Butterworth-Heinemann, Oxford

WHO (1974) *Community Health Nursing*, Technical Report Series 558, World Health Organisation, Geneva

WHO (1985) *Targets for Health for All*, WHO Regional Office for Europe, Copenhagen

8

The contract culture: purchasers and providers

Alison Norman

● **Introduction**

In this chapter, issues involved in the commissioning of community and primary health care services will be explored. Inevitably this will require an examination of the historical provision and funding of services and an exploration of changes, within the National Health Service (NHS), which have transformed the way in which clinical care is organized and purchased.

Community health care nurses may wonder to what extent they should interest themselves in these matters. After all, many practitioners could argue what is important is the interaction between clinician and patient or client, not the bureaucracy that surrounds it. However, today as never before, it is crucial that every nurse, midwife and health visitor has a clear understanding of the organizational background to their specific role within the health service, and the implications this has for patient and client care.

An understanding of the structure and organization enables community health care nurses to influence change as well as demonstrate value and draw attention to deficiencies. In effect, it is essential for practitioners to be professionally, economically and politically aware and thereby better placed to bring about improved and enhanced services, or indeed sustain and protect those services which may be at risk.

● **Community and primary care services**

Traditionally, community services have included the range of professional staff as set out in Table 8.1. The community health professionals identified in the table may be employed by the same NHS Trust or a variety of different providers (see Chapter 2). As well as a range of clinical staff, services such as loan of equipment are provided, in addition to products to assist patients with continence difficulties. Although some

Table 8.1   Community health professionals

Doctors	*Nurses*
Paediatricians	District
Clinical medical officers	Health visitors
Geriatricians	School
Psychiatrists	Community midwife
	Community psychiatric
Dentists	Community mental handicap
Community dentists	Macmillan
	Marie Curie
Professions allied to medicine	Family planning
Occupational therapists	Stoma care
Chiropodists	Continence adviser
Speech therapists	Diabetic liaison
Physiotherapists	Paediatric liaison
Psychologists	Discharge liaison
Dietitians	Clinics
Audiologists	TB
Orthoptists	Nurse practitioner
Health promotion staff	
Community pharmacists	

Source: Audit Commission (1992a).

providers may offer additional professional services, such as community children's nursing, others may offer considerably less than is suggested here, which has obvious implications for the quality of patient care.

Indeed, this variation in range and level of service is common and raises issues about equity for local populations. The question of access to services is particularly acute when neighbouring geographical areas provide significantly different levels of input. A practical illustration of this may be that one provider offers a through-the-night nursing service, whereas the neighbouring organization has a service which finishes at 22.30 hours. For carers, anxious to keep a terminally ill relative at home, the presence, or absence, of a night sitting or nursing service could make the crucial difference between this being a realistic proposition or not. Failure to provide such a service can cause distress to both the carer and the patient (Twigg, 1992).

General Practitioners, whose practice population straddles the geographical boundaries of two or more community provider organizations, not only have some experience of this kind of difficulty but also possible differences in terms of the organizational style of the provider. Examples of this may include community nursing staff working in attachment, within a primary health care team, or geographical patch working. The range of clinical activity undertaken by nursing and health visiting colleagues may also vary – a situation which may appear to have more to do with organizational constraints rather than individual skill and meeting clinical need (NHSME, 1992a).

The report on community services produced by the Audit Commission (1992a) pointed out that

spending on community health services ... varies considerably between districts with some spending twice as much per person as others and the relationship between local provision and the measures of need available is poor. The 'Jarman Under-Privileged Area Score' – a weighted average of eight population factors – can be used to assess demand for community services; but the match between district Jarman Scores and expenditure is weak. A more direct measure of need is the number of elderly people, major users of district nursing services, but people over seventy-five have two or three times as many staff available to them in some districts as those in others.

It is therefore hardly surprising that variations are found in service provision given the uneven pattern of funding which, on the evidence produced by the Audit Commission, appeared entirely unrelated to the health needs of the population. As well as pointing out the variation in provision from district to district, the Audit Commission went on to state that:

- community services had not received priority attention at the District Health Authority level
- integration with other service providers and evidence of joint planning for care groups was poor
- a lack of overall management control had led to significant variations in grade and skill mix and how staff use their time; this problem, in part, was felt to be due to the lack of effective management information systems and underdeveloped quality assessment techniques.

The areas of concern highlighted by the Audit Commission have obvious implications both for the effectiveness of patient care services and the ability of community providers to respond to changing patterns of care. This particularly relates to the move to manage increasing numbers of patients within a non-institutional setting as required within the NHS and Community Care Act (DoH, 1990).

Another more recent report published by the Audit Commission (1994) examined the co-ordination of Community Child Health and Social Services for children in need. The report demonstrated a number of similar themes to those contained within the publication described above. Among other recommendations, key points were:

- there should be an overall assessment of needs, with priorities being agreed and resources redistributed if necessary
- services should be more clearly focused to meet need
- methods of ensuring effectiveness should be developed
- authorities and professionals should work together to plan and deliver services
- role ambiguity between professionals should be reduced.

In setting out what might seem to be a rather harsh commentary on the current state of services provided in the community, it is important to retain some sense of perspective. The criticisms made by the Audit Commission, perhaps particularly those relating to the requirement to ensure that services meet properly identified need and the extent to which these are demonstrably effective, can be, and have been, levelled at many other services and organizations (Netten and Beecham, 1993). Indeed, given another comment from the Audit Commission (1992a) that, 'many argue, with some justification, that community services have always been poor relations of the acute sector, suffering cutbacks when times are hard', it may be a cause of some satisfaction that in many places, services are developing and meeting identified health care needs with a significant degree of success (NHSME, 1992b, 1993). However, despite this fact, it is important for students, practitioners, managers and the purchasers/ commissioners of community services to have a clear appreciation of service reality in order to meet the challenge of providing comprehensive health care to an increasingly aware and demanding population.

In the Foreword to *Working for Patients* (DHSS, 1989), the then Prime Minister reiterated the government's strong commitment to the NHS; the commitment emphasized not only that this would be available to all regardless of income, but also that it would continue to be financed from general taxation. The key principles identified in the document, which saw legislative light within the NHS and Community Care Act 1990, were those of modernization and value for money. The Prime Minister suggested that the proposals were the most far reaching reform of the NHS in its history. Few working with the service would deny, five years on, that this was indeed the case.

The proposals set out two primary objectives:

- to give patients, wherever they live in the UK, better health care and a greater choice of the services available
- greater satisfaction and rewards for those working in the NHS who successfully respond to local needs and preferences.

The objectives were to be secured by seven key measures:

1. To make the health service more responsive to the needs of patients with as much power and responsibility as possible being delegated to a local level.
2. In order to stimulate a better service to patients, hospitals will be able to apply for new self-governing status as NHS Hospital Trusts, an objective which applied equally to community services organizations.
3. To enable hospitals which best meet the needs and wishes of patients to get the money to do so, with the money required to treat patients being able to cross administrative boundaries. This objective reflects the concept of money following the patient, with the intention that successful and busy providers should never run out of money.
4. One hundred new consultant posts to be created.
5. To help family doctors improve their service to patients, large GP practices will be able to apply for their own budgets to obtain a defined range of services direct from hospitals. The GP fundholding scheme, as it has become known, was implemented on the basis of practices with 9000 or more patients registered with them, holding funds to purchase primarily hospital care. In April 1993, the practice size was reduced to 7000 patients and the scope of the fund was increased to include further hospital services and elements of community health services (NHSME, 1992c). These elements included district nursing, health visiting (excluding a 10%

public health component for services provided outside the practice population), chiropody, dietetics, and mental health and mental handicap services. GP fundholders, therefore, have become both purchasers and providers of health care services.

6. To improve the effectiveness of NHS management, regional, district and family practitioner management bodies will be reduced in size and re-formed on business lines with executive and non-executive directors.

7. To ensure that all concerned with delivering services to the patient make the best use of the resources available to them, quality of service and value for money will be rigorously audited.

The impact of the legislation has been to organize the provision of health care through an internal market mechanism and to separate the function of provision from that of purchasing (see Chapter 2).

In 1991, the NHS structure, to support the system of health care, included:

- 190 District Health Authorities (DHAs)
- 8 Special Health Authorities (SHAs) (which manage London's postgraduate teaching hospitals)
- 90 Family Health Services Authorities (FHSAs) which administer the general practitioner services (doctors, dentists, opticians and pharmacists)
- 14 Regional Health Authorities (RHAs)
- the NHS Management Executive (NHSME) within the Department of Health (DoH, 1994).

Figure 8.1 schematically represents the structure, linking the Secretary of State to both the provider and purchaser elements of the service as at April 1993.

Between April 1991 and April 1994, significant change was required of provider units and Trusts and purchasing organizations, including GP fundholders. Baggott (1994) describes the development of an internal market in which health authorities would buy services from doctors and other health care providers on behalf of their resident populations. The internal market was seen by the government as a possible remedy to the problems of the NHS, although over two-thirds of health service managers believed that the internal market alone could not solve the fundamental problems of underfunding (NAHAT, 1992).

Implementing an internal market required the setting up of a much more detailed costing system, so that appropriate charges could be made. Systems to monitor services and test their quality and sensitivity had to be developed and implemented. Initially, largely crude, so-called 'block contracts' were in the majority; these arrangements mirrored existing service provision and priorities and therefore did not produce a means of bringing about dramatic, or even modest, shifts of emphasis in health care. However, GP fundholders, in particular, perhaps due to their smaller size and therefore higher degree of focus, were able to agree more sensitive contracts with providers, and as highlighted by Appleby et al. (1990) to negotiate, on the whole, an enhanced response in relation to waiting times and quality of communication from consultant to referring GP.

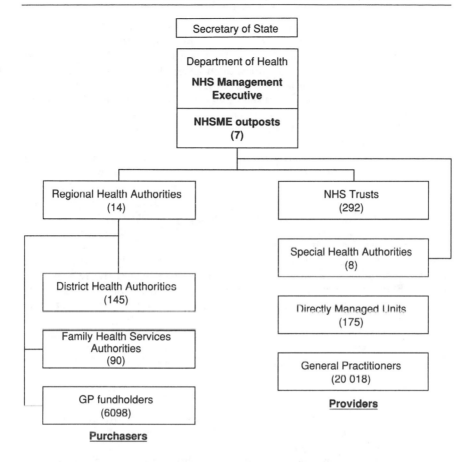

Figure 8.1 Structure of the NHS as at April 1993 (Source: Department of Health, 1994)

Within the community services, many fundholders took the opportunity to invest additional funds and to increase the level of provision for their practice population (Baggott, 1994). They were also able to negotiate the way in which attached and associated staff worked with the practice, for example the composition of the primary health care team and the degree of influence exercised by the practice on the day-to-day activity of staff. In order to achieve their preferred configuration, a minority of practices either moved from their local provider or threatened to do so in order to obtain their preferred organizational model. However, as Baggott (1994) acknowledges, this raises the possibility of inconvenience for the patient, particularly when the chosen hospital is some distance away.

Some controversy exists, in respect of the ability of fundholders to secure a better service from providers, than can be achieved by District Health Authorities purchasing on behalf of non-fundholding practices. A survey by the Association of Community Health Councils in England and Wales (ACHCEW, 1993) found that 20% of CHCs stated that fundholders' patients got priority access to hospital services in their area, while

50% reported that this was not happening. Several CHCs suspected that priority access was occurring though not officially acknowledged. Appleby (1992), also acknowledging that a number of GP fundholders have managed to negotiate quicker treatment for their patients, raises the questions of fairness and equity. The emphasis seems now to have shifted from a denial that a 'two-tier service' exists to that of the requirement for non-fundholders to secure, by means of either becoming fundholders themselves or putting pressure on their DHA, the same benefits for their own patients (Baggott, 1994).

In March 1994 the progress report given by the Secretary of State set out what she believed to be a watershed in the development of the NHS reforms. She stated that in the three years since implementation, a total of 419 NHS Trusts had been established, leading to 96% of hospital and community health service funding being spent with them. Over half the eligible practices were controlling their own budgets, covering some 36% of the population in England.

Butler (1992) observes that it is simply too early to draw a line across the balance sheet and to say unequivocally whether the reforms are good or bad. However, the potential benefits, in terms of responsiveness to patients, flexibility and greater efficiency are, he believes, certainly worth striving for. In order to maintain this momentum, organizational change, at the most senior level of the NHS, was seen to be required, leading to a streamlining of the central management structure and consolidating the joint working between DHAs and FHSAs (DoH, 1994). This new structure is demonstrated in Figure 8.2.

The key objectives for this slimmer organization are:

- to lead the drive for improvement in the health of the nation
- to provide a health service for all, on the basis of clinical need, regardless of ability to pay
- to secure continuous improvement in the quality of patient care
- to ensure that treatment and care are targeted to meet local needs
- to use available resources as efficiently as possible to meet the rising demands and expectations of the public.

It is important to appreciate the connection between purchasing strategy at the local level and the link back to the central management of the NHS. Both DHAs and GP fundholders, as purchasers, are bound to carry out broadly based purchasing priorities and their performance, in this respect, is monitored by the NHS Executive Regional Office. This demonstrates the fact that the internal NHS market is 'managed' in so far as the pursuit of certain key policy objectives and principles are concerned.

During the period of implementation of the NHS reforms, significant other imperatives have also emerged either legislatively or as core components of the change process. Perhaps the most important among these are:

- improving health through *The Health of the Nation* (DoH, 1992)
- securing high-quality care in the community in partnership with local authorities (Audit Commission, 1992b)

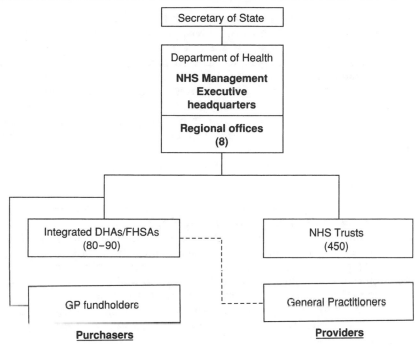

Figure 8.2 New structure of the NHS (1994) (Source: Department of Health, 1994)

- continuous improvement in the quality of services with particular reference to the implementation of *The Patient's Charter* (DoH, 1991) and the needs and wishes of patients
- achieving greater efficiency and effectiveness through the use of resources and organizational development (Audit Commission, 1992a)
- technological and other change, moving the focus of service from secondary to primary care (see Chapter 4).

Primarily DHAs and FHSAs, but also GP fundholders, will have the above five elements as a centrepiece to their purchasing strategy. The NHS Executive (NHSME, 1992c) lays a clear obligation upon particularly the purchasing authorities to act as agents for the public by:

- assessing people's health needs and developing local strategies for improving health
- targeting resources through the contracts they secure with providers of health care, on high-quality, value-for-money services
- bringing pressure to bear on providers to raise the quality of care and efficiency by setting standards, monitoring performance and exercising choice between competing providers
- working with and influencing other statutory and voluntary organizations to improve people's health.

In effect, the NHS Executive is attempting to move the local purchase of health care towards a rather more holistic notion of health commissioning, which takes DHAs and FHSAs away from perhaps historic and traditional patterns of provision, by means of undertaking an assessment of health needs and then formulating and implementing a strategy by which to purchase services to meet those needs within the resources available to them.

A crucial factor here is the requirement to collaborate closely with other agencies, notably the personal Social Services, in order to ensure coherent provision of services for those people whose care needs bridge the health and social care divide. Equally important is the fact that resources available to commissioners of service are finite and therefore choices, informed by national and local priorities, have to be made.

● Making choices or effective rationing?

Commissioners of community services, in order to fulfil their obligation to carry centrally driven policies, must now look carefully at the level of provision in community services. The Audit Commission's (1992a) findings in relation to this and the variations that exist have already been discussed. Purchasers are aware that GPs will not be able to operate successfully in a dynamic health scenario which is moving a range of patient care from secondary to primary care, without access to good-quality nursing therapy services.

New World, New Opportunities (NHSME, 1992a) also pointed out that deficits were to be found, perhaps particularly within urban areas, in relation to the adequacy and appropriateness of primary health care premises for modern health care practice. Therefore, a number of spending opportunities exist for Commissioners, both in terms of the provision of professional staff to work with GPs in primary health care teams, and in the improvement of physical facilities. Alongside these issues, the availability of more sophisticated equipment and enhanced specialist services, to manage more dependent patients at home safely, are often either absent or under pressure, therefore requiring significant investment (Audit Commission, 1992a)

The difficulty for commissioners is the availability of 'free money' which they can spend. Free money in this context is the ability to invest resources which are new, or unattached, to an existing service, rather than having to make hard decisions about shifting money from one service to another. In 1994, Newchurch summed up the opportunity and risk for commissioners as follows:

> *In the development of purchasing – by allowing for the defining of health care choices, by focusing on needs and outcomes and through the increasing empowerment of the consumer – the Government has created a process capable of delivering radical change in the nature and quality of health services. The crucial question is the extent to which this Government, or any Government, will be prepared to restrain their own intervention when Purchasers start making sensible choices for health which have difficult political consequences.*

Commissioners, by means of rigorous health needs assessment and an increasing knowledge of what measures are clinically effective, are now able to make informed judgements on provision. However, many of these judgements are value laden, for example, should a DHA purchase cosmetic surgery, or should those who have contributed to their problems, such as smokers, be treated? High-technology medicine is very expensive and although health economists can assist in comparing the value of a high-dependency intensive care bed set against an immunization programme for preschool children, the problem becomes one of managing the public and press fallout if a ward closure, or adverse publicity in respect of an individual patient, is the consequence of such a decision. Indeed, as highlighted by Harrison and Wistow (1992), there is little evidence that consistent criteria for rationing are being applied.

This all presupposes that the resources available for health care are finite and that some element of rationing is inevitable. In a research paper for the National Association of Health Authorities and Trusts, Hunter (1993) explores three reasons why this is the case, which are:

- the growing pressures on all health care systems to contain costs
- the British NHS, together with many other European health care systems, is undergoing major reform, a central plank of which is to separate the purchasing, or commissioning, of health care from its provision
- a key aspect of the NHS reforms has been an emphasis on consulting the public who, after all, pay for and are the users of health services.

The emphasis, placed by Hunter (1993) on the element of public consultation, is important both in terms of producing public knowledge which is sufficiently informed to assist debate, and in relation to the willingness of purchasers to respond to public demand. Certainly, the public's perceptions of how they should be treated, and in what time span, has increased and no longer can health care providers rely on a compliant and uncomplaining patient care group (NHSME, 1992d).

Commissioners do not depend solely upon their ability to find new funds to develop services. They may also contract, with providers, to bring about improved performance either by changing the configuration of a service or by improved productivity. Providers may therefore be required to undertake additional activity without access to commensurable funds to support the work. This obviously produces some tension and it is key decision, for commissioners, as to how much change they can bring about without also changing the level of resource allocation. It might be easy, given the argument within this section, to assume that the primary function of a Provider Trust or Directly Managed Unit is merely to respond to purchaser demand in a rather reactive way. This would be misleading and in the next section some views will be explored on the future of community services' providers in relation to the commissioning function and policy context.

● **Facing the future**

Community services providers have already faced up to considerable organizational change. In becoming Trusts, an immense amount of work has been undertaken in relation to improving information and other systems which, on the whole, were less well developed than those within the acute sector. Initially it was considered that community services do not do well when managed within acute Provider Trusts. The rationale for this has been that there is a tendency for resource allocation to be biased towards more 'high tech' acute services.

However, commercial realities are now bringing about a somewhat different view. Purchasers are becoming clearer about their priorities and would not wish to see any diminution in their investment in the non-institutional sector (Baggott, 1994). At the same time, as highlighted by Starey *et al*. (1993), acute providers are becoming very conscious of the need to have a good-quality community services network in order to facilitate optimum patient throughput. However, perhaps most importantly, the need to maximize clinical activity at an optimum price makes the need to cut down overhead costs a priority; community Trusts tend to have smaller turnover of funds and therefore relatively high overhead costs making them comparatively expensive. Also, the debate continues as to the possible direct employment of community health care nurses by fundholding practices. Obviously, were this to be the case, community Trusts would become smaller organizations, retaining employees of core and specialist services, such as school nursing and out-of-hours nursing services, but possibly not large enough to be viable as individual Trusts.

Certainly there are considerable uncertainties in terms of the organizational future. The above points would tend to support a view that community service providers should seek to merge with other Trusts in order to become more competitive and share risks. Alternatively, some community providers may see themselves becoming less direct employers rather agents and consultants, ensuring that GPs have access to appropriate qualified staff and a range of specialist services to support patient care. They may also seek to develop social care activity such as some of the elements of personal care currently undertaken by Social Services Departments in order to capitalize on opportunities presented by the community care legislation.

Successful community services providers will need to evaluate their structure and portfolio of services constantly in order to be in the best position to both respond, and if possible act, in advance of changes. In the meantime, they have to run effective services in response to the specifications set by their providers. GP fundholders tend to have high aspirations for their specific practice population, and District Health Authorities require providers to take a more holistic, population-based view. In the middle of these divergent views two perspectives are emerging: first, locality purchasing (for example on the basis of 25 000–30 000 people organized under the auspices of the DHA), and secondly, multi-funds, with a number of practices coming together often covering substantial numbers of people. In addition there is, as yet, an unresolved tension between fundholders and the Commissioning Authorities in relation to their proper functions and linkages, particularly in relation to planning of service development. However, the previous reputation of community services as a backwater is no longer true – it is probably now the most dynamic area of health care.

● **Conclusion**

As practitioners, community health care nurses are undoubtedly entering an area of increasing importance to the success of health care in the UK. There are many challenges to meet, ranging from those involved in working with well people to assist them to maximize their health, to the other end of the health continuum, supporting increasingly dependent and unwell people within the home setting.

As members of primary health care teams, community health care nurses will have influence directly on practice, but also, and increasingly in relation to the team function, as commissioners of services. The growth of fundholding and other schemes aimed at increasing the influence of GPs in purchasing will ensure this. Practitioners may also contribute greatly to the success of their organization, whether a Trust or directly managed unit, by seeking means to assist the commissioning process, for example by demonstrating clinical effectiveness.

Although some organizational change may continue, in relation to the commissioning of community services, it seems likely that many of the themes explored within this chapter will continue as core principles for the foreseeable future.

References

ACHCEW (1993) *The Internal Market and NHS Finances*, Association of Community Health Councils of England and Wales, London

Appleby, J. (1992) *Financing Health Care in the 1990s*, Open University Press, Buckingham

Appleby, J., Robinson, R., Ranade, W. *et al.* (1990) The use of markets in the Health Service: the NHS reforms and managed competition. *Public Money and Management*, **10**(4), 27–33

Audit Commission (1992a) *Homeward Bound*, HMSO, London

Audit Commission (1992b) *Community Care: Managing the Cascade of Change*, HMSO, London

Audit Commission (1994) *Seen but not Heard*, HMSO, London

Baggott, R. (1994) *Health and Health Care in Britian*, Macmillan, London

Butler, J. (1992) *Patients, Policies and Politics: Before and After 'Working for Patients'*, Open University Press, Buckingham

DoH (1990) *NHS and Community Care Act*, HMSO, London

DoH (1991) *The Patient's Charter*, HMSO, London

DoH (1992) *The Health of the Nation: A Strategy for Health in England*, HMSO, London

DoH (1994) *Managing the New NHS: A Background Document*, HMSO, London

DHSS (1989) *Working for Patients*, Cmnd 555, HMSO, London

Harrison, S. and Wistow, G. (1992) The purchaser/provider split in English health care: towards explicit rationing. *Policy and Politics*, **20**(2), 123–130

Hunter, D.J. (1993) *Rationing Dilemmas in Health Care*, Research Paper No. 8, National Association of Health Authorities and Trusts, Birmingham

NAHAT (1992) *Implementing the Reform – A Second National Survey of District General Managers*, National Association of Health Authorities and Trusts, Birmingham

Netten, A. and Beecham, J. (1993) *Costing Community Care: Theory and Practice*, University of Kent, Canterbury

NHSME (1992a) *New World, New Opportunities*, HMSO, London
NHSME (1992b) *NHS Trusts: The First 12 months*, Department of Health, London
NHSME (1992c) *Priorities and Planning Guidance 1993/4*, National Health Service Management Executive, Leeds
NHSME (1992d) *Local Voices.* Department of Health, London
NHSME (1993) *A-Z of Quality: A Guide to Quality Initiatives in the NHS*, Department of Health, London
Starey, N., Bosanquet, N. and Griffiths, J. (1993) General Practitioners in partnership with management: an organisational model for debate. *British Medical Journal*, **306**, 308–310
Twigg, J. (ed) (1992) *Carers: Research and Practice*, HMSO, London

9

Ethics and values

Verena Tschudin

● Introduction

Ethics is about *right* and *good*. It is about 'good' people doing 'right' acts. What is not right will be dealt with by the law. But how people are taught to be good depends on education and the choices which people make about being good. Consequently, doing right is an individual choice which nevertheless affects society as a whole.

Clearly, good and right are not black and white issues, and being a good person is different from being a do-gooder. Since these latter probably do no good but rather irritate people, they could be said to do wrong.

How and why people act ethically depends on their value-basis. For many people this is a religious basis. In the Judaeo-Christian tradition the Ten Commandments stand as that value-basis, and religious people consider it their duty to follow it. The Buddhist tradition has its basis in the Four Noble Truths which are expressed in the Noble Eightfold Path. Other value-systems are based on humanism, politics and, more recently, ecology in its widest sense. Before being able to think in terms of ethics, it is therefore useful to take a brief look at values.

● Values

A value is a personal belief or attitude about the truth, beauty or worth of any thought, object or behaviour.

(Uustal, 1980)

If someone was asked, 'What values to you hold?' it would usually be difficult to give an answer. People do not simply have a set of values which can be displayed like a label. Values are tested against specific situations. What individuals do and say (not only think) shows them up for what they are. People constantly judge themselves, other people and objects against a background of personal values. Most people would say that cars pollute the atmosphere, but few give up owning and driving a car. Nurses say and write much about treating patients and clients as individuals, but care plans and style of care given generally do not fully reflect this philosophy.

A non-judgemental attitude is now often seen to be a basis for helping. But this does not mean that a non-judgemental person has no values; on the contrary, such a person has chosen to refrain from making value-judgements about another so as to help that person more effectively.

These examples show that values have to be chosen, prized and acted on (Raths *et al.*, 1966). Values are not inborn qualities; that is, a person is not simply good because she or he had good parents who passed on the 'right' genes. Similarly, a person is not bad because of 'poor' parentage. Circumstances influence a person's nurture, but that person – once able to reason – has the choice, at least morally, of what to do with the given set of circumstances. Values have to be chosen from among alternatives, freely, and after considering the consequence of each alternative.

Simmons (1982) established a table of 100 value-statements which can be used for teaching. Students are asked to respond either by putting the statements in numerical order, or by giving them high, medium or low marks. A selection of such statements, according to Simmons, may be:

1.   The opportunity to improve my standard of living.
8.   Having happy, healthy children.
26.   Moderation in all moods.
42.   The hope of being wealthy.
57.   Leading a life of freedom.
74.   Being well dressed.
84.   Being thrifty.
98.   Being victorious.

Such lists can stimulate further thinking and awareness, but a disadvantage is that the impression given is that values are static. When people are asked to role-play or demonstrate a declared value, it becomes obvious that what is said and what is done do not always correspond; hence the usefulness of training in value-basis and the making of value-statements.

Values have to be chosen from among alternatives, and in every situation of choice there are at least two alternatives. Sometimes it seems that there is no choice and whichever way one looks at a situation, one is going to lose or suffer. Yet choosing to do nothing is a choice based on value. Perhaps that value is peace rather than struggle, or taking the path of least resistance because that has been the usual mode of action.

Whichever choice is made, the outcome has to be something which is prized; that is, something which is worth having, which gives satisfaction, or which has meaning. The person who prizes a car more than a clean environment demonstrates this by owning a car. The person who considers it more important to lead a quiet life rather than to fight for some rights also shows a value which is prized. The outcome of these choices and the internal prizing are the action: the car stays on the road; a struggle is not put up – effort, time and money is spent, perhaps, in admiring a work of art. For a value to be a value, it has to be seen to be such.

When people ask, 'Who am I?' or 'What makes me unique?', they see that the ways in which they act define who they are, and those ways are marked by the choices made, what is prized, and why.

● **Personal and professional values**

Uustal (1980) says that 'People who feel good about themselves . . . are more willing to take risks and try new and creative approaches. They are more willing to question situations that do not seem to affirm individual rights and values'. She quotes Wilmot (1975) who says, 'It is those with a low sense of self esteem who find it necessary to reject others. It is not that as ye judge so shall ye be judged, but as you judge yourself, so shall you judge others'.

Values and nursing

One of the main aspects of nursing is caring. But what exactly is caring? And is caring the same when there is time and all the necessary resources are available, as when these requirements are not present? 'How you perform as a nurse depends on your values, and these values form your philosophy of nursing' (Uustal, 1980). In other words, professional values are based on personal values. The way in which nurses care for them-selves is the basis for the way in which they care as nurses.

Roach (1987), herself a nurse, describes caring as 'the human mode of being', and the study of caring as a particularly important task for those involved in the education of professional carers. Caring as 'the human mode of being' implies that we express our humanity in and through caring. In this sense, caring is not specific to nursing, but it is specific *in* nursing. How nurses express that caring is how nursing is perceived as a profession, and a profession is judged by its individual members. One caring nurse gives the impression of a caring profession, but the profession of nursing cannot tell individuals how to be caring people. At best, the profession can publish a Code of Professional Conduct, specifying a minimum standard.

Roach (1987) details her caring into five aspects, all starting with the letter C: compassion, competence, confidence, conscience and commitment. Each of these is necessary in a professional relationship if one person is to be cared for, and the other cares. This set of words is not exclusive; other aspects can be important at times, but broadly speaking, the 'five Cs' cover the necessary elements if caring is to take place. The gap between theory and practice begins to close in the light of these aspects.

Professional values in nursing are coloured by the practitioners' attitudes to quality of life, the meaning of illness, health values and dying and death (Uustal, 1980). A nurse's personal values to these issues inevitably influence her or his behaviour towards a patient. Is that as it should be? The case study below will further address this question.

It is becoming more and more recognized that the values of a health care system are not necessarily those of its individual users. Routines and rituals in nursing are giving way to individualized care – but at great cost to the carers and the institution. Menzies (1960) showed clearly that ritual was a defence against individual and corporate anxiety. If the people with those systems are exposed to anxiety, what do they do? The need for personal support has grown tremendously in recent years, but so also has the unacknowledged stress, the disillusionment and apparent loss of values among many health care workers.

Changing values

Values change constantly. What is of value today will be discarded tomorrow. It barely needs repeating that we live in a time of great change.

Beliefs and attitudes, together with values, form the basis for the way in which we express ourselves as human beings. Beliefs are those elements which change least in this trio, with attitudes being seen as more settled behaviours (Tschudin, 1992). Values are the changeable aspects. But values are not changed like clothes – they are tied to an individual's belief and attitudes.

Yet values need to change. In order to grow as human beings and to remain human, adaptation and change must occur; however, a person who can be trusted is recognized as someone dependable and not capricious. Values and attitudes usually change slowly, but sometimes quickly after some significant insight. A person who has always considered it right to be submissive will only become assertive after much personal soul-searching. Not so many years ago, nurses were exhorted always to carry out the doctor's orders without question and willingly. Today, nurses find that they often need to advocate on a patient's behalf against doctors, systems or pressure of any kind (see Chapter 28). As we change, so our values change.

Case study

Mrs W. was a resident in a supported care environment. She had lived with her daughter, Mrs S., until 5 years ago. At that time, Mrs S. had married again and was hoping to have a child with her new partner, although she already had four children. One of these, Charlie, a boy of 9 at the time, had been particularly close to his grandmother. Mrs S. did, in fact, have two other children then, but still managed to visit her mother once a week.

Charlie, now 14, had always visited Mrs W., often on his own, going there straight from school. Mrs W. suffered badly with leg ulcers and the community nurse, Rosie, went to her daily for dressings and heard the whole family history in time. She was pleased that Charlie came to visit Mrs W. so regularly.

In the last year or so Mrs W. had a few times mentioned that she had given Charlie some money to help him buy school books. It was dreadful, she mused, that schools can't even afford books. Charlie had also stayed the night at his grandmother's home a couple of times recently, being too tired to go home. He felt that there was now quite a crowd at home, and he was better off out of it.

On one of these occasions, Rosie had come early to Mrs W. and Charlie hadn't left yet to go to school. Rosie noticed his dishevelled appearance, which surprised her, but most of all she noticed a distinctive smell about him which she recognized as being that of cannabis. Mrs W. had known him to smoke occasionally, but she hadn't realized what he smoked. It was clear that Rosie couldn't say anything there and then, but she wondered if she should say anything – and, if so, what – to Mrs W.

Rosie's personal values are in question here, and her eventual decision (to speak out or not, and what she will say) is an ethical decision. Her values relate to the way in which she views Charlie's quality of life, his health and welfare, his education, the meaning of life in general and of his life in particular. She will also consider issues such as justice, honesty or truth, and freedom or autonomy. With this she is venturing into the area of ethics.

Last, but not least, she has to consider her professional role. What can she, as a health care professional, do in this situation?

By a consideration of ethics, it may become clearer what is involved in this case.

● **Ethics**

Ethics as a study pertains to basic principles of moral behaviour. These principles are not absolutes and cannot be demanded of people; people can only be exhorted to respect them.

The first such principle is that of the value of life (Thiroux, 1980). This principle is generally considered to be pre-eminent because life is what all people have in common and they should therefore revere it, while at the same time accepting death. But life is clearly not an absolute – it is infringed by abortion, euthanasia, suicide, war, and capital punishment.

Although life should be revered, the value put on an individual can vary greatly. People who torture others consider those lives inferior to their own. The life of a fetus is considered in some cultures not to have the same value as that of the mother, hence abortion is tolerated. Some countries may condemn a person to death, thus also declaring that that particular life is not worth sustaining.

The case of Tony Bland, a severely brain-damaged victim of the 1987 Hillsborough football stadium disaster in the UK, has been much debated. In making a decision about whether artificial feeding should be stopped, enabling death to occur, the Law Lords argued that this would be in Bland's best interest because 'when treatment started, decisions that he could not make for himself were made in his best interests'. Subsequently, with the passage of time, it became apparent that recovery was impossible, therefore: 'Although termination of his life is not in his best interests, his best interests in being kept alive have all disappeared, taking with them the justification of the con-consensual regime and the co-relative duty to keep it going' (Bulletin of Medical Ethics, 1993a).

The principle of justice or fairness means 'that human beings should treat other human beings fairly and justly' (Thiroux, 1980). With increasing awareness today that resources are scarce, be this in health care or in the use of fossil fuels, ways have to be found of distributing what is available equitably.

The effects of being good persons doing right actions are seen particularly in this principle. In health care it is recognized that justice does not mean that everyone has equal access to all resources possible, but that everyone has equal access to the resources needed. The determination of need is, in part, dependent upon an honest (or truthful) assessment of need. The principle of truth-telling or honesty underlies all meaningful communication. Indeed, society rests on this principle. Unless a patient gives a truthful description of symptoms, a diagnosis cannot be made, nor treatment be successful. Caring in general, and caring relationships in particular, are based on this principle. It may therefore be somewhat surprising to realize that no nursing or medical code makes any mention of truth. The nearest nursing comes to such a statement is in the UKCC (1989) Advisory Document *Exercising Accountability*, where Section D is entitled 'Consent and truth'. Truth-telling in nursing should not be limited to consent, because truth does not merely imply that what is said is truthful, but rather that vital information is not withheld.

The principle of individual freedom means that 'people, being individuals with individual differences, must have the freedom to choose their own ways and means of being moral' (Thiroux, 1980). Freedom (or autonomy), like the other principles, is not absolute. A person cannot, because she or he is free, drive above the speed limit in an urban area. A further example is given in an editorial of the Bulletin of Medical Ethics (1993b), which describes an incident from a television debate: 'Several young mothers – who had just been complaining loud and long at having had to deliver their babies in a hospital where the midwife was HIV positive – were sitting round smoking. They admitted to having smoked in pregnancy. If they were so worried about the non-existent risks of HIV infection, why expose their infants to known risks from smoking? "Well, its my choice, isn't it", one replied'. The principle of individual freedom supports her, but the principles of the value of life (hers and her baby's) and justice do not support her actions in the same way. Her choice is not so simple. Freedom can only be seen within the context of the other principles.

Similarly, in professional practice, a nurse must have basic training, confidence in her or his ability, and then be given the professional freedom to practise. The nurse, in turn, pledges accountability for her or his practice.

Two theories of ethics

The study of ethics in the West is firmly based in the Greek schools of Plato, Aristotle and Socrates. Two broad schools have, however, emerged which will only be outlined very briefly.

Deontology, or duty ethics, relies on laws and rules – common and personal – to guide people to act rightly. In this theory, the stress is on the action itself; that is, an act has to be right in itself for it to be called ethically or morally right. Hence the appeal to duty. A person's observance of rules, and the moral duty to act rightly are the parameters of this theory.

Teleology, or consequentialism, is concerned with the consequence of any action, not the action itself. Utilitarianism is the best known of its branches, with its slogan 'the greatest good for the greatest number'. The NHS in the UK is firmly rooted in this theory.

In the case study detailed earlier, the nurse would need to decide if she has a duty to say anything about her observation. The duty comes out of laws (religious, personal, professional), and her adherence to these laws would lead her to act rightly. She would have to ensure that her action (speaking up) is in itself right and good, if she follows the deontological model. But following the teleological model, the nurse would think first of all of the consequences of any action. Would speaking out bring good (to whom?) or cause harm (to whom?). Only when she had looked at the possibilities and decided that speaking out would be better for all concerned than not speaking out, could she take such an action.

Response ethics

H. Richard Niebuhr (1894–1962), an American political theologian and ethicist, put forward a theory of ethics which is particularly apt in health care, and which has gained prominence in Britain in recent years. Niebuhr starts his theory, which is outlined in *The Responsible Self* (Niebuhr, 1963), not from duty or goals, but from the idea of co-humanity. What people have in common is their humanity. In order to express their humanity, people use their creativity to respond to each other in various ways. Thus being human is living a dialogue, with one response leading to another response, but each response is interpreted by each individual in the light of what has just been said, and that person's experiences and hopes.

Niebuhr played with the word 'response' to make it apply to different aspects of his theory:

We respond to each other.
People are responsible, i.e. they have the ability to respond.
This leads to responsibility on a personal and communal level.

Whereas deontology and teleology tend to stress the individual and his or her personal choice and decisions – which can lead to great isolation and also to the paternalism of so much past medical practice – response ethics stresses relationships, community and the common human experience. This can be seen clearly in the 'pattern of responsibility' which Niebuhr saw in this approach:

Challenge:

- response
- interpretation/accountability
- responsive action
- social solidarity.

By challenge, Niebuhr means that element which first evokes an ethical awareness. In the case of the community nurse, Rosie, this is seeing Charlie, smelling the distinctive smell of the drug and her awareness as a professional person in this situation.

A challenge may be a telephone call asking a nurse to stay on duty a couple of hours longer; a woman asking a friend for help with thinking about her unwanted pregnancy; or realizing that a particular situation presents a question to the conscience.

Once we are aware of a problem or potential dilemma, our response is first of all physical: one's heart beats faster, one's mouth becomes dry, or one's legs will not move. We are aware in our bodies of feelings and sensations of fear, anger, opposition, hurt, shame, or any other strong emotion.

This emphasis on a response of the body and the emotions is significant. Most other ethical theories appeal mainly to logic and thinking, granting feelings a 'look in' rather grudgingly (hence the isolation which can be experienced). In response ethics, the importance of feelings is restored to the beginning of the pattern. It takes little imagination for nurses to be aware that patients make most decisions on the basis of feelings, and not in the first instance on logic or reason. When feelings are acknowledged, it is also possible to see that this enhances human relationships and the importance of community.

Once the response has been established, the next step is an interpretation. This means that we draw on similar situations which have occurred in the past and recall what happened then. It is then possible to calculate the outcomes if various decisions were made. These possible outcomes are then considered and interpreted in the light of present knowledge and emotion

Conscience will be a guide, so mental decisions will not be arbitrary but principled, depending on values, a sense of responsibility and the ability to respond now. Niebuhr uses the word 'accountability' for this part of the pattern.

Since a decision has to be implemented – there has to be an action for it to be an ethical act – something has to be done. This action is a responsive action, that is, it is the response to how the challenge is interpreted – the bodily response to it.

The outcome of this process is social solidarity. This means basically that for an action to have been an ethical act, something greater has resulted. This is not simply 'the greatest good for the greatest number'. It means essentially that all who have been affected by the original challenge have gained from the responsive action. The community, that is, the family, team or group, will have gained, not just the individual.

In the earlier case of Rosie, this might mean that she, Mrs W., Mrs S. and her family, and Charlie and his friends, will all have gained something from whatever action was taken.

Niebuhr asks two main question in this process: 'What is happening' and 'What is the fitting answer?' An answer has to be given to the first question and thus, says Niebuhr, we recognize 'Man-the-answerer', or put in another way, responding and responsibility are at the heart of this theory of ethics. Instead of asking 'What is my duty?' as in deontology, or 'What is the goal?' as in teleology, this theory asks again and again, 'What is happening?'

The very basic question is perhaps the one asked least. It is all too easy to jump from challenge to solution, thus reacting rather than questioning, and never learning how the process of ethical decision-making really happens. Asking 'What is happening?' is so basic that it is often totally overlooked. We tend to think that we know anyway. Assumptions are made about people's perceptions and there is a belief that we all think in the same way. Individuals ascribe values to people, thoughts and objects. When it was said that being non-judgemental is a value in caring, this is what was being highlighted.

Ethical decision-making

The 'pattern of responsibility' simply means that making deliberate decisions goes through a process which is recognizable at any level. Taking these models then, there is the possibility of asking four questions following the challenge using Niebuhr's (1963) approach. These would be:

What is happening?	*Response*
What would happen if . . .?	*Interpretation/accountability*
What is the fitting answer?	*Responsive action*
What has happened?	*Social solidarity*

Thus it can be seen that response ethics is a way of making decisions for oneself and also for helping others to make decisions.

Rosie, in the case history above, might need to ask herself, 'What is happening here?' What does Rosie see as fact? What is she conjecturing? What feelings are aroused? What values are being questioned? What is happening to each of the individuals involved?

What would happen if she challenged Charlie? Spoke to Mrs W.? Said nothing? Does she have a duty? To whom? Is it a professional duty? Of what does the duty consist? What could be a possible way forward? For her? For Mrs W.?

Which of the ethical principles is mainly addressed here: value of life, what is good and right, justice, truth, freedom? Are other issues involved, such as doing no harm, confidentiality, advocacy, rights, responsibilities?

What might be the fitting answer? Based on this analysis, this is not simply the right or lawful or dutiful answer, but the fitting answer dependent on what is happening and what is involved in terms of ethics.

What will have happened in terms of social solidarity? How would

Rosie benefit or not as the community nurse? Will Charlie have gained in understanding and responsible behaviour? Will Mrs W. feel at ease and be satisfied? Will there be greater understanding all round of the issues, the needs of people and how to be good and act rightly?

Rosie is asking these questions of herself, but a colleague or manager to whom she could have taken the problem may also ask her the same questions. The model is applicable to oneself and also to helping others in making ethical decisions. If the model is used to help someone, two crucially important things need to be done: assumptions must not be made and the other person must be allowed a voice, a space, and the possibility to express himself or herself as a person. A response is asked for and a response which tells a story. Both the main questions – 'What is happening' and 'What is the fitting answer' – are open questions.

Response ethics is therefore firmly rooted in the best principles of communication, and it considers caring for others as 'the human mode of being'.

The UKCC (1992) *Code of Professional Conduct* lays upon nurses, midwives and health visitors the duty (you 'must') always act in the patient's or client's interest and well-being. By asking a few basic questions at strategic moments, this injunction is a great deal less daunting.

● **Conclusion**

For many people the subject of ethics may appear somewhat intangible. 'Don't bother my head with ethics, but let me get on with my job' has been heard to come from one community nurse. The fact is that all her actions are based on values and ethics which affect her life and the lives of all with whom she comes into contact.

This chapter presents only a very simple outline of the most important ethical principles. In applying them, every nurse will come across her or his own problems, challenges and responses. The outline of a model for decision-making may make the subject of ethics less daunting – but it will never make it less demanding.

References

Bulletin of Medical Ethics (1993a) Futile nutrition may be withdrawn. *Bulletin of Medical Ethics*, **85**, 81–84
Bulletin of Medical Ethics (1993b) Editorial. *Bulletin of Medical Ethics*, **86**, 1
Menzies, I. (1960) A case-study in the functioning of social systems as a defence against anxiety. *Human Relations*, **13**(2), 95–121
Niebuhr, H.R. (1963) *The Responsible Self*, Harper and Row, San Francisco
Raths, L.E., Harmin, M. and Simon, S.B. (1966) *Values and Teaching*, Merrill, Columbus, OH
Roach, M.S. (1987) *The Human Act of Caring*, Canadian Hospital Association, Ottawa
Simmons, D. (1982) Value statements. Quoted in V. Tschudin (1992) *Ethics in Nursing: The Caring Relationship*, Butterworth-Heinemann, Oxford
Thiroux, J. (1980) *Ethics, Theory and Practice*, Glencoe Publishing, Encino, CA

Tschudin, V. (1992) *Values: A Primer for Nurses* (Workbook), Baillière Tindall, London

UKCC (1989) *Exercising Accountability*, UKCC, London

UKCC (1992) *Code of Professional Conduct*, UKCC, London

Uustal, D.B. (1980) Exploring values in nursing. *AORN Journal*, **31**(2), 183–187

Wilmot, W. (1975) Dyadic communication. Quoted in D.B. Uustal (1980) Exploring values in nursing. *AORN Journal*, **31**(2), 183–187

10

Levels of care and prevention: implications for practice

Dorothy Ferguson and Lesley Whyte

● **Introduction**

Health care within the UK continues to evolve in response to both international and national influences. As described in Chapter 4, a major response to these influences has prompted a shift in government policy from secondary to primary health care. Despite this shift in policy, the concept of levels of care and prevention continue to play an important role in guiding the framework for practice for community health care nursing. It is therefore important that practitioners have a clear understanding of this concept and consider the implications for practice. Consequently, the first section of this chapter defines and explores the terms primary, secondary and tertiary in the context of health care systems at both an international and national level. The second section discusses the terms in relation to prevention of ill health within the context of nursing in the community.

● **An international perspective: levels of care**

Primary health care

Primary health care is not a new concept within the health care system of many different countries. In 1975, the World Health Organisation (WHO) defined primary health care as the first point of contact for the individual with the physician and secondary health care as being that which fell beyond the resources of the General Practitioner (Hogarth, 1975). Less discussion was given to the concept of tertiary health care at that stage. The reader will note that although definitions at that point in time were medically orientated they involve a progression through first to second points of contact within the caring services. However, it was also at that stage that the WHO recognized the importance of primary health care in promoting the health of communities by developing the global strategy of *Health for All by the Year 2000*. This strategy, conceived at the World Health Assembly in 1977, was endorsed at the 1978 WHO/

UNICEF conference in Alma Ata, as is discussed in more detail in Chapter 3.

The Declaration of Alma Ata recognized that improved primary health care was central to achieving the goal of 'Health for All by the Year 2000'. Primary health care was therefore described by WHO (1978) as

essential health care, based on practical, scientifically sound and socially acceptable methods and technology made universally accessible to individuals and families in the community through their full participation and at a cost that the community and country can afford to maintain at every stage of their development in the spirit of self reliance and self determination.

The key features of a primary health care system can thus be summarised as:

- acceptable
- accessible
- equitable
- cost-effective
- participatory.

This definition widens the concept of primary health care from that of the earlier definition, altering the domination of the medical aspects of care, to health care made available locally to the individual or family. The definition acknowledges the potential influence of policy, finance and culture. The provider of primary health care may be a professional, as is often the case in the UK, a specially trained worker such as paramedics in Bangladesh (Payne, 1993) or indeed a traditional healer (Bastien, 1994). Primary health care remains, however, the first point of contact with the services.

Primary health care as advocated by the declaration of Alma Ata not only extended the range of carers but also the scope of care, with the major focus placed on preventive health care and health promotion. This philosophy is based on the belief that information combined with earlier diagnosis and prompt intervention contributes to the prevention of chronic conditions and degenerative disease. In addition, primary health care must address the main health problems within a community by providing promotive, preventive, curative and rehabilitative services. Thus primary health care, as advocated by the WHO, may include every aspect of health care activity and a variety of workers. Ashton and Seymour (1988) suggest that this broad, public health approach to primary health care forms the basis for the 'Health for All by the Year 2000' strategy, by attempting to eliminate inequalities in health and health care. Indeed, primary health care, as described by the WHO, should apply to all countries from the most to the least developed. All health-related sectors should contribute to primary health care with full involvement from the community. Primary health care should also be integrated within the overall health care system of the country (WHO, 1978).

An example of the effectiveness of implementing a primary health care system such as that recommended by the WHO guidelines is provided in mainland China (WHO, 1983). The high level of primary health care in parts of China reflects such aspects as political commitment to improving the quality of life by treating health goals as priority targets. The decentralization of economic structures led to the integration of health with other aspects of development. The local people were included in the provision of the health care system in which traditional and modern methods combined and utilized appropriate technology. Nugroho *et al.* (1986) summarize further examples of various ways in which primary health care systems may be implemented. In Hong Kong, where new satellite towns have been developed to ease overcrowding, the decentralization of health services has aided effectiveness and efficiency. In Malaysia, a system of village aid responds to local need and maximizes the involvement of the local community. The emphasis on partnership in the Philippines also falls well within the WHO description of primary care.

Primary health care within the global context is then an integral part of the various countries' health care system. It involves the community in all aspects of care and is acceptable to those it serves, since it is compatible with its political and social structures. Although primary health care forms the first point of contact for the individual with the health care system, the qualification of the worker varies with the specific country or community involved.

Secondary and tertiary health care

Just as primary health care forms the first point of contact for the individual in health care provision, so secondary care forms the second stage of that contact and tertiary the third. As previously identified, definitions on tertiary care are less readily available than those for primary and secondary care. Stephen (1980) suggests that tertiary care consists of the 'superspecialist' hospital or department within a general hospital. The definition provided by WHO (1988) seems to support this description. This clearly refers to countries where primary health care includes medical consultation. As with primary health care, the personnel involved and the nature of the care in both secondary and tertiary levels of care will vary with the geographical and national setting.

In developed countries, secondary care generally equates to the definition provided by the WHO (Hogarth, 1975), with care being more complex and sophisticated than could be handled by the General Practitioner. Secondary care in such systems consists of referral to a consultant within a specialized field, based within a hospital setting, although the initial contact may be at a clinic within the community setting. The secondary level of care will be more specialized, hospital based and generally more costly to provide. Tertiary care in such settings will consist of such highly specialized fields as high-dependency transplantation units and specialist oncology units. In such settings, patients following consultations in primary health care have been referred to hospital-based consultants for more specialized advice. Those secondary carers have then requested the care of the more specialized tertiary providers.

In many of the less developed countries of the world, primary health care will have been given by workers with minimal training, so that secondary health care consists of consultations with doctors and nurses. Although a different system, it should not be assumed that the care is necessarily of a lower standard than in the more developed countries, particularly due to the value placed on the local knowledge of the worker and the possibility that his/her advice may be more acceptable to the patient and thus more likely to be adhered to. Therefore, in such countries the secondary care may be the first contact they have with the professionally qualified doctor or nurse, demonstrating that the content of the secondary care may vary with the setting. This will also be reflected in any tertiary care available, where the hospital provision and the facilities available generally reflect the economic conditions in the country. Highly specialized units, such as those available in the more developed countries, may not be available or may only be available within main centres which are not easily accessible to the majority of the population.

There are, however, several features about the secondary and tertiary care which reflect that provided in the more developed countries. The care will be more sophisticated than that available within the primary care setting. It will be more specialized, hospital or clinic based and will be more costly to provide. The expense of providing secondary care has contributed to a large extent to the development of improved primary care. The inequality in provision of and access to tertiary care serves as one example of the inequalities in health which the policy of 'Health for All by the Year 2000' seeks to overcome. Indeed, the use of limited resources to benefit the majority underpins the 'Health for All' philosophy (WHO, 1978). However, to function effectively, all sectors within the health care system must co-operate (WHO, 1991). Indeed, cost-effective primary health care is now high on the political agenda of many countries (WHO, 1993) and through effective implementation of this approach many populations of the world can be helped towards achieving basic health needs by the year 2000.

● The national perspective

In the UK, a major influence on the levels of care resulted from the introduction of the National Health Act 1946 which provided a free national health system offering both curative and rehabilitative services. Although the National Health Service has evolved over time in response to the changing health needs of patients, the most significant reforms occurred as a result of the White Paper *Working for Patients* (DoH, 1989). These reforms were necessary because of escalating health care costs. Indeed, Fry (1986) argues that 'expenditure on health services everywhere has assumed rates of infinite growth'. He goes on to highlight that ' "wants" of services by patients and of facilities by doctors are always going to be greater than "needs" as calculated by planners and administrators, and these will always exceed the resources that are available'.

Although this dilemma of balancing wants with needs is unlikely to be completely resolved by the health care reforms, it has contributed to the shift of emphasis from secondary to primary health care described in Chapter 4. This shift in policy has led the government to adopt the WHO principles of setting health targets which reflect the emphasis on prevention and promotion of health. The following discussion considers the levels of care within the reformed British health care system. The levels will be discussed individually and then the interface between them will be examined.

Primary health care

Primary health care, as discussed earlier, is the 'first point of contact' for patients seeking health care. This should not be confused with the term 'community care', which resulted from the National Health Service and Community Care Act 1990 and is the process by which people are assisted to live in the community. In community care an assessment is carried out, generally by social services, to identify the needs of the individual and to organize an appropriate package of care. Although health care professionals, in particular community health care nurses, have a valuable role to play within community care, it is a complex process and a more detailed discussion of the implications of community care in the context of case management is given in Chapter 30.

Primary health care therefore consists of many services including general medical practice, well-women and family planning clinics, occupational health, nurses (of which there are now eight different community specialties (UKCC, 1994)), physiotherapy, speech therapy, chiropody, dental, accident and emergency departments within community settings. This is a wider remit than first envisaged in the original definition which equated with primary medical care.

Although many health care professionals are involved in the delivery of primary health care, the General Practitioner is seen as the 'gate-keeper' to other services. Approximately 97% of the population are registered with a GP (Haines and Iliffe, 1992). General practitioners are independent contractors who provide care to people living within an identified area of the practice setting. The system of primary health care in the UK, with a named GP providing 24-hour medical care for the population and acting as gate-keeper for secondary and tertiary care is unusual compared to health care systems in other countries (Haines and Iliffe, 1992). It is argued that this controlled access system has contributed to the cost-effectiveness of health care within the UK and is being considered, and in some cases adopted, by other countries (Horder, 1986).

Care is normally delivered by members of the primary health care team. Membership of the team can vary but includes medical, nursing, paramedical staff and administrative personnel (Fry and Hasler, 1986; Naidoo and Wills, 1994). Core membership usually comprises the general practitioner, practice nurse, district nurse and health visitor. Pritchard (1995) advises that the primary health care team is in the unique position of being able to co-ordinate a variety of services for patients and also can act as an informational resource for clients so that they can acquire knowledge of local services. Members bring to the team a broad range of knowledge, skills and expertise. Within the nursing team there will usually be different grades and disciplines of staff who work together with a team leader. Although the wider role of nurses within the team is discussed later in this chapter, there are also implications for nurses within the team since the introduction of GP fundholding. These are discussed in more detail in Chapter 8.

Secondary health care

Secondary health care within the UK is usually seen as 'hospital-based services', reflecting the WHO definition described earlier. These services may be provided by a variety of 'providers' including directly managed units (DMUs), which are under the direct control of health boards/authorities, NHS Trust hospitals (independently managed hospitals) and private hospitals. The majority of referrals for secondary health care come from GPs (Haines and Iliffe, 1992).

The pattern of secondary health care has changed considerably over the past decade, with patients spending much shorter periods in hospital. Many different factors have contributed to this, including developments in medical technology and significant advances in pharmacology. The evolution of day surgery for many minor and intermediate surgical procedures has occurred as a result of changes in clinical practice, technological developments and financial pressures (Audit Commission, 1990). Likewise many chemotherapy treatments and medical investigations can now be carried out within outpatient departments. Other examples of secondary health care offered on an non-admission basis include day hospital provision for the elderly and mentally ill, physiotherapy, dietetic and speech therapy. Treatment advances in the field of psychiatry as well as the implementation of community care legislation have also seen fewer long-term admissions to hospital care. This pattern of care is being actively encouraged by current government policy as these developments contribute to cost-effective health care and reduced waiting times for patients. However, the reduction of in-patient stay within secondary care facilities means that resources will have to be redirected to primary health care in order that patients and carers can be appropriately supported and cared for in the community.

Tertiary health care

The lack of clarity of the definition of tertiary care has led to frequent confusion over its true meaning. The WHO (1988) reinforces its original definition of tertiary care, stating that it comprises services with very specialist characteristics which require highly trained personnel and complex technology. The USA is an example of a country which has invested heavily in this level of health care. The UK, to a lesser extent, provides tertiary health care which includes intensive care, renal care, cardiothoracic and oncology care. One area of concern has been that the development of so many 'specialist' services has blurred the boundary between secondary and tertiary care, making the definition of tertiary care less clear. The WHO (1988) also highlight that this level of care is often the most costly and that 'the investment in tertiary services, as compared with that in primary care, has been excessive'. However, tertiary care in the UK also provides and seeks to develop continuing care and rehabilitative services, which presents a much broader definition of tertiary care. This interpretation demonstrates the interdependent nature of the three levels of health care, since frequently primary health care services contribute to the provision of tertiary care in the form of rehabilitation and palliative care.

The interface between primary, secondary and tertiary health care
The majority of patients remain in the care of primary health care. According to Fry and Hasler (1986), in any one year 65% of the population will consult their GP, 20% will attend an accident and emergency department and only 12% of the population will require admission to either secondary or tertiary care. More up-to-date figures are required to identify the consultation rate with other members of the primary health care team such as practice nurses. Following admission to secondary or tertiary levels of care, most patients will return to the care of the primary health care team. This constant movement of people between these different levels of care has the potential for care to become fragmented; thus good communication networks are necessary to ensure continuity of care. Indeed, the policy document *Working for Patients* (DoH, 1989) emphasized the need for practitioners to prepare patients adequately for discharge from secondary and tertiary care. It is important to note that the term discharge is no longer the preferred option as it creates the impression of cessation of care. The term patient transfer has been introduced to reflect the philosophy of continuity and seamless care.

Although specific information on patient transfer is not provided in the White Paper, implicit in the reforms is the need for improved communication between all professionals for the benefit of patients. This interface is no longer specific to practitioners within the NHS, but also to other agencies such as the private and voluntary care sectors. Practitioners are also being encouraged to devise and utilize formalized written transfer forms. With the increased use of information technology, including fax machines, the transfer of information between different levels of health care should be easier to achieve. Another future consideration is the use of patient-held records which can be shared by practitioners working in the different levels of nursing care. This would significantly assist in the sharing of patient information. The use of patient-held records is one example of the implementation of this approach to care. The Access to Medical Health Records Act 1990 has facilitated this approach, as it has enabled patients generally to have access to their health records.

Prevention
Whereas clear statements of definition of primary, secondary and tertiary care are relatively rare in the context of health care, a rather

different picture is presented within the context of prevention. Caplan's work in the 1960s, in the field of mental health education, was important in the development of the concept of primary, secondary and tertiary prevention (Caplan, 1964). However, Tannahill (cited in Downie *et al.*, 1990) suggests that the range of definitions available in the literature not only demonstrates the lack of standardization among definitions of the three levels of practice, but also significant differences in the concepts identified within these definitions. He goes on to suggest that definitions either implicitly or explicitly relate to the treatment of ill-health rather than promoting health. An example of this focus is demonstrated in the definitions provided by Tones *et al.* (1990) which describe primary prevention concerned with prevention of the onset of disease and reduction in incidence, secondary concerned with preventing the development of existing disease and tertiary concerned with the prevention of deterioration, relapse and complications. Although these definitions are described in the context of the preventive model of health education, which the authors quite rightly criticize as not being an approach to health education, it highlights the complexity of defining levels of prevention in an era where much greater emphasis is placed on the promotion of health than prevention of disease.

Primary prevention

Indeed, the definition of primary prevention provided by authors such as Ashton and Seymour (1988), Butler (1989) and Davies (1991) supports that provided by Tones *et al* (1990), describing it as preventing the occurrence of disease. Immunization programmes are now well established as primary prevention strategies, seeking to prevent the occurrence of disease by stimulating the body's immune system. The low levels of disease notification and absence of deaths from measles and pertussis confirm the efficacy of this primary preventive strategy (DoH, 1992). Many community health care nurses, such as district nurses, health visitors and occupational health nurses, play an important role in immunization programmes. The addition of fluoride to toothpaste, and in some areas to water, serves as another familiar example of primary prevention. The benefits of this strategy are most significant during childhood, in the prevention of dental caries (Jacobson *et al.*, 1991).

Once again, a range of practitioners is involved in promoting dental health. The potential influence of local government through public policy can also be seen in this setting (Naidoo and Wills, 1994), providing an important illustration of how primary prevention can be seen outside the context of merely preventing ill health. In addition, promoting healthy lifestyles and changing behaviours known to be associated with specific risk factors are also important strategies in primary prevention.

Secondary prevention

Secondary prevention seeks to reduce the prevalence of disease and shorten the course of illness (Hall *et al.*, 1990; Holland and Stewart, 1990; Hall, 1991). Methods used to achieve this include early diagnosis and prompt effective intervention and treatment. Screening of people thought to be at risk of disease but who are as yet symptom free is an important strategy used in secondary prevention. Hall (1991) discusses the surveillance of children by screening to detect disease; in particular, issues in the efficacy of this process. Indeed, Holland and Stewart (1990) discuss issues in the efficacy of screening in some detail, in particular the problem of screening programmes being introduced before 'comprehensive and respectable assessment of the benefit is available'. However, with the emphasis placed on screening in the current climate of primary health care practice, nurses and general practitioners generally are involved in screening programmes. Cervical screening programmes using Papanicolaou smears are, however, a good example of an initiative that has clearly demonstrated benefits in reducing mortality and morbidity rates in cervical cancer (Edlin and Golanty, 1992).

Tertiary prevention

Tertiary prevention aims to minimize the effects of the disease for both the individual and society, and also to promote rehabilitation and adaptation to terminal conditions (Kendall, 1989; Downie *et al.*, 1990). The prevention of complications associated with specific conditions and the minimizing of any deformity would be included within tertiary preventive strategies. Educating patients to comply with medication, a frequent task for community psychiatric nurses and district nurses, may be one way to minimize the effects of disease (Ross, 1988). Radley (1994) suggests that coronary bypass surgery may be seen as a tertiary prevention as it 'reduces the progress of an already established disease'. Ashton and Seymour (1988) also argue, in those situations where death is inevitable, that terminal care of a high standard may be interpreted as a form of tertiary prevention.

The similarity between tertiary care and tertiary prevention becomes clear when such examples are considered. Tertiary care may be seen to offer tertiary prevention in that this third 'level' of care provides the services which act as the preventive measure. Rehabilitation is another example of tertiary care and prevention. Such services are offered to individuals who have been through primary and secondary care services with the intention of minimizing the effects of the established disease. The confusion between the boundaries of care and prevention at the tertiary level may have contributed to the lack of specific definitions within existing literature.

Prevention can thus be described as occurring at primary, secondary or tertiary levels, in a similar way to care. Community health care nurses will be involved in prevention at varying stages and levels. Advice about the adverse effects of cigarette smoking is undertaken by many nurses within their practice setting, whether at school, a surgery, a clinic or the home. This constitutes primary prevention where it prevents the client taking up the habit. When a client who does smoke is encouraged to stop because of evidence of early respiratory problems, this could be described as secondary prevention. The client with established and irreversible respiratory disease who is taught to manage their own medication and care will also be encouraged to stop smoking as part of the tertiary prevention, seeking to minimize further deterioration.

● Implications for community health care nurses

The role of the nurse within primary health care is both challenging and dynamic and must be responsive to the key philosophy of providing a service which is acceptable, accessible, equitable, cost-effective and encourages partnership with service users. Community health care nursing has undergone significant change as a result of the Cumberlege Report (Cumberlege, 1986) and more recently in response to the NHS reforms and the NHS and Community Care Act. The role of the community health care nurse caseload manager/team leader in the 1990s incorporates clinical expertise, management and research. Indeed, a recent report acknowledging the valuable contribution of nurses in primary health care (NHSME, 1993) advised that in the future the role may change in respect of responsibilities and client caseloads. Bryar (1994) has suggested that nurses practising in the community may develop their role to that of the 'nurse practitioner' or 'public health nurse'. The 'nurse practitioner' role is seen as autonomous in that the practitioner is accountable for health assessment and initiation of treatments for specified patients, whereas the public health nurse role focuses on the assessment of health needs within a population rather than working with individual clients. Both these roles demonstrate how the experienced community health care nurse may develop his/her professional expertise.

Community health care nurses are involved in providing the range of services advocated by the WHO and described as promotive, preventive, curative and rehabilitative. The degree to which any one practitioner contributes to these individual services will vary according to their specialist skills. While the district nurse and community psychiatric nurse may have a major role in both curative and rehabilitative care of patients with physical or mental health problems, they will also have input into promotive and preventive care with both patients and carers. A study by Minghella (1989) evaluated a specialist community psychiatric service for parasuicide clients attending an Accident and Emergency following a self-harm incident. The findings demonstrated that the CPN service was as safe and efficient as the traditional service offered for this client group. The study also highlighted an important way in which nurses can provide the vital link between primary, secondary and tertiary care. In addition, nurse prescribing is becoming a reality for selected practitioners in community health care nursing. Emmerson (1994) has demonstrated how multidisciplinary working between the community pharmacist, district nurse, nurse practitioner and NHS Trust has resulted in the development of a service for homeless men which includes selective drug prescribing.

For other practitioners, such as the school nurse, health visitor, occupational health nurse and practice nurse, the focus on health promotion and prevention is greater. In addition, Sines (1993) has identified the importance of health promotion activities among clients with learning disabilities. Community health care nurses working with this group in the future will see their role developing more fully in this aspect of care. Within the literature there is ample evidence of community nurses developing innovative activities in health promotion. Newton-Livens and Brown (1994) describe how an occupational health service developed a workplace exercise programme to meet the specific needs of health workers within the NHS Trust. Working with other agencies was a central theme of an education programme set up by a practice nurse to educate teachers on childhood asthma (Edwards, 1994). A collaborative venture between a health visitor, dietitian and members of an Asian community resulted in the development of a successful health promotion initiative aimed at coronary heart disease prevention among Asian women (Redmond, 1993). These are just some examples of how community health care nurses are developing innovative practices in response to health needs within the population.

● Conclusion

Health care has undergone significant changes in response to changing cultural, political and social influences. Levels of health care and levels of prevention are now interwoven in both legislation and service provision. This chapter has shown how boundaries between health care levels are less rigid, thus facilitating greater flexibility across services. It has also highlighted that all levels of prevention are now recognized as being an essential part of modern health care systems. Within the UK, the role of the community health care nurse has evolved in tandem with the developing health care system. The government is now beginning to acknowledge the contribution of practitioners in the development, implementation and evaluation of promotive, preventive, curative and rehabilitative health care services. The participation of community health care nurses in primary, secondary and tertiary levels of care and prevention is therefore essential for the ongoing development of those services.

References

Ashton, J. and Seymour, H. (1988) *The New Public Health*, OU Press, Milton Keynes

Audit Commission (1990). *A Short Cut to Better Services – Day Surgery in England and Wales*, HMSO, London

Bastien, J. (1994). Collaboration of doctors and nurses with ethnomedical practitioners. *WHO Health Forum*, **15**, 133–137

Bryar, R. (1994) An examination of the need for new nursing roles in primary health care. *Journal of Interprofessional Care*, **8**, 73–84

Butler, J. (1989). *Child Surveillance in Primary Care*, HMSO, London

Caplan, G. (1964) *Principles for Preventive Psychiatry*, Tavistock Publications, London

Cumberlege, J. (1986) *Neighbourhood Nursing – A Focus for Change*, HMSO, London

Davies, B.M. (1991) *Community Health and Social Services*, 5th edn, Edward Arnold, London

DoH (1989) *Working for Patients*, HMSO, London
DoH (1992) *Immunisation Against Infectious Disease*, HMSO, London
Downie, R.S., Fyfe, C. and Tannahill, A. (1990) *Health Promotion, Models and Values*, Oxford University Press, Oxford
Edlin, G. and Golanty, E. (1992). *Health and Wellness*, 4th edn, Jones and Bartlett, London
Edwards, M. (1994). Educating schools about asthma. *Community Outlook*, **4**(5), 28–29
Emmerson, P. (1994) Get in on the act. *Community Outlook*, **4**(10), 15–20
Fry, J. (1986) Economics, politics and society. In *Primary Health Care 2000* (eds J. Fry and J. Hasler), Churchill Livingstone, New York
Fry, J. and Hasler, J.C. (eds) (1986) *Primary Health Care 2000*, Churchill Livingstone, New York
Haines, A. and Iliffe, S. (1992). *Primary Health Care in Beck et al 'In the Best of Health'*, Chapman and Hall, London
Hall, D.M.B. (1991) *Health for All children*, Oxford University Press, Oxford
Hall, D.M.B., Hill, P. and Elliman, D. (1990). *The Child Surveillance Handbook*, Radcliffe Medical Press Ltd, Oxford
Hogarth, J. (1975). *Glossary of Health Care Terminology*, WHO Regional Office for Europe, Copenhagen
Holland, W. and Stewart, S. (1990) *Screening in Health Care: Benefit or Bane?* Nuffield Provincial Hospital Trust, London
Horder, J. (1986) Primary health care. In *Primary Health Care 2000* (eds J. Fry and J.C. Hasler), Churchill Livingstone, New York
Jacobson, B., Smith, A. and Whitehead, M. (1991) *The Nation's Health: A Strategy for the 1990s*, 2nd edn, King's Fund Centre, London
Kendall, S. (1989) Maintaining health. In *New Practice and Health Care* (eds S. Hinchliff, S. Norman and J. Scholer), Edward Arnold, London
Minghella, E. (1989) The role of the nurse in the management of parasuicide in the community. In *Directions in Nursing Research* (eds J. Wilson-Barnett and S. Robinson), Scutari Press, London
Naidoo, J. and Wills, J. (1994). *Health Promotion Foundations for Practice*, Baillière-Tindall, London
Newton-Livens, M. and Brown, P. (1994). Fine-tuning at health promotion to local needs. *Occupational Health*, **46**(7), 240–243
NIISME (1993). *New World, New Opportunities*, Department of Health, London
Nugroho, G. Chen, P.C.Y. and Phua, K.H. (1986) Examples of primary health care. In *Textbook of Community Medicine in South East Asia* (eds W.O. Phoon and P.C.Y. Chen), Wiley, Singapore
Payne, P. (1993). Livelihood and survival: a case study of Bangladesh. In *World Health and Disease* (eds A. Gary and P. Payne), Open University Press, Buckingham
Pritchard, P. (1995). Learning to work effectively in teams. In *Interprofessional Issues in Community and Primary Health Care* (eds P. Owens, J. Carrier and J. Horder), Macmillan, London
Radley, A. (1994) *Making Sense of Illness*, Sage, London
RCN (1992) *Powerhouse for Change*, Royal College of Nursing, London
Redmond, E. (1993). Reaching out to the Asian community. *Community Outlook*, **3**(7), 13–16
Ross, F. (1988) Information sharing between patients, nurses and doctors: evaluation of a drug guide for old people in primary health care. *Recent Advances in Nursing* **21**, 159–185
Sines, D. (1993) Promoting health for people with learning disabilities. In *Health Promotion Concepts and Practice* (eds A. Dines and A. Cribb), Blackwell Scientific, London

Stephen, J. (1980). Systems of primary health care. In *Primary Care* (ed. J. Fry), Heinemann, London

Tones, K., Tuford, S. and Robinson, Y. (1990) *Health Education Effectiveness and Efficiency*, Chapman and Hall, London

UKCC (1994) Registrar's Letter CMc/MJW/PG/2/boc, UKCC, London

WHO (1978) *Alma-Ata 1978: Primary Health Care*, World Health Organisation, Geneva

WHO (1983) *Primary Health Care – The Chinese Experiences*, Report on an Inter-regional Seminar, World Health Organisation, Geneva

WHO (1988). *Strengthening Ministers of Health for Primary Health Care*, World Health Organisation, Geneva

WHO (1991). *Primary Health Care Development in Southern Europe*, Report on the 4th WHO Forum, World Health Organisation, Geneva

WHO (1993) *Reforms in Family Medicine or General Practice in the Countries of Central and Eastern Europe*, Report on a WHO meeting, World Health Organisation, Geneva

Part III

Research and using research to develop practice

The role that research and researched-based practice plays in high-quality patient and client care has been recognized for some time both in government reports and the nursing profession (DHSS, 1972; UKCC, 1986). A number of accounts have described the development of nursing research activity in the UK (Goodman, 1989; Lelean and Clark, 1990). These accounts recognize the significance of a series of events in catalysing and facilitating the growth of research activity in nursing. Such events include the publication of a number of government reports recommending research-based practice (DHSS, 1972; DoH, 1989), the growth of educational programmes aimed at developing research skills among practising nurses and the establishment of resource centres for nursing research, including nursing research units attached to academic departments. The more recent setting up of the Taskforce on the Strategy for Research in Nursing, Midwifery and Health Visiting (DoH, 1993) highlights the increasing significance placed on this approach to practice within the government's agenda. The response to the Taskforce from the profession has demonstrated an acknowledgement of the contribution of research to practice by many practitioners, managers and professional organizations. Indeed, the recommendations of the Taskforce also recognize the constraints of the current health care system as well as the education and training of nurses in facilitating research (DoH, 1993).

There remain practitioners who are sceptical not only about the relationship of research to practice, but also about the implementation of findings in practice. Although this situation is not unique to community health care nursing, it is perhaps more apparent than in the acute sector where greater emphasis has been given to the contribution of research over a longer period of time. In part, this situation may have occurred because there is less opportunity for research in the community. Two factors may have contributed to this situation: first, constraints in the implementation of research studies and, secondly, the relative professional isolation of many practitioners.

The development of Nursing Development Units (NDUs) provides a good example of the first factor. NDUs have been well established in the acute sector for many years. However, this development in practice is a relatively recent phenomenon in the community (Boyd *et al.*, 1993). Secondly, the relative professional isolation of many practitioners in the community has contributed to the difficulty of sharing new research-based knowledge and ideas for the implementation of research.

This part of the book provides readers with the opportunity to think about the use of research in community health care nursing. Chapter 11 provides readers with an understanding of the issues involved in the research process and in Chapter 12 the author discusses the issues involved in the implementation of research findings in practice. The significance of practitioners critically evaluating research findings and the implications for practice are considered. In addition, an understanding of the research process is provided for those readers who are interested in developing skills in implementing research. Community research studies are used to illustrate the points raised by the authors, and to some extent the research they have selected reflects their different but complementary professional backgrounds. In this way, as in other parts of the book, the different professional needs of readers are acknowledged. However, there are many principles of practice and research which are common to all practitioners working in the community and these provide the focus for the discussion in the following chapters.

References

Boyd, M., Brummell, K., Billingham, K. and Perkins, E. (1993) *The Public Health Post at Strelley: an Interin Report*, Nottingham Community Health NHS Trust, Nottingham

DoH (1989) *A Strategy for Nursing: Report of the Steering Committee*, HMSO, London

DoH (1993) *Report of the Taskforce on the Strategy for Research in Nursing, Midwifery and Health Visting*, Department of Health, London

DHSS (1972) *Report of the Committee on Nursing* (Chairman Sir Asa Briggs), HMSO, London

Goodman, C. (1989) Nursing research: growth and development. In *Current Issues in Nursing* (eds M. Jolley and P. Allen), Chapman and Hall, London

Lelean, S.R and Clark, M. (1990) Research resource development in the United Kingdom. *International Journal of Nursing Studies*, **17**(2), 123–138

UKCC (1986) *Project 2000: A New Preparation for Practice*, UKCC, London

11

Understanding, use and conduct of research

Sue Davies

● **Introduction**

Skilled and effective community nursing practice requires that practitioners are able to retrieve, interpret and apply research findings appropriately. In line with the Code of Professional Conduct (UKCC, 1992), it also requires community nurses to identify appropriate questions for research relevant to their sphere of work. Additionally, some practitioners should possess the skills to plan and carry out research which will contribute to the knowledge base for community nursing practice.

Recent developments, affecting both practice and education, require community nurses to be more research aware than ever before. Particularly within the current climate of an internal market in health care, community nurses must be able to demonstrate the outcomes of their practice and this requires research skills. Recent changes in government policy affecting the delivery of community health nursing services have tended towards piecemeal introduction, with limited trial or pilot evaluation (for example, the NHS and Community Care Act (DoH, 1990) and the new GP contract (DoH, 1989)): it falls then to service providers and researcher colleagues to produce systematic evidence on the effects of change for both the receivers and providers of the service. This also requires research skills.

Changes in the pre- and post-registration education for community nursing have resulted in an increased emphasis on identifying and developing the research base to practice (UKCC, 1986, 1990, 1993). It is therefore essential that community nurses with responsibility for teaching and supervising students are themselves competent in the evaluation and synthesis of research reports.

While this chapter will not seek to provide practitioners with all the requisite skills to undertake empirical research, it will aim to promote the beginnings of research awareness by providing an overview of research processes and motivating the reader to further study.

● Definitions of research

There are numerous attempts within the literature to define research and a selection is reproduced here:

Research in its broadest sense is an attempt to gain solutions to problems. More precisely, it is the collection of data in a rigorously controlled situation for the purpose of prediction or explanation.

(Treece and Treece, 1986)

Multiple, systematic strategies to generate knowledge about human behavior, human experience and human environments in which the thought and action process of the researcher are clearly specified so that they are logical, understandable, confirmable and useful.

(Depoy and Gitlin, 1993)

An attempt to increase available knowledge by the discovery of new factors or relationships through systematic enquiry.

(Macleod, Clark and Hockey, 1989)

Systematic inquiry that uses orderly scientific methods to answer questions or solve problems.

(Polit and Hungler, 1991)

A number of ideas recur repeatedly within these definitions; for example, the suggestions that research is a sytematic process and that it creates new knowledge. Gilbert (1993) proposes that good research concerns itself with regularities which transcend time and place. In other words, the knowledge generated through research is systematically organized into general laws and theories which can be used to describe, explain and predict events of interest and relevance (to nursing practice).

Research and theory

Theory has been defined by Seaman as:

a statement that explains the interrelationships among propositions, concepts or observations; summarises what is known from past work and predicts what will be found on future observation.

(Seaman, 1987)

In more general terms, a theory represents a set of assumptions that are put forward to explain events in the real world. It represents a summary of existing knowledge in relation to a particular phenomenon. Research which develops the knowledge base for nursing practice is inevitably linked to theory – distinguishing it from activities such as nursing audit which may use the methods of research but do not contribute to theory development. There are two broad processes connecting research and theory: inductive reasoning or *induction* and deductive reasoning or *deduction*. Induction involves developing generalizations and explanations of phenomena from observation of events in the real world. Categories and concepts emerge from the analysis of empirical observation and theoretical propositions are generated. Deduction, on the other hand, involves testing theory by gathering data in the real world and examining it to see if it fits. The theory is then modified accordingly.

Some examples might help to illustrate these two approaches. Chalmers (1992), for example, used conversational interviews with 45 health visitors to begin to develop a theory about how health visitors work with clients in the community during their day-to-day health visiting practice. Using a grounded theory approach, in which categories and themes are developed from the data (Glaser and Strauss, 1967; Strauss, 1987), Chalmers identified a number of processes occurring within health-visitor/client interactions, which converged into a unified theme of 'giving and receiving.' By a process of induction, Chalmers has developed the beginnings of a framework which health visitors can use to reflect upon what they offer and receive from clients during the course of their health visiting practice.

In comparison, Clarke and Khadom (1988) used the process of deductive reasoning to examine differences between the prevention of pressure sores in hospital and community settings. Research has generated a great deal of information about the prevention of pressure sores and the aim of the research was to test whether this knowledge applied equally in community settings as in hospital settings. Using structured research tools, data were collected from hospital nurses and from relatives and nurses in the community who were asked to record pressure area care as it was given onto diary sheets. The researcher also collected data about the patient's appetite, Norton score (Norton *et al.*, 1975), age, sex and diagnosis. The outcome measure was whether or not the patient developed a pressure sore. Findings confirmed that the amount of nursing care devoted to the prevention of pressure sores is significantly related to outcome and also demonstrated that a higher percentage of the hospital patients developed pressure sores than the community patients studied. Although the small sample size is a limitation of the study, it contributes to a confirmation of theoretical knowledge about the most effective prevention of pressure sores.

It is important to recognize also that induction and deduction are not completely separate and may form part of the same research cycle (Figure 11.1). Data gathered through empirical observation can be used to generate theoretical propositions (induction) which can then be developed and tested to see if they fit with empirical observation (deduction). In this way the theory is strengthened and affirmed.

● **Paradigms in nursing research**

In developing and testing nursing theory, research draws upon two broad research traditions or paradigms: positivism and naturalism (or interpretivism). Frequently, the terms quantitative and qualitative research are used to distinguish these approaches. However, these terms imply an emphasis on the methods used to collect data rather than suggesting differences in the basic assumptions underpinning the research process (Bryman, 1984). These assumptions are discussed more fully in Chapter 12.

INDUCTIVE   DEDUCTIVE

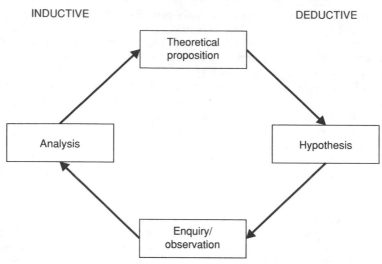

Figure 11.1   Inductive and deductive approaches

The relationship between the two paradigms is the subject of much debate both within nursing circles and within the wider field of social research. Tripp-Reimer (1985), for example, argues that qualitative and quantitative approaches may provide complementary data sets which together give a more complete picture than can be obtained using either approach singly. Goodman (1989) also argues that quantitative and qualitative research approaches lie along a continuum and do not occupy opposing camps. However, others argue against this view on the basis that the two approaches reflect divergent philosophies and are therefore contradictory and mutually exclusive (Moccia, 1988). For a fuller discussion see Bryman (1988), Duffy (1985) and Corner (1991).

The debate is set to continue and, for the moment, examples of both research traditions are to be found in the nursing literature together with an increasing number of studies employing a combination of research perspectives. This approach of combining research methods has been termed triangulation (Denzin, 1978). However, the problems of combining data gathered from diverse methods have also been discussed (Fielding and Fielding, 1986). These include the possibility of increasing the chance of error by using multiple methods and the problem of making valid inferences between different sets of data.

● **The research process**

An overview

Research comprises a series of steps or stages which are usually undertaken in a logical order but which frequently overlap. The initial step in the process is problem identification and most nursing research proceeds from the recognition of something which is a problem for practice, education or management. A review of existing literature and information allows the problem to be refined and focused to a manageable proportion and, at this stage, research aims and questions can be more precisely stated. Depending upon the nature of the research problem and the existing level of knowledge in relation to the topic, it may be appropriate to develop a hypothesis, which is a statement about the predicted relationship between the variables to be studied. The researcher then sets out to test the hypothesis by gathering evidence which will either support or refute the statement.

The next stage in the process is to design an empirical study which will meet the aims of the research, answer the research questions or test the hypothesis or hypotheses. The research design provides a blueprint for action and will incorporate aspects such as the broad approach to be used, the research setting, subjects and sample, methods for data collection and analysis, together with plans for gaining access to the setting and managing ethical considerations. Most researchers will then carry out a pilot study, rather like a practice of the main study, which allows them to test out research instruments and rehearse the logistics of data collection. Necessary adjustments can then be made and the main study can proceed. Final steps in the process will require analysis, interpretation and discussion of the findings and preparation of a full report for dissemination.

In drawing conclusions from a study, most researchers identify new problems and questions for further research, leading Couchman and Dawson (1990) to describe the research process as a cycle (Figure 11.2). In this way, research builds upon existing work to create new knowledge for nursing practice. It is important to recognize that the discrete stages within the cycle do not always proceed in a consistent order. As

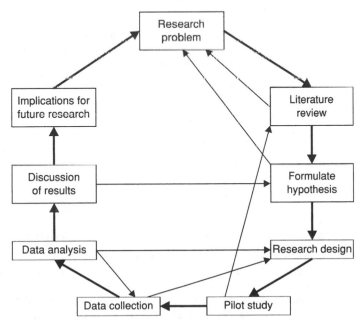

Figure 11.2 The research cycle (After Couchman and Dawson, 1990)

illustrated in Figure 11.2, it is often necessary to return to an earlier stage in the cycle, for example to redefine research questions or to make adjustments to the study design.

Individual stages

Identifying and refining questions for research
Research questions emanate from three main sources (Clark, 1987):

- professional experience
- previous research
- existing theory.

Professional experience provides a rich source of questions for research since there are so many unsolved problems in everyday nursing practice. Community health care services – and preventive services in particular – remain largely unevaluated and in many situations there is insufficient research-based knowledge to inform decisions about practice. This situation highlights the need for further research.

Most research studies will themselves raise questions for further research and will devote a section of the research report to identifying other investigations or studies that need to be undertaken. In this way, researchers build upon existing research to expand and create new knowledge. If the process of knowledge creation has reached the level of theory, then research may be required to test whether the theory is accurate. This involves deriving a hypothesis from theory and designing an empirical study to test whether this relationship appears to exist within the real world.

Having identified a problem or question for research, the next step is to assess whether the question forms a resonable basis for a research study. Polit and Hungler (1991) suggest that there are three aspects of the question to consider in making this assessment:

1. How *significant* is the problem?
   Will the study findings have wide applicability?
   Will they have ultimate implications for patient care?
2. Is the problem *researchable*?
   Some questions of an ethical or moral nature are simply not amenable to study through empirical methods since the answers lie within individual beliefs, values and opinions.
3. Is the proposed study *feasible*?
   Will it be possible to gain access to research subjects?
   Will they be willing to participate?
   Are the resources needed to undertake the study available?

Having decided that the problem is researchable, research questions or aims need to be refined and stated very precisely (Valiga and Mermel, 1985). If the researcher is using a positivist approach, the concepts or variables to be studied must be operationally defined. For example, how will 'stress' be observed? How will 'satisfaction' be measured? Although in a naturalist approach the researcher will generally allow the precise definition of concepts to emerge from the data, it is important that at the beginning of the study the researcher clarifies the interpretation of terms used in the study. Decisions about the adopted research approach and the most appropriate definition of variables, if relevant, will usually be made once the researcher has consulted the literature available on the topic.

Searching the literature

The purposes of the literature review as a step in the research process have been succinctly summarized by Couchman and Dawson (1990).

- to find out what other research has already been conducted on the topic or related topics
- to give ideas on the research design and methodology and tools which could be appropriately applied
- to aid in the definition of the variables in the intended research
- to consider the theoretical framework that will underpin the study
- to put the project into the context of the broader body of knowledge in the field.

There are broadly five categories of literature which may contribute to the achievement of these objectives (Polit and Hungler, 1991):

- facts, statistics or research findings – the results of empirical investigation
- theory or interpretation
- methods and procedures
- opinions, beliefs or points of view
- anecdotes, clinical impressions or narrations of incidents and situations.

With such a range of material available, it is essential that the review of the literature is undertaken using a systematic approach. Pollock (1984), for example, suggests the use of index cards to record the reference and significant points from each piece of literature reviewed. It is also important to recognize that the review of the literature, rather than forming a discrete step in the research process, is ongoing throughout the course of the study. In particular, the researcher will move back and forth between the literature and the research topic in order to formulate research questions and/or hypotheses and to determine the most appropriate research approach and data collection methods. New information which is relevant to the objectives of the study may continue to appear throughout the progress of the research until the point of dissemination of the study findings.

It is essential that the review of the literature should seek not only to describe but to evaluate the body of information available in relation to the research topic. In this way, the literature review contributes to the development and refinement of the aims of the research, by identifying weaknesses and gaps in the knowledge base. Theoretical perspectives within the literature must also be considered in order to recognize the assumptions underpinning previous empirical work. It may be appropriate, for example, to consider a problem or research questions from a different theoretical perspective to see whether new insights can be gained. For examples of published literature reviews, readers are referred to Bergen (1991) and Kelly and May (1982).

Selecting a research approach
Within the two broad philosophical paradigms identified above, several distinctive research strategies have emerged. Lathlean (1989) suggests that it is useful to think about these individual research strategies according to where they fit on each of two polar dimensions. These are:

- the extent to which the researcher attempts to influence reality within the research setting
- the body of theory that is used to inform the research and interpret the findings – this will either be social science theory or probability theory reflecting the qualitative/quantitative continuum.

If these two dimensions are plotted as a matrix, individual research strategies could be located as shown in Figure 11.3. On one dimension, experiments and action research attempt to identify the effects which a particular change will make in a given situation. In contrast, ethnography and survey are both concerned with describing a situation as it exists and attempt to minimize the effects which the researcher has on reality. On the other dimension, experiments and surveys rely on the careful selection of a representative sample of the population under study to allow generalization and theory testing through the application of probability theory. Action research and ethnography, on the other hand,

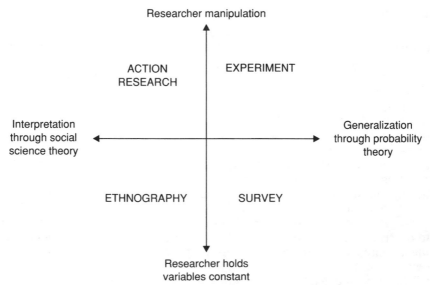

Figure 11.3   The context of individual research designs (After Lathlean, 1989)

rely on careful description of the research setting and events within it in order to generate social science theory and allow the reader to make a decision about the transferability of research findings.

The four exemplary research strategies outlined above are described in more detail below, together with an account of the methods commonly used to identify samples and collect data within each strategy. However, it is important to remember that real research rarely fits neatly within an exemplary strategy. Indeed, many researchers will use elements of more than one strategy within an individual research design.

Survey research.   This attempts to identify population parameters for specific variables. In addition, it may describe the relationship between variables for a given population. Observations are made for a representative sample of the population, allowing generalizations to be drawn.

There are three main types of survey design:

- cross-sectional
- longitudinal
- retrospective.

A cross-sectional survey collects data from all subjects at one point in time and is frequently used to study groups of subjects at various stages of development simultaneously. In comparison, longitudinal surveys collect information from the same group or cohort of subjects at different points in time. Longitudinal surveys have the advantage of controlling for individual differences between subjects but are more costly and time-consuming than cross-sectional surveys. Retrospective surveys collect information relating to subjects' previous experience and are frequently used to make inferences about cause-and-effect relationships in situations where a classical experimental design would be either impossible or ethically inappropriate.

The choice of survey design will be determined to a large extent by the aims of the research and the resources available. Bond *et al.* (1990), for example, wished to examine the knowledge and attitudes of community nurses in relation to HIV and AIDS in order to identify the need for education and support. It was therefore appropriate to undertake a cross-sectional survey of a representative sample of community nurses within the area under study. Rajan (1986), on the other hand, was interested in studying the process of weaning babies on to solid foods and used a longitudinal design to interview mothers when their babies were 6, 12 and 18 weeks old. By using this approach, she was able to describe how mothers' beliefs influenced the weaning process.

Experimental research designs.   These are appropriate when a researcher wishes to establish a cause-and-effect relationship between variables, that is, the researcher wants to demonstrate that by making a change in the independent or treatment variable, they can cause a predicted change in an identified dependent or outcome variable. Seaman (1987) identifies three essential features of a true experimental research design. There are:

- randomization
- manipulation
- control.

Randomization involves the random allocation of research subjects to either the intervention group or a control group(s), so that every subject has an equal chance of being in each group. The researcher then *manipulates* the independent or treatment variable for the intervention group and measures any effect on the dependent or outcome variable(s). Measurement of the dependent variables for both the intervention group and the control group (for whom the independent variable is not manipulated) allows the researcher to be reasonably confident that any observed changes in the intervention group are a direct consequence of changes to the independent variable. An important example of experimental research with relevance to community nursing is reported by Luker (1982). This study evaluated the effects of visits by health visitors on elderly women's health status and was one of the first studies to attempt to demonstrate the effects of health visiting practice on health.

The major limitation of experimental research designs for studying problems of relevance for community nursing is the difficulty of *controlling* all possible *extraneous* or *intervening* variables which may have an effect on the dependent variable. Ethical and logistical issues sometimes render randomization or strict control impossible, leading some researchers to conduct a *quasi-experiment*, where one or more of the essential features of a true experimental design is missing. However, in interpreting the findings of a quasi-experiment, it is important to acknowledge that the extent to which observed change in the dependent variable can be imputed to manipulation of the independent variable is limited.

Ethnography. This approach to social research has a basis in anthropology and seeks to describe and explain the culture of specific groups of people. Hammersley and Atkinson (1983) identify the main aims of the ethnographic approach to research as discovery, description and understanding. Ethnography attempts to understand social action by exploring its meaning for the main participants. Investigation takes place in natural settings and explores multiple perspectives of the topic under study.

Ethnographers use a variety of methods to collect data, but rely mainly upon participant observation and interviewing. Mackenzie (1992), for example, used a combination of observation and informal interviews to gain an understanding of the learning experiences of student district nurses in community placements. Other methods include collecting documentary and physical evidence and audio-recording of naturally occurring talk. Montgomery-Robinson (1986) examined the social organization of health visiting practice by analysing tape-recordings of health visitors interacting with mothers in their own homes.

The process of triangulation is widely used to strengthen the validity of the findings in ethnographic research (Denzin, 1978). Respondent triangulation combines the perspectives of a range of participants within the research setting, whereas methodological triangulation uses a combination of methods for collecting data in order to overcome the weaknesses inherent to each method.

Other methods for enhancing the validity of findings include 'member-checking' – feeding back results of the analysis to individual respondents to see whether the researcher's interpretation of events accords with theirs. Such an approach was used by Field (1983) in a study to explore public health nurses' perceptions of their roles.

Action research. Disillusionment with the limitations of both purely descriptive research and the artificial control of classical experimental design has led many nurse researchers to consider alternative approaches. Action research in particular is being seen increasingly by nurses as an approach which has much to offer (Webb, 1989; Titchen and Binnie, 1993; Meyer, 1993). Action research attempts to effect change in the functioning of the real world (Greenwood, 1984) with the purpose of gaining a better theoretical understanding of a social situation, in particular the part played by the researcher in initiating and managing the change (Lathlean, 1989). Nurse researchers can therefore use action research to problem-solve within a particular setting and make use of their systematic description and evaluation of the change to generate theory about how such a change might be achieved in other settings.

Action researchers frequently use a combination of research methods to gather data within a naturalistic setting. In particular, participant observation together with informal interviews are used to describe the process of change and its effects on the main participants. However, more structured tools may also be used to provide a quantifiable measure of the effects of the change introduced. A number of different roles for the researcher within action research designs have been described, characterized by the extent to which the researcher integrates within the group or culture under study (Titchen and Binnie, 1993). Few explicit examples of action research in community nursing settings have been described; however, Drennan's work, which both implemented and evaluated a new role for the health visitor in working with groups, could be described as action research (Drennan, 1990). Griffin and Speigal (1993) also employ an action research framework within a study to facilitate the effective management of diabetes within primary health care.

Identifying the appropriate research design. Brink and Wood (1988) identify three levels of research question and suggest that the most appropriate research design will be determined by the level of question. Each level is based upon the amount of existing knowledge and/or theory about the topic under study.

At the first level (level I), there is little existing knowledge either on the topic or the population and the purpose is to describe what is found as it exists naturally. Level I studies are exploratory, descriptive and take place in natural settings. An ethnographic approach or perhaps an action research design would be appropriate to study this level of question. At the second level, there is knowledge about the topic and about the population, and the researcher sets out to provide a statistical description of the relationship between variables. In this situation, a survey approach would be indicated. At the third level, there is a great deal of knowledge about the topic and the population and the researcher sets out to demonstrate cause and effect through the direct manipulation of variables. Level III questions require the testing of hypotheses by means of an experimental design. It can be seen then that the selection of the most appropriate research strategy is best determined by the research question and the existing level of knowledge in relation to that question, rather than by the researcher's own particular preferences.

Identifying a sample

The way in which a researcher identifies a sample for study will depend upon the aims of the study. Some research will require a sample which will provide the maximum theoretical understanding of the issues under study, whereas other research will be concerned with obtaining a representative sample to allow generalization to a wider population. In some cases, it is impossible to obtain a full list of members of the population to be studied and the researcher must rely upon a *convenience sample*, that is, a sample of people who are readily available and willing to participate in the research. In some cases, for example in the study of deviant groups, the researcher is forced to rely upon building up a network of contacts by word of mouth. This approach is known as *snowball sampling*.

Sampling methods can broadly be categorized into two types: *probability* sampling and *non-probability* sampling. In probability sampling, each element in a population has an equal and non-zero chance of being selected for the sample. In non-probability sampling, the chance of selection for each element in the population is unknown and for some elements may be zero. The advantage of probability sampling is that it allows the researcher to calculate the likely degree of error in extrapolating findings from the study sample to the wider population. However, probability sampling does depend upon the existence of a full list of the population (known as the sampling frame). In the absence of any such list, researchers have no option but to make use of non-probability sample. Most research within the positivist tradition will make use of a probability sample, whereas most qualitative research uses a non-probability sample since the sample is selected for the data they can provide to the researcher. Purposive sampling is an example. However, for an excellent discussion of sample design see Arber (1993).

Designing tools for data collection

Although the choice of research approach will to some extent determine the degree of structure within research instruments, the researcher still has a fairly wide choice of the methods to be used. Broadly, these methods include asking questions, either by interview or self-completion questionnaire, observation, either as a participant or a non-participant, and the use of existing documentary sources. Interview schedules for example can comprise mainly closed questions for use in a face-to-face survey, or may be semi-structured and open-ended, for use in more qualitative research designs. Observation schedules can also be highly structured in the form of a checklist, or completely open-ended as in the case of observational field-notes.

Rigour

Whatever the research approach and methods adopted, the researcher will be concerned to make the study design as rigorous as possible. The concept of rigour within empirical research comprises two main elements: validity and reliability. Validity is concerned with the extent to which the researcher is observing (or measuring) what they intend to observe (or measure). Validity can be considered in terms of external validity. This is defined as the degree to which it is possible to generalize the study findings to the wider population from which the study sample was drawn. Validity can also be considered in terms of internal validity. This is defined as the degree to which conclusions can be drawn about the causal effects of one variable on another. Reliability refers to the consistency of observation (or measurement).

Although validity and reliability are important issues within both qualitative and quantitative research designs, their achievement usually relies on different design features within the two research traditions. Researchers working within a positivist framework will rely upon control of as many extraneous variables as possible in order to maximize internal validity and upon careful selection of a representative sample to ensure external validity. The reliability of research instruments will be determined carefully during the development and piloting stage. Those carrying out research in the naturalist tradition, on the other hand, will attempt to ensure the validity of their findings by studying research subjects in their natural setting and by very careful description of events. However, issues of reliability remain important and methods such as tape-recording interviews are used to enhance the reliability of a study. Because of the explicit recognition of the influence which the researcher will have on the selection of data, the question of reliability is more complex. The reliability of coding procedures is often checked during data analysis by, for example, having two researchers code the same batch of data.

Waterman (1993) summarizes a number of methods for enhancing the rigour of qualitative research designs. These include:

- being reflexive within the research process
- triangulating research methods
- investing sufficient time in data collection to learn the culture
- undertaking negative case analysis – looking for examples which do not fit into the developing theory
- carrying out data analysis concurrently with data collection
- member-checking – feeding back the researcher's interpretation of the data to respondents to check whether it agrees with their own understanding.

There are indications that nurse researchers operating within a naturalist perspective are acknowledging the criticisms often levelled at this type of research, and are developing ways of demonstrating rigour within a research tradition which is increasingly being seen as relevant to and congruent with the goals of nursing (Sandelowski, 1986; Hinds *et al*. 1990).

Methods of data collection within a quantitative research framework

Within surveys and experiments, data collection instruments are designed to allow measurement and comparison of the variables of interest. Items are usually highly structured and the range of responses is limited and predetermined by the researcher. It is particularly important to avoid ambiguity in the wording of questions, as the researcher will have little or no opportunity to clarify the meaning of a specific question to the respondent. Other issues to be considered in questionnaire design include (Moser and Kalton, 1979; Oppenheim, 1992):

- the provision of clear instructions to the respondent
- the use of language which is easy to understand
- the avoidance of questions which rely on memory, or hypothetical and vague questions
- the avoidance of leading and presuming questions
- the ordering of questions to maintain interest
- phrasing and positioning of embarrassing questions.

The development of questionnaires and interview schedules for use within a quantitative framework requires careful pre-testing in order to establish the validity and reliability of the instrument. A frequent criticism of much nursing research is that often this rigorous testing and piloting of research instruments does not take place and validity and reliability are not established in advance of data collection. Alternatively, instruments are used with respondents who are fundamentally different from those upon which the tool was developed and tested.

Luker (1982) used a structured interview schedule known as the Neugarten Life Satisfaction Index to measure life satisfaction for elderly women who had received visits from a health visitor. However, given that the tool had been developed for use with older people living in the USA, Luker recognized the need to establish validity and reliability for the population she was about to study. She provides a useful account of how she undertook this process (Luker, 1979). Unfortunately, such detailed accounts of the methods used to determine the rigour of structured research instruments are rare within the British nursing press and the consumer of research is left to ponder their accuracy and consistency for themselves.

Methods for data collection within a qualitative framework

Two main approaches to data collection are commonly employed within qualitative research. These are participant observation and un-structured or semi-structured interviews.

Participant observation

Four role types for the participant observer have been identified (Gold, 1958; Pearsall, 1965) and these can be plotted on a continuum in relation to the extent to which participants are aware that they are being observed for the purposes of a research study (Figure 11.4). In practice, although one role type usually predominates, a researcher tends to move between roles at different stages during fieldwork. As Hilton (1987) points out, the important issue for the researcher is to maintain an awareness of his/her role and a consciousness of their social position within the research setting.

An important issue for participant observers to consider is the possible change in behaviour in the setting when the observer is present (Field and Morse, 1985). However, these effects normally diminish once the participants become used to the observer and trust is established. Another potential problem lies in the possibility that the observer, over a period of time, will assume the beliefs and values of the group being studied and will lose the capacity for objective observation. This process, termed 'going native', can be avoided if the observer takes regular breaks from the field and continually reflects upon his/her own reactions to events observed.

Interviews

Qualitative interviews differ from survey interviews in being less structured in approach and in encouraging individuals to expand on their immediate responses to questions. The process depends upon a rapport being established between the interviewer and the respondent, which will allow the person being interviewed to 'open up' about their beliefs, values and experiences. The complex nature of the interview relationship has been acknowledged, reflecting an increasing awareness of the effect which the researcher has on the data collected. Informed by feminist perspectives, some researchers are seeking to develop a more egalitarian relationship between themselves and the researched, as opposed to the detachment and control advocated in some of the more traditional texts on social research (Roberts, 1981). The presence and personality of the researcher are acknowledged as important variables and it behoves the researcher to reflect upon the nature of the interview relationship and its effect upon the data subsequently gathered. Finch, for example, discusses the trust which she was able to establish with her respondents in a sociological study of the wives of clergymen, by revealing that she too was a clergyman's wife (Finch, 1984).

An interview schedule for use within a qualitative framework

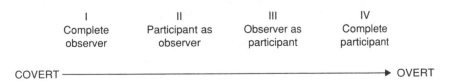

I	II	III	IV
Complete observer	Participant as observer	Observer as participant	Complete participant

COVERT ———————————————————————→ OVERT

Figure 11.4 Observational roles for fieldwork

normally acts as an aide-memoire for the interviewer and comprises a list of topics or a few key questions with areas to be explored or probed. The schedule does not normally dictate the order of questions or include all the questions that will be asked. The specific issues developed within the topics covered are likely to be different for each interview, since different respondents are likely to focus on slightly different areas. Also, the researcher's understanding of the key issues may develop as the study proceeds and new question areas may be introduced accordingly.

Methods for data collection in community nursing research

Because of the nature of community nursing practice, certain methods for collecting data lend themselves more easily to community nursing research than others. Self-completion questionnaires, for example, can reach a wide sample of respondents at little cost. Even within a small locality, district nurses, health visitors and community midwives may be spread over a wide geographical area, making face-to-face interviews time-consuming and expensive. Observation also poses particular problems for the researcher conducting research in community settings where most client contact happens in the client's own home. It is relatively easy for a non-participant observer on a hospital ward to 'merge into the background', whereas a researcher observing community nursing practice cannot help but be obvious to the main participants. The effect which this is likely to have on the behaviour of research subjects must be considered in planning the research design.

On the other hand, interviews are more often easily carried out in community settings, either in clients' homes or at a clinic or health centre. In either case, background noise levels and interruptions are likely to be less than in a busy hospital ward. Once again, it is important to acknowledge that it is the research question that plays the major role in determining the methods of data collection.

Data analysis

Whether analysing qualitative or quantitative data, the overall purpose is the same: to look for patterns in the data that will aid interpretation. However, there are also important differences in the way that different types of data will be presented and analysed (Figure 11.5).

Analysing qualitative data

In qualitative analysis, themes, concepts and hypotheses are derived from the data in order to describe phenomena through narratives and accounts as a way of understanding, explaining and making inferences (Smith, 1992). Data, usually in the form of written field notes and/or transcription of tape-recorded interviews, are repeatedly examined for evidence of recurrent issues and themes. These are coded and categories developed. A number of methods for coding and categorizing

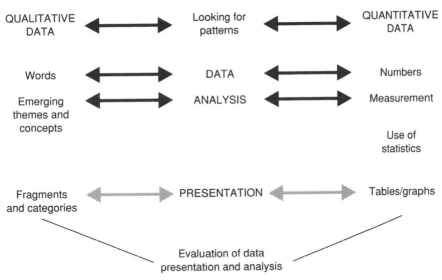

Figure 11.5   Overview of data presentation

data have been described, including highlighting text, colour coding and transferring relevant quotes onto cards representing each category (Riley, 1990). Overlap between categories frequently suggests broader categories or themes which can be used to describe the main patterns within the data. In a series of qualitative interviews with the parents of children with cystic fibrosis, Whyte (1992), for example, identified a number of themes which encompassed the main categories within the data. These included *the assault to self-image* (of the parents – the result of having a handicapped child), *difficult decisions* (about management and treatment options) and *the chronic burden of care* (in relation to the continuous nature of their situation).

White *et al.* (1993) describe the use of a data matrix to analyse semi-structured interviews as part of a qualitative study to explore the supervision of 'Project 2000' students, both in hospital wards and in community practice settings. The matrix consisted of the categories emerging from content analysis of the taped interviews down one axis and individual respondents across the other. Such an organizational approach allows easy comparison between respondent groups and between research settings. The development of computer programs such as ETHNOGRAPH and NUDIST have provided additional methods for analysing qualitative data.

The analysis of qualitative data often takes place concurrently with data collection, in that the researcher will be using their interpretation of evidence previously collected to inform their next excursion into 'the field'. In this way, ongoing analysis can sometimes determine the appropriate sample size, in that the researcher continues to select respondents until no new categories are emerging from the data. This has been referred to as theoretical saturation (Glaser and Strauss, 1967; Morse, 1991).

Analysing quantitative data

Data gathered by the use of more quantitative structured methods is generally transferred into numerical form. Statistical analysis is generally used to interpret the data, particularly where large data sets have been obtained. There are two main types of statistic: *descriptive statistics* and *inferential statistics*.

Descriptive statistics can broadly be categorized into two groups: measures of central tendency, which give a representative or average figure (e.g. mean, mode, and median), and measures of dispersion, which indicate how spread out a set of scores are (e.g. the range and standard deviation). Inferential statistics provide a measure of the likelihood that a certain set of results could have occurred by chance, rather than as a result of a true relationship between observed variables, and are based on probability theory. For example, in most circumstances an apparent relationship suggested by the study data is assumed to represent a true relationship if the findings have less than a 5% chance of having occurred as a result of random variation. A range of statistical tests is available to help the researcher to calculate this probability and the choice of test will be dependent upon features of the study design and the type of data collected, in particular the levels of measurement used. For a clear description of the process of hypothesis testing, in particular selection of the most appropriate statistical test, readers are referred to Hicks (1990) and Reid (1993).

Discussion, conclusions and recommendations

The final steps in the research process require the interpretation of the analysed data and discussion of the findings in the context of existing literature. In this final process, the researcher should discuss the weaknesses and limitations of the study. This is essential in order to allow the reader to assess the generalizability of the findings and their applicability to their own practice. The researcher should also highlight persistent gaps in the knowledge base relating to the topic under consideration and identify questions for further research. Dissemination of the research report is usually the researcher's final responsibility within the research process. However, interpretation for particular areas of practice and application is the responsibility of the reader.

● Ethical considerations

It is generally recognized that the major dilemma in any research involving human subjects is the conflict between the protection of human rights and the generation of new knowledge. The ethics of nursing research are closely tied up with the ethics of nursing practice, where the 'humanism versus science' paradox is also apparent. According to Fry, for example:

The concept of nursing embodies the scientific (competence) values of

technological skills, scientific inquiry, as well as humanistic (moral) values of caring and the promotion of individual welfare and rights.
(Fry 1981)

Nursing practice is based upon the ethic of caring which essentially involves recognizing individuality yet offering a similar level of service to all patients and clients. It is easy to recognize how this ethic might conflict with the wishes of a researcher attempting to evaluate the effectiveness of a particular nursing intervention, whose study design involves withholding this intervention from a particular group of patients or clients. A further drawback in the use of experimental research to evaluate nursing interventions is the potential to raise expectations of a service which cannot be immediately realized. Oakley (1993), for example, reports on a randomized controlled trial to evaluate the effects of midwife-provided social support for women during pregnancy. She describes the distress of both the research subjects and of the midwives providing care, when social support was withdrawn at the end of the intervention period.

Although the ethical issues involved in conducting experiments with human beings are well recognized, the ethical implications of descriptive research are less frequently acknowledged. Nevertheless, the powerful emotions which, for example, in-depth interviewing on sensitive topics can arouse in the subject require recognition and careful handling. Cowles (1988) describes vividly the emotions expressed by her respondents during qualitative interviews to explore the life experiences of the relatives of victims of murder. Several authors also describe the emergence of an almost therapeutic relationship between themselves and their respondents during data collection, particularly in the context of longitudinal studies. These possibilities must be anticipated by the researcher and plans made for suporting respondents both during and following data collection by means of appropriate referral to other agencies. Flatley, for example, in studying the relatives of patients who had suffered a stroke, found enormous areas of unmet need among her respondents. She describes her anguish at having raised expectations of services which were simply not available (Flatley, 1992).

The main guiding principles for protecting the rights of research subjects relate to the issues of informed consent, confidentiality and the duty to care. The Royal College of Nursing has produced guidelines for nurses involved in research or any study/project concerning human subjects, which considers these issues in detail (RCN, 1977). Local Research Ethics Committees also play an important role in protecting the rights and interests of both the researcher and the researched.

●   **Conclusion**

This chapter has attempted to outline the main empirical research approaches and methods used in research likely to be of relevance to nurses working in community settings. In order to be able to utilize research effectively and participate in research appropriately, nurses need to understand the processes involved in identifying topics for investigation and to have an overview of the options available when considering the most appropriate way to explore or answer a particular research question. This chapter is by no means a comprehensive account of research methodology and it is hoped that the reader may have been stimulated to further enquiry. Ultimately, it is the responsibility of each and every nurse to develop skills in retrieving, evaluating and sometimes in undertaking research – only then will community nursing practice achieve its full potential to meet the needs of the communities which it serves.

References

Arber, S. (1993) Designing samples. In *Researching Social Life* (ed. N. Gilbert), Sage, London

Bergen, A. (1991) Nurses caring for the terminally ill in the community: a review of the literature. *International Journal of Nursing Studies*, **28**(1), 89–101

Bond, S., Rhodes, T., Philips, P. and Tierney, A. (1990) HIV infection and community nursing staff in Scotland – 1. Experience, practice and education. *Nursing Times*, **86**(44), 47–50

Brink, P. and Wood, M. (1988) *Planning Nursing Research: from Question to Proposal*, Jones and Bartlett, Boston

Bryman, A. (1984) The debate about quantitative and qualitative research: a question of method or epistemology? *British Journal of Sociology*, **35**(1), 75–92.

Bryman, A. (1988) *Quantity and Quality in Social Research*, Contemporary Social Research Series 18, Unwin, London

Chalmers, K.I. (1992) Giving and receiving: an empirically derived theory on health visiting practice. *Journal of Advanced Nursing*, **17**, 1317–1325

Clark, E. (1987) *Identifying and Defining Questions for Research*, Research Awareness Programme Module 5, Distance Learning Centre, South Bank Polytechnic

Clarke, M. and Khadom, H. (1988) The nursing prevention of pressure sores in hospital and community patients. *Journal of Advanced Nursing*, **13**, 365–373

Corner, J. (1991) In search of more complete answers to research questions. Quantitative versus qualitative research methods: is there a way forward? *Journal of Advanced Nursing*, **16**, 718–727

Couchman, W. and Dawson, J. (1990) *Nursing and Health Care Research*, Scutari, London

Cowles, K. (1988) Issues in qualitative research on sensitive topics. *Western Journal of Nursing Research*, **10**(2), 163–179

Denzin, N. (1978) *The Research Act: A Theoretical Introduction to Research Methods*, McGraw-Hill, New York

Depoy, E. and Gitlin, L. (1993) *Introduction to Research: Multiple Strategies for Health and Human Services*. Mosby, St. Louis

DoH (1989) *General Practice in the National Health Service. A New Contract*, HMSO, London

DoH (1990) *The NHS and Community Care Act*, HMSO, London

Drennan, V. (1990) *Health Visitors and Groups: Politics and Practice*, Heinemann, London

Duffy, M. (1985) Designing nursing research: the qualitative/quantitative debate. *Journal of Advanced Nursing*, **10**, 225–232

Field, P. (1983) An ethnography: four public health nurses' perspectives of nursing. *Journal of Advanced Nursing*, **8**, 3–12

Field, P. and Morse, J. (1985) *Nursing Research: The Application of Qualitative Approaches*, Chapman and Hall, London

Fielding, N. and Fielding, J. (1986) *Linking Data*, Qualitative Research Methods, Series No. 4, Sage, Beverly Hills

Finch, J. (1984) 'It's great to have someone to talk to'. In *Social Researching* (eds C. Bell and H. Roberts), Routledge and Kegan Paul, London

Flatley, M. (1992) *In Depth Interviewing: A Discussion of Ethical Issues*, Paper presented to the Research Advisory Group Annual Conference, Birmingham

Fry, S. (1981) Accountability in research: the relationship of scientific and humanistic values. *Advances in Nursing Science*, **4**, 1–13

Gilbert, N. (1993) Research, theory and method. In *Researching Social Life* (ed. N. Gilbert), Sage, London

Glaser, B. and Strauss, A. (1967) *The Discovery of Grounded Theory*, Aldine, Chicago

Gold, R.L. (1958) Roles in sociological fieldwork. *Social Forces*, **36**, 217–223

Greenwood, J. (1984) Nursing research: a position paper. *Journal of Advanced Nursing*, **9**, 77–82

Goodman, C. (1989) Nursing research: growth and development. In *Current Issues in Nursing* (eds M. Jolley and P. Allen), Chapman and Hall, London

Griffin, S. and Speigal, N. (1993) *Diabetes in Practice*, Report for the Department of Health

Hammersley, M. and Atkinson, P. (1983) *Ethnography: Principles in Practice*, Tavistock Publications, London

Hicks, C. (1990) *Research and Statistics: A Practical Introduction for Nurses*, Prentice-Hall, London

Hilton, A. (1987) *The Ethnographic Perspective*, Research Awareness Programme Module 7, Distance Learning Centre, South Bank Polytechnic

Hinds, P.S., Scandrett-Hibden, S. and McAulay, L.S. (1990) Further assessment of a method to estimate the reliability and validity of qualitative research findings. *Journal of Advanced Nursing*, **15**, 430–435

Kelly, M. and May, D. (1982) Good and bad patients: a review of the literature and a theoretical critique. *Journal of Advanced Nursing*, **7**, 147–156

Lathlean, J. (1989) *Action Research for Nursing*, Unpublished paper, Oxford University Department of Educational Studies, Oxford

Luker, K. (1979) Measuring life satisfaction in an elderly female population. *Journal of Advanced Nursing*, **4**, 503–511

Luker, K. (1982) *Evaluating Health Visiting*, Royal College of Nursing, London

Mackenzie, A.E. (1992) Learning from experiences in the community: an ethnographic study of district nurse students. *Journal of Advanced Nursing*, **17**, 682–691

Macleod Clark, J. and Hockey, L. (1989) *Further Research for Nursing*, Scutari, London

Meyer, J. (1993) New paradigm research in practice: the trials and tribulations of action research. *Journal of Advanced Nursing*, **18**, 1066–1072

Moccia, P. (1988) A critique of compromise: beyond the methods debate. *Advances in Nursing Science*, **10**, 1–9

Montgomery-Robinson, K. (1986) Accounts of health visiting. In *Research in Preventive Community Nursing Care* (ed. A. While), Developments in Nursing Research, Vol. 4, Wiley, Chichester

Morse, J. (1991) Strategies for sampling. In *Qualitative Nursing Research: A Contemporary Dialogue* (ed. J. Morse), Sage, Newbury Park

Moser, C. and Kalton, G. (1979) *Survey Methods in Social Investigation*, Heinemann, London

Norton, D., McLaren, R. and Exton Smith, A.N. (1975) *An Investigation of Geriatric Nursing Problems in Hospitals*. Churchill Livingstone, Edinburgh

Oakley, A. (1993) Giving support in pregnancy: the role of research midwives in a randomised controlled trial. In *Midwives, Research and Childbirth*, Vol. 3 (eds S. Robinson and A.M. Thomson), Chapman and Hall, London

Oppenheim, A. (1992) *Questionnaire Design, Interviewing and Attitude Measurement*, Pinter, New York

Pearsall, M. (1965) Participant observation as role and method in behavioural research. *Nursing Research*, **14**(1), 37–42

Polit, D. and Hungler, B. (1991) *Nursing Research: Principles and Methods*, Lippincott, Philadelphia

Pollock, L. (1984) 6 steps to a successful literature search. *Nursing Times*, **80**(44), 40–43

Rajan, L. (1986) Weaning onto solid foods: mothers' beliefs and practices. *Health Visitor*, **59**(2), 41–44

RCN (1977) *Ethics Related to Research in Nursing*, Royal College of Nursing, London

Reid, N. (1993) *Health Care Research by Degrees*, Blackwell, Oxford

Riley, J. (1990) *Getting the Most from your Data. A Handbook of Practical Ideas on how to Analyse Qualitative Data*, Technical and Educational Services, Bristol

Roberts, H. (1981) *Doing Feminist Research*, Routledge and Kegan Paul, London

Sandelowski, M. (1986) The problem of rigor in qualitative research. *Advances in Nursing Science*, **8**(3), 27–37

Seaman, C. (1987) *Research Methods: Principles, Practice and Theory for Nursing*, Appleton and Lange, Norwalk, Connecticut

Smith, P. (1992) Research and its application. In *Common Foundation Studies in Nursing* (eds N. Kenworthy, G. Snowley and C. Gilling), Churchill Livingstone, Edinburgh

Strauss, A, (1987) *Qualitative Analysis for Social Scientists*, Cambridge University Press, New York

Titchen, A. and Binnie, A. (1993) Research partnerships: collaborative action research in nursing. *Journal of Advanced Nursing*, **18**, 858–865

Treece, E. and Treece, J. (1986) *Elements of Research in Nursing*, C.V. Mosby, St. Louis

Tripp-Reimer, T. (1985) Combining qualitative and quantitative methodologies. In *Qualitative Research Methods in Nursing* (ed. M. Leininger), Grune and Stratton, New York

UKCC (1986) *Project 2000: A New Preparation for Practice*, United Kingdom Central Council for Nursing, Midwifery and Health Visiting, London

UKCC (1990) *Report of Proposals for the Future of Community Education and Practice*, United Kingdom Central Council for Nursing, Midwifery and Health Visiting, London

UKCC (1992) *Code of Professional Conduct*, United Kingdom Central Council for Nursing, Midwifery and Health Visiting, London

UKCC (1993) *The Council's Proposed Standards for Post-Registration Education*, United Kingdom Central Council for Nursing, Midwifery and Health Visiting, London

Valiga, T.M. and Mermel, V.M. (1985) Formulating the researchable question. *Topics in Clinical Nursing*, **7**(2), 1–14

Waterman, H. (1993) *Issues of Reliability and Validity in Reflexive Action Research: a Case Study*, Paper given to the Research Advisory Group Annual Conference, Glasgow

Webb, C. (1989) Action research: philosophy, methods and personal experiences. *Journal of Advanced Nursing*, **14**, 403–410

White, E., Riley, E., Davies, S. and Twinn, S. (1993) *A Detailed Study of the Relationship Between Teaching, Support, Supervision and Role Modelling in Clinical Areas, within the Context of Project 2000 Courses*. Report for the

English National Board for Nursing, Midwifery and Health Visiting (unpublished), King's College, London and the University of Manchester
Whyte, D.A. (1992) A family nursing approach to the care of a child with a chronic illness. *Journal of Advanced Nursing*, **17**(3), 17–27

12

Using research to inform practice

Ann Mackenzie

● Introduction

It is the equal responsibility of researchers, educators and practitioners to contribute to the implementation and utilization of research findings and to move nursing towards becoming a profession that has a body of knowledge based on research (DoH, 1993). An appreciation of the epistemological issues surrounding research will enhance evaluation of research reports and help community health care nurses to make decisions about the utilization of research findings. Practitioners have a clear responsibility for promoting health (DoH, 1992). Their contribution to promoting health for identified community populations will be reliant on their ability to identify appropriate knowledge and define relevant questions about practice.

● Nursing knowledge

The move towards greater professional autonomy emphasized by *The Scope of Professional Practice* (UKCC, 1992a) and underpinned by the *Code of Professional Conduct* (UKCC, 1992b) means that nurses must have justification for their decisions about changes in professional practice. Some of this justification will come from knowledge drawn from research. However, there are many philosophical and ethical questions involved in nursing practice for which research-based knowledge does not provide clear-cut answers. Indeed, philosophy is concerned with raising questions and not with answering them. An example of philosophical knowledge is the work of Schrock, which contributed to the development of the principles of health visiting which have been fundamental in guiding health visiting practice (CETHV, 1977).

Many of the dilemmas of practice are those related to everyday decisions, such as how much information to give patients about their terminal illness against the wishes of close relatives. While the knowledge from research will help community health care nurses to take ethical decisions, these decisions will inevitably be influenced by the nurses' own values and experience as to what is right in the circumstances. Research does not necessarily provide all the answers but does offer a point of reference when ethical decisions have to be taken.

According to Clark (1987a), the authority from which nurses draw their knowledge about nursing practice may be based on tradition, trial and error or science. In this context science refers to research. Most nursing research is empirical, in that it is carried out in the real situation and involves researchers collecting data through not only observing, but also talking and listening to individuals and practitioners in the practice setting. Philosophical knowledge, on the other hand, is 'second order knowledge' (Schrock, 1981) and does not use the methods of scientific investigation such as empirical research to find answers. Rather it contributes to understanding and knowledge by conceptual analysis, by clarifying thinking and definitions and by removing ambiguities. The development of nursing models has been likened to this conceptual process. Nursing theorists such as Orem (1985) and Roy (1984) have attempted to examine and analyse concepts of nursing and to contribute to the clarification of nursing practice and the distinctive features of nursing in relation to other disciplines. Nursing models are still to be tested for their effectiveness in professional practice and do not provide a complete knowledge base for making judgements (Field, 1987). However, by distinguishing nursing from other disciplines, models indicate the parameters of nursing and have the potential to help community health care nurses explicate their contribution to primary health care.

The beginnings of all practice-based knowledge are the questions that practitioners ask about their work, whether it be in the field of education, management or clinical practice. Such questions may arise from enquiry about traditional practices, many of which are indulged in by community nurses. Examples of traditional practices are routine visiting of elderly people or of children under 5 years or routine screening procedures across all age groups, carried out without a clear understanding of their health-related purpose or concern for health-related outcomes. Trial and error has also contributed to the development of questions for practice. The whole range of treatments administered by district nurses in managing wounds and promoting wound healing, particularly those wounds which are intractable such as fungating malignant wounds, provides an example of raising questions from trial and error. Sims and Fitzgerald (1985) discovered that district nurses used a wide range of local applications to promote comfort and reduce unpleasant odour. Further examples are provided by the range of parenting advice given by health visitors or bereavement counselling undertaken by community psychiatric nurses (Brooker and White, 1993).

It is not that practitioners should disregard trial and error or tradition, but that they should use the best available knowledge they have at the time. Indeed, some of the answers to nursing questions may not have been researched or may be at an early stage of investigation. Although some aspects of practice may be well thought out and tested, if practitioners do not continue to question practice it may once again become traditional and ritualized.

However, in attempting to answer some of these practice-based questions, nurses will need to draw on the disciplines of the natural and social sciences, each with its own distinctive approach to the development of scientific knowledge. Consequently, nursing research is influenced by the development of knowledge from this broad continuum of sciences which have distinct ways of developing scientific knowledge through empirical research (Robinson *et al.*, 1992).

● **Epistemological issues**

Research from disciplines such as psychology, sociology, biology, pharmacology and epidemiology come to address their research questions with a set of assumptions about the source and nature of knowledge. Such epistemological issues will influence the orientation of the researcher and guide research strategies and design, resulting in debates between those involved in quantitative or qualitative research. The characteristics and assumptions of each approach are summarized in Table 12.1.

The dichotomy between quantitative and qualitative research arises mainly from the debate about epistemological issues of what constitutes scientific knowledge. Positivism, as ideally portrayed, encompasses the philosophy of the natural sciences, which in turn is taken to be the benchmark for all scientific research, including that of the social sciences (Hammersley and Atkinson, 1983). Central to positivism is the concept of scientific method modelled on the natural sciences and concerned with the testing of theories. Such theories are open to testing by the scientific community by confirmation or falsification, and by the application of a set of procedures and rules which guide research strategies, such as structured interviews or experiments.

Table 12.1   Characteristics and underpinning assumptions of quantitative and qualitative research

Quantitative	Qualitative
Hard science: natural science	Soft science: human and social sciences
Focus: concise, narrow	Focus: complex, broad
Reductionist	Holistic
Objective	Subjective
Researcher's stance: outsider	Researcher's stance: insider
Theory: tests, confirms	Theory: develops, emergent
Research design: structured controlled, predetermined	Research design: unstructured flexible, indeterminate
Nature of data: precise, numerical, hard	Nature of data: explanatory, contextual, rich
Elements of analysis: number, statistical	Elements of analysis: words, interpretation
Scope of findings: nomethetic – establish rules, laws, generalizable, representative	Scope of findings: idiographic – specific to location, time, context, individual
Reasoning: deductive	Reasoning: inductive
Assumptions drawn from positivism	Assumptions drawn from naturalism

POSSIBLE RESEARCH DESIGNS

Experimental	*Survey*	*Ethnographic*

After Bryman (1988) and Burns and Grove (1987).

However, major concerns in the natural sciences, such as numerical measurement, causality, generalization and replication, do not fit the assumptions identified as appropriate for qualitative research, particularly for many of the more complex investigations required of nursing research (Pollock, 1991).

In contrast to this view, naturalism is concerned with understanding, process, meaning and holism. Individuals respond according to their interpretation and understanding of the social world and therefore actions and events must be studied in the natural context and not in a controlled 'laboratory' setting. Supporters of naturalism would argue that standardized procedures in no way ensure comparability or eliminate different interpretations.

It is obvious that the research method, and the underpinning assumptions which together comprise the research methodology, must be made clear in order that practitioners can evaluate the relevance of the research method and findings to practice. Indeed, a greater understanding by practitioners of the utilization of nursing research would be gained if researchers indulged in critical appraisal of their methodology and shared some of their dilemmas about methodological issues (Webb, 1985; Reid, 1991). Through these types of debates ideas may be clarified and developed. This seems particularly important in nursing, where research is a developing skill and where studies drawing on both the natural and social sciences are equally important (Corner, 1991).

It is now becoming clear that in nursing research the defence of these extremes in research methodology is irrelevant. This is particularly so if health care is to be examined in the present climate with its emphasis on the interactive nature of participation, consumer choice and client satisfaction (Wilson-Barnett, 1991). Research then is not just a mechanical set of steps which are undertaken without thought – it is underpinned by assumptions about how knowledge is generated, about the nature of the discipline and about the values and beliefs of the scientific community.

However, whatever design is chosen, the development of new knowledge will be acquired by a process of systematic and scientific enquiry; a process common to all empirical research. As with all other disciplines, nursing uses scientific enquiry to carry out research within the scientific method, the steps of which are described by Robinson *et al.* (1992) as:

systematic observation of some aspect of the world around us, the generation of scientific theories, the systematic testing of theories and, where necessary, their modification in the light of new data.

Few individual research projects, however, will move through all these steps. It will take a number of projects, building on previous work, to get to the stage of testing out theories which can be said to be able to predict and control the effects of clinical practice. The descriptive research about pressure sores carried out by Norton *et al.* (1962) was an early step in the UK in developing knowledge of this common patient problem. Nursing knowledge in this area of practice has now reached a stage of prediction, and to some extent control, in the prevention of pressure sores (Gould, 1986). Similarly, investigation into hospital discharge was described 27 years ago (Hockey, 1968). This was the beginning of research-based information about the difficulties that patients experienced when discharged into the community. Further research over two decades has offered some explanations of why these difficulties occur (Marks, 1994; King and Macmillan, 1994). To some extent practitioners can now predict the circumstances that are most likely to offer a smooth transfer of patient from hospital to community care. As a result of current knowledge about discharge planning, different models of practice are being examined with groups such as elderly people (Ryan, 1994) and those suffering severe mental illness (Rainsford and Caan, 1994).

These different stages of measurement – description, explanation, prediction and control – will use different research designs drawn from both the quantitative and the qualitative domains. The research questions, together with the initial clinical problems, should be stated by the researcher to allow the practitioner to evaluate the validity and relevance of the findings to practice.

● **Research questions in community nursing**

There is a dearth of research in community settings which can be said to control or predict the results of practice, with the exception of that drawn from the biological sciences. Perhaps this is not surprising, as nursing in the community is pervaded by uncertainty and indeterminate human problems, which do not always lend themselves to the problem-solving of the hard natural sciences. Indeed, there will always be a need to explain and thereby increase understanding of the problems encountered by practitioners in the community.

The prevailing view of scientific knowledge, drawn from the positivist school, assumes that human beings can be studied according to the application of laws through experimentation and rigorous application of empirical method to explore the physical world. Schon (1983) describes this approach as a technical rationality model. Some of the questions are not answerable by a positivist methodology and the challenge for practitioners is to transfer problems into researchable questions without losing their relevance. Community nurses are dealing with what Schon (1983) refers to as the 'messy but crucially important problems' of professional practice. His analogy of the high ground of technical rationality and the swampy low ground of practical human problems graphically demonstrates the dilemmas of researching nursing practice in the community (Figure 12.1).

The real problems of practice are those raised and addressed by practitioners themselves, such as the work by Ross (1989). This study concentrates on prescribed medication for elderly people and highlights the problems of maintaining accurate records in primary care and the implications for teamwork. The demand for new ways of working by practitioners has also raised questions about the roles of community nurses, and studies have looked at various aspects of community nursing

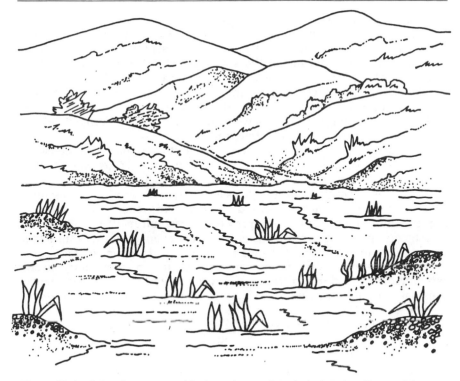

Figure 12.1 Schon's topographical analogy of technical rationality and human problems

practice in health visiting (Davies, 1990), practice nursing (Ross and Campbell, 1992) and community psychiatric nursing (Ferguson, 1993).

These examples, from an increasing number of small-scale studies, individually raise further questions and produce useful findings that help to clarify practice problems. Hunt (1981) argues that although they offer indicators that nurses could try out in practice, on their own they do not offer enough evidence for guiding practice. However, if the practice area is examined further from a similar or different perspective, or the study replicated, theoretical knowledge will be developed to offer valuable guidance for practice. It is crucial in community nursing that there is some drawing together and synthesis of research into cognate and practice-related areas. This is particularly important, since the scientific research knowledge in community nursing is sparse and therefore at this stage it is not useful to disperse knowledge superficially across broad areas.

However, community health care nursing is not context free and much of the research undertaken in the community setting is driven by policy. The majority of explicit policy research is not undertaken by nurses, but by social scientists carrying out contracted research on behalf of policy-makers and health planners. The problem for practitioners is that it may seem unrelated to practice, since it has the clear-cut purpose of answering policy questions. This approach comes much more from the high ground of predetermined clear-cut questions than the low ground of human problems of practice. The requirement for measurement of practice outcomes is also influencing the sorts of questions that purchasers are asking about community nursing (Barriball and Mackenzie, 1993). This in turn will influence the type of research that is likely to be funded. The targets set out in the strategy document *The Health of the Nation* (DoH, 1992) provide another example of policy-driven research by demanding research to measure outcomes of practice. However, practitioners will, no doubt, look further than the prescribed key areas and use the strategy as a framework for identifying priority areas for research in their own practice populations.

While the findings of policy research studies may have considerable influence on community health care nursing, even to the extent of reducing numbers of staff (NHSME, 1992), such studies have to be evaluated by practitioners with the same rigour as any other research. The criterion that single studies do not provide enough evidence for implementation and utilization prevails (MacGuire, 1990). Policy research can point to the problems and suggest change, but it is up to the practitioners to validate that change in relation to the practice area.

The introduction of the contract culture in community health care nursing has led to a plethora of new ideas and demands for change. This has prompted research into practice which is not well understood, or well established, such as the role of nurse practitioners or the use of dependency levels in assessment. This is likely to lead to research of which the findings will not be utilized, because questions informed by practice are impossible to formulate. However, before questions are raised, the practitioner has to experience the phenomena in order to conceptualize the problem. In addition, exploration of the problems of health through carefully designed pilot or descriptive studies are a prerequisite of large-scale research if practitioners are to examine areas such as those in subcultures which are difficult to access due to language or cultural differences. To achieve health for all cultural groups, it is important to understand the consumer's viewpoint about health care – consumers such as homeless people or carers of the elderly in black populations.

Even with good research evidence to guide practitioners, it is still important that evaluation of specific practice-based findings is made. The extensive research into carers recently escalated by policy requirements has provided community nurses with strong guidelines about the needs of carers. Twigg *et al*. (1990) state that focusing on the instrumental aspects of services has not been comprehensive enough to direct appropriate utilization. The findings that carers need information and support has led, in some areas, to a plethora of incomprehensible information being produced and inappropriate carer support groups being established. The complex relationships between informal carers and dependents also determines need (Lewis and Meredith, 1988; Grant and Nolan, 1993). The research also needs to be ongoing and to involve community nurses who are aware of the practice problems. It seems that in this area of knowledge practitioners are in danger of overload (MacGuire, 1990). This situation occurs when there is too much information which has not been synthesized or in some respects is contradictory. The results might be that practitioners either do nothing or implement services that are not effective.

● Implementation and utilization of research findings

Implementing and utilizing research findings is not easy. In the past, the majority of research studies have, as Wilson-Barnett *et al.* (1990) suggest, 'involved "nurse-watching" rather than evaluation of care'. As a result there is a dearth of studies that have applied clinical changes in practice and therefore few studies from which direct recommendations for care can be confidently made. This viewpoint implies that researchers are not addressing the problems of clinical practice, nor are they actively involving nurses in evaluating and applying research findings. However, such views are not new. Indeed, the early philosophical work of Schrock (1981) debates the problems of aligning appropriate questions with answers that practitioners can use. As Schrock states, if the researcher is not asking the right questions then the findings will be inappropriate and have little relevance to practice. Given that relevant research is available, then enquiring practitioners must take steps to evaluate what knowledge is available in their area of practice, or more usefully, in their area of interest or specialization. Even within community nursing, specialties such as district nursing, community psychiatric nursing, school nursing or health visiting involve a complexity of practice. Therefore, practitioners cannot be expected to have up-to-date research knowledge about every area of practice and must specialize in specific areas, sharing their specialist knowledge within the team.

There is some research knowledge, such as that in health promotion or communication, which is relevant to all practitioners and about which community nurses must keep up to date. There will also be specific areas which may have been researched in hospital settings, but may not be directly applicable to the community. Pressure sore indicators developed in hospital provide an example and further discussion on this topic is provided in Chapter 11.

Exhorting community health care nurses to become more research based in their practice is not helpful unless one can offer some synthesis about research that has been done. Hunt (1987) suggests that this lack of synthesis of known research findings is one reason why nurses do not implement research findings. This observation seems relevant to the context of community health care nursing research. However, it is not that there is overwhelming research by community nurses, but rather that the nature of the work cuts across broad areas of practice. Therefore, the problem is illustrated by one community health care nursing student stating 'where do I start'? Perhaps the first point is practice itself and the areas of practice which are of specific interest or where the work is concentrated.

● Framework for raising questions about practice

In an attempt to help practitioners decide where to start in researching their practice, the following questions provide a framework:

- What particular aspect of practice is important in the locality or prevalent in the caseload?

- Is it of broad interest such as teamwork, communication or health promotion with patients or clients, or is it specific, such as rehabilitating people following a stroke or the prevention of sudden infant death?
- What sort of questions does this area of practice raise?
- What is already known?
- What is the source of this knowledge?
- What is the level of research-based knowledge, if any?
- What is not known?
- In the light of further knowledge, do I need to refine and focus my question further?
- Do I have enough information about my question to implement and utilize research-based findings?
- Would it be useful to share the information I have discovered so far?

In using this framework, for example in district nursing practice, the district nurse may respond thus about pressure sore prevention:

Pressure sore prevention is certainly an important area of practice for the district nursing team and others involved in short-term or long-term rehabilitation.

It is a specific area of interest to those who are involved in pressure sores and their prevention, but knowledge of the subject is concerned with other areas such as general wound healing.

The specific questions may be about prevention – how can pressure sores be prevented in the community? This is a very broad question which would need to be refined if the district nurse was intent on identifying a question for research (Clark, 1987b).

A great deal is already known about pressure sores and their prevention (Gould, 1986). Certainly, as previously described, it is a well-researched area in the UK and it can be argued there are a number of known predisposing factors in pressure sore development related to activity, mobility, age, chronic illness, mental status, medications, skin moisture, nutrition and hydration (Torrance, 1983).

The source of knowledge about the above factors and other factors relating to nursing activities is research based. A synthesis of information is also available, based on research literature (David, 1982).

Knowledge is at a level of explanation and to some extent prediction, in that practitioners can explain causes of pressure sores and predict that some categories of patient are more likely to develop pressure sores than others, particularly in institutional settings and in the older age groups.

As far as the district nursing team is concerned there is not a great deal known about the validity and reliability of instruments that will calculate the pressure sore risk in the community setting. Indeed, the predictive value of such as the well-known scores developed by Norton *et al.* (1962) and Waterlow (1985) have been questioned.

The question then may be refined to consider the validity and reliability of pressure sore risk calculators as part of the assessment and rehabilitation of patients who have suffered a stroke.

There is certainly enough knowledge in the general area of pressure sore prevention to incorporate into practice at the level that Hunt (1981) describes as being an indicator for what nurses 'should do'. This compares to a level of research knowledge which indicates 'What nurses could try or which practices and procedures have no sound basis' (Hunt, 1981).

This is a fairly easy area to take as an example since there has been research into pressure sores for 35 years. However, the majority of nurses are still not taking such findings into account (Gould, 1986). Hunt (1981) identified some reasons for such situations existing because nurses 'do not know about them, understand them, believe them, know how to apply them or are not allowed to use them'. The first two reasons are very much linked to the responsibility of the practitioner to evaluate research reports and to the researcher in disseminating research findings. The remainder are to do with changing practice. Other authors have suggested that nurses themselves are resistant to, or unable to read, published research and therefore research findings are not accessible to them (Greenwood, 1984; Hunt, 1987; MacGuire, 1990).

● **Evaluating research reports**

The relevance of research to practice can only be assessed by practitioners if they are able to carry out informed evaluation of written reports and discuss, and become involved in, practice-based research projects with researchers. Both practitioners and researchers have responsibilities in this critical appraisal of published research. As noted above, the nature of questions raised by community nursing practice requires a range of research designs, and the combinations of such approaches make evaluation of research reports a complex undertaking.

Practitioners' evaluation

There are a number of research texts which give a framework for evaluating research reports (Burns and Grove, 1987; Clark, 1991; Cormack, 1991). It is fair to say that all these texts and many other nursing texts emphasize a quantitative approach and use this as a framework for their analysis. The strong influence of quantitative methodology in nursing is obvious and one has to turn to general education for good guidance on assessing qualitative research in the UK (Hammersley, 1990). Practitioners therefore often take a quantitative stance which leads to undervaluing of qualitative or mixed approaches to practice-based research. Table 12.2 summarizes the stages of evaluation which take into account both qualitative and quantitative approaches. The evaluation of research is not just a question of methodology, but equally important is a judgement about relevance to practice (Hammersley, 1990). It should also begin with the significance of the research problem and its refinement into a researchable question.

All practice-based research begins with a problem which should be

Table 12.2   Guidelines for critically evaluating qualitative and quantitative research reports

The following questions can be used as a set of criteria against which an evaluation of the relevance of the report to practitioners can be made:

INTRODUCTION
Is there a clear abstract which covers the substantial areas of the research?
Are the author's qualifications and background relevant?
Is the source of funding, if any, stated?
Is the report clearly presented and comprehensible?

RESEARCH PROBLEM
Is there a clear statement of the problem to be investigated?
Is the problem significant to professional practice?
Is the rationale for the research identified?

LITERATURE REVIEW
Is there a comprehensive summary of appropriate, differentiating research from other literature?
Does the review select relevant material?
Does the review establish a theoretical framework or a rationale for the research?
Does the review demonstrate what is known and what is not known about the research problem?

RESEARCH QUESTIONS
Are the research questions defined and linked to the literature review?
Are the aims and objective or the research hypothesis clearly stated together with the variables to be investigated?

RESEARCH DESIGN
Is the study design appropriate to the research question?
Is the level of measurement clear?
Are the key concepts or terms clarified and defined?
Is the study population clearly identified?
Is the sample described and appropriately selected for the level of measurement and the design, e.g. key informants or random sample?
Has adequate consideration been given to ethical issues, including ethical approval?
Has validity and reliability been addressed appropriate to the design?
Was a relevant pilot study carried out and are any changes to the study noted?
Are data collection methods appropriate to the design?
Is the analysis clearly described and appropriate to the level of measurement and the design?
Is there evidence of rigorous analysis using appropriate conceptual strategies or statistical tests?

RESEARCH FINDINGS AND CONCLUSIONS
Are the findings precisely and concisely stated?
Is there substantial evidence from the data to support the findings?
Are the implications of the findings for nursing practice discussed?
To what extent do the findings answer the research question?
Are the contributions to the current state of knowledge discussed?
Are further research questions raised?
Are the limitations of the study discussed?

significant to practitioners and to the area of practice. The extent to which the problem is driven by practice or, as is frequently the case in the community at present, policy initiatives, is of crucial importance. Policy initiatives may be local, but may also have broader applications such as that undertaken by Ross and Campbell (1992). Others may be carried out by policy-making bodies such as the recent skill mix research into district nursing (NHSME, 1992). The purpose of the research and motives of the authors and funding authority must be questioned. Questions such as whether the researchers are nurses or social or biological scientists and whether this gives the research a specific focus need to be considered. It is perhaps naive to anticipate that all research in the community in such a time of political change is carried out for the good of the profession or even for the good of the consumer. The skill mix report (NHSME, 1992) is a good example. The purpose of the research has been questioned, with some practitioners suggesting that it was merely to reduce the grades and numbers of district nurses. This argument has been extended further to suggest the research was merely a cost-cutting exercise initiated by health planners with little relevance to practice in the form it was presented (Cowley and Mackenzie, 1993). Equally important is the ability of the researcher to carry out the research. Small-scale research carried out by unqualified or unsupervised researchers is generally inappropriate in practice terms and unethical in research terms.

The literature review will help to refine and define the problem into a researchable question. The review should also be substantial enough to provide a theoretical base for the research. In doing so it will demonstrate the gaps in the literature and enable the reader to see the rationale for the research. It should be clear to the reader whether or not this is a new area of investigation or is contributing to previous knowledge or testing out previous theories. This will lead the practitioner to an expectation about the method of investigation to be used and the level of measurement and investigation that might be expected.

The aims, objectives or hypothesis to be tested shall be described, together with clarification and definition of key terms and concepts.

The research design, which includes sampling, ethical procedures, data collection methods and analysis, will be addressed in the light of knowledge of research methods. These are addressed in some detail in Chapter 11. The crucial aspects of assessing relevance to practice are the concepts of validity and reliability.

For instance, sampling is an issue of validity and must therefore be described with reference to the research question. In qualitative research, sampling of people, both in terms of time and place, is carried out with the purpose of developing categories from which theory may be developed. Indeed, sampling may be a continuous process throughout the period of data collection (Mackenzie, 1994). Quantitative sampling, on the other hand, has a different purpose and is to ensure a representative sample from the study population, thus enabling generalizations and theory testing through the examination of relationships between specified and predetermined variables. The practitioner will be looking for evidence of random or stratified sampling in quantitative research and purposive sampling in qualitative studies.

An estimation of whether the findings are relevant will take into account all the above concerns, but will also be a judgement about whether or not the results are clinically significant. Practitioners should consider whether or not the findings will make a significant and positive difference to health care and provide appropriate answers to the original problem. This frequently depends on the theoretical basis of the analysis. For instance, if learning environments in the community are examined using organizational theory, then the findings might be concerned with managerial or organizational changes such as alterations to the practice base of placements or changes in responsibilities. If, on the other hand, adult learning theory is used, then the findings may result in changes to teaching practices or opportunities for learning. Research that is carried out with no understanding of real practical problems and which is set up to answer predetermined problems may well be irrelevant to community nurses.

Researchers' responsibilities
While the practitioner has a major part to play in evaluating research reports as part of the process of assessing the appropriateness of implementing research findings, the researcher has an equally important part to play. Such responsibilities cover not only clear accounts and analysis of the methodology, but also a commitment to work with practitioners in educating them about research methods and in undertaking research co-operatively in the practice situation (Wilson-Barnett *et al.*, 1990).

The responsibilities of researchers can be summarized as follows:

- make research accessible through national journal publications, local seminars and conferences
- work with practitioners to identify appropriate research questions and offer relevant findings
- resist jumping on the bandwagon merely to raise research funding
- resist small-scale studies that are not building on or replicating previous research
- publish critical literature reviews that can inform practitioners and contribute to the synthesis of research findings
- disseminate findings in numerous forms that can be used in practice and educational settings such as videos, poster display or teaching packs
- ensure that policy research has relevance to local practice and has generalizability
- contribute to teaching programmes about research appreciation and critical appraisal of research reports.

It is quite clear that not all research is well reported and a useful critique of quantitative research is to be found in Clark (1991). Insight into qualitative methodology such as ethnography is helped by critical appraisal of the method by researchers themselves, thus helping others to understand the criteria against which qualitative research may be measured (Reid, 1991).

Changing practice

Barriers to implementation and utilization have been well re-hearsed in the literature. These include well-known and accepted reasons such as the need for practitioners to acknowledge their own responsibility to search out and critically evaluate appropriate research (Hunt, 1981; Greenwood, 1984; Gould, 1986). More recently, issues such as the relevance of the research to practice and the difficulties of carrying out research in clinical areas have been added (Wilson-Barnett *et al.*, 1990). In addition, the drive to investigate innovative phenomena that are not well understood, and information overload, have been highlighted (MacGuire, 1990).

● Conclusion

Although practitioners are becoming more research aware and skilled in critical evaluation and researchers are attempting to disseminate their findings, there remains the difficulty of motivating nurses to change. The work of Hunt (1987) provides a valuable insight into the resistance of practitioners to adopting well-understood and clear research findings. Despite organizational barriers to change being overcome and support from other professional colleagues being provided, nurses on the ward were not prepared to change their individual practice to implement well-substantiated and relevant findings that stated that patients did not normally need to be subjected to the practice of 'nil-by-mouth' for long periods.

From studies such as these it would seem that change is not just about knowing or understanding research findings, described by Bennis *et al.*, 1976 – but the rational empirical approach is far more complex. Interestingly, the involvement of practitioners in the much advocated bottom-up approach of normative or problem-solving approaches to change was not successful here either. Indeed, Closs and Cheater (1994) argue that changes in thinking, or in practice, as a result of research, require a positive culture that supports change, promotes interest in research and values research-based knowledge.

Generally, community health care nurses are well versed in change and may have accomplished many of the known strategies to maintain stability where change in nursing is most rife. Given that there is a wealth of literature about change, some of which is discussed in Chapter 29, and about barriers to utilization of research findings in nursing, the most appropriate people to accomplish utilization of research to inform practice in the community are community health care nurses themselves.

References

Barriball, K.L. and Mackenzie, A. (1993) Measuring the impact of nursing interventions in the community: a selective review of the literature. *Journal of Advanced Nursing*, **18**, 401–407

Bennis, W.G., Benne, K.D., Chin, R. and Corey, K.E. (1976) *The Planning of Change*, 3rd edn, Holt, Rinehart and Winston, New York

Brooker, C. and White, E. (1993) *Community Psychiatric Nursing: A Research Perspective*, Vol. 2, Chapman and Hall, London

Bryman, A. (1988) *Quantity and Quality in Social Research*, Unwin Hyman, London

Burns, N. and Grove, S.K. (1987) *The Practice of Nursing: Research. Conduct, Critique and Utilization*, W.B. Saunders, Philadelphia

CETHV (1977) *An Investigation into the Principles of Health Visiting*, Council for the Education and Training of Health Visitors, London

Clark, E. (1987a) *Sources of Nursing Knowledge*, Module 2, Research Awareness, Distance Learning Centre, South Bank Polytechnic, London

Clark, E. (1987b) *Identifying and Defining Questions for Research*, Module 5, Research Awareness, Distance Learning Centre, South Bank Polytechnic, London

Clark, E. (1991) *Evaluating Research*, Module 10, Research Awareness, Distance Learning Centre, South Bank Polytechnic, London

Closs, J.S. and Cheater, F.M. (1994) Utilization of nursing research: culture, interest and support. *Journal of Advanced Nursing*, **19**, 762–773

Cormack, D.F.S. (ed.) (1991) *The Research Process in Nursing*, 2nd edn, Blackwell Scientific, Oxford

Corner, J. (1991) In search of more complete answers to research questions. Quantitative versus qualitative research methods: is there a way forward? *Journal of Advanced Nursing*, **16**, 718–727

Cowley, S. and Mackenzie, A.E. (1993) *Nursing Skill Mix in the District Nursing Service*, District Nursing Association UK Newsletter, Vol. X, No. 1, Spring, District Nursing Association, Edinburgh

David, J. (1982) Pressure sore treatment: literature review. *International Journal of Nursing Studies*, **19**, 183–191

Davies, S. (1990) An approach to case-finding the elderly. *Nursing Times*. Occasional Paper, **86**(51), 48–51

DoH (1992) *The Health of the Nation. A Strategy for Health in England*, HMSO, London

DoH (1993) *Report of the Task Force on the Strategy for Research in Nursing, Midwifery and Health Visiting*, HMSO, London

Ferguson, K.E. (1993) A study to investigate the views of patients and their carers on the work undertaken by nurses to prepare the patient for discharge from hospital. In *Community Psychiatric Nursing. A Research Perspective*, Vol. 2 (eds C. Brooker and E. White), Chapman and Hall, London

Field, P.A. (1987) The impact of nursing theory on the clinical decision making process. *Journal of Advanced Nursing*, **12**, 563–571

Grant, G. and Nolan, M. (1993) Informal carers: sources and concomitants of satisfaction. *Health and Social Care*, **1**, 147–159

Gould, D. (1986) Pressure sore prevention and treatment: an example of nurses' failure to implement research findings. *Journal of Advanced Nursing*, **11**, 389–397

Greenwood, J. (1984) Nursing research: a position paper. *Journal of Advanced Nursing*, **9**, 77–82

Hammersley, M. (1990) *Reading Ethnographic Research. A Critical Guide*, Longman, London

Hammersley, M. and Atkinson, P. (1983) *Ethnography Principles in Practice*, Tavistock Publications, London

Hockey, L. (1968) *Care in the Balance – A Study of Collaboration Between Hospital and Community*, Queen's Institute of District Nursing, London

Hunt, J. (1981) Indicators for nursing practice: the use of research findings. *Journal of Advanced Nursing*, **6**, 189–194

Hunt, M. (1987) The process of translating research findings into nursing practice. *Journal of Advanced Nursing*, **12**, 101–110

King, C. and Macmillan, M. (1994) Documentation and discharge planning for elderly patients. *Nursing Times*, **90**, 20

Lewis, J. and Meredith, B. (1988) Daughters caring for mothers: the experience of caring and its implications for professional helpers. *Ageing and Society*, **8**, 1–22

MacGuire, J.M. (1990) Putting nursing research findings into practice: research utilisation as an aspect of the management of change. *Journal of Advanced Nursing*, **5**, 614–620

Mackenzie, A.E. (1994) Evaluating ethnography: considerations for analysis. *Journal of Advanced Nursing*, **19**, 774–781

Marks, L. (1994) *Seamless Care or Patchwork Quilt? Discharging Patients from Acute Hospital Care*, King's Fund Centre, London

NHSME (1992) *The Nursing Skill Mix in The District Nursing Service*, HMSO, London

Norton, D., McLaren, R. and Exton-Smith, A.N. (1962) *An Investigation of Geriatric Nursing Problems in Hospital*, Churchill Livingstone, Edinburgh

Orem, D.E. (1985) *Nursing Concepts of Practices*, 3rd edn, McGraw-Hill, New York

Pollock, L.C. (1991) Qualitative analysis. In *The Research Process in Nursing* (ed. F.S. Cormack), Blackwell Publications, Oxford

Rainsford, E. and Caan, W. (1994) Experience of supervising discharges. *Journal of Clinical Nursing*, **3**, 133–137

Reid, B. (1991) Developing and documenting a qualitative methodology. *Journal of Advanced Nursing*, **16**, 544–551

Robinson, K., Robinson, H. and Hilton, A. (1992) *What is Research?*, Research Awareness, Module 3, Distance Learning Centre, South Bank University, London

Ross, F.M. (1989) Doctor, nurse and patient knowledge of prescribed medication in primary care. *Public Health*, **103**, 131–137

Ross, F.M. and Campbell, F. (1992) Inter professional collaboration in the provision of aids for daily living and nursing equipment in the community – a district nurse and consumer perspective. *Journal of Inter Professional Care*, **16**(2), 109–118

Roy, C. (1984) *Introduction to Nursing: An Adaptation Model*, Prentice Hall, Englewood Cliffs, N.J.

Ryan, A. (1994) Improving discharge planning. *Nursing Times*, **90**, 20

Schon, D. (1983) *The Reflective Practitioner. How Professionals Think in Action*, Avebury, Aldershot

Schrock, R.A. (1981) Philosophical issues. In *Recent Advances in Nursing* (ed. L. Hockey), Churchill Livingstone, Edinburgh

Sims, R. and Fitzgerald, V. (1985) *Community Nursing Management of Patients with Ulcerating/Fungating Malignant Breast Disease*, Oncology Nursing Society, London

Torrance, C. (1983) *The Aetiology, Prevention and Treatment of Pressure Sores*, Croom Helm, Edinburgh

Twigg, J., Atkin, K. and Perring, C. (1990) *Carers and Services: A Review of Research*, HMSO, London

UKCC (1992a) *The Scope of Professional Practice*, United Kingdom Central Council, London

UKCC (1992b) *Code of Professional Conduct*, 3rd edn, United Kingdom Central Council, London

Waterlow, J. (1985) The Waterlow Card for the prevention and management of pressure area sores: towards a pocket policy. *Care, Science and Practice*, **6**(1), 8–12

Webb, C. (1985) Gynaecological nursing: a compromising situation. *Journal of Advanced Nursing*, **10**, 47–54

Wilson-Barnett, J. (1991) The experiment: is it worthwhile? *International Journal of Nursing Studies*, **28**(1), 77–78

Wilson-Barnett, J., Corner, J. and DeCarle, B. (1990) Integrating nursing research and practice – the role of the researcher as teacher. *Journal of Advanced Nursing*, **15**, 621–625

Part IV

Patterns of living and working: implications for health

Community health care nursing is much more than nursing practised in the community. As McMurray (1993) states: 'It is a unique and continually evolving specialized area within the profession which considers the *context* of people's lives as paramount to attaining and maintaining health.' This part focuses on how the differing context of individuals' lives influences not only their health status but also their response to health promotion and illness prevention as well as to treatment, care and rehabilitation. An important focus in all the chapters are the implications of these contextual influences for the health care provided by practitioners.

Boundaries of community health care nursing are not distinct and each of the chosen settings are those in which, although there may be a primary input from one group of practitioners with a specific area of expertise, teamwork is essential to high-quality care. The five settings chosen are those which influence the individual, family and community, as these are places where they live, learn and work; indeed, the places where individuals spend the major part of their lives. These therefore are seen as the key influences on health and lifestyles, although it is recognized that even a short visit to a health care setting such as a general practice or health centre can have a lasting impact on an individual.

The part begins with Chapter 13 which focuses on the home, since this is the setting which has a major influence on people's lives. Particular attention is paid to the vital contribution of carers, and the needs of some specific vulnerable groups are considered.

Chapter 14 addresses the important setting of the school. In the UK, children spend a minimum of 12 years in school and it is during these years that children are particularly receptive to health care advice and where healthy lifestyles are formed. As adults spend a large part of their life at work,

Chapter 15 provides a logical continuation from school and offers an insight into health in the workplace. However, it is important to remember those who, for whatever reason, are not employed and the possible effects of this on their physical, social and mental wellbeing. The interdependent effects of work on health and health on work are debated and the implications for practitioners involved with the adult population highlighted.

It may seem inappropriate in a book on community health care nursing to include a chapter on residential care. However, as community health care nurses are making an increasing contribution to care in the many small institutions which are part of the community, Chapter 16 addresses this situation. The final chapter in this part recognizes the important context of homelessness. The authors argue that the many different definitions of home and the provision of health care in the community are equally important to those who are homeless and live in alternative accommodation.

This part considers the influence of various environments on health and how within these contexts a level of health appropriate for the individual may be attained and maintained. The editors recognize that there are many innovative schemes that provide support for people either at home, at school, in the workplace, in residential institutions or indeed for the homeless. Some examples of such schemes are provided by Lynch and Perry (1992) who give case studies of innovations in the UK for supporting the frail elderly, ethnic minorities, those with learning disability and those with mental health problems. The NHSME (1993) also gives many examples of special schemes, including liaison work and specialist areas of work linking hospital and home.

It is anticipated that this part will help readers to recognize that the context of an individual's life and work has a great influence on their health status, their acceptance of health advice and on the way in which health care is delivered.

References

Lynch, B. and Perry, R. (1992) *Experiences of Community Care*, Longman, London

McMurray, A. (1993) *Community Health Nursing: Primary Health Care in Practice*, 2nd edn, Churchill Livingstone, Melbourne

NHSME (1993) *The A–Z of Quality: A Guide to Quality Initiatives in the NHS*, Department of Health, London

13

Health at home

Barbara Roberts

● **Introduction**

Although at least 90% of all health care in the UK is carried out at home or, at least, outside large institutions (Baggott, 1994), it is interesting that so little has been written about the home as a context of care. This chapter therefore considers the concept of home and the provision of care by family and other carers, followed by a discussion on whether clients have a choice about their place of care. The health care needs of specific groups are explored and some special schemes for home care are introduced. Finally, the role of the community health care nurse in the provision of care in the home is addressed.

● **Home**

Carboni (1990) describes home as being more than a physical environment – it is also an experience that emerges from many complex relationships between the individual and his environment. The concept of the home has a particular meaning for each individual, which will vary with the person's experience. The concept of home should be considered as a whole, and cannot be broken down into parts without losing some of the sense or meaning of the whole. Home is unique to each person, and not necessarily consistent with the physical surroundings. How a person perceives home will depend largely on expectations, experience and social influences. Where one makes one's home is very much dependent on socio-economic and political influences, with many individuals having little choice.

Carboni (1990) sees home and homelessness on a continuum: at one extreme is home, where a strong relationship exists between the individual and the environment; at the other end of the continuum she sees homelessness, where the relationship between the individual and the environment is tenuous and severely damaged (see Chapter 17 for detail on the concept of homelessness).

For example, because of the multiplicity of losses that older people suffer in terms of physical, social, economic and impairment or severance of their relationship with the environment, it is suggested that the residential or nursing home in no way represents home. In fact, at the extreme it may represent homelessness, with all the attributes of insecurity, non-personhood, placelessness, disconnectedness, powerlessness and lack of choices. This is an important concept to consider, as frequently people entering residential care are told that this is a good alternative to home or, indeed, that this is now 'home'. It is important to recognize the losses such a move may incur if effective management of the move into such an environment is lacking.

Home is a place that people have usually known for many years before the majority of practitioners have contact with them. It may be a bed-sit, a flat in a high-rise block, or an owner occupied dwelling. The community health care nurse has to see beyond the building and to get some indication of the lifestyle of the individuals. This may be done by not only observing the environment but also by analysing the dynamics between those living together or visiting the home. The home may be full of treasures, a place of pride, a place of rest and retreat, a place of hospitality to others. There may be animals, a garden, grandchildren and friends may visit. However, the home may have none of these things, but this does not necessarily mean that it is a place of loneliness and isolation. Conversely, the outsider may see the leafy suburb but not recognize the situation as described by Glancey (1994):

> *a house, a lawn, nice neighbours, but for the women left there during the day, the suburban dream has become a nightmare of isolation.*

Flaskerud (1980) describes cultural variations as those occurring wherever a group of people remains isolated from the majority of society as a result of discrimination, geography or choice. This is in addition to cultural differences that may be the result of regional, religious, urban/rural, occupational or social class factors. Individuals are not always aware of their stereotyping, but Cameron *et al.* (1988), in research carried out in the city of Birmingham, describe the stereotype and myth that give rise to the assumption that black elders are cared for by the extended family.

The attributes that make a living place a home can inform practitioners about the lifestyle of the individual and are an essential component to planning sensitive needs led care in the home.

Family

The relationships that make a house a home revolve to a greater or lesser degree around the family or close friends. In the early 1980s, authors such as Clark (1984) still quoted the family as being the basic social unit despite major societal changes; however, she indicated that the technological and sociological changes that have provided the impetus for alternative lifestyles probably lead to the need for a redefinition of family.

Orr (1992) notes that the idea that families should care for their needy such as handicapped and elderly is not new; what is new is the return to the vision of the family unit and home as the desirable place for care, not necessarily because it is best but because it will soon be the main, if not the only, place for many people in line with the proposals of the NHS and Community Care Act (DoH, 1990a). Professional community workers must therefore use the home as the focus for their endeavour. Indeed, Florence Nightingale, in a letter to H. Bonham Carter, 4 July 1867 (Baly, 1986), wrote:

> *My view, you know, is that the ultimate destination of all nursing care is the caring of the sick in their own homes. . . . But it is no use to talk about the year 2000.*

All this implies that there is a family but, as McMurray (1993) argues, many families in the developed world find themselves in the process of questioning and redefining their role in contemporary society and this has very strong implications for the health care professionals attempting to guide them. The most dramatic changes in family described by Eastman (1989), and since shown in the annual national statistics collected by the Central Statistics Office (CSO), have included the escalating rates of divorce, the blending of families through remarriage, a decline in those choosing to marry, marriage being delayed and small numbers of children.

For example, statistics drawn from the CSO *Annual Abstract of Statistics* (CSO, 1994a) show for the UK:

	Single ('000)	Married ('000)	Divorced ('000)	Widowed ('000)
1971	12014	13976	200	762
1981	11860	13563	606	749
1991	12306	13071	1149	818

Source: Central Statistics Office.

- the number of marriages in 1990 was 375 410 compared with 418 446 in 1980, including remarriages
- the number of divorces per 1000 couples in 1990 was 12.9 compared with 12.0 in 1980.

Another CSO publication, *Social Trends* (1994b), gives further information:

- more than a quarter of households in 1991 consisted of one person living alone – this is almost double the proportion in 1961
- there were over 5 people, on average, living in each Bangladeshi household, this being more than twice the average for all ethnic groups
- of the 7 million mothers with dependent children in 1991, just over 1 million were lone parents
- nearly 1 in 5 unmarried men and women aged 15–59 were cohabiting in 1992
- for every two marriages in the UK in 1991 there was one divorce

- over the past decade, the proportion of births outside marriage has more than doubled to almost 1 in every 3 births in 1992 – three-quarters of these were registered with both parents being named.

The traditional definition of family brings to mind the nuclear family composed of mother, father and children. However, as Orr (1992) contends and as clearly indicated from the statistics above, the nuclear family can no longer be viewed as the norm and by implication therefore all other groupings should not be measured by this standard.

Friedmann (1986), in redefining family in American society, argues that it needs to allow a variety of heterosexual and homosexual partnerships and communal arrangements to be accepted. In the UK it is increasingly common for groups of people related by birth and marriage to be separated by geographical and social distance.

In view of these constantly changing dynamics of family life and thus the constitution of 'home' for individuals, it is as McMurray (1993) states imperative that nurses working with families gain an appreciation of the changes confronting the family in today's society and issues which society must deal with as a consequence.

As stated earlier, the majority of health care is carried out within the home and the people who take the major responsibility for this are the carers, and their role and needs are now considered.

Carers

Who are the carers?
The Carers' National Association (1988) defines a carer as

anyone whose life is in some way restricted because of the need to take responsibility for the care of a person who is mentally handicapped, physically disabled or whose health is impaired by sickness or old age.

Significant words in this definition are *restricted* and *responsibility*. Twigg *et al.* (1990), in reviewing the research on carers and services, noted that the point is frequently made that many carers do not recognize themselves as such, the term is unfamiliar to them, and they found some would argue that the term is at odds with how they perceive their actions. These carers regard what they do as an extension of family or personal relationships rather than in terms of being a carer with its formal, quasi-employment overtones. This again shows the need to treat each situation with clients and carers as unique and to identify their perceptions and needs.

In May 1986 a debate on carers was held in the House of Commons. In summing up, the then Minister for Social Security said:

In the past, the people about whom we have been talking have had inadequate recognition ... such people are worthy not only of the admiration that has been expressed by every honourable member who has spoken but the support of the whole community for what they do.

Griffiths (1988), in developing the plans for community care, asserted that the first task of public services was to support carers and that service providers should start by identifying such actual and potential carers, consulting them about their needs and those of the people they are caring for.

Statistics about the number of carers vary, but the most comprehensive figures are those collected in the General Household Survey in 1985 (OPCS, 1989a). This provided, for the first time, information from a nationally representative sample about the extent and nature of informal care in the community, and the characteristics of carers and their dependants. These showed that approximately 6 million people in Britain were, at that time, carers. An update of some of the factors was included in the 1990 census and this suggested an increase of 15% since 1985 to 6.8 million carers, of whom 2.9 million were men and 3.9 million women. A more recent report from the Carers' National Association (1994), while not a full survey, indicates that the numbers involved in caring are increasing, which is inevitable with the increasing numbers of elderly and the philosophy of community care. This survey also showed that the concern of the carers is still as acute as ever. Twigg (1992) disputes the General Household Survey figures and states that these are an overestimate, but she distinguishes between *informal* and *main* carers. However, whatever statistics are used, the numbers are high and will never be an absolutely true representation as many will not identify themselves as carers.

The GHS (1985) statistics demonstrate that 4 out of 10 carers are men, thus breaking the stereotype of the female carers. The peak age for caring is 45–65 and therefore the lives of one-fifth of people in this age group are restricted by their caring responsibilities. Of the 6 million, 57% spent more than 20 hours per week providing care and had not had a break of more than 2 days since commencing giving this care. In addition, 25% had been caring for over 10 years. The data demonstrates there is no typical carer, caring is not exclusive to either sex, age, socio-economic status or racial group. Carers are ordinary people consisting of husbands, wives, partners, daughters, in-laws, parents, friends and neighbours. Young carers, that is those of school age, have become increasingly recognized as enduring a considerable burden of caring (Carers' National Association, 1993).

Identification of carers

A key problem is the identification of carers and this is a major responsibility for practitioners. A project in Croydon, planned by the London Boroughs Training Committee (1988), discussed the problem of identifying carers and found four key reasons for this phenomenon:

- professionals may fail to identify carers because their focus is the person being cared for and the carer's role is not recognized
- carers may fail to identify themselves through feelings of pride or independence or simply not knowing that such a role exists or applies to them

- isolation, that is, carers may not come into contact with the people, organizations or information that might help them to define what is happening to them
- gender role – the cultural expectations that wives and daughters will perform the caring role may lead to women not identifying themselves as carers

Carers' needs

The Carers' National Association (1994) developed a carers' code containing eight key principles which should underpin good practice for health and social care personnel working with carers. These principles, providing benchmarks against which to measure the services available to carers, are as follows:

1. Recognition that carers have rights of their own and that services should be tailored to their individual needs. Furthermore, professionals should acknowledge that carers possess expertise and skills which are complementary to professional knowledge.
2. Choice of whether to become or remain a carer and about how much and what care to provide.
3. Equity: access to services regardless of gender, culture, age, sexual orientation, race or disability.
4. Consultation through representation, participation and action, thereby developing a voice for carers.
5. Information provided in an open and honest fashion before, during and after caring.
6. Practical help that is assessed using timely, well-thought-out and accessible assessment procedures that focus on carer-specific services, with such services being flexible and available when required.
7. Minimize the cost of caring by ensuring that carers receive all the benefits to which they are entitled and by keeping charges for services to a minimum.
8. Co-ordinated services to ensure that agencies work together and communicate effectively so that hospital discharge procedures involve carers at all stages. Also, voluntary and private sector agencies need to be involved in planning and service development.

Many carers and/or dependants have written about their experience of caring. *Sweet Adeline: A Journey through Care*, written by Adeline's daughter and son-in-law (Slack and Mulville, 1988), provides an example of the good and the bad times in caring for a frail mentally confused lady, and the novel *Have the Men had Enough?* (Forster, 1989), based on factual experiences, gives further insight into the needs of carers and those cared for. Although not all negative experiences, the majority of carers suffer stress to a greater or lesser degree and it is a responsibility of all agencies to consider means of reducing this stress.

Stress in carers

The consequences of not providing help and support to carers need to be considered. A 1990 survey by Crossroads using a sample of 790 found the following:

- 1 in 20 admitted they had been violent to their dependants
- nearly half said they were at breaking point
- 13% often felt like being violent
- 23% often felt hate
- 5 had seriously contemplated suicide
- 54 had given up full-time work
- 60% had been caring for more than 5 years.

This survey only touched the tip of the iceberg in terms of numbers of carers. If the above facts are extrapolated across 6 million carers, some indication of the burden imposed on carers can be contemplated.

Nolan (1993) identified significant factors causing stress in carers. Interestingly, he found that stress was not correlated with performing major activities of daily living, the presence of incontinence or confusion. His findings showed the significant factors for stress to be:

- carer's response to the caring situation
- the nature of the carer–dependant relationship
- the perceived adequacy of family support
- the carer's financial situation.

A study by the Carers' National Association (1992) showed that out of a sample of 2916, 65% of carers reported their health had been adversely affected. In addition, King (1993) says

The tightrope of suppressed emotion which carers must walk every day makes them easy scapegoats for society's growing problem of elder abuse.

Support of carers

Carers must therefore be supported to relieve their stress and to make their caring role easier. This is an important role for practitioners. The Department of Health Policy Guidance (DoH, 1991a) directly encourages the statutory authorities to consider the views of 'informal carers' when carrying out assessments of older or disabled people. The overall provision of care is seen to be a shared responsibility, with the relationship between the carers and the statutory authorities being one of mutual support.

The GHS (1985) found that one-third of all carers received no help from statutory or voluntary agencies. This was endorsed by Nolan and Grant (1989) who also found that addressing the needs of carers is a neglected area of nursing practice. They found that most services for carers are based on expediency and more often than not designed to maintain their caring role rather than addressing their wider needs. Atkinson (1992) considered that there is scope for practitioners to make greater contribution to the support of carers. These comments about nursing, could, no doubt, equally apply to other statutory health and social services.

Costs of caring

Glendenning (1992) cites work undertaken by the Family Policy Studies Unit in 1989 which, using the GHS (1985) data, put the value of the help given by those caring for more than 20 hours per week at between £11.5 billion and £15.2 billion, a considerable saving on public expenditure by the largely unpaid and uncosted work of those involved in providing 'informal' care. Indeed, Glendenning (1992) cites research that demonstrates that community care is both cheaper and a more effective alternative to residential or institutional care. This is because the costs of care being considered are only the public expenditure costs and not the costs incurred by the carer and/or the patient.

Netten (1993) argues that the contribution of the carers needs to take account of costs both to the carers and to society as a whole. She highlights five types of costs:

- direct financial expenditures on goods and service
- non-waged time
- waged time
- future costs
- accommodation.

The costs of caring cannot be measured in current financial terms only. Indeed, having to give up work, take part-time work or have considerable time off may have an adverse influence on job prospects for the carer. Carers also suffer from a loss of personal space and privacy.

The House of Commons Social Services Committee (1990) noted that within the current social security system the income replacement system considered essential for pensioners and disabled people does not operate for carers. For the first time this issue is being addressed and some financial allowances are now available for carers. It is therefore essential that community health care nurses are aware of current benefits and ensure carers have this knowledge.

Provision of support

The voluntary sector

A wide range of organizations, groups and individuals provide valuable help and support for carers. There are national organizations such as the Carers' National Association and many local groups providing carers' groups, befriending schemes, listening services, day care and a variety of other activities to meet the local, specific needs of different carers and those they care for. It is important that the community health care nurse identifies such groups within the locality to enable relevant support and advice to be provided.

The NHS and Community Care Act (DoH, 1990a) states that local authorities must consult voluntary organizations which appear to represent the interests of persons who use or are likely to use any community care services within that locality. The Department of Health Policy Guidance (DoH, 1991a), on the implementation of community care under the Act, stipulates that Social Services should contract out 85% of their home care services to the independent and voluntary sectors.

However, the notion of voluntary is often seen to imply 'do-gooders', and sometimes it is more appropriate to use the term non-statutory to give a clearer understanding of the organization. Handy (1988) records that there are over 150 000 registered charities in the UK and over 350 000 voluntary organizations of all types. He described various types of organizations – service providers, research and advocacy, self-help groups, mutual interest groups, and intermediary bodies. Many obviously span these divisions.

Crossroads care

Crossroads provides an example of a non-statutory UK organization and will be used to demonstrate how the voluntary sector can support carers of people of all age groups. This is primarily a service delivery organization which, using Handy's (1988) definitions, exists to meet a need and to provide help to those who need it. It takes pride not only in being professional, effective and low cost but also in being selective in recruits and demanding in standards.

The Association of Crossroads Care Attendants Schemes Limited started its first scheme in 1973 with the aims to relieve stress in the family and to avoid admission to hospital of the disabled should a breakdown occur in the family. There are now over 200 schemes in the UK, with others also in Holland. It is a national organization with local autonomous schemes. Although it includes all age groups within its remit, the 1992–93 annual statistics showed that 50% of clients were over the age of 50.

Schemes are managed by a voluntary management committee who are Trustees and care is provided through co-ordinators and care attendants who are paid employees. The key aims remain the same, but over the years the work has escalated from being a voluntary organization with all that entails in terms of fund-raising, to most schemes now receiving their major funding from Social Services under the terms of the NHS and Community Care Act (DoH, 1990a). So, as Handy (1988) points out, it is increasingly like a business and therefore requires structured organization and management. Since staff are appointed for the hours that meet carers needs, flexibility of the organization is required. In a survey undertaken on behalf of Crossroads in 1986, it was found that contrary to popular belief and prejudice, carers need only a very minimal amount of support, but the help had to be at times requested by individuals and agreed with the staff. It also had to be ongoing, reliable and flexible. As one carer said:

I can rely on Crossroads coming at an agreed time and I am able to plan for that day.

Care attendants are carefully selected for their understanding of the philosophy of the scheme and their adaptability, and in the early days of the scheme were described as a hybrid between a nursing auxiliary and a home help. With the increased dependence of the elderly and disabled in the community, the skills of the care attendants are being developed to take on more sophisticated tasks. Indeed, there have been times when the suitability of tasks for a care attendant has been challenged by nurses, yet for many hours a day, seven days a week, 52 weeks of the year, these tasks are undertaken by carers with little or no training. Practitioners have to analyse nursing practice and determine what must be done by a nurse and what can, in appropriate circumstances, be equally well be done by the carer and/or care attendant.

Crossroads has been used to provide one example of the role of a voluntary organization providing help and support to carers and their dependants, thus alleviating some of the stress of caring described earlier. However, there are many other organizations that could equally have been used to describe the need for the statutory and voluntary sectors to work alongside one another, complementing each other's work.

The challenge to all health care professionals and to community health care nurses in particular is to recognize the needs of carers and to determine who are the best people to provide care and support for them and their dependants. True partnership requires imaginative planning between statutory and voluntary services, and with the carer and cared for being fully involved – to achieve this practitioners must acknowledge the contribution of non-professionals.

Respite care

Strang and Neufeld (1990) define respite care as planned, inter-mittent, short-term care that is designed to provide periodic relief to the family and care-giver. They propose that respite care can be considered an illness prevention and health promotion activity for both care-givers and for persons dependent on them. The purpose of respite care is to prevent the breakdown of carers and to promote their quality of life. A report from the House of Commons Social Services Committee (1990), *Community Care: Carers*, stated that adequate and appropriate respite care is perhaps the single biggest need for carers. The Carers' National Association (1992) found that 20% of carers had never taken a break from their caring activities and 75% of carers felt the need for more help which 38% of this sample felt should come from respite services.

The NHS and Community Care Act 1990 states that enabling people to live independently in their own homes requires a broad range of support services and close co-ordination of health and social services. The demand for respite and domiciliary care is likely to increase if more people are cared for in the community. An Office of Population Censuses and Surveys study (OPCS, 1989b) found that the main service valued by carers was respite care, which ranged from admission to hospital for periods of up to two weeks to occasional visits in clients' own homes. An important finding of the study was that people wanted choice and would prefer respite care at home.

A survey of respite care carried out by the (then) Spastics Society and the RCN (1993) described the absence of choice and flexibility in the provision of respite care services. They found various types of respite care which included clients with private families, small cottage hospitals, respite units, residential/nursing homes, night sitting and day care.

The Spastics Society/RCN study listed the value of respite care as follows:

For clients	For carers
Encouraged to be more independent	Time to relax without feeling
Opportunity to air feelings to	guilty
someone else	Time to rest
Can feel a burden to carers, so want	Be themselves
to provide them with a break	Avoid burnout
Relief from dominant carer	Helps to keep going
Chance for reassessment	

However, the report also highlights that respite care can have disadvantages in that it may upset the client, and in particular that the carer frequently cannot 'let go' continuing the visit, so negating the benefits of a period of respite. Homer and Gilleard (1994) found that dependent older people are admitted to hospital for respite care in order to give their carers a break, despite there being little evidence of any benefit of such care for either the carers or the patients. Out of 77 carers in their study, 39 experienced significant emotional distress during the respite period and most did not show any significant improvement in their physical state. Many carers visited the relative regularly, despite being encouraged to stay away, and many felt guilty about using respite services. The clients, however, in this study revealed a significant reduction in overall dependency during the respite stay, with a marked reduction in physical disability and social disturbance. Perhaps not surprisingly, the greatest improvement in function was achieved by those with the most stressed carers, but those with dementia did not show this significant improvement. In spite of the problems, most of the carers felt that respite care was worth while but wanted different respite, for example, day care or sitter services. There is an obvious need for more research into the effects of respite care.

Smith (1994) discusses the situation of respite care for older people with learning disability and their carers. As these people survive into older age they may outlive their carers. This research in Scotland shows how this group of older people are being cared for within specialist services rather than in services for older people because of the need for the specialist knowledge. Respite care needs to develop to help with the inevitable transition from parental care to another form of care.

Day care

George (1993) describes the enormous variation in the availability of day care services between different localities. Overall he highlights a lack of suitable day care services. Rickford (1993) reports that English Social Service Departments supported nearly 117 000 day care places in 1991. This figure had grown by 25% over the previous decade in response to demographic change and the closure of long-stay NHS facilities for all adult client groups. She stresses that there is still a large shortfall related to need. She further highlights the dearth of places for those with a learning disability leaving about 20 000 people without a day care place. However, Rickford (1993) cites examples of alternative ways of providing day support for the disabled which, dependent upon client need, may include work experience, education facilities and access to leisure activities.

George (1993) considers the role of day hospitals and sees them as providing short-term physical rehabilitation programmes. Clients then may well need to be transferred to another form of day care. One topic that is always raised when looking at day care services is the problem of transport. This may be provided through social services or by voluntary agencies. Cameron (1993) describes two projects carried out into the needs of carers of those attending a day hospital. These showed that carers shouldered a heavy burden of care both physically and emotionally. They also confirmed previous studies by Nolan and Grant (1989) and Wade (1991) that many carers are unaware of the services available to them or of whom to contact concerning such services. This led Cameron to set up a carers' group at the day hospital. She planned the group by drawing on work by Atkinson and McHaffie (1992) which identified four areas in which carers constantly needed more support – information, skill training, emotional support and respite care. So, in this example both the dependent person and their carer are helped by services of the day hospital.

Rickford (1993) considers the variety of other day care facilities for the elderly which range from lunch clubs for the active elderly people to intensive personal support for the very frail and dependent. She enters a debate about funding of day care and cites a director of a social services department who points out that day care services can be funded more easily if they are provided through the voluntary or private sectors, as it is a requirement of the NHS and Community Care Act 1990 that 85% of the money must go to these sectors.

Once again these few examples of day care highlight the importance of practitioners exploring facilities in the locality in order to match the provision with the client need. Above all, the provision of appropriate day care will facilitate keeping people in their own homes by providing relief for the carers and a change for the person being cared for. However, the pitfalls of day care need to be recognized. For instance, a very confused person may find the change of environment to be distressing; the more mentally alert may get disillusioned with seemingly meaningless activity. It takes considerable creative planning to arrange day care that is appropriate for people with a range of physical, mental and emotional needs. The question may well need to be asked as to whether five days spent in day care and two at home is really preferable to being in permanent residential care, albeit not 'home'.

Although day care provides cost-effective provision for the government, the quality needs to be addressed. In addition, day care should be one of a range of options from which people choose according to their particular circumstances. Above all, clients and carers need to be involved in expressing their needs and choosing between alternatives for care.

● Choice

The White Paper *Caring for People* (DHSS, 1989a) states

Government's intentions for community care development describe the prospect for service development which could promote the independence of users, as well as securing for them greater control over their lives.

It also states that 'the decision to take on the caring role is never an easy one'. The *Policy Guidance* (DoH, 1991a) states

... the preferences of carers should be taken into account and their willingness to continue caring should not be assumed.

These statements suggest an element of choice for both the carer and the client, yet the study involving 2916 carers (Carers' National Association, 1992) showed that 79% of carers felt they had no choice.

Barnes (1992), discussing the professional relationship with clients, states that this requires partnership and negotiation, yet lack of flexibility denies patients the care they would choose at the times they would prefer. She argues that ceding control of situations to the patients and carers may be a painful process for the professional, but holding on to control denies the very people for whom professionals care the ability to make decisions and to control their lives.

Barnes (1992) cites criticism expressed by disabled people and their carers which frequently focuses on the inability or unwillingness of professionals to provide appropriate and flexible services. *A Framework for Local Community Care Charters in England* (DoH, 1994a) stresses the involvement of users and carers and in relation to service provision makes pertinent additions to *The Patient's Charter* (DoH, 1991c). The document states:

Appointment Times
There are nurses, health visitors and midwives working in the community. From April 1995, if you require a home visit from one of these professionals, you can expect to be consulted about a conveni-

ent time. You can then expect a visit within a two hour time band.
Exceptionally, your community nurse, health visitor or midwife may
be unable to make this appointment. In such cases, the community
nurse, health visitor or midwife should let you know and make
another appointment with you.

Although many community health care nurses have been working in this
way, for some it will require a more systematic way of organizing their
work. The key reasoning behind this requirement for appointment times
is for the client and carers to be able to plan their day.

Johnston and Brown (1993) contend that once clients have been
transferred home from hospital the power relationship should shift in
their favour. Some do not like the word 'client', preferring the label
'patient', whereas others use 'consumer'. Consumer implies active partnership with people exercising choice in health care. A more recently
introduced term is that of 'users' of the service which links with the
concept of advocacy and people's rights.

The introduction of *The Patient's Charter*, although not without its
critics or problems, has heightened awareness both among health service
users and health care providers of the overt need for acceptable standards
of care.

Caring for People (DHSS, 1989a) proposed that local authorities
would have the responsibility to purchase and manage packages of care
for people who are elderly, mentally ill, have learning disabilities, or are
disabled. The report argued that such vulnerable people and their carers
deserved greater choice in their care and, in particular, alternatives to
institutional care allowing people to be supported in their own home
should be provided.

Yeo (1993), in debating the implementation of the NHS and
Community Care Act 1990 said:

the reforms will bring a number of benefits to service users. They will
benefit from the wide options and flexibility that the new arrange-
ments will offer. Services will be tailored to need, rather than need to
services, so clients will have more control over their lives and a
greater say in what happens to them.

The principle directed under this Act that care will be co-ordinated by
one person is important. Carers have complained for many years about
the host of professionals entering their homes, asking the same questions
and rarely involving the client in the process.

Shields (1985) suggests that few inroads have been made in
psychiatric consumerism. He proposes three reasons why user views must
be sought:

• the moral reason because these are often vulnerable, anxious,
  frightened, unassertive, and inarticulate people
• the technological and economic reasons – that more effective
  treatments may be provided
• political reason – that democratic society must devolve power to
  the ordinary citizen.

Lindow (1990) similarly argues that a false notion of real choice is conveyed. In mental health terms he feels that people diagnosed and treated with a serious mental illness are seen as difficult to reach and incapable of making sensible decisions. Winkler (1987) advocates the partnership model and criticizes the frequent reinforcement of patronizing attitudes to vulnerable people. She argues that there is a danger of only listening to the articulate and assertive groups of users. But, as Davis (1991) asserts, consumers provide professionalists with a source of wisdom.

Booth (1994) discusses the implications of The Children Act (HMSO, 1989) and says that rights are at the heart of the Act and there is a necessity to obtain consent for examination when the child is able to make an informed choice. That leads to a debate on when does the child acquire sufficient understanding of the concepts of language. Franklin (1994), in discussing organ transplantation and children, suggests that the children themselves are often excluded from the discussion with professionals and parents making decisions in the belief that they know what is best for the child. Indeed, it is important when discussing client choice to include the carers within that choice. For example, the choice of one family member, the dependent person, may become a 'sentence' for the carer. Decisions also have to be made about what risks can be taken to give a person their choice – questions need to be asked about the safety of the person and their right to choose their actions. Client choice is a concept that all practitioners need to acknowledge as well as recognizing that this may involve them in a shift in the perception of their role and a change of power base.

● Families with special needs

Travellers

Travellers are an example of a group with special needs. Tyler (1993) describes travellers' access to basic health care provision as tragic. Surveys in the Kent region (Pahl and Vaile, 1993) reveal that the infant mortality rate among travellers is twice that of the settled community and some 75% of traveller children do not complete immunization courses. Travellers, they contend, face insurmountable problems in gaining access to the most basic services, particularly since the introduction of the GP Contract in 1992 and the need for the doctors to achieve health promotion targets. According to Tyler (1993), the problem is not so much one of how travellers choose to live their lives as the fact that providers and professionals involved in the provision of health care have been unwilling to respond to specific client needs, in particular greater and easier access and the follow-up of families.

Jones (1991) found that travellers rarely move from choice, but eviction was forcing them onto sites without clean water and proper sanitation. These conditions were responsible for ill health and early death. The 1991 reform of The Caravan Sites Act 1968 gives greater eviction powers and fewer official sites which will cause an increase in the movement of families and a return to unsuitable and unhealthy stopping places. Rose (1993) noted a change in the health of travellers since their being forced to settle on sites, with less exercise being taken and smoking becoming more common. When she first became involved with a group of these families, not only were immunization rates as low as 5% but children also missed the opportunity of developmental screening and mothers missed antenatal checks. By taking a health mobile to the travellers, in 5 years the immunization rate had risen to 95%. In addition, Jones (1991), describing a project working in partnership with the Save the Children charity involving a specialist health visitor working with the travelling families, highlights the paramount importance of a good relationship with the travelling community themselves.

● Home care of people with special needs

People with mental health problems

The closing of large psychiatric hospitals has stimulated the development of innovative services for people with severe mental health problems who previously would not have been cared for in the community. Gatula and Morris (1993) maintain that people with severe mental health problems can live in the community provided they receive the right support. They describe the work of one community rehabilitation home which is jointly managed by the local authority sector and the mental health unit of the local NHS Trust. The staff in the home, which is a house in an ordinary street known by its number like any other house, also provide support to residents in nearby group homes and to some in their own homes.

As Thomas (1993) states, patients become residents when outside the large institutions, and this requires staff to take on wider roles such as helping with cooking and cleaning, and also to cope with behavioural disturbances more openly in the community. However, as Gatula and Morris (1993) note, staff are more isolated and there may be initial difficulties for the residents with their new freedom, some having lived as long as 40 years in a large institution. Thomas (1993) recognizes that staff working in community homes are expected to reverse the sick role which residents have been encouraged to adopt in a residential institution. He also found, in his experience of working in a residential home in the community, that institutional practices can flourish there just as they did in the old institutions, particularly with entrenched staff who are custodial and resistant to change. There is an obvious need for staff to learn about new philosophies and modes of care, as indeed that is a need to increase public awareness, thus reducing resistance to people with mental health problems being their neighbours.

People with learning disabilities

McCormack (1992) describes the two extremes of situations facing a family who have a child with a learning disability – a son or daughter with learning disabilities can either be a mainly negative, or a positive, experience for these parents and family. Some gain inner strength from the caring involved, but sometimes for other the effects are detrimental.

The Social Services Inspectorate (1991) draws attention to the fact that the central feature of care management for the client group is the participation of the service user, families and carers throughout the process of enabling care to be provided in their own homes for as long as possible. Barr (1993) stresses that nurses need to pay closer attention to issues such as relationships, values and dynamics displayed by the families they are working with. They need to look at how these are integrated into the family's coping strategies if they are to work successfully alongside the person receiving care and his or her family. She shows how some parents cope and others cannot, but as McCormack (1992) says, even for those parents who appear to be coping well 'life never gets easy'. In addition, as previously mentioned Smith (1994) recognizes the problems that occur when people with learning difficulties survive into older age and outlive their carers. Alternatives to home care need to be discussed and tried before the situation occurs.

Children

Webb and Colson (1993) state that family-centred nursing of children implies either caring for the child or assisting a family member to care for the child who is developmentally healthy or may deviate from norms. This family-centred concept for care of the child is important to maintain whether the child is cared for in hospital or at home.

Well children

A large proportion of the work of the community health care nurse working in the field of health promotion and public health (health visiting) involves providing advice and reassurance to the parent(s) on child care, child behaviour, feeding and nutrition. Undertaking an initial assessment within the home is important to allow the practitioner to observe factors such as the home environment and dynamics which may affect the child's development. Subsequent contacts will frequently be made in a clinic setting; however, if a child is found not to be achieving his/her potential, visits may again be made to the child in the security of the home. In this way, child development can be noted and any deviations from the normal or any suspicion of the child being at risk recorded, as outlined in Chapter 19.

Vulnerable children

Home visits are invaluable in the assessment of any child whose development is considered not within normal limits or who is deemed to be at risk, since it is in the home setting that a true picture can be established. Luker and Orr (1992) give an example of focused work with families through the national Child Development Programme based at

Bristol University. This focuses on altering the human environment surrounding of the disadvantaged child during the early years of life. The NHSME (1993) gives information on home monitoring of infants at risk of sudden death syndrome. Schemes have also been developed to enable many infants who might otherwise have needed to stay in a neonatal unit to go home earlier. This has been to the advantage of both the babies and their parents. In addition, there are schemes which provide help for the physically and emotionally deprived child as well as those at risk in some way. An important factor in helping these children and their families is for the community health care nurses to have an insight into the home and the relationships therein.

Sick children

The idea that sick children should be cared for at home has been accepted since the Platt Report (Central Services Council, 1959), which stated that children should be admitted to hospital only if the care they required could not equally well be provided at home. The Court Report (DHSS, 1976) also identified children as a priority group for whom community and preventive care should be the main focus of care provision. *The Charter for Children in Hospital* (NAWCH, 1984) stated that children should only be admitted to hospital if care cannot be provided at home. These facts were further reinforced by the DoH (1991b), but until recent years the development of specialist teams to care for the sick child at home has been slow. Fradd (1993) reports that although in 1980 there were only 7 schemes in the UK, this had increased to 52 paediatric community nursing teams by 1992, with a further 30 teams caring for children with specific conditions such as diabetes and cancer. However the Audit Commission (1993) found that wide variations in hospital stays for children still exist and that many could be discharged earlier.

Catchpole (1989) lists benefits to the child of having intravenous therapy at home for treatment of cystic fibrosis. These benefits can be applied to any sick child being cared for at home. They are:

- reduced hospital admission
- continued schooling
- minimal disruption of family routine
- minimized cross-infection
- cost-effectiveness.

Hughes (1993) states that the partnership between a parent and nurse is widely accepted and its practice is increasing in paediatric services. Casey and Charles-Edwards (1992) point out the importance of allowing parents and children to make their own decisions. Parents should have a choice of shared management since some cope with procedures such as intravenous therapy at home, whereas others prefer this to be done in hospital. Whyte (1992), in a study analysing the experiences of four families caring for a child with cystic fibrosis, describes the experience of crises and the chronic burden of care.

The older person

An increasing amount of time is spent in the care of older people by the community health care nurse – this is both with the well elderly and with those who are sick. Luker (1982) attempted to evaluate the effect of health visiting intervention on a group of elderly women in Scotland. Interestingly, although up to 43% of health problems improved with intervention there was no clear improvement in life satisfaction and the elderly in the study generally saw the health visitor as someone to call in when they were ill or had a particular need, rather than as an agent of preventive health care who could give advice. This finding is supported by Victor and Vetter (1985) who describe many schemes for visiting the elderly at home and found a marked increase in the use of the health visiting service by elderly patients who had been discharged from hospital. This finding has implications for the service, with the trend for earlier hospital discharge or, indeed, preventing older people from being admitted to hospital.

Dunnell and Dobbs (1982) showed that 75% of the district nurses' time was spent with patients who were aged over 65. Victor and Vetter (1985) found that not only did health visitor visits increase following hospital discharge, but the district nurses' visits increased threefold compared to the period before hospitalization.

Blanchard et al. (1994), in a study of 96 people of pensionable age in Inner London, found that there is substantial hidden psychiatric morbidity among older people that requires identification and treatment. They suggest that the current annual health screening required from the age of 75 could be used to identify these depressed older people. This then poses the question of not only whether the early signs of depression would be more readily picked up in the home environment, but also who is the most appropriate practitioner to make this assessment?

People with chronic illness

Kratz (1978) found that chronic illness and long-term care are not necessarily synonymous; many people learn to cope with their illness without the help of others. Werner-Beland (1980) vividly describes the problems of continually living with chronic health problems and the associated problem of grief not only in the sick person but also in those closely involved. McMurray (1993) describes the long-term nature of some care in the community for those with chronic illness. The family, often the partner only, are called upon to provide extended periods of care and need to manage this care within the routine of the family. This may also require managing the visiting of a dependant in a nursing home which again disrupts family routine. As described earlier, this can impose an intolerable burden on the carers and the family need to adapt to the disruption for all the family which inevitably accompanies this care.

Coping with the long-term contact required by these families demands practitioners to use to the full their skills of relationships, provision of quality care and constant evaluation.

The terminally ill patient at home

Hector and Whitfield (1982) state that one of the great advantages for the patient with a terminal illness being cared for at home is the range of activity that can continue. At home the patient, family and nurse can consider the convenience of care, in particular patients' changing wishes and needs. The authors state that one of the greatest advantages of providing care at home for the dying person is the central role of the relative in care. However, it must be recognized that all relatives cannot cope with such a role and many patients who spend most of their terminal illness at home may go into hospital to die.

Indeed, Copperman (1983) noted that the majority of people die in a hospital or a hospice and questions whether the majority would really prefer to die in their own homes, surrounded by their own belongings, and with family and friends around them. However, she found that both patients and relatives were more frightened of the process of dying than of death itself and identifies the need for anticipation of these fears by practitioners. This is discussed in more detail in Chapter 22.

● **Special schemes for care at home**

Acute home health care

Various schemes have been developed which enable patients to be cared for at home in the acute stages of an illness when they are generally more dependent than normally appropriate for home care. This may be, for instance, in early stages following a stroke or following surgery such as hip fracture or hysterectomy. Such schemes were initially known as 'Hospital at Home' (HAH), but some of the newer schemes have titles such as 'intensive care in the community', 'rapid response' and others, as described by the NHSME (1993).

Mowat and Morgan (1982) describe the first HAH scheme developed in 1978 in the UK in Peterborough which at that time was the third fastest growing city in Europe. The scheme was based on the concept and framework developed in France in 1961. They suggested that, if adopted, generally shorter waiting lists and the use of fewer hospital beds would result. Few (1991) identifies the criteria for being cared for by HAHs as

● without HAH the patient would be admitted to, or remain in, hospital
● the consultant agrees with discharge from hospital
● the GP accepts medical responsibility
● the patient and carer wish it to happen.

The requirements for the scheme include the need for a 24-hour community nursing service with support from paramedics including occupational therapists and physiotherapists. Referral to the team may be from hospital, GP or specialist nurse.

Allen (1991) describes a pilot study in Peterborough where hysterectomy patients are admitted to HAH on the second postoperative day. Prior and Williams (1989), in a study of rehabilitation after hip fracture, have shown that patients return from their pre-traumatic state quicker by early discharge from hospital. Hollingsworth *et al.* (1993) reveal that cost analysis of early discharge after hip fracture shows that patients who were discharged early spent a mean of 11.5 days under HAH care. The total direct care cost to the health service was significantly less for those patients with access to early discharge than those with no early discharge option. The savings accrue largely from shorter stays in orthopaedic and geriatric wards. However, costs must not be seen as the only reasons for admitting someone to the HAH scheme. The HAH is in line with the government White Paper *Working for Patients* (DHSS, 1989b) since it offers patients and their carers a greater choice of service and therefore is responsive to client need.

The community health care nurse (district nurse) is the key worker in the HAH service and care is available for 24 hours. The team leader identifies the quantity and quality of care required and this is provided by the qualified community health care nurse and patient aides whom Allen (1991) describes as combining the role of community care assistant, nursing auxiliary and physiotherapy helper. Roper (1983) describes a new post in Rugby of 'supplementary nursing sister' (district nursing), mostly for those with terminal illness but also for those with chronic conditions. The purpose is to supplement care provide by the Primary Health Care Team and to allocate longer time with each patient.

The Audit Commission (1992) cites similar services, more recently developed in South Derbyshire and West Glamorgan. Other schemes quoted by Baker *et al.* (1987) include 'augmented' home care for acutely or sub-acutely ill elderly patients in Edinburgh and an innovative scheme in Norfolk involving local people as well as professionals. However, the HAH service in Peterborough is a good example of how an idea that started in one place can be replicated and developed in others using slightly different models to meet local need.

Liaison between hospital and home

Liaison which ensures a smooth transfer of care from one setting to another is essential and fits with the government's demands of a seamless service. This is of particular importance for vulnerable groups such as those people with long-term illness, terminal illness or children as well as those receiving day care. Without good liaison, 'seamless' care is not possible. Concern about the transfer of patients between hospital and home was first highlighted by Skeet (1970) when she showed that only a minority of patients on discharge from hospital received advice on medication, activity, diet and pain management. Further research has shown that similar problems continue to occur (Gay and Pitkeathley, 1979; Marks, 1994). Indeed, a report in 1994 shows that the discharge of patients into the community from London hospitals is in 'chaos' (GLACHC, 1994). This report gives illustrations of people being sent home without warning and carers being unaware that discharge was imminent. It provides a list of commonsense recommendations on discharge procedures for hospital staff, health authorities, local authorities, general practitioners and community health care nurses. The DoH (1994b) has also published checklists for hospital and community staff of core issues which must be addressed to check the effectiveness of the discharge process.

Waters (1987) emphasizes the continuous nature of discharge when she argues that the discharge process does not begin on the day a decision is made to send a patient home. Jewell (1993) stresses the need for a careful assessment of need and adequately arranged aftercare. She examines the process of discharge which facilitates the transition of the patient from one environment to another. She urges that community personnel enter the discharge process early, ideally with the discharge process starting on admission to hospital. It should also include patients and relatives as appropriate.

Worth *et al*. (1994) describe the increasing importance of careful discharge planning following the implementation of the NHS and Community Care Act (DoH, 1990a). They suggest that elderly patients are being discharged quicker and sicker which has implications for the amount and type of care for the community health care nurse. Farès (1993) stresses the need for nursing staff and social services to work closely together to provide patients with seamless care when they leave hospital.

Transfer is not only from hospital but also from community to hospital. This is generally not seen to be such a problem, yet for a person to leave a loved one in the unfamiliar hospital environment can provoke considerable anxiety. This is particularly true for a carer who provides care on a long-term basis. Shannon (1993) describes how when she has to take her physically and mentally disabled daughter to hospital, six pages of notes go with her. The notes describe in detail the care and routine her daughter is used to and requires. By doing this, Shannon's daughter gets care that is comparable to that she receives at home and her parents are more confident when leaving her. It is regrettable that many professionals do not encourage such an approach, as so much can be learned from the carer who normally provides care for 24 hours a day, seven days a week.

● **The contribution of the community health care nurse**

A person receiving care in hospital or indeed from the general practitioner is described as the patient. Johnston and Brown (1993) argue that patients in hospital are viewed as dependent, passive and usually sick, whereas in the community they are more commonly described as clients, with the power relationship shifts in their favour.

Freeman and Heinrich (1981) describe the visit by the community health care nurse as that of 'professional guest'. Barnes (1992) sees this professional relationship as an expression of the expertise and skill of the practitioner which focuses on a partnership with the individual and his/her carers. At the same time, practitioners must remain skilled professionals and exert sufficient influence to establish their own authority in respect of nursing care and advice for the client.

Andrews (1990) describes research into the nature and quantity of district nursing practice which highlights the complex and valuable skills of district nurses. High value is placed on the relationship between the nurse and the patient and the ability of district nurses to act as a friend as well as practitioner. The nurse is a guest, albeit usually a welcome guest, but nevertheless there may be a conflict of roles and the nurse needs to enable the relatives and patients to feel they remain in control of their own home.

McMurray (1992) describes research undertaken in Australia with 37 community health care nurses. The main aim was to identify the characteristics of expertise in community health management. She noted that the vast wealth of knowledge used by community health care nurses was in their interactions with clients. She concludes that they are required to

- judge an individual's capacity for self-care and self-monitoring
- understand individual functioning, family dynamics, patterns of human responses in the face of illness and disruption, and how emotional states either inhibit or potentiate health.

McMurray (1992) argues that this behavioural knowledge, together with the knowledge of health and illness and an understanding of social and economic conditions, forms the essential components of the community health care nurse's knowledge base for practice. An interesting finding was the value experts placed on using previous experiences to evaluate current situations. Benner and Tanner (1987) describe this as *deliberative rationality* which entails integrating the data in the present situation with memory of previous cases and trusting in their intuitive judgement.

Effective care in the home involves three phases – preparation, the visit and relevant documentation following the visit. The preparation, which includes being conversant with previously gathered data, referral information and medical information, allows the client to be more confident in the practice of the community health care nurse. These data will include an understanding of the community in which the client lives, including the social groups, networks and support. Community health care nurses need to undertake a profile of the community in which they work not only to develop a picture of the people who make up that community, but also other health, social and cultural needs, as well as the resources and services available to meet those needs (see Chapter 23). The practitioner must enter the home prepared to encounter a variety of situations, some of which will be totally unexpected. The final stage, post visit, involves documentation (UKCC, 1993) and relevant referrals.

The Audit Commission (1992) states:

The community health services meet the health care needs of people living at home that are beyond the scope of self-help, but do not require the centralised services of hospitals.

Although a rather idealistic statement, it perhaps provides a goal for practitioners to strive towards. Indeed, the developing role of the community health care nurse as outlined by the UKCC (1994) is that of expert clinician, team leader and care manager. The community health care nurse needs to acquire new knowledge and skills to meet the changing health needs of people at home, whether well or sick. The challenge to all community health care nurses is to provide, with others, optimum care with the available resources.

● **Conclusion**

This chapter has explored some of the attributes that make a living place into a home. Some of the people who provide care in the home have been identified, with particular emphasis being laid on the role and needs of the informal carers. With the increasing numbers of people being cared for at home, following the implementation of the NHS and Community Care Act (DoH, 1990a), the contribution of the community health care nurse in the management of health care at home assumes greater importance. The UKCC (1994) proposals for the post-registration education of the community health care nurse will ensure that the practitioner has the necessary knowledge and skill to undertake this demanding yet fulfilling role. The Chief Nursing Officers in the UK, in taking a visionary look at the health services and the contribution of nursing in the year 2010 (Chief Nursing Officers, 1994), state:

> It is envisaged that more will be done in families and the general community to maintain health. More people will care about their health and be willing to take control. Home care, supported by peripatetic staff, telemonitoring and portable equipment, will be commonplace. More births will occur at home. When people look to expert help the greater part of their care needs will be met by general (family) care teams.

All community health care nurses need to be prepared to meet these challenges.

References

Allen, L. (1991) The manager's view. In *Hospital at Home. A Selection of Conference Papers*, District Nursing Association, Edinburgh

Andrews, S. (1990) Nurse you are wonderful. *Journal of Distric Nursing*, **9**(3), 16–23

Atkinson, F.I. (1992) Experiences of informal carers providing nursing support for disabled independents. *Journal of Advanced Nursing*, **17**, 835–840

Atkinson, I. and McHaffie, H. (1992) Shared cares. *Health Services Journal*, **102**(5302), 24–25

Audit Commission (1992) *Homeward Bound: A New Course for Community Health*, HMSO, London

Audit Commission (1993) *Children First: A Study of Hospital Services*, HMSO, London

Baker, G., Bevan, J.M., McDonnell, L. *et al*. (1987) *Community Nursing: Research and Recent Developments*, Croom Helm, London

Baggott, R. (1994) *Health and Health Care in Britain*, Macmillan, London

Baly, M.E. (1986) *Florence Nightingale: the Nursing Legacy*, Croom Helm, Kent

Barnes, E. (1992) District nurses fail patients over appointment times. *British Journal of Nursing*, **1**(13), 640

Barr, O. (1993) Caring teams. *Nursing Times*, **89**(35), 58

Benner, P. and Tanner, C. (1987) How expert nurses use intuition. *American Journal of Nursing*, **87**, 23–31

Blanchard, M.R., Waterreus, A. and Mann, A. (1994) The nature of depression among older people in inner London and the contact with primary health care. *British Journal of Psychiatry*, **164**, 396–402

Booth, B. (1994) A guiding act. *Nursing Times*, **90**(8), 30–31

Cameron, E., Badger, F. and Evers, H. (1988) Old, needy – and black. *Nursing Times*, **84**(2), 38–40

Cameron, S. (1993) The group that cares. *British Journal of Nursing*, **2**(18), 909–910

Carboni, J.T. (1990) Homelessness among the institutionalised elderly. *Journal of Gerontological Nursing*, **16**(7), 32–37

Carers' National Association (1988) *Publicity Leaflet*, CNA, London

Carers' National Association (1992) *Speak Up, Speak Out*, CNA, London

Carers' National Association (1993) *Annual Report 1992–1993*, CNA, London

Carers' National Association (1994) *Community Care: Just a Fairy Tale*, CNA, London

Casey, A. and Charles-Edwards, I. (1992) Parental involvement and voluntary consent. *Paediatric Nurse*, **4**(1), 16–18

Catchpole, A. (1989) Cystic fibrosis: IV treatments at home. *Nursing Times*, **85**(12), 40–42

Central Health Services Council (1959) *The Welfare of Children in Hospital* (Platt Report), HMSO, London

Chief Nursing Officers (1994) *The Challenges for Nursing and Midwifery in the 21st Century (The Heathrow Debate)*, Department of Health, London

Clark, M.J.D. (1984) *Community Nursing: Health Care for Today and Tomorrow*, Prentice-Hall, Virginia

Copperman, H. (1983) *Dying at Home*, John Wiley, Chichester

Crossroads (1986) *Cause for Concern*, Crossroads, Rugby

Crossroads (1990) *Caring for Carers – A Survey*, Crossroads, Rugby

CSO (1994a) *Annual Abstract of Statistics – Number 130*. HMSO, London

CSO (1994b) *Social Trends 24*, HMSO, London

Davis, A. (1991) User's perspective. In *Psychiatry in Transition* (ed S. Ramon), Pluto Press, London

DHSS (1976) *Fit for the Future: Report of the Committee on Child Health Services* (Court Report), Cmd. 6684, HMSO, London

DHSS (1989a) *Caring for People: Community Care in the Next Decade and Beyond*, Cmd. 849, HMSO, London

DHSS (1989b) *Working for Patients*, Cmd 555, HMSO, London

DoH (1990a) *The NHS and Community Care Act*, HMSO, London

DoH (1990b) *Community Care in the Next Decade and Beyond: Policy Guidance*, HMSO, London

DoH (1991a) *Caring for People – Policy Guidance*, HMSO, London

DoH (1991b) *Guidelines on the Welfare of Children and Young People in Hospital*, HMSO, London

DoH (1991c) *The Patient's Charter*, HMSO, London

DoH (1994a) *A Framework for Local Community Care Charters in England*, Department of Health, London

DoH (1994b) *The Hospital Discharge Workbook: A Manual of Hospital Discharge Policy and Practice*, Department of Health, London

Dunnell, K. and Dobbs, J. (1982) *Nurses Working in the Community*, OPCS, London

Eastman, M. (1989) *Family: The Vital Factor*, Collins Dove, Melbourne

Farès, S. (1993) A smooth path home. *Nursing Times*, **89**, 21

Few, S. (1991) The district nurses's view. In *Hospital at Home. A Selection of Conference Papers*, District Nurse Association, Edinburgh

Flaskerud, J.H. (1980) Perception of problematic behaviour by Appalacians, mental health professionals and lay non-Appalacians. *Nursing Research*, **29**, 140–149

Forster, M. (1989) *Have the Men had Enough?* Penguin, Middlesex

Fradd, E. (1993) Meeting a need. *Nursing Times*, **89**(39), 36–37

Franklin, P. (1994) Straight talking. *Nursing Times*, **90**(8), 33–34

Freeman, R.B. and Heinrich, J. (1981) *Community Health Nursing Practice*, W.B. Saunders, Philadelphia

Friedmann, M. (1986) *Family Nursing: Theory and Assessment*, 2nd edn, Appleton Century Crofts, Norwalk, Conn.

Gatula, D. and Morris, I. (1993) Learning independence. *Nursing Times*, **89**(32), 58–60

Gay, P. and Pitkeathly, J. (1979) *When I Went Home: A Study of Patients Discharged from Hospital*, King's Fund, London

George, M. (1993) Honing support. *Nursing Standard*, **7**(20), 20–21

GLACHC (1994) *London Hospitals – Discharging their Responsibility*, Greater London Association of Community Health Councils, London

Griffiths, R. (1988) Chairman. *Community Care: Agenda for Action*, HMSO, London

Handy, C. (1988) *Understanding Voluntary Organisations*, Penguin, Middlesex

Hector, W. and Whitfield, S. (1982) *Nursing Care for the Dying Patient and the Family*, Heinemann, London

HMSO (1989) *The Children Act – Guidance and Regulation*, HMSO, London

Hollingsworth, W., Todd, C., Parker, M. *et al*. (1993) Cost analysis of early discharge after hip fracture. *British Medical Journal*, **307**, 903–906

Homer, A.C. and Gilleard, C.J. (1994) The effect of inpatient respite care on elderly patients and their carers. *Age and Ageing*, **23**(4), 274–276

House of Commons Social Services Committee (1990) *Community Care: Carers*, 5th Report, House of Commons Paper 410, Session 1989–90, HMSO, London

Hughes, S. (1993) Meeting a need. *Nursing Times*, **89**(39), 36–37

Jewell, S.E. (1993) Discovery of the discharge process: a study of patient discharge from a care unit for elderly people. *Journal of Advanced Nursing*, **18**, 1288–1296

Johnston, C. and Brown, K. (1993) *Community Health Care, London*. Macmillan Magazines, London

Jones, V. (1991) *An Inter-agency Model*, Walsall District Health Authority, Walsall

King, J. (1993) Walking a tightrope. *Community Care*, 24 June

Kratz, C. (1978) *Care of the Long-term Sick in the Community*, Churchill Livingstone, Edinburgh

Lindow, V. (1990) A consumer's view. *Openmind*, No. 47, London

London Boroughs Training Committee (1988) *Action for Carers: A Guide to Multidisciplinary Support at Local Level*, Training Package, LBTC, London

Luker, K. (1982) *Evaluating Health Visiting Practice*, Royal College of Nursing, London

Luker, K. and Orr, J. (1992) *Health Visiting: Towards Community Health Nursing*, 2nd edn, Blackwell, Oxford

McCormack, M. (1992) *Special Children, Special Needs. Families Talk about Mental Handicap*, Thorson, London

McMurray, A. (1992) Expertise in community health nursing. *Journal of Community Health Nursing*, **9**(2), 65–75

McMurray, A. (1993) *Community Health Nursing. Primary Health Care in Practice*, 2nd edn, Churchill Livingstone, Melbourne

Marks, L. (1994) *Seamless Care or Patchwork Quilt? Discharging Patients from Acute Hospital Care*, King's Fund Centre, London

Mowat, I.G. and Morgan, R.T. (1982) Peterborough Hospital and Home scheme. *British Medical Journal*, **284**, 641–643

NAWCH (1984) *The Charter for Children in Hospital*, National Association for the Welfare of Children in Hospital, London

Netten, A. (1993) Costing informal care. In *Costing Community Care: Theory and Practice* (eds A. Netten and J. Beecham), University of Kent, Canterbury

NHSME (1993) *The A–Z of Quality: A Guide to Quality Initiatives in the NHS*, Department of Health, London

Nolan, M. (1993) Carer-dependant relationships and the prevention of elder abuse. In *The Mistreatment of Elderly People* (eds P. Decalmer and F. Glendenning), Sage Publications, London

Nolan, M. and Grant, G. (1989) Addressing the needs of informal carers: a neglected area of nursing practice. *Journal of Advanced Nursing*, **14**, 950–961

OPCS (1989a) *General Household Survey (1985) – Supplement on Informal Carers*, HMSO, London

OPCS (1989b) *Disabled Adults: Services, Transport and Employment*, HMSO, London

Orr, J. (1992) *Health Visiting: Towards Community Health Nursing*, 2nd edn (K. Luker and J. Orr), Blackwell, Oxford

Pahl, J. and Vaile, M. (1986) *Health and Health Care among Travellers*, University of Kent and Canterbury, Kent

Prior, G.A. and Williams, D.R. (1989) Rehabilitation after hip fracture – home and hospital management compared. *British Medical Journal*, **71**(3), 471–474

Rickford, F. (1993) Conflicting interests. *Community Care*, 12 August

Roper, M. (1983) District nurse plus. *Journal of District Nursing*, **1**, 8

Rose, V. (1993) On the road. *Nursing Times*, **89**(33), 31

Shannon, J. (1993) How can I leave my child with strangers? *The Carer*, November

Shields, P. (1985) The consumer's view of psychiatry. *Hospital and Health Services Review*, pp. 117–119

Skeet, M. (1970) *Home from Hospital*, 4th edn, Macmillan Journals, London

Slack, P. and Mulville, F. (1988) *Sweet Adeline: A Journey through Care*, Macmillan, London

Smith, K. (1994) A lifetime for opportunity. *Nursing Times*, **90**(44), 14–15

Social Services Inspectorate (1991) *Care Management and Assessment Managers Guide*, HMSO, London

Spastics Society/RCN (1993) *Day in, Day out. A Survey of Views of Respite Care*, Royal College of Nursing, London

Strang, V. and Neufeld, A. (1990) Adult day care programs. A source for respite. *Journal of Gerontological Nursing*, **11**, 16–19

Thomas, A. (1993) No room for change. *Nursing Times*, **89**(16), 34–36

Twigg, J. (ed.) (1992) *Carers: Research and Practice*, HMSO, London

Twigg, J., Atkin, K. and Perring, C. (1990) *Carers and Services: A Review of Research*, HMSO, London

Tyler, C. (1993) Travellers' tale. *Nursing Times*, **89**(33), 26–27

UKCC (1993) *Standards for Records and Record Keeping*, United Kingdom Central Council for Nursing, Midwifery and Health Visiting, London

UKCC (1994) *The Future of Professional Practice – the Council's Standards for Education and Practice following Registration*, United Kingdom Central Council for Nursing, Midwifery and Health Visiting, London

Victor, C.R. and Vetter, N.J. (1985) The use of the health visiting service by the elderly after discharge from hospital. *Health Visitor*, **58**, 95–96

Wade, S. (1991) Support for carers. *Journal of District Nursing*, November, pp. 13–19

Waters, K.R. (1987) Outcomes of discharge from hospital for elderly people. *Journal of Advanced Nursing*, **12**, 347–355

Webb, S. and Colson, J. (1993) *Nursing Practice and Health Care* (eds S. Hinchliff, S.E. Norman and J. Schober), Edward Arnold, London

Werner-Beland, J.A. (1980) *Grief Responses to Long-Term Illness*, Prentice-Hall, Virginia

Whyte, D.A. (1992) A family approach to the care of a child with chronic illness. *Journal of Advanced Nursing*, **17**, 317–327

Winkler, F. (1987) Consumerism in healthcare: beyond the supermarket model. *Policy and Politics*, **15**, 1

Worth, A., Tierney, A. and Lockerbie, L. (1994) Community nurses and discharge planning. *Nursing Standard*, **8**(21), 25–30

Yeo, T. (1993) Community care and mental health: the Stanley Moore memorial lecture. *Community Psychiatric Nursing Journal*, April, pp. 13–17

14

Health at school

Mary Pearce and Kate Saffin

● **Introduction**

The focus of this chapter is on the health of children in the context of school. It is not about the health at school of children. This approach presented the authors with a dilemma; it is difficult to take a holistic view of a child's health when focusing on only one specific area of their life. On the other hand, all aspects of children's health will affect their ability to learn and enjoy school. There is an increasing opinion that the school health services should adopt an occupational health role which aims to provide support for children whatever their health needs at school. Although the school health service is complementary to services provided by primary health care teams, it can be argued that school health services rightly fall into the domain of primary health care.

This chapter briefly explores the background to health care in schools and then addresses the role of the community health care nurse in the promotion of health, the prevention of disease and health education in the school. These issues are linked to government policies in relation to health and education. Cameos are used to provide practical examples to illustrate the discussion. This chapter links with Chapter 10 in considering the levels of prevention within the context of the school.

● **Historical development of health care in schools**

A brief historical background of the school health service in the UK gives insight into the development of health care and education in the school in the 1990s. Compulsory education in the UK was introduced in 1880 and for the next 50 years the main health input to schools was the inspection of children's heads and feet and the provision of school meals. The service gradually expanded in the 1930s with a proliferation of school-based clinics dealing with most of the common childhood disorders of health.

With the implementation of the NHS Act 1946, a wider range of health services became available to families. The number of school-based clinics dwindled steadily once access to General Practitioners was free of charge and specialist services more readily accessible. Stacey (1988) argues that the school health service kept a broad public health focus until the 1974 reorganization of the NHS. This reorganization accounted for a significant change in the service as it became led by the more dominant medical approach to health care. However, by the 1980s school nurses were increasingly being asked to contribute to health education, handle concerns about child abuse, deal with enquiries from parents and answer a multitude of queries about the health of pupils and staff. The professional organizations began to demand proper training and the first school nurse courses were introduced. These equipped the school nurse with the skills to develop the particular role of a community health care nurse working to promote health in the school. In many areas, routine medical examinations have been replaced with health interviews carried out by nurses (Mattock, 1991). In addition, nurses have taken responsibility for immunization which was once the province of the doctor (Saffin, 1992), as well as developing collaborative ways of working with teachers, parents, children and other health and social agencies.

Legislation of the 1980s was extensive and far reaching. The Education Act 1981 probably marks the watershed in many ways as it affected schools, children, parents and teachers. In particular, it provided for any child with suspected special needs to have a full multi-professional assessment and a statement of his or her educational needs and provisions in school. The Education Act 1988 is best known for introducing the National Curriculum into schools, but it also provided for local authorities to buy in additional services for children with special needs such as nursing, physiotherapy, occupational and speech therapy. Government policies during the 1980s increasingly emphasized the role of the individual as opposed to society. The Children Act 1989 illustrates this well, with its emphasis on parental responsibility rather than rights.

Professional associations began to produce guidelines for the service and for practice (RCN, 1991; HVA, 1991). Indeed, as the NHS changed, organizations saw a need for guidance, not only for those delivering the service but perhaps even more importantly those who were responsible for purchasing it, many of whom had no experience of health provision within schools.

The NHS and Community Care Act 1990 and the creation of an internal market (see Chapter 8) has presented District Health Authorities (DHAs) with an interesting dilemma regarding the purchasing of school health services. If the service is essentially an occupational health service, aimed at optimizing a child's health in order to take advantage of the education on offer, it raises questions about whether it is the responsibility of the DHA to buy it. On the other hand, a child's health for the purposes of education and a child's health for any purpose can hardly be separated. Furthermore, there is considerable political rhetoric about investing in the health of children as citizens of the future. In practice, this dilemma is being addressed in many different ways and some areas face severe reductions or abolition of school health services (Health Visitor Journal, 1994). At the same time there are also areas that are developing services and taking a creative approach to joint commissioning in partnership with Family Health Service Authorities (FHSAs) and education departments in local authorities.

The Health of the Nation (DoH, 1992) made a clear commitment to preventive health care. Although its targets address the whole population, there are several which focus on adolescent health, for example those relating to reducing unwanted teenage pregnancies and smoking among 13–15 year olds. Many health professionals saw the report and its recommendations as an important endorsement of their role in health promotion.

Today's school children are less likely to die before the age of 15, face a longer life than their predecessors, an average of four more years than in 1961, and are twice as likely to live in a one-parent family (OPCS, 1994). Some of the issues facing young people and some possible responses are now explored.

● Children and their health at school

School is only a part of the structure of the lives of children, albeit a significant part. Their essential attributes and personalities, needs, hopes and fears are shaped as a result of many influences such as the family and social and economic factors, but may be significantly changed by what happens to them at school. Most adults can recall experiences, good or bad, at school which have profoundly influenced their lives long after what they actually 'learned' has been forgotten. As stated earlier, an approach gaining in popularity is that the school health services should adopt an occupational health role. An alternative view is that school is the place for the provision of total health care for children. In the USA, for example, many of a child's health needs may be met in school by clinics and specialist school medical personnel. This is in contrast to the situation in the UK where the principal providers of health care are the Primary Health Care Teams (PHCTs). This system of care has many advantages: family doctors and community health care nurses know families within their care well and as a consequence are able to offer high levels of support and help in times of need. Knowledge of the family background and circumstances, as well as identifying the need for preventive work, is also more likely to result in speedier intervention when health problems occur.

There are, however, circumstances when this system does not work to the best advantage of children. Some families, notably travellers (see Chapter 13), may not be registered with a GP at all, while highly mobile families may never be registered with a practice long enough to receive the full range of services. Not all families choose to take up the services offered by their GP practice; developmental screening programmes may be declined and immunizations refused. Inevitably some children will 'slip through the net' and arrive at school with undetected and/or un-treated problems. Examples include children with severe speech and language problems, hearing defects, continence problems and develop-mental delay.

Young people at the other end of the school age spectrum may find it difficult to access the health services via the PHCT. Although one study found that 31% of teenagers had consulted their GP in the previous

3 months (MacFarlane *et al.*, 1989), health centres may not always be user-friendly places for young people even if they have the confidence and skills necessary to present themselves for treatment or advice. This poses several questions for schools and the school health services of the 1990s:

- To what extent can children's health needs be identified at school?
- Is it appropriate to attempt to meet those needs via the School Health Services?
- How can adequate provision be resourced, given the diversity of need within the population?

The British Paediatric Association report *Health Services for School Age Children* (BPA, 1993) recognizes that the school environment possesses unique characteristics, challenges and opportunities to which school health services can respond. The report offers the following factors in support of this view:

- the population is 'captive'
- the environment is educational
- the focus is child centred
- health and lifestyle are open to influence through curriculum and example
- health may be promoted in partnership with teachers and the wider community (the Health Promoting School)
- the effects of ill health and disability may be minimized in co-operation with teachers
- services for children in need may be initiated
- health monitoring may be offered
- ill health, including infectious diseases, in the individual and the child population as a whole may be prevented.

Furthermore, the authors of this report believe that the school health services are in a unique position to develop strategies to address the targets set out in *The Health of the Nation* (DoH, 1992) in the five key areas – coronary heart disease and stroke; cancers; mental illness; HIV/ AIDS and sexual health; and accidents. Specific targets such as the reduction by one-third of smoking, the reduction of teenage pregnancies and the reduction of childhood accidents present major challenges to community health care nurses working with school age children.

The broad remit of health promotion, to which the majority of school health services now work, lends itself well to the provision of a needs-based service which takes full advantage of the factors outlined above. An exploration of the concept of health promotion is worth while at this stage in order to justify these statements.

● Health promotion

Health promotion is described by the World Health Organization (WHO, 1986) as

the process of enabling people to increase control over, and to improve, their heatlh. To reach a stage of complete physical, mental and social well-being, an individual or group must be able to identify and to realise aspirations, to satisfy needs and to change or cope with the environment. Health is, therefore, seen as a resource for every-day life, not the object of living. Health is a positive concept emphasising social and personal resources, as well as physical capacities. Therefore health promotion is not just the responsibility of the health sector, but goes beyond healthy lifestyles to well-being.

Hall (1991) defines health promotion as consisting of three interlinking components – health education, health protection and disease prevention. It could be argued, however, that both health education and health protection are themselves components of disease prevention. This notion of disease prevention provides a useful framework within which to consider both individual and public health issues. This framework will be used for the remainder of this chapter to explore the health needs of the child at school.

● Disease prevention

Discase prevention can be undertaken at three levels, as illustrated in Table 14.1 (see also Chapter 10).

Primary prevention

The most striking example of primary prevention in the context of school is the preclusion of disease by immunization. The effectiveness of

Table 14.1 The three levels of disease prevention

Primary prevention	*Secondary prevention*	*Tertiary prevention*
Reduction of incidence of disease; action taken to prevent a problem occurring	*Early detection of abnormality/deviation from normal; reduction of prevalence of disease*	*Reduction and minimization of disability and handicap*
EXAMPLES Immunization	EXAMPLES Surveillance and screening	EXAMPLES Management of asthma in school
Advice on nutrition, contraception, lifestyle	Observations by parents, school staff	Management and care of children with chronic conditions
Advice of normal development	Health interviews	Management and care of children with neurological problems
Child protection	Follow-up of high-risk situations	
Accident prevention		

school immunization programmes is due to two factors:

- In many cases the pool of infection is within institutions, and schools provide ideal breeding grounds for infection. Arresting the process of infection at school therefore not only protects the children themselves, but also conveys a protection via herd immunity to the rest of the population.
- Uptake of immunization at school is consistently high. It is relatively easy to target the appropriate age group, to educate them about the importance of immunization, given parental consent, and then to hold immunization sessions. The co-operation of school staff and the fact that the school population is 'captive' are also important factors.

An excellent example of this was seen in the measles–rubella campaign undertaken in schools in the UK in November 1994 following an initiative by the Department of Health in response to the expectation of a measles epidemic in 1995. Mass immunization campaigns are currently the strategy recommended by the World Health Organisation for dealing with predicted epidemics. Throughout the UK, in excess of 90% of 5–16 year olds were immunized (Wiltsher, 1995), a sufficient uptake to ensure herd immunity and, it is hoped, to eradicate the diseases, at least in the short/medium term. Certainly the two factors as outlined above were in large part responsible for the success of the campaign. It must be remembered, however, that the success of the campaign has been measured in terms of the uptake of the immunization. Until data on the future incidence of both diseases are available, it is impossible to say whether it was successful or cost-effective in terms of disease prevention.

It was not a straightforward campaign, however, and the following cameo illustrates some of the dilemmas that faced parents, children and teachers:

The headteacher of a school in Oxfordshire, noticing that a significant number of consent forms for the MR immunization had not been returned, mentioned her concern to one of the parents. It became evident during the course of the conversation that many of the parents were confused by what they saw as conflicting media messages. On the one hand, the strong imagery of the death of a child in a hospital casualty department conveyed via the government's TV campaign exhorted them to agree to the immunization; on the other hand, they were hearing accounts of children brain-damaged by previous vaccines. Some accounts, notably those in the tabloid press, caused particular distress. The headteacher and the school health nurse after discussing the situation agreed to offer an open meeting to the parents as a forum for their concerns. About 30 parents attended the meeting. The school health nurse took with her all the relevant statistical data both on immunizations and on the diseases in question. Parents were encouraged to express their fears, and were given open and honest answers to their questions. It was evident that the leaflet issued by the Department of Health for the purpose of giving parents the information they needed, was, for a significant number of adults, difficult to read and understand. The outcome of the meeting was favourable; in the end all the parents gave consent for the injection, and a 100% uptake was achieved in that school. No adverse reactions were reported.

● Health education

In the early 1970s alarm was already being expressed at the perceived increase in the incidence of drug abuse among young people. Experimentation with drugs was described as one aspect of the teenage school years which required particular attention because of its increasing incidence and potentially sinister significance (Mitchell and Court, 1977). By the early 1990s, surveys collated by the Institute for the Study of Drug Dependence revealed that 22% of pupils aged 15–16 had tried illegal drugs or solvents (Balding, 1992). There is evidence, 20 years later, that drug-taking is occurring on an even greater scale. Local surveys suggest that as many as 57% of 15 and 16 year olds have tried using illegal drugs (Coggans *et al.*, 1991). Some recent reports claim that up to 70% of young people have been offered drugs. Anecdotal evidence suggests that teenagers can obtain drugs with ease, very often on or just outside the school premises.

Schools face a dilemma in dealing with this problem; drug use is illegal and as such must not be condoned by the authorities. As Strasburger (1989) argues, it is useless simply to exhort teenagers not to use drugs – they need information to help them make their own decisions. They also need knowledge about the effects and side-effects of drugs to enable them to cause the least possible damage to their own health if they do decide to experiment. Many secondary schools use the expertise of the police to deal with this subject in the curriculum, involving officers who have valuable knowledge to share with the teenagers and who are able to share the information in a sensitive and thoughtful way. Yet this method of dealing with the issue could be criticized for conveying the covert message *'don't do drugs – it's against the law'* rather than the preferable *'think about it – do you really want this for your body?'* The following is an example of an approach made by a teenager to the community health care nurse providing an open access facility in the school:

A 15-year-old boy had on several previous occasions used the drop-in facility to discuss minor and trivial health concerns with the school nurse. It is quite a common feature of drop-ins that young people broach only 'safe' subjects until they have 'tested the water'.

His latest visit, however, was different – he seemed anxious and rather agitated. He told the school nurse that he was worried about his friend, who he said was taking some sort of drug. He implied that this was cannabis, and seemed to be seeking reassurance that such drugs were harmless. The school nurse talked to him about the effects and side-effects of drugs, but suggested that it would be much better if the boy could persuade the friend himself to come and visit her. She strongly suspected that 'the friend' was the boy himself and wanted to make it easier for him to be open about his fears. When the boy returned a week later, however, he was still expressing concern for his 'friend', this time asking 'what if' he were using stronger drugs such as 'E's.

The school nurse was very concerned. At a recent community liaison meeting, the local police officer had expressed his belief that children were being given a quota of drugs to sell by a teenage pusher, the pusher himself being manipulated by someone else. The police officer was very anxious about the potential harm the children could do themselves or others. The school nurse faced a dilemma, should she discuss this boy with the police officer and identify him? What would be the consequences of that action?

In the event, she did not report the conversations but continued to see the boy at approximately weekly intervals and to offer advice and counselling. The discussion never progressed beyond the stage where it was the 'friend's' problem.

This illustration demonstrates the community health care nurse working within the guidelines offered by the UKCC (1987) document *Confidentiality*.

Alcohol is an even greater problem. A study of almost 25 000 young people aged from 12 to 16 years was carried out by the Schools Health Education Unit at Exeter University in 1991. This study revealed that almost 50% of 15- and 16-year-old boys had drunk beer or lager in the previous week and it was estimated that 10% of these drank a pint or more a day. Paradoxically, the fact that alcohol is *not* illegal poses problems for schools equal to but different from those mentioned above in relation to drug use. Society in the main, as well as the law, condones the recreational use of alcohol over the age of 18. Therefore, it is difficult for young people to understand the logic of this, given not only the potential health hazard of drinking, but also the potential for causing serious harm to others as a result of, for example, drunken driving. Understandably, many young people feel confused and angry by what they see as society's dual standards.

There is a growing belief that greater priority should be given to addressing issues relating to drug and alcohol abuse in the school curriculum, beginning at the primary school level. It is evident from discussion with children in primary schools that they already have a considerable awareness of drugs; a commonly expressed fear about the move to secondary school is the possible pressure from peers to take drugs.

Research carried out into the smoking habits of young people shows little evidence that school-based programmes of health education have any impact (Flay *et al.*, 1989; Vartiainen *et al.*, 1990). The only programme to date to report significant reduction in smoking among teenagers is the Minnesota Heart Health Campaign (Perry *et al.*, 1992), where a community campaign was mounted simultaneously with the school campaign. *The Health of the Nation* (DoH, 1992) clearly recognizes the importance of this wider approach in its recommendation that inter-agency Healthy Alliances should be established (see Chapter 3). However, there continues to be little enthusiasm at government level to ban tobacco advertising, considered by many to be an essential ingredient of a successful anti-smoking strategy (Michell, 1994).

If health education is apparently so ineffective, it raises questions as to the way forward, given that the school provides a good base to address issues of health. The ethos of the school itself plays a major part in the success or otherwise of health education. In *Swimming Upstream* (Whitehead, 1989), the author suggests that a wider view of health education should replace the traditional one in which transmission of information and acquisition of knowledge are paramount. The health-promoting school defines health in terms of the interaction of physical, mental, social and environmental factors, and values the development of the school as a caring community. Health authorities and education authorities should work together to develop health-promoting schools (HVA, 1991); the resulting powerful 'Healthy Alliance' could have enormous potential to improve the health of tomorrow's adults.

Many of the activities of the community health care nurse in the field of health promotion and health education in schools can be described as primary prevention. Accident prevention is one example, advice on the importance of a healthy diet is another. So many factors influence the lifestyles and habits of young people, however, that it is unrealistic to expect the acquisition of knowledge alone to change their attitudes and behaviour. Using the example of diet, for instance, poverty is a very potent cause of poor standards of nutrition, while peer pressure to conform to the 'norm' by eating junk food is powerful.

The role of the school health services in health education is diverse. School health nurses are frequently involved in planning programmes with school staff of which they may participate in the delivery. In many cases they supply teaching staff with relevant and up-to-date information and resources, and offer support to enable the teachers to deliver the programme themselves. All health education, regardless of the topic, should be underpinned by a philosophy which aims at improving the self-esteem of the young people involved. Information and knowledge alone are of limited value unless the young people are helped to value themselves, to develop a belief in their own judgement and to possess the skills to assert those beliefs, thus empowering them to make appropriate choices.

The following cameo illustrates this point:

As part of the activities for 'No Smoking Day', a secondary school was targeted by a group of school health nurses and health visitors. Sessions were held in several classes of 14–15 year olds. Using the strategy of an 'Agree/Disagree' continuum placed across the classroom, the team read out statements about smoking and asked the pupils to stand on the line according to their feelings about the statement. Lively and illuminating discussions ensued from this activity. Discussions were facilitated and guided by the team, who also ensured that correct information was passed on. The most powerful non-smoking messages, however, came from the young people themselves. In the evaluations completed after the sessions, several pupils commented that they had really enjoyed being able to state their point of view, and that they felt their views had been valued. One pupil commented that no one had ever previously asked them what they thought.

Secondary prevention

Secondary prevention is defined as identifying that which impedes the progress and development of disease through early detection. Although screening programmes are, in many cases, the vehicle for early detection, they must be continuously reviewed in terms of outcomes, cost-effectiveness and value to the client. Wilson and Jungner (1968) devised a set of criteria for screening programmes (reproduced in Hall, 1991, p. 10). These include the assertion that the condition being sought should be an important health problem for the individual and for the community. The authors emphasize the need for an acceptable form of treatment for those discovered to have a disease or disability.

In some areas of the country, school-based programmes of screening for hypertension have been considered (Kelsall and Watson, 1989), the aims of such programmes being to detect children with mild elevation of blood pressure who may be at risk of developing essential hypertension in adulthood. It would also detect a small number of children suffering from hypertension secondary to, for example, renal disease and in whom no other symptoms have yet appeared. In order to identify those cases, however, Kelsall and Watson argue that many children with mildly elevated blood pressure would need to be investigated and the anxiety produced by those investigations would not justify the small number of cases of secondary hypertension likely to be discovered. Furthermore, a study of 10 000 children screened as part of a community programme in America failed to discover one case of secondary hypertension. For the small number of children with primary hypertension found, no drug treatment was deemed to be necessary (Fixler and Pennock, 1983).

Routine screening for scoliosis is advocated by some authorities and is still carried out in a number of schools nationally. This screening programme is not supported by Hall (1991) because the current test is too sensitive, resulting in 2–15% referrals, of which two out of three are false positive. Again the resultant anxiety and unnecessary treatment does not justify the numbers of children found to have a treatable condition.

Therefore, routine screening in most schools is now limited to the detection of vision and hearing defects. Children are usually screened on entry to school for distance and near vision, and in many cases for squint. However, there are no national data to suggest that this is in any way universal, although it is generally agreed that screening at this age is of value. Likewise, there is no evidence to suggest that pre-school screening results in a better outcome than if screening, referral and diagnosis are carried out at school entry (Catford *et al.*, 1984). Furthermore, amblyopia is difficult to detect before the ages of 5 or 6 using existing tests (Hall, 1991).

Subsequent screening usually concentrates on distance vision alone, colour vision being tested prior to entry into secondary school. Hall (1991) argues that screening for visual defects in children should be carried out at school at 3-yearly intervals at 5, 8, 11 and 14 years of age 'as myopia may appear at any age'. Stewart-Brown, however, questions 'Could we do better by doing less?' (Stewart-Brown and Haslum, 1988). Research carried out in Oxford suggested that the numbers of new cases of vision defect discovered at 13 and 15 were too low to justify the continuation of the screening programme at these ages (Jewell *et al.*, 1994). The trend in many areas now (although not yet reflected in the literature) is to explore ways in which to raise teenagers' awareness of the importance of good vision. This, together with a method of self-testing or self-referral, may provide a way of empowering young people to take responsibility for one aspect of their health, and as such is probably more valuable than a screening programme which, even if it produces appropriate referrals, often results in non-compliance with suggested treatment.

Screening for hearing problems was at one time carried out routinely in all schools either by school nurses or audiology technicians. There has in recent years, however, been a tendency for authorities to move towards a selective policy of audiometry. This has in the main been a response to financial constraints and to the difficulty of justifying so large a programme in terms of successful outcomes. Audiometry in some areas is now available via the school health service only if a specific concern is raised about a child's hearing. It remains common practice, however, to offer such screening to children with learning difficulties in order to eliminate hearing problems as a contributory factor.

With the virtual cessation of routine school medical sessions, there has been a growing trend towards the use of health interviews in which children and young people are offered an individual appointment with the school nurse. These interviews address issues of both primary prevention (individual health education) and secondary prevention (screening and follow-up of problems). The age at which the interviews are carried out varies, but at, or shortly after, school entry, on transfer to secondary school and prior to leaving school, is common. This provides a very useful opportunity for the school nurse to link health advice to screening procedures, for example by discussing healthy eating while measuring growth. The HVA (1991) recommended the strategy of using health interviews, commenting that 'The role of the school nurse in assessment is extremely important . . . [the interview] . . . gives the school nurse the opportunity to obtain a holistic view of the child, discuss any concerns and form a care plan in partnership with the child, family and others'. The HVA (1992) issued more specific guidance on health assessment for school nurses in which a health assessement is defined as 'a systematic, holistic assessment of a child's health status taking into account his or her age, development and ability'.

In spite of the fact that routine individual health interviews have now been in use for some time in some areas, there is little evidence to show that they are an effective method either of primary or secondary prevention in terms of outcomes. Indeed, very little evaluation is available on the subject, although many school nurses have expressed the opinion that the interviews are highly effective, and that they result in increased job satisfaction (Wade et al., 1989). Although routine interviews are costly in terms of time, health interviews can be seen to form a framework in which the community health care nurses can identify and plan to meet the needs of the school population.

An alternative strategy, which has the advantage of being more child-centred, is the use of 'drop-in' sessions. Here the school nurse makes herself available for individual consultations in school at set times. Pupils are invited to self-refer for specific advice or counselling, but may also be referred by a member of staff. It seems likely that the requests by school staff for the provision of drop-in sessions will increase, in response to the government's guidelines on sex education in schools, published in May 1994 (Department for Education, 1994). These guidelines altered the provision of sex education, taking all but the teaching of the biological facts of reproduction and sexually transmitted diseases out of the national curriculum. Parents have the right to withdraw their children from sex education lessons if subjects other than those which fall within the national curriculum are included. The new guidelines also make it clear that it is not within the remit of teaching staff to offer individual advice or counselling to young people on sexual matters. Critics of the government's approach argue that this undermines attempts to achieve the 'Health of the Nation' target to reduce the rate of teenage pregnancies. It also comes at a time when 18.7% of women and 27.6% of men report having had sexual intercourse before the age of 16 (Welling, 1994).

Teachers are advised that only doctors and nurses working within the health service should counsel young people on sexual matters. It is likely, therefore, that teachers who may suspect a young person is sexually active will encourage the use of the drop-in sessions by pupils as the most appropriate way to obtain advice. Interestingly, research evidence demonstrates that sex education delays onset of sexual activity (Aggleton et al., 1993). This study also showed that school programmes which promote the postponement of sexual intercourse and the use of condoms when sex occurs, were more effective before young people become sexually active.

Tertiary prevention

Tertiary prevention is defined as 'that which impedes the progress of established disease or disability by appropriate treatment' (Hall, 1991). In the context of school, tertiary prevention aims to minimize the effect of illness and disability in order to maximize the child's education potential. This sometimes requires that changes are made in the environment to enable a child to benefit from and enjoy as many aspects of school as possible. Examples include:

- the provision of wheelchair ramps to enable the child to move more freely about school
- adapted toilet facilities
- accessible medical room facilities, with provision made for the privacy of the child who needs to carry out procedures such as self-catheterization
- special learning aids such as computer-aided equipment or communication devices
- removal from the classroom of materials or animals which 'trigger' asthma symptoms in a particular child or children, for example, pets (gerbils, hamsters).

In addition to changes in the physical environment, however, in many cases there will be a need to provide human resources to enable the child to benefit fully from school. This is particularly true in primary schools where children with disabilities, like their able-bodied peers, have not reached independence. Children who need help either coping with physical disabilities or with learning difficulties can be aided in school by Learning Support Assistants (LSAs). Depending on the level of support needed, the LSA may work with one child or several.

The Education Act 1981 made radical changes to the ways in which children's disabilities were categorized. Children who had formerly been defined by disability for the purpose of education are now described as having special educational needs and a 'descriptive analysis of each child's strengths and weaknesses' informed the provision of appropriate education for each child (Hall, 1991). The intention of the 1981 Act is the integration of children with special needs into mainstream school wherever possible. So complex are the issues surrounding the provision for children with profound and multiple disabilities that they cannot be covered fully here, but further detailed information is provided by Roche and Stacey (1991).

In order to explore the concept of tertiary prevention in the school setting, it may be useful to focus first on an example of a specific medical condition and secondly on the issues which must be addressed for children who may need emergency medication in school.

Asthma is one of the commonest diseases in childhood, affecting an estimated 1 in 10 children (Asthma Society, 1991; OPCS, 1994). The effectiveness of modern treatments is such that, given compliance with prescribed treatment, children suffering from all but the most severe forms of asthma should be able to live normal lives. The data collated by the Asthma Society (1991) indicates, however, that a significant number of children undergoing treatment are still regularly experiencing unnecessary symptoms such as night-time coughing and exercise intolerance. There are probably many explanations for this, with poor inhaler technique, lack of understanding of treatment on the part of parents and children, lack of compliance with prescribed treatment and undertreatment by GPs being perhaps the most significant. The cumulative effects of poorly controlled asthma may have a potentially serious impact on the child's education. The child whose sleep is regularly disturbed at night by coughing will find it difficult to maintain concentration at school. The child who experiences wheezing or shortness of breath on exercise will tend to avoid activities such as PE, games and cross-country running, consequently missing out on an important part of the school curriculum. In many children, this situation results in a vicious circle: they become overweight, which compounds the problems of asthma, making them even more reluctant to participate in exercise.

It is of very great importance, therefore, that all those working in schools have an understanding of asthma and its treatment. Inhaler storage poses a dilemma for school staff and for the school health services whose advice on the matter is often sought. Teachers are concerned about the potential for abuse of the medication should children be allowed to carry their inhalers with them; they fear not only that the sufferer may overdose, but also that they may share their medication with friends. It is of great concern that in response to this fear many schools have maintained long-standing policies of locking inhalers away as they would with any other medication. In the event of an acute attack this is potentially very dangerous. If the child has need for the inhaler and the member of staff who holds the key cannot be found, or if the child is experiencing acute symptoms on the far side of the playing fields, at best the child will be caused unnecessary distress. At worst, it could present a life-threatening situation. Work with the school staff therefore needs to focus on this issue to find a solution that takes account of the child's needs and the level of responsibility she/he can reasonably be expected to take. Age is not always the key factor; since levels of maturity vary greatly between children of the same chronological age.

Children themselves, whether sufferers from asthma or not, should be the target for health education on this subject. For those who are not sufferers, understanding the condition demystifies the use of asthma inhalers and makes it less likely that they will either tease their users or try them out for themselves. Children with the condition benefit from being given information which reinforces that given by the GP or practice nurse and places it in the context of school; for example, the suggestion that they use their inhaler before PE if their asthma is triggered by exertion. The observations of teaching staff are very helpful in the treatment of asthma. A child who is noted to be using his inhaler more frequently than usual may need a change or adjustment of treatment; it is important, therefore, that parents are made aware of any changes noticed by school staff.

Lastly, asthma provides a good example of the differing but complementary roles each professional, whether education or health, whether primary health care team, school health service or specialist, can play, as the following cameo shows:

School staff were worried about Billy M. He was frequently absent from the small village primary school he attended. The absences were always explained in notes sent by his mother as being due to illness. Billy was considered by his teachers to be under-achieving at school. He was also very overweight, which had resulted in some teasing and alienation by his peers. Billy was known to have suffered from asthma before starting school.

The headteacher invited Billy's mother into school to discuss all the concerns; the school nurse was also invited to this meeting to give advice about Billy's weight. Mrs M. admitted that she was having difficulty getting him to school, particularly on days when the class did PE because he was teased about his size. When asked about Billy's asthma, Mrs M. said she felt it wasn't a problem for him any more. She was, however, concerned about a cough which disturbed his sleep and which she thought was the continuing after-effect of the flu he'd had last term. The school nurse explained that this cough might be a symptom of asthma and that Billy should be seen by his doctor for assessment.

Mrs M. agreed to take Billy to the surgery, although she expressed concern about the 'fashion' for prescribing inhalers. With Mrs M.'s permission, the school nurse spoke to the GP, and to the practice nurse who ran the asthma clinic, about Billy's problems in school, and about Mrs M.'s confusion about asthma and its treatment.

After investigation, Billy was prescribed prophylactic medication in the form of an inhaler to be used three times a day. A reliever inhaler was prescribed for use when necessary and the practice nurse suggested that Billy should take a puff 5 minutes before games or PE since his asthma appeared to be exercise induced.

Mrs M. continued to feel ambivalent about the regular use of Billy's preventive medication, and had a tendency as soon as his symptoms were well controlled to withhold it. The communication between GP, practice nurse, school nurse and school staff was of enormous importance to ensure that relevant information about Billy was shared and that both Billy and his mother could receive appropriate support.

Billy has gradually taken responsibility for his treatment and is finding that use of the inhaler before sport does make a difference, although he feels he will never really enjoy games. His weight is still a problem. The school nurse is encouraging him to eat healthily and to swim regularly, an activity which he does enjoy. She regularly communicates with his mother and with the practice nurse about both his diet and his asthma, and makes sure that school staff are informed if there is any change in treatment.

The issues of medication in school are broader than that of asthma medication. Parents may want or need a child to return to school after an illness, but before a course of antibiotics is completed. Children may be on long-term medication or need access to emergency medication in school. Local Education Authorities issue Health and Safety guidelines to schools on many areas including child health issues, and these are formulated in conjunction with child health and school health workers. The school then develops its own detailed policy.

Wherever possible, long-term treatment regimens should avoid the need for medication during the school day; however, this is not always possible and detailed protocols for managing the medication for a named child need to be developed. For example, as intervention may be necessary for the child with epilepsy it is important that some treatment is available in school should a fit occur and fail to be self-limiting. Rectal diazepam is frequently prescribed for emergency treatment of such a situation. School staff should have no difficulty in administering the medication should the need arise. However, this presents teachers with a dilemma because, although the actual administration of the medication may be straightforward, there are issues of accountability and responsibility which make many teachers reluctant to carry out such emergency treatment. However clear-cut the guidelines are, the decision as to whether or not to administer the medication, for instance, would be the teacher's; this would, in effect, amount to a requirement that they 'diagnose' the problem before instituting appropriate treatment. This, they believe, leaves them very vulnerable in the eyes of the law, as does the potential for accusations of assault because of the nature of the administration of rectal medication. All the teaching unions, recognizing these potential problems, recommend that teachers do not administer medication.

Posing similar problems are the children who suffer from severe life-threatening allergies. These children, should they come into contact with the allergen which affects them, need adrenaline administered by injection within minutes of the contact. Adrenaline is produced for this purpose in a 'mini-jet' – a device with a $\frac{1}{4}$-inch (6mm) needle which can safely be injected into any fleshy part of the body. No special knowledge or technique is necessary and the device is very easy to use. For the same reasons that they are concerned about the use of rectal diazepam, however, many teachers are reluctant to take responsibility for the administration of adrenaline.

The question is therefore raised that if school staff are not able to administer medication to children in life-threatening situations, who will? It is not practical, nor is it in a child's best interest, for a parent to be present in school for the entire school day in the event that the child needs medication. School health services are already seriously under-resourced and overstretched and school nurses, who are almost always peripatetic, would not be able to undertake to be available at the very short notice such a situation would demand.

Local policies and protocols, including training for school staff, have gone some way towards addressing the problems (DTB, 1994). Written 'contracts', signed by parents, paediatricians, GPs and teachers, document the procedure for each individual child. Local authorities have, in many cases, taken legal advice on providing appropriate indemnity for teachers who have agreed to be trained to carry out the procedures. This remains, however, a very contentious issue in the realm of tertiary prevention in schools, and one for which there does not appear to be an obvious or easy solution.

● Child protection

Many of the health issues and available school-based services for children and young people can be addressed through the framework used here. There are those which span all three levels of prevention and which would become fragmented if forced into a framework of convenience. Child protection is a good example and is therefore addressed separately to illustrate this range of work and issues involved (see Chapter 19).

Teaching staff in many schools carry out important preventive work using programmes such as KIDSCAPE (Elliott, 1986). This is a programme intended for use with children from 5 to 11 years, which aims to help them understand the difference between 'good touches and bad touches', between 'good secrets and bad secrets' and to develop assertiveness skills to empower then to tell a trusted adult if they are being abused. The acquisition of such skills may also contribute to the empowering of children to deal with the growing problem of bullying.

Children spend more than 6 hours of every day at school during term time; school staff therefore come to know individual children well and are able to recognize changes of health, behaviour or demeanour. For this reason, school staff play an important role in the detecting of abuse. Once there is concern, clear-cut, local shared policies exist for dealing with child protection issues. Detailed records are kept describing any incidents which raise concern, and well-defined links with social services departments are forged to facilitate reporting of suspected physical, emotional and sexual abuse. The school health service has a responsibility to monitor children at risk to liaise with members of the PHCT. The NSPCC (in its Training Project 7193) argues that the school nurse has a potentially important role in the detection and prevention of child abuse.

When a child's name has been placed on the child protection register, decisions about the frequency and nature of monitoring at school are made at a case conference. The surveillance undertaken is usually aimed to give an overview of the child's general health. An important component of the surveillance is weighing and measuring, plotting the results on a growth chart to determine whether the child's growth is satisfactory. It has long been understood that pattern of growth is a very useful indicator of a child's wellbeing. Growth may be affected not only by physical disease, but also by emotional upset (Mitchell, 1977).

● Conclusion

This chapter has attempted to explore some of the health issues that are relevant to school, such as ill health or special needs, or those which can be addressed within the curriculum such as health promotion. It has been impossible to be completely child-centred, as to do so would immediately shift the focus away from school which is the context of the chapter. However, it is to be hoped that it has provided an introduction to a large and complex area and one that the reader will continue to probe.

References

Aggleton, P., Baldo, M. and Slutkin, G. (1993) Sex education leads to safer behaviour. World Health Organisation Global Programme for AIDS. Reported in the Newsletter for WHO Global Programme on AIDS, 1993, no. 4. In MacFarlane, A. (ed.) *Adolescent Health Monitor*, Radcliffe Medical Press

Asthma Society (1991) *Asthma: Who Cares?*, The Asthma Training Centre, Stratford-on-Avon

Balding, J. (1992) *Young People in 1991*, Schools Health Education Unit, University of Exeter

BPA (1993) *Health Services for School Age Children*, Consultation Report of the Joint Working Party, British Paediatric Society, London

Catford, J.C., Absolom, M.J. and Mill, O.A. (1984) Squints – a sideways look. In *Progress in Child Health*, Vol. 3 (ed. J.A. Macfarlane), Churchill Livingstone, Edinburgh

Coggans, N. *et al*. (1991) *National Evaluation of Drug Education in Scotland*, ISDD, London

Davidson, Y. (1994) Health policy for school children in the state of Israel. Paper presented to the European Society for Social Paediatrics Congress, Jerusalem

Department for Education (1994) *Sex Education in Schools*, Circular 5/94

DoH (1991) *The Children Act 1989: An Introductory Guide for the NHS*, HMSO, London

DoH (1992) *The Health of the Nation*, HMSO, London

DTB (1994) Using medicines in schools, *Drug and Therapeutics Bulletin*, **32**(11), 81–83

Elliott, M. (1986) KIDSCAPE – Primary Kit Prevention Programme for 5–11 yr olds. Kidscape, 82 Brook St., London

Fixler, D.E. and Pennock, W. (1983) Validity of mass blood pressure screening in children. *Pediatrics*, **72**, 459–463

Flay, B.S., Worden, J.K., Secker-Walker, R.H. *et al*. (1989) Prevention of cigarette smoking through mass media intervention and school programs. *American Journal of Public Health*, **82**(6), 827–834

Hall, D. (1991) *Health for all Children: A Programme for Child Health Surveillance*, 2nd edn, Oxford University Press, Oxford

Health Visitor Journal (1994) Trust threatens to axe posts [news item]. *Health Visitor Journal*, **67**(4), 116

HVA (1991) *Project Health*, Health Visitors' Association, London

HVA (1992) *Health Assessment and the School Nurse*, Health Visitors' Association, London

Inglis, J. (1989) Health interviews for school children. *Midwife, Health Visitor and Community Nurse*, **25**(5), 202–204

Jewell, G., Reeves, B., Saffin, K. and Crofts, B. (1994) The effectiveness of vision screening by school nurses in secondary school. *Archives of Diseases of Childhood*, **70**, 14–18

Kelsall, J.E. and Watson, A.R. (1989) Should blood pressure be measured by school nurses, paper presented to the British Paediatric Association Annual Meeting, York, mimeo

MacFarlane, A., McPherson, A., McPherson, K. and Ahmed, L. (1989) Teenagers and their health. *Archives of Disease in Childhood*, **62**, 1125–1129

Mattock, C. (1991) Stepping off the medical treadmill. *Health Visitor Journal*, **64**(5), 154–156

Michell, L. (1994) *Smoking Prevention Programmes for Adolescents: A Literature Review*, Commissioned by Directorate of Health Policy and Public Health, Anglia & Oxford Regional Health Authority with The National Adolescent & Student Health Unit

Mitchell, R. (ed.) (1977) *Child Health in the Community*, Churchill Livingstone, Edinburgh

OPCS (1994) *Population Trends: 78*, Office of Population Census and Surveys/ HMSO, London

Perry, C.L., Kelder, S.H., Murray, D.M. and Klepp, K. (1992) Community wide smoking prevention: long-term outcomes of the Minnesota health program and the class of 1989 study. *American Journal of Public Health*, **82**(9), 1210–1216

RCN (1991) *Standards of Care for School Nursing*, Royal College of Nursing, London

Roche, S. and Stacey, M. (1991) *Overview of Research on the Provision and Utilisation of Child Health Services in the Community*, University of Warwick, Warwick

Saffin, K. (1992) School nurses immunising without a doctor present. *Health Visitor*, **65**(11), 394–396

Stacey, M. (1988) *The Sociology of Health and Healing*, Unwin Hyman, London

Stewart-Brown, S. and Haslum, M. (1988) Screening of vision in school: could we do better by doing less? *British Medical Journal*, **297**, 1111–1113

Strasburger, V.C. (1989) Prevention of adolescent drug abuse: why 'Just Say No' just won't work. *Journal of Pediatrics*, **114**,4(1), 676–681

UKCC (1987) *Confidentiality*, United Kingdom Central Council, London

Vartiainen, E., Fallonen, U., McAlister, A.L. and Puska, P. (1990) Eight year follow up results of an adolescent smoking prevention program: the North Karelia Youth Program. *American Journal of Public Health*, **80**, 78–79

Wade, J., Sinclair, E. and Bennett, J. (1989) Health care interviews in secondary schools – a review of the first two years' experience in the Brighton health district. *Public Health*, **103**, 467–474

Welling, K. (1994) *Sexual Behaviour in Britain: The National Survey of Sexual Attitudes and Lifestyles*, Penguin, London

Whitehead, M. (1989) *Swimming Upstream: Trends and Prospects in Education for Health*, King Edward's Hospital Fund for London, London

WHO (1986) *Charter for Health Promotion*, World Health Organisation, Geneva

Wilson, J.M.G. and Jungner, G. (1968) *Principles and Practice of Screening for Disease*, Public Health Paper No. 34, WHO, Geneva

Wiltsher, A. (1995) Learning the lessons. *Health Visitor Journal*, **68**(2), 52–53

15

Health in the workplace

Cynthia Atwell

● **Introduction**

Occupational health is a much neglected area of health care, but one which has a major influence on the health status of the entire adult working population, a large proportion of whom spend a quarter of their life at work. Workplace exposure to hazards such as dusts, gases, noise, poor ergonomic design and stress will therefore have a detrimental effect on the overall health of the individual.

Ramazzini (1713) was the first to refer to the effects of occupation on health and he decreed that all physicians, when examining patients and before making a final diagnosis, should ask the question, 'What is your occupation?' The relevance of that question is just as important today, although the type of occupational health hazard has changed. Occupational health is twofold: it is concerned with the effects of '*work on health*' and '*health on work*'. This chapter will primarily concentrate on workplace hazards and their effects on health, and includes the responsibilities of the occupational health nurse within this context.

● **Legislation**

Occupational health is part of community practice and it is important that every nurse working in the community has an understanding of the complexities of occupational health. When assessing the needs of the patient or client, information about occupation must be acquired and, furthermore, acknowledgement made of the importance of this on the overall health status and care of the individual. *The Health of the Nation* (DoH, 1992) failed to recognize the significance of ill-health caused by workplace hazards. Although targets for reducing accidents at work and improving the mental health of the workforce are referred to, acknowledgement is not given to the fact that many of the causes of mental ill health can be attributed to stress at work.

The first Factories Act was introduced in 1833 and there is now a plethora of legislation controlling health and safety in the workplace. In 1992 there was an influx of European Community led legislation which both complemented and strengthened the UK Health and Safety at Work Act 1974. These were:

- Management of Health and Safety at Work Regulations 1992 (HSE, 1992a)
- Workplace Health and Safety Regulations 1992 (HSE, 1992b)
- Workplace Equipment Regulations 1992 (HSE, 1992c)
- Personal Protective Equipment Regulations 1992 (HSE, 1992d)
- Manual Handling Operations Regulations 1992 (HSE, 1992e)
- Display Screen Equipment Regulations 1992 (HSE, 1992f)

The last of these was completely new to the UK, but the others specified that which was previously implicit in UK legislation, namely risk assessment and hazard control. *Hazard* is defined as being something that has the potential to cause harm, whereas *risk* is the likelihood that it will cause harm in the circumstances in which it is found.

● The working environment and the effects on health

Nurses need to be aware of the type of working environment to which the patients or clients may be exposed. For ease of identification these will be discussed under five distinct headings – physical hazards, chemical hazards, biological hazards, psychological factors and ergonomic hazards – although it should be appreciated that an individual may be exposed to one or more of these at any one time.

Physical hazards

These are hazards that may cause physical damage or injury and include exposures to noise, vibration, radiation (ionizing, microwave and laser), or to excesses of heat, cold and physical trauma.

Noise

Exposure to high levels of noise – 90 decibels (dB) for an 8-hour period or more – is likely to cause noise-induced hearing loss (NIHL), which is damage to the sensory hair cells of the cochlea resulting in permanent deafness. Such damage is irreversible and hearing aids cannot help, as the effect is not one of reduction in sound levels as in presbycusis, but actual distortion in reception of the speech frequencies, thus causing a major social handicap. The Noise at Work Regulations (HSE, 1989) which came into force on 1 January 1990 set specific standards for assessing noise levels and exposure times, reducing exposure and risk of hearing damage, the use of personal ear protection and the development of hearing conservation programmes.

Vibration

Vibrating tools such as pneumatic implements, chain saws, riveters and similar rotating tools may give rise to injury to soft tissue and the digital circulation of the hand and arm which may result in a condition known as hand–arm vibration syndrome (HAVS), which has symptoms similar to those of Raynaud's syndrome – blanching of the fingers, particularly in cold conditions, tingling and numbness and in severe cases gangrene.

Radiation (ionizing, laser and microwave)

The use of sources of radiation in both industry and health care has increased over the past few years. It is a very specialized area with specific statutory regulations controlling its use (HSE, 1985) and therefore is not appropriate to discuss in detail in this chapter. It would, however, be reasonable to expect that nurses should be aware that such exposures can also happen in the workplace outside the hospital setting and that long-term effects may manifest themselves as malignant tumours, blood disorders, cataracts, dermatitis and genetic damage (Harrington and Gill, 1992).

Heat and cold

Excess of both heat and cold can be found in a number of workplaces. Metal production, glass-making, baking and similar processes can be extremely hot. In settings where metal or glass is being melted down, the furnaces may be operating at temperatures in excess of 2000 °C and the radiant heat and the heavy manual nature of the work cause excessive sweating and loss of body fluid. In some cases, workers may develop symptoms of muscle cramp and heat stroke and in extreme cases may collapse due to the raised body temperature and loss of body fluid. In this situation, emergency treatment will be one of reducing body temperature and rehydration. However, the main concern must be to prevent this situation arising. The ambient temperature of the work area would need to be reduced by improving ventilation and air flow rates, as well as implementing regular rest breaks for the workers, with access to fluids to maintain levels of hydration.

There are also occupations requiring people to work in extremes of cold. This is always a problem for those who predominantly work outdoors such as farmers, road workers, builders and others who are exposed to the natural elements in winter. Mackie (1992) also states that outdoor workers are at higher risk of skin cancer in the form of malignant melanoma, due to sun exposure. He records that malignant melanoma accounts for approximately 20% of all skin cancers, but is responsible for 80% of deaths due to skin cancer.

In the industrial situation, producers of frozen foods employ people to work in deep-freeze storage warehouses in similarly cold environments, and frostbite and circulatory problems may occur among this group of workers. Prevention is achieved by ensuring that suitable clothing is provided and worn, together with rest breaks and/or work rotation.

Physical trauma

Any type of physical injury may occur in the workplace, caused by accidents with machines, tools or the general work environment such as floors and stairs. As identified by the Health and Safety Executive (HSE, 1993), the main causes of accidents in industry are handling and lifting, closely followed by slips, trips and falls. All nurses should be familiar with accident prevention procedures and be able to recognize potential hazards. In the majority of organizations, safety and accident prevention are dealt with separately, but with the rationalization of industry, many occupational health nurses are expected to take on a safety role which requires additional specialist training.

Chemical hazards

These are hazards in which, when an individual is exposed to them, a chemical reaction or change may take place in the exposed individual. Such hazards can be broadly categorized as follows:

- paints
- plastics
- dyes
- solvents
- metals
- drugs
- dusts
- pesticides/herbicides/fertilizers
- wood, plant and organic dusts.

To understand how these hazards affect the body it is important to appreciate the concept of 'target organs'. The modes of entry for chemicals to enter the body are through inhalation, ingestion and absorption through the conjunctiva and skin – broken and unbroken. A substance inhaled or absorbed into the body in this way may not necessarily affect that particular organ directly, but will be absorbed into the bloodstream and affect other organs. Some examples are shown in Table 15.1.

The inhalation of coal dust particles and asbestos fibres are well-documented examples of damage occurring directly to the lung (Parkes, 1994). The dust or fibres deposited in the alveoli cause hardening of the air sacs and consequently impair the interchange of oxygen and carbon dioxide. The long-term effects cause reduced lung function and conditions such as pneumoconiosis, asbestosis and chronic

Table 15.1   Examples of chemical hazards affecting organs

Substance	Mode of entry	Target organ
Mercury	Lungs, skin, ingestion	Brain/central nervous system
Lead	Lungs, skin, ingestion	Blood, bone, brain
Cadmium	Lungs, skin, ingestion	Kidney
Trichloroethylene	Lungs, skin, ingestion	Liver

respiratory disability. In the case of asbestos inhalation, carcinoma of the lung or mesothelioma may occur.

Exposure of chemicals on the skin may cause a breakdown in the natural protective barrier resulting in dermatitis or sensitization. Some chemicals penetrate unbroken skin, for example mercury which can be absorbed through the skin and be transported by the bloodstream and can pass the blood–brain barrier and cross the placenta causing damage to the fetus (Waldron, 1990).

Controlling chemical hazards is a major role for the occupational health practitioner. The introduction of the Control of Substances Hazardous to Health Regulations (HSE, 1988) placed additional responsibilities on employers to carry out assessments of all hazardous substances used, document the assessments and introduce measures to remove and/or control the hazards. The nurse should be involved in the assessment process, advising management on hazard control and carrying out health surveillance on those employees identified at high risk of exposure to a recognized hazard. The control of hazards must be a structured methodical procedure, taking account of all aspects of the problem, and started by asking the question, 'Can the hazard be eliminated or substituted or redesigned?' Figure 15.1 details the process diagrammatically.

Biological hazards

Biological hazards at work include infections and parasites which are derived from both human and animal sources. These may be contracted through normal social contact, but for the purpose of this chapter they will be discussed as an occupational hazard. Table 15.2 shows some examples of infections and parasites and the occupational groups at risk. These occupational groups have a higher risk than the average person due to their direct, and in many cases, intimate contact with the human or animal source of infection.

Prevention of exposure to occupational infections is difficult. In the case of health care workers, for example, they may be caring for an individual who has one of the infections identified in Table 15.2. The

Table 15.2   Examples of infections and parasites affecting various occupations

Infection	Occupational group
Hepatitus 'B', human immunodeficiency virus (HIV), tuberculosis, rubella	Health care professionals, laboratory staff, dentists, morticians, police, prison officers
Leptospirosis, tetanus	Sewer workers, farmers, miners, veterinary workers
Anthrax, brucellosis	Farmers, slaughterhouse and veterinary workers
Salmonella, listeria, typhoid	Food handlers, food manufacturers
Scabies, head lice	Teachers and school support workers, home carers, migrant workers who live in poor conditions

Can the hazard be:

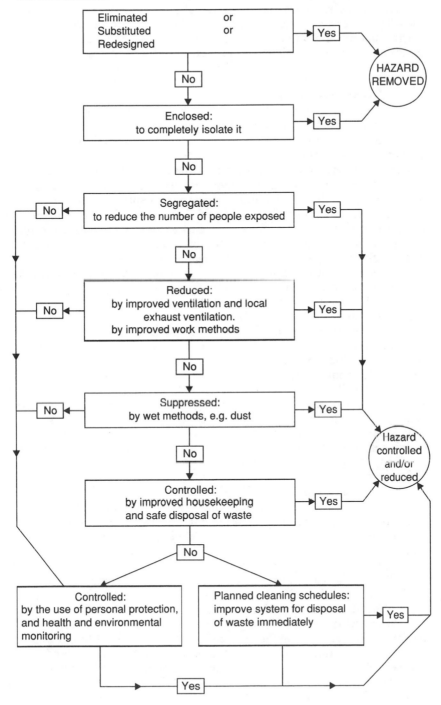

Figure 15.1 Hierarchy for effective hazard control

main focus must therefore be on control through vaccination for those at high risk from tuberculosis, hepatitis 'B', rubella, typhoid and tetanus. Developing safe systems of work, including the safe disposal of clinical waste, sharps and other waste, is a prime factor, together with the education of staff in hygiene and prevention procedures.

Psychosocial factors

There are many situations which affect the mental and social health of the worker. Long working hours, shift work and redundancy/ unemployment are some of the major problems affecting many organizations today (Sutherland and Cooper, 1993). The fluctuating political and economic climate and pressure on organizations to reduce overheads and to 'downsize' to improve productivity are having a major impact on local government, the National Health Service and central government owned organizations (Bamford, 1995). In addition, many of these organizations are being privatized. A recent survey carried out by the Confederation of British Industry (1993) indicated an increase in absenteeism within these organizations compared with other private companies.

There has also been an increase in both verbal and physical abuse of people at work, particularly those involved in service provision such as council workers, social workers, police and ambulance staff. Post-traumatic stress disorder (PTSD) is a major problem for the frontline emergency services – police, fire and ambulance – all of which have to deal with major incidents of multiple deaths/injury (see, for example, Stewart and Hodgkinson, 1992).

Prevention of stress under these circumstances is often difficult. The nurse will need to be involved in 'post-incidence debriefing' and possibly even longer term counselling. There are no easy answers to reducing workloads; therefore, most of the emphasis must be on individual stress management and control, including education and training in stress management techniques, as well as support counselling.

Ergonomic hazards

According to the Health and Safety Executive (HSE, 1993), muscular skeletal injuries accounted for the loss of 3.5 million working days in 1992. These included back injury, general strains and sprains, and work-related upper limb disorder (WRULD), much of which could have been prevented by good workplace design, layout and safe work procedures. Until the introduction of the Manual Handling Operations Regulations (HSE, 1992e), the main emphasis for controlling and preventing handling and lifting accidents was on employee training on safe lifting procedures. These regulations now place a requirement on employers to carry out an assessment of all manual handling procedures. The assessment must be documented and where hazardous handling and lifting procedures are identified, remedial action must be implemented to remove that hazard. This may mean redesigning the job and/or using mechanical equipment.

WRULD such as tenosynovitis and carpal tunnel syndrome are conditions that appear to be associated with the increased use of computers and word processors. The problem is also found in electronic and mechanical assembly workers, poultry processors and many other occupations which require dynamic and static forces to be applied. Dynamic forces arise when muscles and tendons are applying force for brief periods, as in pushing, pulling, holding and gripping. Even more important are the static forces which occur when part of the body is held in a particular position for extended periods without the muscles, tendons and other soft tissues being allowed to relax. Static loading can cause the muscles and tendons to be held in a constant state of tension, thus restricting their blood supply and hampering their recovery.

Prevention of these conditions requires workplace assessment and the introduction of flexible work procedures in order to facilitate sufficient changes in activity and rest periods. 'Piece work' (work paid at a per item rate) also contributes to these problems, particularly where workers are encouraged to carry out high-speed, repetitive work using dynamic and static forces. The Display Screen Equipment Regulations (HSE, 1992f) came into force on 1 January 1993, requiring employers not only to assess computer workstations, but also provide a suitable ergonomically designed workstation, implement procedures for eyesight checks and ensure regular changes in activity and rest breaks.

● **Effects of health on work**

Occupational health practice requires the practitioner to understand the effects of 'health on work' as well as 'work on health'. Standards of health are important in many occupations, particularly in safety-critical posts where the health of the individual could have devastating effects on other people or the environment. Airline pilots, train drivers, road tanker drivers are just some examples of occupations that require strict health standards in order to safeguard the safety of both passengers and public. In the case of tanker drivers, who may be carrying highly toxic, flammable or explosive materials on road networks, an accident could endanger the lives of the local community as well as damage the general environment.

Before setting standards of health for any group of workers it is important to know exactly what the job entails – the physical and psychological demands that will be made on the worker in carrying out that job, together with information on hours of work, shift patterns, location, level of supervision and welfare facilities.

However, health standards are often used as an excuse for rejecting an applicant who has a disability. Standards must therefore be set, taking full account of the needs of the job, and then each individual should be assessed on their capabilities. People with known health problems should not be rejected without being given a full assessment, which should include information on the clinical condition, prognosis and treatment from the individual's family doctor. Only then, with this information and knowledge of the job requirements, can the occupational health nurse or doctor make an objective assessment of the person's suitability for a job.

Recent figures produced by the Department for Health (DoH, 1991) on alcohol and drug abuse indicate that this is an increasing social problem in our society. Jenkins and Warman (1993) record that over £1.3 billion is lost each year due to alcohol-related problems alone in the UK. Employers are implementing drug and alcohol policies in an attempt to minimize the workplace effects of abuse. Most policies set out the organization's philosophy on drinking and drug-taking and offer advice, support and treatment for those who are identified as abusers, either because of poor work performance or through self-referral.

The railway industry and London Transport are just two examples of companies which have gone further with their policies and carry out pre-employment and random drug screening on their employees. They also undertake 'for cause screening', which is testing for both alcohol and drugs following any critical incident involving loss of life or serious injury and/or damage to property, equipment or the environment.

Mental health is one of the government's targets in the 'Health of the Nation' Document (DoH, 1992). Occupational stress and mental illness can have detrimental effects on an individual's employment prospects. Mental illness is stigmatized by many employers who are reluctant to employ people with a history of it (Floyd *et al.*, 1994). However, occupational health nurses and doctors can do much to alleviate this problem by undertaking objective assessment of such people and educating employers. The findings of Clothier *et al.* (1994), relating to a nurse with Munchausen's syndrome, seem to have done little to improve employers' attitudes towards mental health, but with proper assessment, medical history and knowledge of the job the risks of situations such as this arising should be minimized.

● **Nursing in the working environment**

Education

Nurse education in the UK has changed rapidly over the past 10 years. With the introduction of 'Project 2000' the emphasis is on community care, independence and rehabilitation. Occupational health nurse education has developed in line with this and has moved into higher education, achieving Diploma and First and Higher degree status. The curriculum is frequently based on the Hanasaari conceptual model (Figure 15.2), developed by a group of occupational health nurses at a workshop in Hanasaari, Finland in 1989, and now used as the basis for practice and education.

The model encompasses an outer circle which represents the total global concept, covering all aspects of health and safety affecting the total population in the general environment. Extending out from the centre of the model are social, political, ecological, organizational and economic factors which influence the environment. The political and social policies of the country, together with the organization's culture and strategy, make the biggest impact. An example is provided by the economic climate in the 1990s which brought about a complete change in social

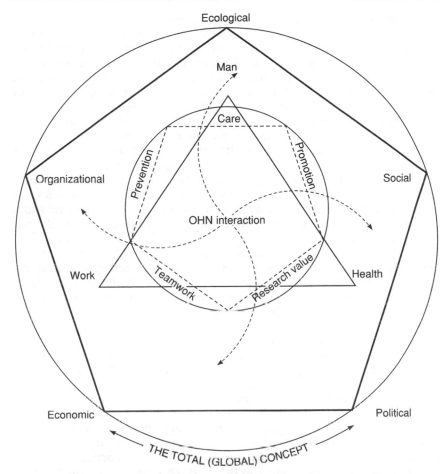

Figure 15.2 The Hanasaari model for occupational health nursing (From Alston *et al.*, 1989, by permission)

policy, and organizations were forced to make major savings in order to survive. Much of this has resulted in cutbacks in occupational health care and welfare provision. This highlights the need for the occupational health nurse to be fully conversant with the organization, basing occupational health provision on business needs and contributing to the aims and profitability of the business.

The Man–Work–Health concept is represented by a triangle pointing outwards, indicating how aspects of the total environment can influence health. Finally, the centre of the model is a circle containing five major concepts of occupational health nursing. The arrows represent movement which is the occupational health nurse's interactive role, and indicate the continuous developing and changing role of practice, pushing out from the centre, encompassing all parts of the model.

Professional accountability and responsibilities

The occupational health nurse's primary responsibility is to the worker as the client or patient, aiming to safeguard the health and wellbeing of the employee, while ensuring that the interests of the employing organization are met. The nurse has a responsibility to the employee, employer, trades unions and the public at large to ensure the highest standard of professional practice. A considerable number of occupational health nurses work alone, without other professional support, and so professional standards must be exemplary.

Within the occupational health team in larger organizations, nurses may work with doctors, occupational hygienists, safety advisers and others. However, where the nurse is the only occupational health practitioner, she or he will need to work closely with managers and trades unions to develop health and safety policies. In addition, she or he will be expected to lead on all aspects of health and in some instances take on a safety role as well.

Occupational health practice is unique in that the nurse does not have the support of the wider health team which is generally available in other health care settings. It is the responsibility of the nurse to educate the employer regarding professional accountability and responsibility. The UKCC Code of Professional Conduct (UKCC, 1992), requiring nurses to 'maintain and improve professional knowledge and competence', is often a sticking point for employers, particularly where the nurse identifies a need for personal development and training.

A study by Dorward (1993) found that only 34% of managers considered the continuing educational needs of the occupational health nurse to be necessary. Furthermore, they did not see the need for continuing education on 'professional issues'. It is imperative that nurses discuss with their employer not only issues involved in professional competence to practise, but also the requirements of the Code which include the employer's vicarious liability for the nurse's actions.

Ensuring confidentiality in the workplace setting is a major ethical issue for the occupational health nurse. The employer should only be informed of personal health details with the employee's informed consent. However, the nurse must be mindful of the responsibility for the health of others and accountability to the employer. If it is considered that to withhold information may endanger the health and/or safety of others, then releasing information without consent may be necessary, as detailed in Section 10 of the Code, but these situations will be exceptional.

The introduction of the Access to Medical Reports Act 1988 gave individuals the right of access to medical reports obtained for employment and insurance purposes from the medical practitioner responsible for their clinical care. Reports are sometimes requested to assist with pre-employment health assessment and more frequently to assist in the assessment of an employee with a health problem, who may need redeployment or restrictions on work. During the assessment process the occupational health nurse or doctor may contact the family or hospital doctor for a report on the condition, treatment and prognosis of an individual. This will enable an informed, objective assessment to be made of the suitability of the individual for work or to continue in a specific job. At all times in this situation, the occupational health nurse or doctor is acting on behalf of the employer and must gain written informed consent from the employee for the release of such a report to them.

Assessing and controlling the working environment

The specialist aspects of occupational health nurse practice require the nurse to have the knowledge and skills to assess the working environment. The latest health and safety legislation (HSE, 1992a) emphasizes the requirements for hazard identification and risk assessment. Where the nurse is the only occupational health specialist in the organization, this will form a major part of his or her function, and requires the nurse to be a source of expertise to the managers in carrying out assessments. Knowledge of the workplace, its hazards and work procedures form the basis of such assessments.

Questions which must be asked include:

- What is the job and what are the hazards to health – physical, chemical, biological, psychosocial, ergonomic?
- How will the hazard affect the worker – mode of entry?
- Who is exposed to the hazard? – male/female; young/old; how many are exposed?
- What are the likely health effects? – short/long term.
- Can the hazard be removed/controlled (see Figure 15.1)?
- Is health surveillance appropriate?
- Should environmental monitoring be carried out?

All this information should be documented and a final recommendation made on the action that must be taken to remove or control the identified hazards. However, advice on control measures must be practical and attainable, taking account of the nature and severity of the hazard. The risk must be quantified before the control measures can be decided upon.

Assessment of health

An important component of the practice of occupational health nurses is to carry out health assessments in the workplace. A qualified occupational health nurse will undertake assessments as an autonomous practitioner and will be able to certify those who are fit for employment. Those people whose fitness for a particular job is questionable should be referred for a medical opinion. However, in small organizations where there is no occupational physician employed, the person may have to be referred to their General Practitioner. This can sometimes cause difficulties, particularly when the GP has no knowledge or experience of occupational health practice and is anxious to see the 'patient' in employment.

Assessments may be carried out for pre-employment screening; following illness/injury; monitoring of the effectiveness of control measures; in order to comply with legal requirements; and monitoirng those with known health problems. When undertaking health assessments and screening, the nurse must be concerned with the holistic care of the employee as well as identifying signs of disease and disability. The assessment process may require the nurse to carry out physical measurements such as lung function tests, visual screening, audiometry, electrocardiography, urinalysis and height/weight ratio (body mass index). The individual nurse must also accept responsibility for ensuring that she or he has adequate training to carry out these activities and where there are deficiencies, arrange for further training. Competence in these activities must be updated and reassessed periodically.

Health promotion

All activities carried out by the occupational health nurse will have an element of health promotion within them. The nurse should also lead by example, such as by wearing protective clothing and using specific equipment in designated areas.

The workplace is an ideal place for health promotion activities. People are at work for approximately 8 hours a day, 5 days a week, and the opportunities for education are numerous and the benefits to the employer can be enormous. The benefits to the employer include:

- improved productivity/work performance through improved standards of health
- reduced absence attributed to illness/injury
- improved employee morale and therefore improved employee relations
- improved company image as a caring employer and therefore reduced labour turnover

The benefits to the employee are equally important and include:

- increased knowledge of factors leading to ill-health and injury
- changes in lifestyle leading to improved general health standard
- improved wellbeing and feeling valued by the employer.

When planning formal health promotion programmes the nurse must identify the organization's health needs. This should be agreed jointly with the employer and employees, with clearly defined objectives and most importantly a means of evaluating the programme. If the programme is not achieving its objectives, then it must be changed or modified. Health promotion can be very expensive, taking account of the cost of educational/promotional materials, staff resources and time away from the job for employees. It is therefore vital that the nurse demonstrates the benefits to both the employer and employees for this financial outlay.

Identifying health promotional topics should be based on relevant research findings such as local and national statistics, the company's sickness absence statistics, occupational health records and the types of hazards within the organization, particularly where specific occupational health education is necessary such as handling and lifting, noise, skin care, stress. Programmes that are co-ordinated with national campaigns can also be very successful. 'Drinkwise Day' and 'No Smoking Day' provide examples. If these can be linked with local community health centres and clinics they can have a considerable impact on the workforce, their families and the community as a whole.

Counselling

All nurses require counselling skills in order to be able to support their clients and patients through difficult times and situations. The occupational health nurse may be the only source of support within an organization and will need to gain the confidence of the workforce, taking an impartial stance and ensuring confidentiality. There will be many situations where the counselling skills of the occupational health nurse will be required.

D'Auria (1993) states that PTSD following major incidents involving death, serious injury or assault is now a recognized psychological problem. People witnessing and/or involved in such incidents require support to help them come to terms with the horrors they have experienced. Employees affected by PTSD can be in any job. The police, ambulance and fire services, by the very nature of their work, experience all types of incidents and many of these services have well-organized support networks for their employees. Assaults on local government staff and other service providers is a relatively frequent occurrence and requires action and understanding from the employer (Goldman, 1994). Other workers who experience a high incidence of PTSD are train drivers and operational railway staff. Suicide by jumping in front of a fast moving train is horrific for the driver and those who have to investigate the incident and deal with the remains. 'Debriefing' by the line manager, within 72 hours of the incident, with back-up counselling from the occupational health nurse is essential. Referral to specialist help may be necessary in order to minimize the possible long-term psychological effects of these incidents on the employees.

According to the 'Health of the Nation' document (DoH, 1992), alcohol and drug abuse continues to increase and has been identified as a target for action by the government. The occupational health nurse will frequently be involved in the initial counselling of employees who recognize that they have a problem and ask for help, or who have been referred by management because of absenteeism or poor performance. The nurse will need to develop good relationships with outside agencies and other health specialists in order to have the necessary support network for referring these cases. When dealing with alcohol- and drug-related problems, it is important that the nurse plans and sets targets for the programme with the employer and employee. Monitoring of progress is vital both for the employee and employer, particularly where the employer is financially supporting a treatment programme. However, confidentiality must be maintained while keeping the employer informed of the key aspects of the case.

● **Treatment of illness and injury at work**

Originally, nurses were employed in industry to carry out treatments on employees injured at work. Over the past 20 years occupational health nursing has moved away from this approach into a pro-active role, where prevention and control of hazards which cause ill-health and injury is the prime aim. It should be recognized, however, that in companies with specific high-risk operations, or who are located in areas where access to emergency services and departments is difficult, a treatment service may be appropriate. Before deciding on the type of service required, it is necessary for the nurse to know the hazards in the workplace and to become familiarized with the local emergency services and hospitals.

Where a treatment service is necessary, it should be for emergency treatment only, with referral to the employee's GP or hospital as soon as possible. Follow-up treatment should only be continued with the GP's agreement and so liaison is essential.

The main role for the occupational health nurse in relation to emergency treatment in the workplace is to ensure that adequate first-aid provision is available, in compliance with legal requirements set down by the Health and Safety Executive (HSE, 1981). The nurse will advise management on the level of service required, assist with and/or carry out special training for first aiders, monitor the standard and arrange and carry out training for specific hazards, e.g. cyanide, hydrofluoric acid.

● **Conclusion**

In conclusion, occupational health is practised in a range of different settings, for example in hospitals, local government, industry, farms and oil rigs – wherever people work there is a need for occupational health care. Hazard identification involves complex issues; and the occupational health nurse has to be ever vigilant in helping to identify and control them. Indeed, the role of the occupational health nurse will continue to change as work patterns change. With new technology being introduced, many of the traditional occupational diseases, such as lead poisoning, will disappear, but will be replaced by others, many of which will be related to social and psychological issues. As industry and commerce becomes more competitive, there will be more cutbacks in services for employees. The occupational health nurse must ensure that the care given to her or his employing organization meets their needs, is business led and demonstrates that there are benefits to all concerned.

References

Alston, R.M. *et al*. (1989) Workshop for Occupational Health Nursing, Hanasaari, Finland (quoted in Harrington and Gill, 1992)

Bamford, M. (1995) Work and health: an introduction to health care. In *The Quality of Working Life* (eds P. Spurgeon and F. Barwell), Chapman and Hall, London

Clothier, C., MacDonald, C.A. and Shaw, D.A. (1994) *The Allitt Inquiry Report*, HMSO, London

Confederation of British Industry (1993) News. *Occupational Health Review*, **43**, 1–3

D'Auria, D. (1993) Emergency services and post traumatic stress disorder. *Occupational Health Review*, **43**, 30–32

Department for Health (1988) *Access to Medical Reports Act*, HMSO, London

DoH (1991) *The Health of the Nation, Consultative Document for Health in England*, HMSO, London

DoH (1992) *The Health of the Nation. A Strategy for Health in England*, HMSO, London

Dorward, A.L. (1993) Managers' perceptions of the role and continuing education needs of occupational health nurses, Research Paper 34, HSE Books, HMSO, London

Floyd, M., Povall, M. and Watson, G. (1994) Mental health at work. *Disability and Rehabilitation*, Series 5, 'Some personal experiences', pp. 20–27

Goldman, L. (1994) Violence in the workplace. *Occupational Health*, **46**(5), 166–167

Harrington, J.M. and Gill, F.S. (1992) *Occupational Health, Pocket Consultant*, Blackwell Scientific, Oxford

HSE (1981) *First Aid at Work Regulations*, HMSO, London

HSE (1985) *Ionising Radiations Regulations*, HMSO, London

HSE (1988) *Control of Substances Hazardous to Health Regulations*, HMSO, London

HSE (1989) *Noise at Work Regulations*, HMSO, London

HSE (1992a) *Management of Health and Safety at Work Regulations*, HMSO, London

HSE (1992b) *Workplace Health and Safety Regulations*, HMSO London

HSE (1992c) *Workplace Equipment Regulations*, HMSO, London

HSE (1992d) *Personal Protective Equipment Regulations*, HMSO, London

HSE (1992e) *Manual Handling Operations Regulations*, HMSO, London

HSE (1992f) *Display Screen Equipment Regulations*, HMSO, London

HSE (1993) Key fact sheet on handling injuries to employees between 1986/87 and 1990/91, HSE Statistical Services Unit, HMSO, London

Industrial Relations Services (1993) News. *Occupational Health Review*, **43**, 1–3

Jenkins, R. and Warman, D. (1993) *Promoting Mental Health Policies in the Workplace*, HMSO, London

Mackie, R. (1992) Screening for skin cancer. *Occupational Health Journal*, **44**(7), 202–206

Parkes, W.R. (1994) *Occupational Lung Disorders*, 3rd edn, Butterworths, London

Ramazzini, B. (1713) *De Morbis Artificum*, translated by W.C. Wright (1940), Chicago University Press, Geneva

Stewart, M. and Hodgkinson, P. (1992) *Coping with Catastrophe: A Handbook of Disaster Management*, Routledge, London

Sutherland, V.J. and Cooper, C.L. (1993) *Understanding Stress: A Psychological Perspective for Health Performance*, Psychology and Health Series 5, Chapman and Hall, London

UKCC (1992) *Code of Professional Conduct*, 3rd edn, United Kingdom Central Council for Nursing, Midwifery and Health Visiting, London

Waldron, H.A. (1990) *Lecture Notes on Occupational Medicine*, 4th edn, Blackwell Scientific, Oxford

16

Health in residential care

David Sines

● **The policy context**

No informed discussion or debate on the provision of social or health care to clients in the community may be undertaken without due consideration of the policy context within which care is provided. There are a range of external social and policy issues that shape and influence the pattern of service delivery and these in turn will be influenced by historical forces. As Wagner (1988) states:

> *No informed conclusion about the future of residential care can be reached without paying careful attention to the kinds of external changes that are likely to determine its scale and character. That, in turn, cannot be done satisfactorily without some understanding and appreciation of those forces that have shaped its history.*

Societal attitudes and beliefs towards the more dependent members of society have dictated the nature of the models of service delivery that have been provided over the last century and beyond. The deployment of staff skills, the philosophy of care applied and the environments within which people have been cared for are influenced by changes in public attitude, the allocation of resources and by changes in social policy.

Until the mid-nineteenth century, care was provided in villages and towns within the context of the family. At a time characterized by the lack of technological development, when families were encouraged to be self-sufficient, rural and tribal societies have tended to display a greater acceptance of responsibility for their few severely handicapped members (Malin *et al.*, 1980). Similarly, in the UK prior to the industrial revolution, the problems associated with the care of people with mental health, learning disability or physical needs were not publicly evident and most members of the village community were able to contribute to the life and economy of the local society in some form or another.

With the industrial revolution came new expectations of the labour force. Large towns developed and labour was attracted from villages, with the result of mass migration to the towns and the erosion of close-knit ties in the villages (Schofield, 1968; Laslett, 1971). Value was placed on an individual's ability to produce for independent employers rather than to contribute to a self-sufficient community, and people were judged by ability to cope with increasing demands of new technology in mills and factories. There also came an increase in recognition of the importance of education, with literacy skills becoming a requisite if any form of social status was to be achieved.

The emergence of the institution may be seen as an attempt to meet the increasing problem of pauperism and the need for more stringent forms of social control and regulation. The workhouse appeared to be the answer and developed after 1834 with the explicit aim of providing social relief to the working classes within the confines of an institution.

With the passing of the rural community, dependent members of the family became more prominent. Families faced increasing demands on their time to work for landlords and had little opportunity to devote to the needs of dependent family members. Poverty, low intelligence and handicaps were regarded as indicating a weakness of moral character.

The ideas of social Darwinism, with its doctrine of the survival of the fittest in a competitive society, reinforced the work ethic principle (Bendix, 1956). Consequently, at this time many dependent people were encouraged to leave their families and to live with other, less fortunate, members of society in workhouses where, subjected to some degree of social control, they were cared for by the state and were able to contribute to the economy of the daily life of the workhouse community. By the end of the nineteenth century a major building campaign was embarked upon and a proliferation of asylums for the mentally ill and the mentally handicapped was introduced, although the major increase in admissions into these hospitals was to follow later between 1920 and 1950.

Following the enactment of the Mental Deficiency Act 1913 in the UK, the provision of additional hospital/asylum provision to meet the increasing demands of people for admission under the relevant sections of the Act was witnessed. The tendency to build institutions for over 2000 people in isolated parts of the country continued from the Victorian era, and in terms of economy the conversion of many workhouses and lunatic asylums became the nation's answer to an escalating problem (Tredgold and Soddy,1963).

● **The nature of the institution**

The nature of such total institutions has been well documented and described by Goffman (1961) in his writings on the social situation of mental patients. The principles expounded in his writings apply equally to other residential client groups with whom community nurses meet during their work.

Two basic features distinguish these total institutions from other social establishments. According to Goffman (1961):

> their 'encompassing or total character' and the fact that the staff 'in their work, and hence their world, have uniquely to do with people. This people-work is not quite like personnel work or the work of those involved in service relationships; the staff, after all, have objects

*and products to work upon, but these objects and products are
people'.*

Goffman states that these features make the total institution a social
hybrid – part residential community, part formal organization – and as
such this unique combination provides a special area for sociological
investigation and interest.

Goffman provides an account of the characteristics of such
institutions in terms of the staff and inmate worlds and identifies three
distinct elements of an individual's life. These are, the tendency to sleep,
work and play in different places under normal circumstances. These
activities usually take place with different co-participants and without an
overall, rational plan. The total institution does not distinguish between
different activities and breaks down the naturally occurring boundaries
that separate these three spheres of life. Other authors (Morris, 1969;
King *et al.*, 1971; Oswin, 1976) have also demonstrated that all aspects of
institutional life are conducted in the same place and under the same
single authority. Daily activities are also carried out in the company of a
large number of other people, all of whom are treated alike and required
to do the same thing together at the same time, without reference to
individual choice or interest. Systems operate to control the schedule of
daily activities which are imposed and regulated by senior staff in
complex, rigid hierarchies. Systems appear to be introduced to impose a
degree of social control, as described by the National Children's Bureau
(cited in Wagner Development Group, 1988):

> *Control was (and is) a remarkably complicated thread running
> through the history of institutions and if we are to understand its
> significance it is necessary to appreciate that complexity. . . . Or how
> does one gauge the contribution of institutions to the more general
> processes of social control when, for instance, a person in care could
> say in 1971: 'I always used to be threatened with being put away in a
> home where they are always nasty to you, that's the general
> impression everyone outside has'.*

● **The advent of community care**

In 1946, with the coming of the Welfare State in the UK, the
asylums were handed over to the National Health Service and were
renamed as hospitals. Henceforward, care for people with mental
handicaps and mental health needs were integrated within a medical
model of care and the medical and nursing professions became highly
influential in service planning and determining appropriate models of
care. Changes in public attitude and levels of public expenditure have also
determined the pattern of care that has been afforded to all specialist
client care groups and in turn these have been embedded within social
policy.

However, a consistent pattern of care provision based on the
hospital model persisted throughout the UK. By the 1980s the com-
placency was over and a significant period of change and challenge to the

postwar consensus on the way in which social care policy was to be discharged was placed firmly on the policy agenda. The effective end of protected status for public expenditure was noted by the government (Jenkin, 1979) which resulted in the virtual residualization of the role of the health and social services as a major residential community care provider (Walker, 1989). Walker argues that the main thrust of recent welfare policy has been influenced by the following four dimensions that dominated the conservative governments since 1979:

- antagonism towards public expenditure on the welfare state
- increasing emphasis on self-help and family support
- extension of the market and commodification of social relations
- the general breakdown of the social demographic consensus.

The Thatcher government challenged the consensus view of community care and the notion of the Welfare State and was able to exploit the fact that the concept of community care has almost always escaped formal or agreed definition. Hence the government was able to build on the accepted statement that community care means 'care in the community' and to replace this by the statement 'care by the community' (Walker, 1989). This subtle but important distinction may be seen as the cornerstone to recent policy initiatives. Similarly, the government has been able to take advantage of the lack of agreement about the most effective and desirable model to adopt in the provision of care for client groups in the community. Power struggles among consumers, pressure groups, psychiatrists, nurses, administrators, social workers, voluntary groups and politicians provided for the perfect scenario to introduce a new direction of care for client groups.

In keeping with government policy, the need for radical reform and overhaul of the social security and health systems was undertaken (NHS and Community Care Act 1990). Reliance on large, expensive hospitals was seen to be not only an outdated model of care but also to be more expensive than models of family-based care in the community. Success had also been witnessed in the USA through the introduction of private insurance to pay for health care and a prolific system of private enterprise was challenging the statutory services' franchise on care (Strong and Robinson, 1990). Thus began the promotion of the private sector in the UK, which doubled between 1979 and 1984 (Walker, 1989).

Recent changes in funding arrangements have transferred responsibility for the payment of residential care from the Social Security Agency to the social service departments (NHS and Community Care Act 1990). Clients may be expected to make a contribution to the cost of their care from their own means if they are in receipt of care outside the health service system in the future. This subtle but important difference reflects a new dimension on the way in which care is provided for clients in the community.

The attraction of the choice of securing cost-effective packages of care in the private sector provided many hospital managers with the incentive to embark on major hospital closure programmes. As a result many learning disability, mental health and elderly care hospitals have embarked on rapid closure programmes and admissions to long-stay care have reduced dramatically (DoH, 1991). Other influencing factors in reducing admissions into long-stay sector care, thus encouraging people to remain in their own homes for longer, appear to have been additional support provided to families from specialist Community Learning Disability and Mental Health Teams and increases in social security benefits.

It may be argued that the residualization of health authorities and social service departments as main care providers, the centralization of government control over expenditure, the fragmentation of care provision and increased marketization of care enterprise have all played their part in the realization of the UK government's policy of reducing dependence on institutional solutions for residential care provision. In its place has followed a policy of care in the community, thus reducing state sponsorship and expenditure. Consensus now appears to have been accepted by most of the major stakeholders involved in receiving, providing and commissioning residential care solutions.

The reasons for the growth and promotion of community care have been defined by Knapp and Renshaw (1986):

Thus the emphasis on community care is based on three premises:

normalization (which relates to the criterion of justice or equity)
cost (related to the criterion of economy), and
the preferences and wellbeing of mentally retarded persons and their relatives (related to the criterion of efficiency).

Knapp and Renshaw have, in one statement, identified the driving forces behind the government's policy for care in the community. In addition, emphasis on inter-professional teamwork and the central role of consumers in determining their own futures has pointed the direction in which nursing for this client group must follow, as the outcomes of community care are set and measured in terms of the quality of life experienced and desired by service users.

● **Residential care practice**

Following the publication and introduction of the NHS and Community Care Act 1990, local authorities have assumed responsibility for the assessment and co-ordination of most community-based residential services. For the majority of elderly persons, and those with mental health and learning disability needs, care will be provided in the community and clients will receive residential care from a range of providers in both the statutory and independent sectors. Primary health and social care practitioners will support individuals in their own homes and, while most clients will benefit from relatively simple service responses, a significant number will demand more specialist and complex packages of care.

To date, the extent to which relevant services have been received by individuals and families has been largely determined by fitting people into services rather than by designing specific services to meet the needs of individuals. The case management approach (adopted as a key principle within the legislative framework supporting the NHS and

Community Care Act) places emphasis on the provision of individualized services for people and requires that systems are designed to take account of each person's needs (see Chapter 30 for a detailed account of the case management process).

The case management function must not cease once a client enters any form of residential care, since the needs of each client will continue to change and should be subjected to continuous evaluation and review. This function becomes all the more important as contacts for residential care are assigned to one or more service providers who may be selected from statutory, voluntary or independent sector agencies who may, or in some cases may not, employ nurses to deliver front-line services to their clients. In such situations the role of the community nurse is broadened to encompass all clients living in residential care. The importance of ensuring that care packages are evaluated against a set of common standards and their effectiveness are judged in accordance with the extent to which they meet the actual needs of users (Brandon and Towe, 1989).

Consequently for case management to operate successfully it will be necessary for health and social care agencies to work closely together at both a planning level, where major service decisions and strategic plans are made, and at the point of service delivery. In support of this approach, it will also be necessary to demonstrate that multi-agency systems are in place to assess client need and to measure their effectiveness. Shared learning opportunities for nurses and social workers and for joint participation in the design of both care packages and service systems will become an important feature of provision for clients in the future.

The context of community care is therefore changing and artificial boundaries between home-based care and residential care appear to be eroding in favour of the design and implementation of a seamless service that demands community nurses provide their skills flexibly to their clients wherever they live. This, then, is the true meaning of a community-based service.

● **Philosophy of community health care nursing**

The main aim should be to provide practical and responsive support to individuals and their families wherever they live, with the aim of enabling them to live valued and purposeful lives in homes of their choice. In so doing, specialist advice and assistance should be offered in association with family and other carers and other professionals in response to identified needs of service users, to their carers and to others working with them.

Nursing services should be provided in such a way which respects the rights and wishes of individuals. Services should aim to offer a range of real choices and opportunities to assist individuals in participating in the care and in the design of the services they require and receive in order to widen their horizons and to facilitate the development of their wellbeing and skills.

Community nurses will practise as knowledgeable, safe, competent professionals. The following values underpin the provision of services:

- clients have the same rights as other members of society, and should have the opportunity to live in the same way as other people
- services should be planned in partnership with service users to enable them to achieve their maximum potential and to lead full and purposeful lives
- the provision of specialist nursing care must respond to the expressed needs of individuals and should follow an inter-professional and multi-agency approach
- nursing care should be provided in such a way as to enhance the quality of life experienced by individuals.

These values are central to the role and function of all community health care nurses; the next section demonstrates their application to supporting people in residential care settings.

● Maintaining valued and integrated lifestyles

One of the principal aims of residential services in the community should aim to provide facilities which are as fully integrated into local neighbourhoods as possible. Staff care practices should emphasize the importance of involving service users in the planning of their lives and should aim to promote the concept of advocacy to encourage their participation in all decision-making processes.

Essentially most people's lives revolve around their homes, friends, work and families, and the ways in which they choose to spend their time depend on their personal choices and the demands made on their 'free time' by others. O'Brien and Lyle (1987) have identified five key determinants or accomplishments that they consider are necessary for the successful provision of quality-based services:

- choice for individuals
- opportunities for integration in the community
- opportunities for active participation as equal members of the community
- the acquisition of competence
- the formation of new friendships and relationships.

This accomplishments model provides a most useful framework for the assessment of needs and for the evaluation of service quality. However, in order to ensure that clients are involved in determining their own needs, a systematic approach to care planning will be necessary.

One model is known as individual programme planning (IPP), which is described by Wilcock (cited in Sines, 1988). This model emphasizes the importance of planning for people within the context of service management structures and supports:

The increasing emphasis on providing individualised services for people demands the development of service systems that will help identify the person's needs and plan to meet them ... approaches are designed to ensure that staff make decisions that are relevant to a person's life.

The following principles underpin the IPP system and need to be activated in the provision of residential care:

- people with learning disabilities should be involved in planning their own futures
- desirable futures should be planned for people with learning disabilities
- all relevant people should be involved in the planning process
- services should be co-ordinated to meet people's real needs
- service deficiencies should be identified and used in the planning of future services.

Brechin and Swain (1987), in a rather more participative model, introduce the concept of shared action planning which emphasizes the importance of relationships 'being the heart of the matter'. They start their analysis of the skills involved in the shared action planning process with the following quote:

They are used in friendships, family living, relationships at work and in mutual helping and caring. Such skills grow and develop through and within personal relationships. Relationships are, in this sense, the heart of the matter.

Brechin and Swain (1987) introduce a new dimension into the personal planning process which is based on the principle of the importance of the interactions that take place between the client and the carer (and his/her friends). They talk of compassionate and supportive caring relationships, with reference to their place in determining the context of successful care planning and life experiences:

Shared Action Planning happens when there is coordination, organisation and people know who is responsible for doing what.

Consequently individualized approaches to care should provide a framework for people to express their wishes and desires through a shared process with named workers which in turn should lead to valued outcomes for the individual. The IPP system is not a purely nursing method, but builds on inputs from every relevant discipline and carer on the basis of equality. It pays particular attention to clarifying the client's unique needs as she or he sees them. Evidence for the success of this approach is described in Mansell *et al*. (1987).

The shared action planning model affords clients opportunities for empowerment which aim to ensure that maximum control is provided for self-determination and advocacy. However, increased choice may also be accompanied by exposure of vulnerable clients to increased risks in the community. Risk-taking and risk analysis has formed a central part of the debate and it should be acknowledged that an environment which allows an appropriate degree of personal choice and privacy can never be risk-free. Issues relating to freedom of expression, whistle blowing, sexual freedom and refusal to comply with medical instructions are but a few of the issues that might present themselves as challenges to professional carers and support staff caring for people in residential care (Brechin and Swain, 1987).

The delicate balance that must be forged between the provision of an over-protective (perhaps the worst possible scenario which may be characterized by abuse factors) and a facilitative environment will require careful deliberation and this process might well involve multi-professional decision-making. Individual case review, often using the shared action planning approach introduced above, is the most appropriate forum for seeking agreement on issues that might involve calculated risks. Services should ensure that negotiated risk-taking processes and guidelines are available to staff to support them whenever such decisions must be made.

● Assuring quality

This section considers the application of quality assurance methods to residential care provision. Having considered that the most fundamental service objective is that each service user will have access to a personal plan describing their needs and wants, the next stage of the process must be to ensure that service inputs and outcomes are evaluated effectively and systematically. Such systems should form an integral component of the care management process described earlier in this chapter. This process will provide care managers with the opportunity for objective review of the degree to which individual service agreements and contracts are being achieved. This requires that systems are agreed across statutory, voluntary and independent sectors and will require the development of a joint agreement on the standards of care that are to operate in the care situation.

Guidelines should be established which describe criteria for high-quality services, and arrangements for independent audit and inspection should be in place. The starting place is the shared action plan. This provides a detailed summary of the expected outcomes for clients in the form of achievable action targets which can be inspected during professional audit visits. Such objectives should be shared with all members of inter-professional teams which will often include members of the community nursing professions who should encourage feedback from clients and care managers on their own performance. In order to ensure that the values of the organization are integrated with practice, evidence of appropriate and coherent policies and procedures must be provided. In particular, care must be taken to ensure that such policies do not conflict with client-focused objectives or with the value principles of the organization.

Organizationally, clear agreements should be reached in respect of the contribution that each person will be expected to make towards achieving the organization's goals and objectives. These should define each person's scope of decision-making, authority and responsibility.

Information must be provided for all service users and to their carers to encourage active participation and a partnership in achieving the aim of high-quality services. This requires that responsibility for services is shared with service users and that together agreements are reached as to how service quality will be monitored and evaluated. The NHS and Community Care Act 1990 makes provision for the independent inspection of residential care services by arm's length inspectorate teams employed and accountable to social service departments. As part of their brief they will make planned and unannounced visits to all registered care and nursing homes. During these visits, members of the inspection team will discuss issues relating to quality of care and life as perceived by the residents themselves and will also seek information from community staff involved in care provision. Occasionally, community nurses will be invited to join inspection visits on either a formal or informal basis.

The importance of involving all staff in monitoring is emphasized by the inspectorates, and staff should be involved and feel confident to set their own goals and targets through the processes of the staff supervision, training and development performance reviews identified above. Quality will clearly depend on the motivation and commitment and skills of staff who will require personal leadership from their managers.

Service users and their families will provide a vital source of feedback of a quality of services and on their effectiveness. Above all, services must be open to constructive criticism and an independent inspection should provide clear statements of intent against which the quality of their service can be evaluated; in so doing services require management systems to reinforce the value base of the service in practice.

Quality assurance is not a phenomenon that can be managed discretely, but needs to be built in at every level of the service and should be reflected in each professional carer's job description. In order to achieve such aims and objectives, all managers should provide firm guidance and support to staff to ensure that a consistency of service is achieved throughout their service.

● Providing a motivated workforce

The final section of this chapter considers the needs of staff in residential care settings and suggests that staff require an investment in staff training to develop their skills, competences and knowledge in order to make them feel secure and to ensure that they feel that they have a purposeful role to play.

The case management approach advocated throughout this chapter suggests that staff skills must be contracted to support the needs of individual clients. People's needs change and if services are to respond flexibly to emergent demands from users, professionals must be prepared to deliver their skills in different ways to meet changing circumstances.

A mix of skills will be required in most workforces and managers should ensure that they possess adequate knowledge about the abilities and competences of their staff. Competence is defined (NCVQ, 1989) as

the pursuit of a senior occupation or profession – as an employee or as a self-employed person – including the ability to apply a significant range of fundamental principles and techniques to diagnosis, planning and problem solving.

The competence-based model places emphasis on the 'ability to do' and is based on the principle of defining the actual quality and outcome of staff interventions. In residential care, such an approach lends itself to the provision of a multi-skilled workforce which will have the capacity to provide a mix of skills and competences to clients. The role of community nurses will be to provide support, encouragement and development opportunities to residential care workers through the provision of:

- educational and training opportunities at both a formal and opportunistic level
- mentorship and supervision
- informal network support in order to avoid the problems associated with professional isolation witnessed in some community residential services.

The advent of an inter-sectoral approach between health and social service agencies and their personnel provides new opportunities for community nurses. Such opportunities for change have been witnessed among a number of residential care groups. Changes envisaged in the role of the mental handicap nurse confirm that radical approaches to shared learning and working between health and social care agencies might well become a more generalized feature of all community care in the UK by the end of the present decade (Sines, 1993).

Finally, staff will require opportunities for personal and professional advancement and career progression. Managers should provide staff with personal development and education plans which are informed by systematic feedback on personal performance.

● **Conclusion**

This chapter has considered the development and evolution of residential care services in the community. The mixed economy of care facilitated by the enactment of the NHS and Community Care Act 1990 has resulted in the provision of a matrix of opportunity for clients who were otherwise dependent on hospital-based models of care provision.

It is suggested that there is no one blueprint for the ideal residential service model of the future. Instead, a range of basic service principles have been postulated that are regarded as being fundamental to the provision of quality-based services to a range of clients throughout the UK. Underpinning these is the process of case management and shared action planning.

Traditional methods of preparing nurses for practice in the community have also been challenged (Sines, 1993) and a more collaborative approach to care delivery between health and social care agencies will undoubtedly further change the boundaries that currently exist between community nursing staff and social workers.

However, in response to these challenges community health care nurses have extended the traditional boundaries of their home-based practice to include the delivery and monitoring of care to people living in a range of residential services in the community. In so doing they have demonstrated their flexibility and ability to respond to a continuously changing health care agenda. Consequently, the challenge for professionals in the future will be to ensure that their skills are not dependent upon any one facility, but are accessible to clients wherever they live and whenever they need them.

References

3 & 4 Geo. V., C.28. *Mental Deficiency Act* (1913)

43 & 44 Eliz. II., C.19. *The National Health Service and Community Care Act*

Bendix, R. (1956) *Work and Authority in Industry: A Study of Changing Managerial Ideologies in the USA, Britain and in the USSR*, Harper, London

Brandon, D. and Towe, N. (1989) *Free to Choose – An Introduction to Service Brokerage*, Good Impressions, London

Brechin, A. and Swain, A. (1987) *Changing Relationships – Shared Action Planning for People with a Mental Handicap*, Harper and Row, London

DHSS (1988) *Residential Care: A Positive Choice and the Research Reviewed – Report of the Independent Review of Residential Care*, Vols 1 and 2 (Chairman Lady Wagner), Department of Health and Social Security, London, HMSO

DoH (1991) *Statistical Review*, HMSO, London

Goffman, E. (1961) *Asylums: Essays on the Social Situation of Mental Patients and Other Inmates*, Anchor Books/Doubleday, Washington D.C.

Jenkin, P. (1979) Speech to the Social Services Conference, Bournemouth, 21 November

King, R., Raynes, N. and Tizard, J. (1971) *Patterns of Residential Care*, Routledge and Kegan Paul, London

Knapp, M. and Renshaw, J. (1986) *Criteria in Planning Social Services For Mentally Retarded Adults*, Discussion Paper 429/2, Personal Social Services Research Unit, University of Kent, Canterbury

Laslett, P. (1971) *The World We Have Lost*, Methuen, London

Malin, N., Race, D. and Jones, G. (1980) *Services for the Mentally Handicapped in Britain*, Croom Helm, London

Mansell, J., Felce, D., Jenkins, J., de Kock, U. and Toogood, S. (1987) *Developing Staffed Housing for People with Mental Handicaps*, Costello, Tunbridge Wells

Morris, P. (1969) *Put Away: A Sociological Study of Institutions for the Mentally Retarded*, Routledge and Kegan Paul, London

NCVQ (1989) *Extension of the NVQ Framework Above Level IV – A Consultative Document*, National Council for Vocational Qualifications, London

O'Brien, J. and Lyle, C. (1987) *Framework for Accomplishment*, Responsive Service Systems Associates, Georgia

Oswin, M. (1976) *Children Living in Long-Stay Hospitals*, Heinemann, London

Scofield, R.S. (1968) The measurement of literacy in pre-industrial Britain. In *Literacy in Traditional Societies* (ed. J. Goody), Cambridge University Press, London

Sines, D.T. (ed.) (1988) *Towards Integration – Comprehensive Services for People with a Mental Handicap*, Harper and Row, London

Sines, D.T. (1993) *Opportunities for Change – A New Direction for Nursing for People with Learning Disabilities*, Department of Health, London

Strong, P. and Robinson, J. (1990) *The NHS Under New Management*, Open University Press, Buckingham

Tredgold, R. and Soddy, K. (1963) *Tredgold's Textbook of Mental Deficiency*, 10th edn, Baillière, Tindall and Cox, London

Wagner Development Group (1988) *Report of the Independent Review of Residential Care*, Vol. II *The Research Reviewed*, Wagner Development Group, London

Walker, A. (1989) Community care. In *The New Politics of Welfare – An Agenda for the 1990s*? (ed. M. McCarthy), Macmillan, London

17

Health and homelessness

John Dreghorn and John Atkinson

● Introduction

It is highly appropriate that a book about community health care nursing should contain a chapter on the care of homeless people, who form a significant body of the population with specific health needs. Since their origin, community health care nurses have been involved not only in actual nursing care of those without homes but have acted as powerful advocates for better conditions and developers of innovative practice in this area. Lees, an early district nurse, writing at the end of the last century, describes her battles with landlords (Baly, 1987). In recent times both a political and a professional focus has been placed on homeless people. In 1987, the International Year of the Homeless coincided with the centenary of the Queen's Nursing Institute and during the celebrations two projects by community health care nurses which explored the health needs of this group of people were highlighted (Atkinson, 1987; Burke Masters, 1988). In 1993, for the first time, the Royal College of Nursing (RCN) Research Advisory Group National Conference held a session demonstrating nurses' work with rough sleepers, families in bed and breakfast accommodation and single homeless men. In the same year the theme of the RCN Annual Congress was 'Homelessness'.

The authors of this chapter are district nurses who have recently completed a government-funded project examining district nursing intervention with single homeless men (Alexander *et al.*, 1994; Atkinson, 1994). The chapter will describe definitions of homelessness, problems which individuals and groups encounter, some of the social and political implications, and examples of practical strategies to help homeless people gain access to, and receive, health and nursing care.

The chapter will not tell the reader 'what to do', but will highlight the relevant literature and set out strategies that might be useful. The reason for this centres on the fact that each nurse has to examine particular local problems and view the situation of homeless people in their specific context. The authors, who worked in Glasgow, found problems particular to that area, different from those identified by their colleagues in London and Liverpool. It is hoped that nurses interested in this area of community health care nursing will follow up the references and contact the authors.

● **The nature of homelessness**

Popular concepts of homelessness are of the 'cardboard city' or people sleeping in doorways. These are the images of homelessness most often portrayed by the media which present a powerful picture of deprivation within a developed and prosperous society.

However, these images give a distorted view of homelessness when compared with the experience of the larger numbers of people who are not in fact 'roofless' but who live in hostels, boarding houses or multi-occupancy flats (where two or more families live in a dwelling designed for one). Such homeless people are commonly found in urban areas, but may also be found in a country district where overcrowding, inappropriate shelter and lack of suitable housing, particularly for people of working age, has occurred (HHARP, 1993).

Definition

The United Nations General Assembly Resolution, in 1984, defined the homeless as

> *Those who have no home and who live either outdoors or in emergency shelters or hostels, and people whose homes do not meet UN basic standards. Those standards include adequate protection from the elements, access to safe water and sanitation, affordable prices, security of tenure and personal safety and accessibility to employment, education and health care.*

If universally applied, this definition would cover large numbers of people who would not consider themselves to be homeless; nevertheless it is important as it recognizes that there is more to being homeless than the mere lack of shelter, and it allows for the identification of different categories of homelessness. Community nurses look after people in various forms of housing, and may view homelessness as part of a continuum, with the safely, adequately housed client at one end and at the other end the roofless, frequently ill client unable to maintain a safe abode. In between the two poles the community nurse may meet clients with every combination of housing deprivation combined with health and social need.

Who are homeless people?

Much of the literature of homelessness emphasizes that there is no single definition of 'the homeless'. The stereotype of the destitute, middle-aged, male alcoholic, which to some extent is still accepted, resulted from research carried out in the UK in the 1950s and 1960s. (BBC 2, 1987; Marshall and Reed, 1992). Since then, evidence has emerged both in Britain and in the USA that as the numbers of homeless people increase so does the diverse nature of the group (Hondnicki, 1990; Barry *et al.*, 1991). Drake *et al.* (1982) describe the homeless as a 'heterogeneous and ill defined target population' which includes the single homeless who may live in hostels or sleep rough; homeless families who are temporarily residing in bed and breakfast accommodation, and the young homeless who have left the parental home and may be living in a squat. Even within these groups there are numerous subgroups, such as the chronic or traditionally homeless, the de-institutionalized, and the 'dishoused' or temporary homeless (Doolin, 1986).

Single homeless hostel dwellers

Studies in the USA and Britain have found that single men account for between 75% and 90% of the homeless population (Bassuk *et al.*, 1984; Shanks and Smith, 1992). This fact is reflected in the number of available hostel places (in Glasgow there are approximately 250 places in women's hostels compared with 1700 places in men's hostels (Laing, 1993). There is growing evidence that the number of homeless women is still on the increase (Hondnicki, 1990; Marshall and Reed, 1992). However, they are less likely to become hostel dwellers or rough sleepers as women are more likely to become homeless with their children and therefore are found in bed and breakfast and multi-occupancy flats (Thomson and Atkinson, 1989).

Children

Lack of fixed abode provides particular problems for children who often spend a transient life going from place to place and miss out on school and regular contact with health professionals such as a health visitor (Drennan and Stearn, 1986; Billings, 1993). Although they make up the largest percentage of *registered* homeless people in the UK, about 65% of children are registered as homeless with their parent(s) (Shelter, 1990). An individual cannot be registered as homeless, in their own right, until they are 16 years old. There are many children, commonly between the ages of about 10 and 16, who have become separated from their families and live informally with friends and other family members. These children are often 'lost' to the services, apart from people like health visitors who visit children at home and may come across other children living in a house (Macmillan *et al.*, 1992).

Ethnic minority groups

It is appropriate at this stage to highlight people from ethnic minorities as those who suffer from marginalization in many ways, including homelessness. In multi-ethnic areas, being non-white or from another culture or language group can exacerbate other social problems discussed in this chapter which lead to homelessness (Shelter, 1990). Also found are larger proportions of some ethnic groups in certain types of homeless accommodation. O'Meachair and Burns (1988) describe the large proportion of Irish men among the London homeless. The treatment of individuals from ethnic minorities who have mental health problems and are homeless is also a cause for concern and political advocacy (Black Housing, 1989). Workers in the field, including the authors, have also noticed how individuals for whom English is not their first language often find themselves even more disadvantaged than others. The reader is advised to take particular notice of the ethnic profile in their own area, as there are many differences throughout the country. Being from an ethnic minority is seldom the primary cause of being homeless, but is often a cumulative, secondary factor.

● **Homelessness and health**

Problems for the homeless individual
Barry *et al*. (1991) state: 'There is a close relationship between homelessness and poor health.' Many of the health problems experienced by homeless people can be partly explained by poor living environments. Overcrowding, in hostels and bed and breakfast hotels, increases the risks of accidents and fires, as well as the spread of infectious disease. Insanitary conditions to be found in large hostels again encourage the spread of disease. Those who sleep rough experience more respiratory problems and musculoskeletal disorders than those who occupy secure accommodation (Shanks and Smith, 1992). The authors, working with the Tuberculosis (TB) Surveillance Unit, encouraged 100 men to attend for a chest X-ray. Ten were found to have abnormal X-rays, six associated with tuberculosis, four with carcinoma. Bearing in mind the fact that the prevalence of TB (up until 1993 when pockets of resistant TB were found in the UK) has in recent years been so low in the general population that statistics are not given and regular screening is considered unnecessary, the figure is considerable (CD(S)U, 1993; Atkinson, 1994).
A recent study by the charity Crisis at Christmas (Keyes and Kennedy, 1992) found that people sleeping rough were

150 times more likely to be fatally assaulted, 34 times more likely to kill themselves, 8 times more likely to die in an accident, 3 times more likely to die of pneumonia or hypothermia than the population average.

Barry *et al*. (1991) cite a number of studies which report higher incidence of respiratory problems; malnutrition; pulmonary TB; physical handicap; alcohol and drug abuse. A study of hostel dwellers in Glasgow (Macmillan *et al*., 1992) found that 27% had obvious physical disability or illness. These problems are not new: Stewart (1975) and Hewetson (1975) both reported a variety of physical and mental problems associated with homelessness. What is new is that a large and increasing number of people are being affected by the unhealthy lifestyle and living conditions associated with homelessness.
The Health Visitors' Association and the General Medical Services Committee (HVA/GMSC, 1989), in an examination of homeless families, found similar physical morbidity along with development delay, accidents and vulnerability among homeless children.

Mental illness

The high incidence of psychiatric morbidity within homeless populations is well documented (Lamb and Talbot, 1986; Timms and Fry, 1989). In general terms, between 30% and 40% of the homeless population have a history of mental illness compared with between 5% and 10% in the general population. Atkinson (1994) reported similar results based on a study of two large hostels in Glasgow, by using the Hospital Anxiety and Depression (HAD) scale developed by Zigmond and Snaith (1983). Of those interviewed, 34% were found to suffer from anxiety, or depression, or both.

De-institutionalization and its effects

The term de-institutionalization refers to the process by which the large custodial institutions built in the nineteenth century to house those deemed to be insane have gradually (in the UK) or rapidly (in the USA) been reducing their capacity and closing. The resulting de-institutionalization occurs when the former patients are transferred or discharged into the community. In America during the 1960s, a combination of the emergence of civil rights movement and the realization by State governments that considerable sums of money could be saved by closing down State-run hospitals led to a rapid run-down and closure of mental hospitals. In the UK, the move towards de-institutionalization has been a more gradual process: between 1954 and 1983 the number of people residing in long-term stay psychiatric hospitals was reduced from 154 000 to 70 000 (Morris, 1984).

There is considerable controversy regarding the effect that de-institutionalization has had on the composition and numbers of homeless people. In America between 1955 and 1980, the State hospital population fell from 559 000 to 132 000 (Roth *et al.*, 1986). There has been criticism of the policy, with Lamb and Talbot (1986) concluding

With the advantage of hindsight, we can see that the era of deinstitutionalisation was ushered in with much naiveté and many simplistic notions about what would become of the chronically and severely mentally ill.

What seems to have happened is a failure to provide alternative community care for those discharged from hospital. Indeed, Daly (1989) argues: 'Once released from institutions, and without adequate support services, these individuals are effectively adrift in a sea of confusion.'

In the UK, where this process has not been quite so dramatic, there are those who are concerned that the mistakes made in America are being replicated. Williams and Allen (1989) found that 1 in 6 of those who had been in hospital in the previous five years had been discharged onto the street. Quick (1990) states that 'one has only got to look at the American experience . . . to appreciate one possible consequence of the route mapped out by Griffiths'. Similar concerns are expressed by Hollander (1990) who goes on to urge for a slowdown in hospital closures. There have been no clear resolutions to the effects of de-institutionalization and attempts at community integration either in the USA or Europe including the UK.

The social consequences of homelessness

The social consequences of homelessness can be as damaging to individuals' health as the fact of being homeless. The stigma of homelessness further marginalizes a group who are set apart from the rest of society because they do not fit into society's vision of an acceptable lifestyle. Therefore, to be homeless in a society where the majority of the population are owner-occupiers (as in the UK) leads to a loss of status and feelings of inadequacy.

The problem of being homeless is compounded by the fact that the loss of a permanent house frequently follows a series of social difficulties. These may include: loss of employment and income, break-up of marriage or permanent relationship, loss of contact with family, alcohol or drug abuse and a prison record. Many of those living on the streets or in hostel accommodation have a combination of these experiences.

Once someone becomes homeless their problems increase, as an important element of citizenship in the UK is to have a registered address. For example, a homeless person has difficulty registering for employment or benefits, registering with a GP, registering to vote, opening a bank account, applying for a loan and many other practical difficulties associated with modern living which are accepted as rights of citizenship.

Community health care nursing interventions

To provide care for homeless people requires a change in patterns of practice for the majority of community nurses. The move from a reactive referral-based model of community nursing practice to a pro-active case finding approach is the first and most important step to take. Since many community nurses rely on GP and hospital referral for the bulk of their case load, there will therefore be a failure not only to meet the needs of the homeless but a potential failure even to appreciate the level of unmet need.

Atkinson (1994) found that of 106 male hostel dwellers interviewed, 66 required some form of nursing intervention, despite being registered with a local GP. This high level of unmet need can only be recognized if community nurses actively seek it out by providing an outreach service to hostel dwellers, rough sleepers, those in bed and breakfast accommodation and other vulnerable clients in homeless situations. Every kind of community nurse may be involved, depending on group and individual health needs, using a range of strategies for nursing action.

The main benefits for the homeless client occur when she or he receives an appropriate assessment from a community nurse which identifies health and social needs followed by specific and appropriate referral. A measure of success of the intervention is reflected by reductions in the so-called inappropriate use of accident and emergency departments by homeless people who self-refer for health care in the absence of any other available service (Powell, 1987a).

One of the major barriers to the adequate provision of care stems from professional and contextual assumptions which exist with regard to those in homeless accommodation. There exists the belief that their ill-health, both physical and mental, is a direct result of their living conditions and therefore in some way they are less worthy of treatment because the root cause cannot be altered. This attitude may also be found, and parallels can be drawn, with current thinking and practice relating to heart surgery for cigarette smokers, examples of which were given a high profile in the UK press and television media in 1993. Some people are unwilling or unable to cease smoking and are occasionally denied access to treatment on the grounds that their health problem (heart disease) will return unless the root cause (smoking) is resolved.

Similarly, the authors and other community nurses find health professionals who are unwilling to help homeless clients because there is a belief that little may be achieved in improving the health of this population group while they remain homeless. This assumption has been disproved in a recent study by Atkinson (1994), which found that although high levels of physical and, importantly, treatable psychiatric morbidity existed, the majority of participants perceived themselves well. It is important to recognize that a homeless client presenting with health needs is just as relevant to a health professional as any other member of society.

Costs and benefits of intervention

Increasingly health interventions are being determined in relation to the measurable health gains to be achieved. Difficult choices are to be made regarding the provision (or withholding) of a specific treatment where the criterion for provision is not simply 'how ill is she or he?' but also 'by how much will she or he benefit?'. If this criterion is applied universally, it is clear that those with the least healthy lifestyles may lose out when choices have to be made. This will have a direct effect on the already inadequate provision of care for the homeless.

Rationality of being homeless: the individual's choice

It is important to accept that *some* people choose their lifestyle. The authors found that some of the single homeless men chose to live in hostel-type accommodation. They had a warm bed and company which they did not have to provide for themselves. Interestingly, many of these men had lower anxiety levels and were physically better than the other men who did not see the hostels as 'home' and who were highly anxious and unhealthy (Atkinson, 1994). However, it would be quite wrong to assume that *all* homeless people are homeless by choice. Whatever the circumstances, this should not stop the community nurse striving to assist clients achieving full health potential.

● **Strategies for nursing care management**

This section suggests areas where the community nurse may make changes to her practice and ways in which the primary health care team may become more efficient and effective without enormous cost.

Inter-agency working

It is essential to make clear at the beginning of this section on strategies that nurses working with homeless people are often working as the lone health care provider. However, other services have a key role in the care of the homeless, particularly social work and housing departments, many of whom have special units for homeless clients. To get the best client care outcomes, co-operation between nurses and these services are essential and recommended on interpersonal and management strategy levels.

Integration of homeless clients into mainstream practice

In theory, homeless people should have equal access to primary health care services. In practice, people who are homeless face a number of difficulties in gaining access to service. Perhaps the first strategy to suggest is that community nurses refine their role and become *community* nurses. At present, many nurses see their role as strictly to provide services for the case load they derive from referrals from GPs, hospitals and other professionals. It is suggested that their role is also to serve their community by ensuring that homeless people and other marginalized clients have access to appropriate health services. For a discussion of assessment of health needs, see Chapter 23.

Registration with a General Practitioner

Many homeless people are not registered with a GP and considerable numbers no longer reside in the area of registration, having moved to another part of the country. Helping people to register with a sympathetic local GP is probably the single most helpful first act the nurse can instigate. This may be achieved through temporary registration where no hostel or other address is available. Registration may also be effected by using the health centre or surgery address in lieu of a 'home' address for registration purposes, or where prescriptions for medicines are requested. Having emphasized the importance of being registered with a GP, the nurse must also be aware that a number of individuals will not be registered. Even when registered, there is a reluctance to attend the surgery, although some of these individuals may require special attention with GPs visiting them where they reside.

Setting up screening and assessment programmes

As stated above, a limiting factor is the reluctance of many homeless people to attend their GP. Serious illness can go undetected, with chronic conditions often accepted as something to be tolerated. Health visitors, community psychiatric nurses, district nurses, community mental handicap nurses and practice nurses can all bring their particular talents to the screening and monitoring of different types of homeless client. Together with their GP colleagues, community nurses can all play an important role, ensuring that homeless people receive regular health screening when they attend primary health care services for any reason, in the same way that opportunistic screening is conducted for others presenting for health care.

By the nature of their work, community nurses become known to the community at large and develop contacts well beyond the limits of their case load at any given time. This familiarity within the community may be extended to areas where large numbers of homeless people are to be found, for example, hostels, day centres and food distribution centres. By spending time in these areas the nurse will become known and accepted, and as trust develops, opportunities for active intervention will present themselves. In this way the nurse can develop a network of contacts within the homeless population. This approach takes time, since trust cannot develop overnight. To work in this way requires the support of management and colleagues, particularly in the early stages when success cannot be judged on the basis of numbers of client contacts, by numbers of action interventions or by obvious practice outcomes. However, in the longer term this form of pro-active nursing has a number of benefits for the client group, community nursing and the wider health service.

Physical and psychiatric morbidity screening and monitoring

The authors have found that by combining the use of validated assessment tools with an individual needs assessment process, a strong knowledge and database can be accumulated about needs of the homeless individuals within a locality. This ensures comprehensive service planning, including appropriate resourcing for this special group.

For example, the authors used the Barthel Index of Physical Function (Mahoney and Barthel, 1965), the Hospital Anxiety and Depression Scale Questionnaire (Zigmond and Snaith, 1983), a 26-question questionnaire containing personal, health and demographic detail, as well as a needs assessment based on Activities for Daily Living (Roper et al., 1990). This package produced interesting statistical data as well as detailed information which made the nursing interventions known as Treatment, Referral and Advocacy possible (Atkinson, 1994). Nurses working with families and young children would use a different combination, containing tools for assessing levels of development and vulnerability as well as the child's immunization history for instance.

Pro-active nursing

Perhaps the biggest decision for the individual nurse is when she or he decides to take part in pro-active nursing or case finding which requires the commitment of purchasing authorities as well as the support of management within the provider organization in which she or he is working. Having made the decision to help a group, such as homeless men or families, the rewards are sometimes few and the problems difficult. However, those who take part find it worth while and empowering for themselves as well as their clients (Atkinson, 1994).

Packages of care/case management

With the implementation of the NHS and Community Care Act 1990 and the development of NHS Trust areas throughout the UK, accountability has assumed corporate as well as professional meaning. Nurses are increasingly being asked what *specific* needs patients and patient groups have, and what level and grade of nursing support is required to fulfil these needs. Also they are required to identify *exactly* the outcomes of particular interventions and procedures. The community nurse must also influence the purchasers of community care (including social work departments) to ask for the appropriate service, at the same time as providing the highest standard of care possible within the resources available (see also Chapter 8).

Balancing these demands is difficult, to which must be added the challenge of ensuring parity and equity of provision to everyone, including those who are marginalized from mainstream services. The problem of negotiating what may be seen as new or extra services in an already tight budget is particularly problematic and community nurses must not only demonstrate the moral rightness of setting up and maintaining services for the homeless but also the practical benefits to the community which results from the work.

What follows are some of the areas which the authors, in their own work and with reference to others, have found the most effective way of providing high-level nursing care at the same time as providing accurate clinical data and political leverage (Norman and Parker, 1990; Norman *et al.*, 1992; Atkinson, 1994).

Recording nursing care and patient outcomes

Nursing care may be divided into the four main areas of assessment, treatment, referral and advocacy. Detailed documentation is important to enable some continuity of care and advice.

Assessment is particularly important when caring for people with temporary or transient lifestyles as it gives them a bureaucratic existence, fundamental for any service being received regularly. In a sophisticated society, where people have documents such as driving licence and bank accounts, this fact is often forgotten. Making up individual case notes based on assessment of the individual's needs is a vital first act. Where possible registering a person with a GP and their residence with the Department of Social Security ensures that the person officially exists. In many cities, social work departments have dedicated teams who are expert at getting homeless clients into the welfare system. Liaison with these departments increases the client's chance of receiving services.

These measures may not always be possible (for rough sleepers, for example) but it is the ideal. Assessment provides the foundation to all nursing and community care and facilitates continuity of care.

Treatment is any intervention the nurse makes to improve the client's physical safety, health or wellbeing. It is important to record not only the actual procedure such as a dressing, but also the outcome of that treatment. This is both the physical outcome (the wound healed) and the effects on lifestyle. The combination of physical effect and quality of life outcomes is essential to the professional and political case to secure resources. Treatment also has the important function of providing an entry into the client's life and confidence. The great advantage of nursing intervention is the response to physical problems with tangible, practical help, combined with wider socio-economic and psychological support.

Referral is another important area for community nurses. As an expert generalist she or he has a wide clinical knowledge and is also an integrated member of the health and social care system. Frequently this is just the contact the homeless people lack. The clinical knowledge is invaluable, as the nurse can make highly specific referral to medical, nursing and other agencies, and again recording outcomes is important.

Advocacy occurs when a nurse acts on behalf of a client to further their cause or physically accompanies them to give support. In the author's experience this often has profound effects. A supporting telephone call or letter or accompanying a client to a hospital appointment can sometimes 'tip the balance' for the client. Advocacy also involves bearing witness, that is, recording (physically and morally) the person's situation, views and wishes and representing them to those in authority, to others in the professions and to the public. This may be giving evidence to a health authority committee, but it is also the basic human action of saying to the person: 'I may not be able to solve your problems, but you are not forgotten and I am going to tell as many people as will listen what is going on here.' (For more information on the nurse as advocate, see Chapter 28).

Synthesizing practice

Accurate, concise documentation is crucial in planning care for individual – it is of particular importance for this transient group of clients. The process of recording, collating and presenting information may be assisted by using a critical incident diary; that is, writing down in short, clear sentences, comments on events, interactions and interventions as they happen. When collated the comments produce patterns of practice, client morbidity, client response and other phenomena which can be sorted into themes. Themes can then be exemplified with paradigms or short stories which demonstrate an example of what happened to a particular client. The combination of clinical data, which may be statistically analysed if necessary, with the more qualitative themes and paradigms to give a picture of the range of need and nursing activity in a short report is a powerful ally when seeking resources and maintaining a project.

Managing strategy

The process of providing quality nursing intervention for homeless people may be assisted on a management level by designating health centres and personnel to specific hostels, bed and breakfast hotels, streets and any other sites used by these clients, and in this way develop an area community strategy. This requires the nurse to find out, as accurately as possible, exact numbers of individuals and residences. Local authority and environmental health information on homelessness will be helpful in developing a profile of needs. Most importantly, information may be gained from the observations of community nurses who, in the process of the normal duties, get to know where multi-occupancy flats are or where a child is sleeping in a strange house or where the rough sleeper is. This can be formalized by performing a survey, over a designated period of days, by all the community nurses in a particular area recording on a simple form any homeless clients they have seen or treated and where they were. In Glasgow, this was achieved city-wide over a period of a week (Macmillian *et al.*, 1992).

Specialist input

Over the past few years, a number of schemes have been developed to try to tackle the problems faced by the homeless. These include specialist teams of health care professionals who only work with the homeless, the provision of medical clinics within hostels, and having a named doctor for a specific hostel (Powell, 1987b; El Kabir *et al.*, 1989; Hamid and McCarthy, 1989). Schemes such as these have had varying degrees of success in terms of meeting some of the health care needs of homeless people. There are arguments for and against specialist intervention, the main disadvantage being that clients remain outside the mainstream system. However, in some areas the problems may be so numerous or complex that they warrant specialist interventions. These projects work best when there is close liaison between the specialist team and the primary health care, social work and housing teams, the specialists acting as agents of integration as well as providing specialist care.

Benefits to the health service of improved services for the homeless

The homeless as the client group benefit from nursing intervention by gaining direct access into primary health care and a means of communication with GPs. Contact with community nursing also gives improved access to other community services. The development of expertise in this area could be extended to involve other marginalized groups within the community.

Benefits to the health service as a whole may not seem immediately obvious. It may be expected that increased nursing activity would generate a significant number of referrals for medical treatment at a time when resources are limited. However, there are benefits, as increased use of primary care services reduces the inappropriate use of acute services.

Similarly, earlier detection and treatment of morbidity prevents hospital admissions at a later date.

● **Conclusion**

In conclusion, emphasis is given to the following points.

Diversity and depth of the problem

Almost any mental picture one may have of a homeless person is, paradoxically, at once bound to be typical *and* not necessarily representative at the same time. Because the registered homeless numbers are made up from homeless families registered with local authorities, the largest number is made up of children, about 65%. Single homeless people are not centrally registered: the Campaign for the Homeless and Rootless (CHAR) estimate that 2 million people may be in this category. Similarly, numbers of people in overcrowded, unsuitable housing such as multi-occupancy flats are not recorded.

The place for nurses

Throughout this chapter the authors have demonstrated nursing projects with homeless people. These include district nurses (Atkinson, 1994), health visitors (Drennan and Stearn, 1986; Billings, 1993), community psychiatric nurses (Hamid and McCarthy, 1989), surgeries (El Kabir *et al.*, 1989) and nurse practitioners (Burke Masters, 1988; Stern and Stilwell, 1989). It is anticipated that this has demonstrated the need for the different groups within community nursing to be involved both on an individual level and a strategic management level.

Community asylum

Effective provision of primary health care for homeless people rests with the recognition that nurses must take account of the patient's context as well as their mental and physical needs. Nightingale in the Crimea, and one of the first district nurses, Lees, emphasized the importance of holism (Baly, 1987). The negotiation and provision of protection, social context and safe environment of care, sometimes called 'community asylum', demands all the expert advocacy skills of the community nurse (Atkinson, 1993). It is hoped that this chapter has helped prepare readers for this increasingly vital function.

References

Alexander, M.F., McIntosh, J.B., Walsh, D. *et al.* (1994) *A descriptive and evaluative study of district nursing intervention with single homeless men from a private hostel in Glasgow.* Research project funded by the Health Services and

Public Health Research Committee of the Scottish Office Home and Health Department. Department of Nursing and Community Health, Department of Social Sciences, Glasgow Caledonian University (unpublished report)

Atkinson, J. (1987) 'I just exist'. *Community Outlook*, **11**, 12–15

Atkinson, J. (1993) Homeless and marginalised – a case for community asylum? *Integrate News*, **40**, 6–7

Atkinson, J. (1994) A descriptive and evaluative study of district nursing intervention with single homeless men from a private hostel in Glasgow. Department of Nursing and Community Health, Glasgow Caledonian University (unpublished thesis presented for consideration for PhD)

Baly, M. (1987) *A History of the Queen's Nursing Institute*, Croom Helm, Beckenham

Barry, A.M., Carr-Hill, R. and Glanville, J. (1991) Homelessness and health: what do we know?, what should be done? Centre for Health Economics, Health Economics Consortium, University of York

Bassuk, E., Rubin, L. and Lauriat, A. (1984) Is homelessness a mental health problem? *American Journal of Psychiatry*, **141**(12), 1546–1550

BBC 2 (1987) A nice way to treat people: an open space film about health care and homelessness. *Transcript of Programme 12/8*

Billings, J. (1993) Comparing the expressed child health belief hierarchies of families living in bed and breakfast accommodation in Thanet with health visitors' perceptions of these hierarchies. Paper presented Royal College of Nursing Research Advisory Group Annual National Conference, Glasgow

Black Housing (1989) Black people and housing. *Black Housing*, **5**(11), 5–8

Burke Masters, B. (1988) The nurse practitioner's surgery. *Self Health*, **18**, 22–23

CD(S)U (1993) Information from the Communicable Diseases (Scotland) Unit, Glasgow

Doolin, J. (1986) Planning for the special needs of the homeless elderly. *The Gerontologist*, **26**(3), 229–231

Drake, M., O'Brien, M. and Biebuyck, T. (1982) *Single and Homeless*, Department of the Environment, HMSO, London

Drennan, V. and Stearn, J. (1986) Health visitors and homeless families. *Health Visitor*, **59**(11), 340–342

El Kabir, J., Nyiri, P., Ramsden, S.S. *et al.* (1989) A mobile surgery for single homeless people in London. *British Medical Journal*, **298**, 372–374

Hamid, A.W. and McCarthy, M. (1989) Community psychiatric care for homeless people in Inner London. *Health Trends*, **21**(3), 67–69

Hewetson, J. (1975) Homeless people as an at risk group. *Proceedings of the Royal Society of Medicine*, **68**, 9–13

HHARP (1993) *Presentation of projects work with the rural homeless in Yorkshire, funded by Shelter*, Harrogate Housing Action Resource Project, Royal College of Nursing Congress, Harrogate

Hollander, D. (1990) Mentally ill and nowhere to go. *Community Care*, **802**, 16

Hondnicki, D.R. (1990) Homelessness: health care implications. *Journal of Community Health Care Nursing*, **7**(2), 59–67

HVA/GMSC (1989) *Homeless Families and their Health*, Health Visitors' Association and General Medical Services Committee, BMA, London

Keyes, S. and Kennedy, M. (1992) *Sick to Death of Homelessness: An Investigation into the Links between Homelessness, Health and Mortality*, Crisis at Christmas, London

Laing, I. (1993) *Single Homelessness and Mental Health Issues in Glasgow*, Glasgow District Council City Housing, Glasgow

Lamb, H. and Talbot, J. (1986) The homeless mentally ill: the perceptive of the American Psychiatric Association. *Journal of the American Medical Association*, **256**, 498–501

Macmillan, D., Miller, H. and Wormsely, J. (1992) *Homelessness and Health: A Needs Assessment in the Greater Glasgow Health Board Area*, Health Information Unit, Department of Public Health, Greater Glasgow Health Board, Glasgow

Mahoney, F.I. and Barthel, D.W. (1965) Functional education: the Barthel index. *Rehabilitation*, **22/23**, 61–65

Marshall, E. and Reed, J. (1992) Psychiatric morbidity in homeless women. *British Journal of Psychiatry*, **160**, 761–768

Morris, P. (1984) Mentally ill and homeless. *Nursing Times*, **80**(35), 16–18

Norman, I. and Parker, F. (1990) Psychiatric patients' views of their lives before and after moving to a hostel: a qualitative study. *Journal of Advance Nursing*, **15**, 1036–1044

Norman, I.J., Redfern, S.J., Tomalin, D.A. *et al.* (1992) Developing Flanagan's critical incident technique to elicit indicators of high and low nursing care from patients and their nurses. *Journal of Advanced Nursing*, **17**, 590–600

O'Meachair, G. and Burns, A. (1988) *Irish Homelessness: The Hidden Dimension. A Strategy for Change*. City of Westminster CARA, London

Powell, P.V. (1987a) The use of an accident and emergency department by the single homeless. *Health Bulletin*, **45**(5), 225–262

Powell, P.V. (1987b) A house doctor scheme for primary health care for single homeless in Edinburgh. *Journal of the Royal College of General Practitioners*, **37**(303), 444–447

Quick, R. (1990) Lost in America. *Nursing Times*, **86**(30), 44–47

Roper, N., Logan, W.W. and Tierney, A. (1990) *The Elements of Nursing*, Churchill Livingstone, Edinburgh

Roth, D., Bean, G.J. and Hyde, P.S. (1986) Homelessness and mental policy: developing an appropriate role for the 1980's. *Community Mental Health Journal*, **22**(3), 203–214

Shanks, N. and Smith, S.J. (1992) British public policy and the health trends of homeless people. *Policy and Politics Journal*, **20**(1), 35–46

Shelter (1990) *Homelessness in England: The Facts*, Shelter, London

Stern, R. and Stillwell, B. (1989) From margin to mainstream. *Health Service Journal*, **99**, 5169

Stewart, J. (1975) *Of no Fixed Abode: Vagrancy and the Welfare State*, Manchester University Press, 104

Thomson, R. and Atkinson, J. (1989) Homelessness and health. *Nursing Standard*, **3**(48), 30–32

Timms, P.W. and Fry, A.H. (1989) Homelessness and health. *Health Trends*, **21**(3), 70–71

Williams, S. and Allen, I. (1989) *Health Care for Single Homeless People*, Policy Studies Institute, London

Zigmond, A. and Snaith, R.P. (1983) The Hospital Anxiety and Depression Scale: Scandinavia. *Acta Psychiatrica*, **67**, 361–370

Part V

Lifecourse: implications for practice

All community health care nurses must be aware of normal development throughout the life span in order to detect potentially important deviations and offer advice drawn from a sound knowledge base. Because much health advising is opportunistic, this understanding is needed even if the community health care nurse works primarily with a specific age group or with those with particular health needs. For example, the practitioner when visiting an older person could be asked for advice on a specific health need of a child within the family. The community health care nurse, if properly prepared, can use such occasions to respond when information is sought and, if necessary, to refer the enquirer to a practitioner with appropriate specialist expertise.

Chapter 18 covers the significance of preconception care for life development. Some of the problems in early pregnancy are addressed. However, it was not considered appropriate to include the immediate postnatal period which generally falls within the remit of the midwife.

Chapter 19 focuses on the child, encompassing a wide age range. Issues of health promotion, the prevention of ill-health and some key health problems that may occur in childhood are discussed within the chapter. The important topic of child protection is addressed and finally the support and guidance required during times of ill-health are included.

A milestone in an individual's development is that of adolescence. Although a separate chapter has not been devoted to it, this does not imply a lack of recognition of the importance of the delights and difficulties of this significant stage in the life span. Indeed, Chapter 19 follows the child's progress into adolescence and Chapter 20 sees this as the beginning of adulthood, since in real life there is no clear beginning or end point to adolescence. Some specific problems relating to the adolescent at school are discussed in Chapter 14.

Adulthood occupies the largest part of an individual's life span. Chapter 20 explores different theories of adult development, using these to illustrate the complex inter-relationship of biological, sociological and psychological factors which determine the nature of developmental change.

A positive approach to ageing is taken in Chapter 21 and the targets for health promotion set out in *The Health of the Nation* (DoH, 1992) are used as a framework to debate key issues. Ageing is also seen as a process without a clear starting point, but the end of the process leads into the final chapter of this part. Chapter 22 considers the sensitive issues of coping with death, the process of dying at home and the support needed for the patient, family, friends and others as well as the community health care nurse. Alternatives to home care and the important developing role of palliative care are discussed.

The authors in this part have each taken a different approach to debate the lifecourse issues of a particular age group. However, a key theme that runs through this part is the need to acknowledge every person as a unique individual regardless of their sexual orientation, culture, lifestyle or age group. There are no hard-and-fast rules about lifecourse, merely guidance through which the community health care nurse can gain an understanding of the complexity of the development of an individual and the implications for relevant intervention.

Reference

DoH (1992) *The Health of the Nation. A Strategy for Health in England*, HMSO, London.

18

Preconception and early pregnancy

Faye Doris

● Introduction

Preconception care is that provided for a woman prior to conception. It aims to achieve optimum health for the woman prior to, and around conception, providing an opportunity for optimal physical, mental and emotional development of each individual conceived (Hollingsworth *et al*. 1984). It has become increasingly important not only as women delay starting a family but also their increased expectations of the outcome of the pregnancy. Jones (1992) reports the increase in fertility rates in the over thirties and Hollingsworth *et al*. (1984) also confirm that the increase is occurring in women aged 30–44 years.

A successful pregnancy begins with a healthy ovum and healthy sperm. Consideration therefore needs to be given to the health of the man and factors that affect the production of healthy sperm as well as those that affect the development of healthy ova in the woman.

The emphasis within health care is that of general population targeting as embodied in *The Health of the Nation* (DoH, 1992a). An increased awareness in the general public of the effects of a healthy lifestyle on the outcome of a pregnancy should result in couples seeking reproductive counselling, screening and a measure of planning for each pregnancy. The rationale for preconception care, its scope and the role of the health professional is set out below.

● Rationale for preconception care

The embryonic period is that during which morphogenesis (development of shape) and organogenesis (formation of organs) occur (Moore, 1988). This period is commonly accepted to take place between 2 and 8 weeks of gestation. A woman may be unaware that she is pregnant or just beginning to acknowledge this, while major structural and development changes are taking place within the developing embryo. At this time there is a risk of many developmental abnormalities occurring as a result of environmental factors such as rubella infection and social habits such as excessive alcohol (Moore, 1988). Drugs such as tetra-cyclines taken during pregnancy are deposited in growing bone and teeth, resulting in staining (British National Formulary, 1994).

A knowledge of the importance of good health during this period and attention to lifestyle may contribute to reducing the incidence of abnormalities. Advice, investigations and treatment are aimed at preven-tion of conditions such as rubella infection in the population as a whole through screening and immunization, and helping both men and women to be more aware of the conditions that may have an adverse effect on the outcome of pregnancy.

● The scope of preconception care

There are many approaches that may be used in the provision of preconception care. Jack and Culpepper (1990) suggest that care is best provided as part of ongoing primary health care, thus making it accessible to everyone. There are two general approaches that may be used; the first being advice on lifestyle issues and the second providing specialist information and guidance for groups with risk factors associated with conception or pregnancy.

The generalist approach

This is mainly concerned with advice on lifestyle and includes information on the effects of smoking, excessive alcohol, diet, exercise and occupational risks to pregnancy.

Smoking

Economides and Braithwaite (1994) suggest that smoking may influence the reproductive ability of a woman by adversely affecting fertility, the early embryo and the fetus. The relationship between smoking and low birth weight has been known for some time: Butler *et al*. (1972) demonstrated that the birth weight of a smoker's baby may be 150–400 g lighter than that of a non-smoker. Pearson (1994), in reviewing the evidence in relation to smoking and its effect on pregnancy, cites studies which show that smoking may also result in preterm delivery and placental abnormalities. The consensus is that evidence is available to show that smoking may affect the ability of women to conceive and increase risks of miscarriage and the delivery of a healthy infant (Wynn and Wynn, 1987; Economides and Braithwaite, 1994; Pearson 1994). 'Foresight' (the Association for the Promotion of Preconceptional Care), in a recent newsletter (Foresight, 1994), reported on the effects of smoking on sperm count and sperm normality. They suggest that a man should give up smoking prior to attempts of conception. The effect of smoking on sperm count and sperm normality is also supported by Wynn and Wynn (1987). In addition, the smoking of cannabis has been shown to have similar effects to cigarette smoking on both men and women (Wynn and Wynn, 1987). It is therefore important to help prospective parents be aware of the effects of smoking on their reproductive health and this information should be included in general lifestyle information provided by all health care workers.

One of the 'Health of the Nation' (DoH, 1992a) targets for smoking is '*at least a third of women to stop smoking at the start of their pregnancy by the year 2000*', and this should be a key motivator for midwives and members of the primary health care team when giving advice to both men and women in those age groups where fertility is significant (DoH, 1994).

Alcohol

Jones *et al*. (1973) describe the effects of excessive alcohol intake during pregnancy which may result in the malformation known as the 'fetal alcohol syndrome'. At birth, the child may have growth retardation, microcephaly, cardiac abnormalities and in the long term may be found to have a learning disability. Pearson (1994) and Wynn and Wynn (1987) consider the evidence on alcohol consumption and its effects on pregnancy. Pearson (1994) found that the evidence showed an association between lower levels of alcohol intake in the mother (two to three drinks per day) and low birth weight. Wynn and Wynn (1987) also found evidence to show that alcohol consumption could cause sperm abnormality in men.

Advice on alcohol consumption should be provided for the whole population, with increased emphasis for couples who may be planning a pregnancy. Women may seek guidance on how much they may actually drink before the fetus is affected. The general aim is to enable women to reduce alcohol intake during a known preconception phase and to abstain during pregnancy. Balen and Challis (1993) support the need to reduce alcohol intake and say that a sensible limit preconceptionally is less than 6 units of alcohol per week.

Diet

There are many dietary factors which have an influence on a woman's fertility, conception and the developing fetus. It is necessary to understand the significance of these factors in order to give appropriate advice and meet individual needs.

Wynn and Wynn (1994) consider body weight and the effects of slimming diets on a woman's reproductive hormones, particularly luteinizing hormone and progesterone, as well as the effects on the menstrual cycle and fertility. The evidence demonstrates a reduced diet of up to 1000 kcal/day may affect the endocrine system and stop reproduction. When consuming a normal diet there is a progesterone surge during the second half of the menstrual cycle. However, this was not evident in a woman volunteer on a diet of 1000 kcal/day. Wynn and Wynn (1994) examine the evidence closely and conclude that dieting during the preconception period could be associated with failure of ovulation and amenorrhoea. When the effects on the reproductive hormones are less severe, a women may ovulate and conceive but may have a miscarriage.

The Department of Health recommends a diet with a calorific value of up to 1940 kcal/day prior to pregnancy and an increase of 200 kcal/day during pregnancy (DoH, 1991). The detailed recommendations are set out in Table 18.1.

Once a woman conceives she is at an increased risk of having a low birth weight baby if she is underweight – a relationship clearly demonstrated during the Dutch famine of 1944–45 (Gray and Buttriss, 1994).

In relation to diet and weight, the Body Mass Index (BMI) (that is, weight in kilograms divided by height in metres squared), has been used as an indicator of pregnancy success. Wynn and Wynn (1994) suggest that fertility begins to decline with a falling BMI of below 23 kg/m, these levels being based on Swedish and American studies. Balen and Challis (1993) consider the normal range to be between 20 and 25 kg/m. The BMI is one index for assessing a woman's preconception health and should be considered within the context of her full clinical picture.

Vitamin A

The DHSS (1990) recommends that women who are pregnant or who might become pregnant should not have excessive amounts of vitamin A, and avoid taking vitamin A supplements (DoH, 1993a). There is a potential risk of teratogenicity associated with excessive intakes of vitamin A. Supplementation with medical supervision was not ruled out by the Medical Officer of Health, but women should be advised not to increase the recommended dose (DoH, 1993a). Liver is known to have increased levels of vitamin A and women should be discouraged from eating it or liver products prior to and during pregnancy.

Table 18.1 Estimated average daily requirements for energy in the non-pregnant and pregnant woman (Adapted from the Department of Health, 1991)

	Non-pregnancy (19–50 years)	Pregnant
Energy (kcal)	1940	+200*
Protein (g)	45	+6
Thiamine (mg)	0.8	+0.1*
Riboflavin (mg)	1.1	+0.3
Niacin (mg)	13	–
Vitamin B_{12} (μg)	1.5	–
Folate (μg)	200	+100
Vitamin C (mg)	40	+10
Vitamin A (mg)	600	+100
Vitamin D (μg)	–	10
Calcium (mg)	700	–
Phosphorus (mg)	550	–
Magnesium (mg)	270	–
Zinc (mg)	7.0	–
Copper (mg)	1.2	–
Selenium (mg)	60	–

*During the third trimester of pregnancy.

Folic acid

There has been a suggested link between a deficiency in folic acid and the occurrence of neural tube defects (anencephaly, encephalocele and spina bifida) since the 1960s (Hibbard, 1964; Hibbard and Smithells, 1965). A vitamin study undertaken by the MRC Vitamin Study Group (1991) showed that folic acid supplementation significantly reduced the risk of a neural tube defect occurring, although supplementation with multivitamins was not as effective.

On examination of the evidence, the Department of Health's Expert Advisory Group (DoH, 1992a) recommended that:

- couples with spina bifida themselves, or with a history of a previous child with a neural tube defect, should be counselled about the risk of future children being affected
- folic acid supplements should be advised preconceptionally for all women who may become pregnant and continued until the twelfth week of pregnancy
- and the dose of folic acid should be 400 μg per day.

The Expert Advisory Group (DoH, 1992a) highlighted the risk of women consuming an excess of other vitamins when trying to achieve the recommended dose of folic acid by using vitamin supplements. In addition, it advised that women with epilepsy on anticonvulsant therapy should be counselled individually by their doctors priors to starting folic acid, as it may affect the drug control on their epilepsy. Whole population targeting is encouraged, as over 95% of pregnancies with a neural tube defect are first pregnancies (DoH, 1992b). With a number of pregnancies being unplanned, an improvement in the nutritional status of the general population can reduce the risk of neural tube defects occurring. Some sources of folic acid are identified in Table 18.2.

Exercise

It is useful to consider exercise and its significance prior to and during pregnancy, as women often seek guidance on this topic during pregnancy. Pearson (1994), following an examination of the relevant literature, concluded that the degree of physical fitness in pregnancy was not shown to have any significant effect on the outcome of pregnancy and that the effects preconceptionally were not known.

Occupational risks

This is one of the most difficult areas to provide preconception advice that can be supported by sound research findings. Much of the evidence is conflicting and health professionals need to consider the potential occupational risk for a woman or man on an individual basis. Vessey and Nunn (1980) looked at the evidence concerning the hazards of anaesthesia and concluded that there was a 40% increase in miscarriages in women exposed to anaesthetic gases and identified nitrous oxide as the potential agent. Female health professionals should be alerted to this potential risk prior to conception.

Table 18.2 Some sources of folate/folic acid (Adapted from the Department of Health, 1992b)

Food	Folate/folic acid per serving (µg)
VEGETABLES	
Broccoli	30
Brussels sprouts	100
Cabbage	25
Carrots	10
Cauliflower	45
Green beans	50
Peas	30
Potatoes, old	45
Potatoes, new	40
Spinach	80
Sweetcorn	10
Lettuce	15
Tomatoes, raw	15
Cucumber, raw	2
FRUIT	
Bananas	15
Grapefruit	20
Oranges	50
Orange juice	40
CEREALS AND CEREAL PRODUCTS	
Rice, white, boiled	5
Spaghetti, boiled	9
White bread, average	25
Wholemeal bread, average	40
Cornflakes, fortified with folic acid	100
Branflakes, fortified with folic acid	100
OTHER FOODS	
Bovril	95
Yeast extract	40
Milk, whole/semi-skimmed	35 (1 pint)

Although there has been concern about paternal exposure to radiation and the risk of leukaemia, evidence is conflicting (Pearson, 1994). Foresight (1994) reports on the possible risks of miscarriage to women who work with visual display units (VDUs) and suggests ways in which women could reduce the level of radiation from these screens. Chemicals such as lead have been implicated as a potential risk to the fetus. Fletcher (1987) states that the evidence suggests that lead points more clearly to reproductive damage to men than to women. Indeed, many chemicals have been linked to the fertility of men and women and the list is too long to include within this discussion. Further debate on this topic can be found in Fletcher (1987) and Foresight (1994).

Prospective parents can be advised to discuss potential hazards with occupational health staff at their place of work and with their health and safety representative. For example, in an occupation such as sheep farming, women may need to discuss the potential risk of *Chlamydia psittaci* with their doctors to reduce the potential risk of a chlamydial infection in pregnancy and one of the possible outcomes of miscarriage

(Department of Health, 1992c; HEA, 1994). Fletcher (1987) suggests that men and women can informally gather information about hazards from their workmates as well as contacting their safety representative or occupational health nurse, or other health professionals.

● **Specialist at-risk group**

Diabetes mellitus

The benefits of preconception care is perhaps best seen in the management of insulin-dependent diabetes mellitus. Diabetes mellitus has been associated with a poor pregnancy outcome for many years. Cousins (1983) cited evidence which showed a two or three times increase in congenital abnormalities in this group, and Steel (1985) produced further evidence of a four to ten times increase. These studies showed an association between diabetes mellitus and congenital abnormalities. Steel (1985) listed the common abnormalities as cardiac anomalies, neural tube defects, and caudal regression syndrome, and said that developmental disorders were often multiple and often fatal, and commonly occurred before the seventh week of gestation. She suggests that because pregnancy was often not confirmed before 6 weeks of gestation, it was then too late to take preventive action. She developed a pregnancy clinic in Edinburgh in 1976, with one of its aims being

> to obtain optimum control before conception using intensive educa-
> tion and blood glucose monitoring. Partners were instructed about
> the management of hypoglycaemia, including the use of subcutaneous
> glucagon.

In reporting on the first eight years of the clinic the benefits were clearly seen, with a reduction of congenital abnormalities in regular clinic attenders. Improvements in the diabetic condition were seen to take place before conception. In addition, patients appreciated the opportunity for discussion and advice prior to pregnancy; in particular, contraceptive advice reduced the number of unplanned pregnancies, infertility was identified earlier and patients booked earlier at the antenatal clinic and were more sure of their dates of conception. It was found that even the non-attenders at the clinic sought antenatal care earlier and had improved diabetic control because of their increased awareness of the need. The work of Fuhrmann *et al.* (1983) is widely cited as further evidence of the benefits of prepregnancy diabetic care.

The key health educators of insulin-dependent diabetics may be the physician and diabetic specialist nurse, but as many nurses work in diabetic clinics within general practice the opportunity and responsibility to undertake preconception care involves a wide range of community health care nurses. There is a need to recognize that preconception care of the diabetic woman involves more than good diabetic control; it also involves education about pregnancy and its effects, treatment of diabetic complications such as retinopathy prior to conception and good and appropriate family planning advice until stability is achieved. The principles of preconception diabetic care are clearly set out in the aims of the preconception clinic described by Steel (1985).

Phenylketonuria
Phenylketonuria is an inborn error of metabolism (Simpson, 1989) which is characterized by high levels of phenylalanine which may damage the developing brain of the fetus and young children (Simpson, 1989; Hensman, 1989). It is a genetic condition which is managed by a diet low in protein phenylketonuria. High levels of phenylketonuria prior to conception and during pregnancy may result in a baby being born with congenital abnormalities including heart defects, microcephaly and mental retardation (Hensman, 1989). The risk of this is reduced if the woman is aware of the need to have a strictly controlled diet prior to conception and monitoring of her phenylalanine levels.

● **Specific health risks in pregnancy**

Listeriosis
Listeriosis is an illness caused by the bacterium *Listeria monocytogenes*. The organism is found in soil, water and vegetation and up to 1 in 20 people carry it in their gut without apparent ill effects (Acheson, 1989). Infection may occur through consumption of contaminated food and when it occurs in pregnancy it may result in miscarriage, stillbirth or neonatal death (Acheson, 1989). The Chief Medical Officer at the Department of Health in 1989 issued advice to pregnant women which stressed the need to avoid eating certain types of soft cheeses, such as Brie, Camembert and blue vein types. They were also advised to reheat cooked chilled meals and ready-to-eat poultry until piping hot. General hygiene precautions were also advised. More recent advice (DoH, 1992c) relates to women involved with sheep farming, who should avoid lambing as aborted or sick lambs may also carry the organism.

Although the Department of Health states that there is no need to avoid the at-risk foods before pregnancy or after a baby is born (DoH, 1992c), it is prudent to provide this information to women prior to conception, thus reducing the risk of acquiring an infection during pregnancy.

Toxoplasmosis
Toxoplasmosis is an infection by the organism *Toxoplasma gondii*. The organism has been found in the tissue of most vertebrae (Ritter and Vermund, 1985) and the host of this parasitic organism is the cat (Pope, 1992; Pearson, 1994). Infection may be acquired through many sources such as raw or undercooked meat, contact with cat faeces and by eating vegetables and fruit soiled by animal carriers (Pope, 1992; Pearson, 1994). Primary toxoplasmosis infection occurring between 8 and 24 weeks may result in a severely affected fetus. An infection in pregnancy may

lead to an abortion, stillbirth or preterm labour (Pope, 1992). Some of the manifestations that may be seen when fetal infection has occurred include chorioretinitis, hydrocephaly, microcephaly, hepatosplenomegaly and brain damage with cerebral calcification (Pope, 1992).

Preconceptionally, women who have had contact with cat faeces may be offered serological testing for immune status so that if susceptible to infection they could take precautions to prevent them becoming infected (Pearson, 1994). The Department of Health issues clear guidelines on the protection from such an infection during pregnancy for those women in contact with cats (DoH, 1992c).

Rubella

Rubella infection during the first 12 weeks of pregnancy may result in a baby being born with a cataract, deafness heart anomalies and mental retardation (Bennett and Brown, 1993). Rubella infection in pregnancy is largely preventable with childhood and adolescent immunization, as described in Chapter 14, and the opportunity to identify a woman's immunological status prior to conception through serological testing. With the introduction of the measles, mumps and rubella vaccine at the age of 12–18 months for all children, the risk of someone being non-immune in the future should be minimal. However, health professionals will always need to consider new immigrants on an individual basis, as their immunological status may be unknown. Opportunities for screening and vaccination are available for those occupation groups working with pregnant women and young children. Screening is available at family planning clinics, well-woman clinics and fertility clinics, with women being referred to their general practitioners for vaccination where appropriate. It is important that women who are vaccinated are provided with a reliable contraceptive method to prevent pregnancy occurring for at least three months.

Sexually transmitted diseases

Some sexually transmitted diseases such as *Chlamydia trachomatis* may cause a pelvic infection in a woman and may result in a blockage of her uterine tubes and an inability to become pregnant. Syphilis may cross the placenta and infect the fetus and other conditions such as gonorrhoea may infect the baby during a vaginal birth. Infection in a man or woman is best treated as soon as possible and may improve the fertility of the individual. Guidance also needs to be given about safe sex while a couple are receiving treatment. Couples should be referred to the genitourinary medicine clinic for treatment, but attendance at such clinics carries a stigma. The community health care nurse and midwife need to approach the entire subject of sexually transmitted diseases with sensitivity and need to feel comfortable discussing it with prospective parents. Bowles (1994) supports the need for early referral and treatment of genitourinary infections and says such infections are likely to contribute to infertility, miscarriage and preterm birth.

*Human immunodeficiency virus (HIV) and acquired immune
deficiency syndrome (AIDS)*
A woman who is known to be HIV positive may consider planning
a pregnancy. Her needs should be recognized and the need for specialist
counselling acknowledged. This may include counselling about becoming
pregnant; her health during pregnancy; the risk of her child acquiring
HIV infection and many other aspects of her care. Health professionals
should advise her to discuss the above issues with the health adviser at the
genitourinary medicine clinic. The community health care nurse and
midwife need to be aware of the support agents available to the woman
and her partner locally, and liaise with the support groups and health
advisers when providing support and guidance to couples at the preconception stage.

Genetic disease
Preconception counselling and care is of great value to couples
who are at risk of having a child with a genetic condition allowing
examination of medical history and any necessary investigations to take
place. It enables couples to be informed about specific conditions, risks
and the screening services available to them prenatally, such as an
anomaly ultrasound scan, chorionic villi sampling and amniocentesis
which ultimately assist couples making informed choices with specialist
support.
    This form of counselling is also important to women who are at
risk because of their ethnic background. Conditions that need to be
considered within this group are the haemoglobinopathies: sickle cell
trait, sickle cell anaemia and the thalassaemias. The community health
care nurse and midwife need to recognize the groups at risk of these
conditions, identify the counselling available to them and liaise with
specialist counsellors such as the genetic counsellor specializing in the
haemoglobinopathies. Information about such services may be obtained
from groups such as the Sickle Cell Society; the Organisation of Sickle
Cell Anaemia and Research (OSCAR) and the United Kingdom Thalas-
saemia Society.

Drug exposure
Pearson (1994) says that women should be advised to avoid
unnecessary drugs during pregnancy, particularly during the first 12
weeks when organogenesis is taking place. She argues that specific
counselling is required for women on prescribed drugs such as anticonvul-
sants. Women may continue to take drugs in early pregnancy because
they may be unaware of their pregnancy or their doctor may be unaware
of this when prescribing medication. Health professionals need to
continue to make women aware preconceptionally of the potential
hazards of taking medications during the first 12 weeks of pregnancy.

Contraception

A woman may ask about the most appropriate time to stop taking the oral contraceptive pill, have an intrauterine device removed or stop a contraceptive method to start planning a family. Whatever method of contraception is being used, the aim is for the woman to establish her menstrual cycle prior to conception. This is easier with some methods such as the intrauterine device than with others such as the injectable method, medroxyprogesterone acetate (Depo Provera). Women are commonly advised to wait two or three cycles following discontinuation of oral contraceptives before trying to conceive. However, there is conflicting evidence relating to this practice, with authors such as Guillebaud (1993) disputing the need as ultrasound scanning enables pregnancies to be dated. Guillebaud (1993) declares there are no detectable changes from normal in vitamin and mineral metabolism about two months after stopping the oral contraceptive and the Family Planning Association recommends that women wait for one natural period before trying to conceive.

● **When should care begin?**

Lifestyle issues should be part of the everyday life of the general population and the 'Health of the Nation' initiatives (DoH, 1992a) should ensure an increased awareness of the effects of alcohol, smoking and diet. Fertility clinics, family planning clinics and health centres are some areas where information should be available. Midwives and health visitors would also have opportunities with new mothers when some of this information could be shared in preparation for future pregnancies. There is no predetermined time when preconception care should begin, but information, advice and guidance should be available and accessible to all sexually active couples.

Multidisciplinary care

The community provides the ideal setting for effective multidisciplinary care. The roles of the nurse, midwife, health visitor and general practitioner should be interlinked, for preconception care is not the remit of any one group. The primary health care team may also find that a collaborative approach with health promotion units, family planning, well-women and well-men clinics best meet the needs of the community. There are therefore no role boundaries when providing preconception care, but a need for professionals to communicate and share information, thus making the best use of resources.

Health professionals have to acknowledge the need for preconception care, recognize that it is largely preventive care and work co-operatively to achieve optimum health for the couple prior to conception.

● **Cultural and ethnic considerations**
Within a multi-ethnic society, care needs to be appropriate and thus meet the need of all ethnic and cultural groups. Groups may misunderstand each other and communication may be poor. The 'Health of the Nation' document *Ethnicity and Health* (DoH, 1993b) reinforces the need for health professionals to consider these groups. Many Department of Health publications are also available in different languages and it is worth enquiring about this when requesting health education leaflets.

● **Conclusion**
Preconception care focuses on health, and much of the information about such care is widely available. The health professional needs to recognize that it is available; that it is part of the general principle of a healthy lifestyle for the whole population; and that such care should be introduced during the adolescent period and emphasized to women and men who may be contemplating starting a family. The important role that all community health care nurses play in offering this care should be recognized.

References
Acheson, D. (1989) Listeriosis. *Midwives Chronicle and Nursing Notes*, April, 129

Balen, A.H., and Challis, J.D. (1993) Dietary advice for women wishing to conceive. *British Journal of Midwifery*, **1**(5), 238–241

Bennett, V.R. and Brown, L.K. (1993) Jaundice and infection. In *Myles Textbook for Midwives* (eds V.R. Bennett and L.K. Brown), Churchill Livingstone, Edinburgh

Bowles, A. (1994) Getting fit for conception. *Practice Nurse*. 13 October–3 November, 381–384

British National Formulary (1994) British Medical Association and Royal Pharmaceutical Society of Great Britain, March, No. 27, London

Butler, N.R., Goldstein, H. and Ross, E.M. (1972) Cigarette smoking in pregnancy: its influence on birthweight and perinatal mortality. *British Medical Journal*, **11**, 127–130

Cousins, L. (1983) Congenital anomalies among infants of diabetic mothers. *American Journal of Obstetrics and Gynaecology*, **147**(3), 333–338

DHSS (1990). Vitamin A and pregnancy. Letter from the Chief Medical and Nursing Officer, PL/CMO(90)11, PL/CNO(90)10. Department of Health and Social Security, London

DoH (1991) Dietary reference values for food and energy and nutrients for the United Kingdom. *Reports on Health and Social Subjects*, **41**, HMSO, London

DoH (1992a) *The Health of the Nation. A Strategy for England*, HMSO, London

DoH (1992b) *Folic Acid and the Prevention of Neural Tube Defects: Report from the Expert Advisory Group*, Department of Health, London

DoH (1992c) *While You Are Pregnant: Safe Eating and How to Avoid Infection from Food and Animals*, Department of Health, London

DoH (1993a) Vitamin A and pregnancy. Letter from the Chief Medical and Nursing Officer: PL/CMO(93)15, PL/CNO(93)7. Department of Health, London

DoH (1993b) *The Health of the Nation: Ethnicity and Health*, Department of Health, London

DoH (1994) *The Health of the Nation: An Introductory Booklet for the Primary Care Team*, Department of Health, London

Economides, D. and Braithwaite, J. (1994) Smoking, pregnancy and the fetus. *Journal of the Royal Society of Health*, August, 198–201

Fletcher, A.C. (1987) Industrial hazards and preconception care. In *Preconception Care: Proceedings of a One Day Symposium*, City University, London

Foresight (1994), *Spring Newsletter*, Foresight Association for the Promotion of Preconceptual Care, Godalming, Surrey

Fuhrmann, K., Reiher, H., Semmler, K., Fischer, F., Fischer, M. and Glockner, E. (1983) Prevention of congenital abnormalities in infants of insulin dependent diabetic mothers. *Diabetic Care*, **6**, 219–223

Gray, J. and Buttriss, J. (1994) *Maternal and Fetal Nutrition*, National Dairy Council Nutrition Service, Fact File, **11**, London

Guillebaud, J. (1993) *Contraception: Your Questions Answered*, Churchill Livingstone, Edinburgh

HEA (1994) *New Pregnancy Book*, Health Education Authority, London

Hensman, S. (1989) Phenylketonuria. *Paediatric Nursing*, June, 12–13

Hibbard, B.M. (1964) The role of folic acid in pregnancy. *Journal of Obstetrics and Gynaecology, British Commonwealth*, **71**, 529–542

Hibbard, E.D. and Smithells, R.W. (1965) Folic acid metabolism and human embryopathy. *Lancet*, **1**, 1254

Hollingsworth, D.R., Jones, O.W. and Resnik, R. (1984) Expanded care in obstetrics for the 1980s: preconception and early postconception counselling. *American Journal of Obstetrics and Gynecology*, **149**, 811–814

Jack, B.W. and Culpepper, L. (1990) Preconception care. *Journal of the American Medical Association*, **264**, 1147–1149

Jones, C. (1992) Fertility in the over thirties. *Population Trends*, **67**, 10–16

Jones, K.L., Smith, D.W., Ulleland, C.N. and Streissguth, A.P. (1973) Pattern of malformation in offspring of chronic alcoholic women. *Lancet*, **1**, 1076–1078

Moore, K.L. (1988) *The Developing Human*, W.B. Saunders, Philadelphia

MRC Vitamin Study Group (1991) Prevention of neural tube defects: results of the medical research council vitamin study. *Lancet*, **338**, 131–137

Pearson, V. (1994) *Preconception Care*, Health Care Evaluation Unit, University of Bristol

Pope, E. (1992) Toxoplasmosis. *Midwives Chronicle and Nursing Notes*, October, 300–303

Ritter, S.E. and Vermund, S.H. (1985) Congenital toxoplasmosis. *Journal of Obstetric, Gynaecologic and Neonatal Nursing*, November/December, 435

Simpson, D. (1989) Phenylketonuria. *Midwives Chronicle and Nursing Notes*, February, 37–41

SMA Nutrition. *Planning for a Pregnancy, A Guide for Health Professionals*, SMA Nutrition, Taplow

Steel, J.M. (1985) The pre pregnancy clinic. *Practical Diabetes*, **2**(6), 8–10

Vessey, M.P. and Nunn, J.F. (1980) Occupational hazards of anaesthesia. *British Medical Journal*, **281**, 696–698

Wynn, A. and Wynn, M. (1987) Preconception hazards of alcohol, smoking and cannabis. In *Preconception Care: Proceedings of a One Day Symposium*, City University, London

Wynn, M. and Wynn, A. (1994) Slimming and fertility. *Modern Midwife*, **4**(6), 17–20

19

The child

Liz Porter

● Introduction

The health and development of the child is dependent upon the interplay of the environment in which the child lives and the social forces around the child. During the lifecourse of the child, decisions will be taken for them that will influence their lifestyle into adolescence and beyond. Family, peer attitudes and behaviour, education and government policies will impact on their lifespan development. This chapter will focus on some of the recent research findings and policies which, in part, determine lifespan development and intervention from community health care nurses. In this context the chapter will look at three main issues: health promotion, health maintenance and health management. The section on health promotion will focus on accident prevention, nutrition, dental care and exercise. In the section on health maintenance, topics covered will be child protection, screening, chronic illness and behaviour problems affecting the lifecourse of the child. The chapter will conclude with a review of health management issues, including the changing organization and delivery of services for children. In order to work with the child and his/her family the community health care nurse develops a framework within which to assess the nature of the psychological, sociological and environmental consequences on health and ill-health.

By exploring issues around promoting health, maintaining health and managing health it is possible partially to determine the appropriate interventions needed in the lifecourse of the child.

● Promoting health and preventing illness

The essence of promoting health with the child is to work in partnership with the parents, teachers and others to keep the child healthy, detect signs of abnormality or illness, and facilitate the management of chronic illness. One of the primary responsibilities of community health care nursing is in promoting health (DoH, 1993a). The major settings for action include hospitals, schools, homes and other community groupings. There is particular concern for health promotion among minority communities in relation to the type of health education material available to them (Bhatt and Dickinson, 1992). Health visitors make a particular contribution to the prevention of illness and promotion of health, but all nurses contribute to the 'Health of the Nation' objectives (DoH, 1992a), ensuring that healthy alliances are developed with key players in other organizations. Together, decisions are made which affect the lifestyle and environmental factors that influence the child's health.

Accidents

Accidents are not only a leading cause of death in children but also of admission to hospital (HASS, 1991). Whether measured in terms of morbidity or mortality, accidents in children are among the most important health problems encountered in child health after the first year of life, with socio-economic factors being a more important predictor of accidents than ethnic origin (CAPT, 1989; Graham, 1993). Accidents are related to the developmental maturity of the child and therefore each one requires a different approach in prevention (Levene, 1990). Accidents in the home are common in children under 5 years of age and are particularly common in 2–3 year olds – the mobile toddler (Hall *et al.*, 1990). Boys are more often injured than girls and the incidence of accidents is higher in social classes IV and V (CAPT, 1989).

By school age, young children are experiencing fewer accidents at home and more at school, sport and play. Accidental death as a pedestrian in a road traffic accident is a particular problem. Between 10 and 14 years of age children are 'nearly twice as likely to attend hospital as a result of an accident than children in the 1–4 range' (OPCS, cited in CAPT, 1989). Accidents are the commonest cause of death among children over the age of 5, causing 1 in 6 children to attend a hospital accident and emergency department every year. Road accidents account for about a quarter of all deaths among school children and about two-thirds of all accidental deaths in the same age group (DoH, 1992a).

Reducing the number and severity of accidental injuries is one of the key area targets of the 'Health of the Nation' strategy (DoH, 1993b) in which community health care nurses play a major role. A major component of this role is to influence local policies and priorities of Health Commissions and Trusts through collecting, analysing and making available relevant data on which accident prevention programmes can be based. This helps to raise public awareness and to educate parents, children and teachers to take responsibility for the care and protection of the child. Within General Practice, nurses can influence other team members to be aware of safety issues and undertake opportunistic health promotion, with children and parents attending the practice. Through an interdisciplinary approach at a local level, community health care nurses help to develop effective strategies for dealing with major causes/ problems of accidents in the immediate locality. Co-ordinated prevention programmes are vital to ensure that all practitioners are giving the same message to parents, children and teachers. By influencing behaviour, providing advice and education, child accident rates can be reduced (Roberts, 1991) and a simple, quick and practical system to promote child safety implemented (Adams, 1993).

Nutrition

Nutrition must be adequate if children are to reach their full potential. The child has a need for nutrients and dietary energy (calories) in order to maintain and repair the body and its metabolic machinery, and to provide for day-to-day activity. This allows the achievement of optimal growth, metabolic development and nutritional wellbeing (Turner, 1993). In a multi-racial society, community health care nurses need to be informed about traditional diets of children from different communities in order to give appropriate help and advice and this must be understood in the context of the growing child. Foods are complex mixtures of basic constituents and it is often difficult for the community health care nurse to translate the individual child's diet back into protein, carbohydrate, fat, minerals and vitamins. There are situations in which it is necessary and important to do so, especially as there is increasing evidence suggesting links between diet and health, and between poor diet and under-achievement at school. Iron deficiency anaemia can mean time out from school through illness, junk food has been linked with hyperactivity and violent behaviour in school children (Mason, 1992) and there is increasing concern about developing coronary heart disease in later life as a result of a high fat intake in the child's diet (COMA, 1989). Studies carried out by the Medical Research Council's Environmental Epidemiology Unit in Southampton suggest that heart disease and stroke, and associated hypertension and non-insulin dependent diabetes, initially result from impaired growth and development during fetal life and infancy (Barker, 1992).

Over the past decade there has been a shift towards eating more fibre-rich, starchy foods and less fat (particularly animal fat). Children are eating less butter and consuming more wholemeal bread, but their fat intake, as a percentage of dietary energy intake, remains high. Most of the studies carried out on the eating habits of children also suggest that there are differences between the older and younger children, boys and girls, and between higher and lower socio-economic groups. Meal skipping is particularly common among girls (Balding, 1989) and 6 year olds show a preference for strong tastes, hard crispy textures and interesting shapes of food (Rousseau, 1983). By promoting healthy eating, the community health care nurse can help children and parents increase control over their own health and wellbeing.

The challenge is convincing the children and their families of the benefit and importance of a healthy diet and the long-term investment of health in later life. Opportunities for the community health care nurse to carry out effective and successful interventions include easy accessibility and credibility among parents, teachers and children, their basic nutritional knowledge and their involvement with preventive health care. Primary health care offers a setting for regular monitoring and follow-up of the effectiveness of healthy eating advice. In addition, there is evidence of improvements in the quantity and quality of health promotion activities in the Primary Health Care Team (PHCT) when nurses and medical practitioners work together as a team (Solberg, cited in HEA, 1993).

Where the child is living in poor or hostel accommodation, healthy eating is frequently a low priority for parents. The diet of the child may suffer if a combination of adverse factors exist which may include low income, lack of access to cooking and secure food storage facilities and distance from shops. Bradshaw and Morgan (1987) found that in terms of total nutrients per day, children of low income families had grossly inadequate diets with severe deficiencies. The importance of identifying failure to thrive is identified by Batchelor (1990) who states that 'children can suffer retarded physical and intellectual development'. While acknowledging that potential indicators of failure to thrive are poverty and environment, Hall (1991) recommends community health care nurses use centile charts to monitor children's growth. The importance of discussing food hygiene is also an important issue where there is the use of communal kitchens, since this situation predisposes to food-borne infections. Drennan and Stern (1986) identified the problem of repeated outbreaks of gastroenteritis and more seriously outbreaks of hepatitis B in houses in multiple occupation in London. The community health care nurse should develop an awareness of the child's eating patterns and needs, acknowledging the individual, psychosocial aspects of eating and the effects of income. Establishing good dietary habits in the young lays the foundations for healthy eating in adulthood. What is learned in the early years, good or bad, may be difficult to unlearn and will form the basis on which eating and living habits, and social and intellectual performance throughout life, will be built.

Dental care

This principle of early learning also applies to dental care, where the results of early intervention through health education help prevent tooth decay. Dental decay remains one of the most common childhood diseases, causes pain and discomfort, affects wellbeing and appearance and is a prime example of preventable morbidity (DoH, 1991). Much of the disease occurs in children long before they come into contact with the dental profession (Todd and Dodd, 1985) and therefore it is important for the community health care nurse to teach parents about dental care from birth. The issue of adequate fluoridization of drinking water throughout the country remains contentious and dental caries remain prevalent among children. Although it is unrealistic to expect the complete eradication of sugar from the diet, it is important for the community health care nurse to teach the child the importance of reducing the frequency of sugar intake to avoid tooth decay (HEA, 1991).

Physical activity and disease prevention

Other important elements in the lifecourse of the child are physical activity and disease prevention. The physical activities involved in play provide the young child with a good source of exercise, progressing from pushing toys to walking, running and climbing. With the increased understanding of the importance of exercise on health in later life (DoH, 1992a), studies are looking at promoting physical activity in the child. The recent Allied Dunbar national fitness survey (HEA, 1992) demonstrated that lifelong physical activity is most likely to start in childhood. The community health care nurse is in an ideal position to increase the parents' and children's awareness of the importance of physical activity in maintaining a healthy lifestyle, and schools are ideally placed to encourage children to take physical exercise (Armstrong, 1993). Community health care nurses working alongside teachers in class as part of a health education programme foster the formation of better relations with children, parents and teachers (Johnson, 1991). Moon (1985) has shown that children are particularly interested in their health, growth and development and Williams *et al*. (1985) explain how they influence their parents to lead a healthier lifestyle.

● **Maintaining the health of the child**

The journey through childhood holds many dangers for the health of the child, and there are times when the hereditary traits and disabilities handed down from earlier generations reveal themselves. This, coupled with adverse lifestyle and environment, may influence the lifecourse of the child. Interventions which maintain health, prevent deterioration of health and facilitate an improvement in the quality of life may be of benefit to the child. The needs and welfare of the child are an integral part of the work of the community health care nurse within the context of child protection.

Child protection

The family provides the main basis for protecting children and helping them develop into complete adults. By providing parents with information on health and development and what to expect at different stages of development, the community health care nurse develops a partnership of care which enables parents to take control of their own lives and those of their children. The cultural and ethnic background of the family will influence parenting styles, as will the social and environmental factors surrounding the family. Child protection involves providing families with essential necessities which make good parenting possible, such as clean air, safe housing, a sound nutritional basis and good health (Whitehead, 1988).

The Children Act 1989 emphasizes parents' responsibilities for the moral as well as physical development of their children, and a number of ways of working with children and their families have developed as a means of facilitating this (House of Commons, 1989). The Cope Street project aims to work with parents to improve child care and family health in families (Billingham, 1989). It is situated in a multi-racial, working class inner city community and works towards increasing self-confidence, improving material conditions and providing opportunities to learn: 'A woman who has a sense of self worth is better able to meet their child's needs and to provide appropriate child care' (Billingham, 1989). The implementation of the Child Development Programme in disadvantaged areas, with the use of Community Mothers, offers parents the help of skilled local mothers in assessing the health needs of children and their families and the means towards maintaining health. Suppiah (1994), in evaluating such a scheme, highlights how Community Mothers use their own life experience and understanding to provide support and skills based on the principle of client empowerment. Obviously it is important that community health care nurses work with these workers and children and their families, particularly at times of greatest need in the child's formative years.

Screening and surveillance

Through screening and surveillance, parents and professionals work in partnership to detect disorders in children and to diagnose disabling childhood conditions from as early an age as possible (Hall, 1991). This surveillance and monitoring of child health, growth and development includes a descriptive analysis of each child's strengths and weaknesses in order to determine the most appropriate course of action for the child's physical, social and educational needs in the future. Current thinking is severely critical of the role of screening tests and checklists for assessing developmental status (Barker, 1988; Hall, 1991). However, while acknowledging that developmental checklists have limitations, other authors would argue they provide a substantial amount of information about a child's development which can be observed and recorded. This information can be used by the community health care nurse as a basis for planning and delivering services to children (Wolfendale, 1989).

Sickle cell anaemia, a disease which carries a high morbidity and mortality rate in early childhood, justifies the overwhelming case for early identification of children at risk from the disease (Bittles and Roberts, 1990). Indeed, about 1 in 10 of Britain's African and Afro-Caribbean population has sickle cell trait, while 1 in 400 of the same population has the disease (Mares et al., 1985). The role of the community health care nurse here is one of education, counselling and advice at times of greatest need in the child's life. According to Hindmarsh, growth is one of 'the most sensitive indexes of health in childhood' (cited in McCarthy, 1990). Once again, the use of centile charts provides an immediate visual comparison of previous attainments and allows for continuous comparison over time in relation to height and weight.

As infectious diseases of childhood are brought under control, growth disorders are claiming an increasing share of the General Practitioner's and paediatrician's time (Child Growth Foundation, 1993). Prominent among the treatable disorders of growth is growth hormone deficiency. The incidence is estimated at about 1 in 3000 male births and 1 in 5000 female births in the UK, and the condition is four times as common in boys as in girls (Tanner et al., 1985). In addition, there is little evidence that the advantages of regular weighing justify the resources required (Hall, 1991). While parents value regular weighing, further research into the evaluation of its relevance in detecting psychosocial deprivation and preventing unexpected death in infancy needs to be undertaken.

Speech and language development

The development of speech and language represents the evolution of a fairly complex set of skills, and community health care nurses have a key role to play in the early identification of children with language impairment. This is one of the most common of all developmental problems (Drillien and Drummond, 1983). Because language development is intimately related to general intellectual development and to the use of language in the home, an effective way of identifying speech delay is essential. Profile packs such as those developed by Wolfendale (1989) and the Child Development Programme (Barker and Anderson, 1988) are two of many initiatives currently used by health professionals to help identify speech and language delay. However, in a recent study of parents' views of child health surveillance, 26% (17) of a sample of 66 respondents did not recall being asked about their child's speech at three-year developmental checks (Boyle and Gillam, 1993). This could be an indication that further work is needed in this area. However, the methods appropriate in identifying language impairments are complex and may require the involvement of more community health care nurses in special interest groups to promote the early identification of language impairment in order to keep this important area high on the agenda of future surveillance programmes (Law, 1990).

Immunization

Immunization is one of the most important preventive measures taken to protect the future health of children. Given from an early age, it provides high protection in later life against killing and debilitating diseases, with enormous benefits to the general health of the population. A team of nurses provides a comprehensive immunization/vaccination programme to identified groups within the PHCT, and in the population not registered with the practice (NHSME, 1993).

Between 1948 and 1987 tuberculosis declined tenfold, but there are now about 5000 new cases reported each year (DoH, 1992b). However, in recent years there has been some discussion about the BCG immunization policies for tuberculosis (Smith, 1993). Many Health Authorities/Trusts no longer routinely immunize school children, but of those maintaining a policy, vaccination is offered to children aged 10–14 years who have been identified as having tuberculin-negative Mantoux or Heaf test (Sefi and Macfarlane, 1989). Community health care nurses are increasingly taking on the total responsibility for immunizing school children against rubella (at 11 years) and monitoring the uptake of primary immunization as children enter school (Saffin, 1992).

As the government places more emphasis on the prevention of ill-health, it is important that nurses undertake statistical analysis and epidemiological assessment of need for the immunization of the child (Reid, 1991).

Changes in behaviour patterns and chronic illness

Changes of this sort can have a significant impact on the development of the child and on the family. They can disrupt activities at home, affect school attendance, academic achievement and peer relations (Paton and Brown, 1991). The community health care nurses play a key role in developing an appropriate care plan to facilitate the management of chronic conditions to promote individual coping strategies and ensure that nursing interventions develop the intellectual, social and emotional wellbeing of the child.

Behavioural problems. Children who have *behavioural problems* need a lot of time and understanding. They are frequently a major source of anxiety to their parents and family and need a positive approach to care, with an emphasis on self-help and education. This is particularly so for the child with learning disabilities.

An emphasis on behavioural techniques that help teach parents how to instil a positive change of behaviour in the child can have a profound impact. Quine *et al.* (1991) describe the positive outcomes of such an approach on children with severe sleep problems. Alongside sleep problems, temper tantrums, aggressive behaviour, bedwetting, refusal to eat, stammering and hyperactivity are the most common behavioural problems identified in the literature (Polnay and Hall, 1985; Forfar, 1988). By adopting and using appropriate checklists to identify and help parents deal with behavioural problems as soon as they manifest themselves, it is possible to prevent the problem from escalating as well as building up the confidence of parents to deal with the child's adverse behaviour (Stallard, 1993).

Chronic illness. Children are greatly debilitated by chronic illness, which affects, in particular, their ability to learn. This is markedly so in the school child for whom continued absence through illness, and loss of concentration and motivation while at school, leads to gaps in their education – a structure which ultimately affects the development of their learning. Riley (1987) describes how these children often assume a role in school of being delicate, and where treatment interferes with their ability to learn they frequently become less eager to go to school as they find themselves struggling academically.

Asthma is one such debilitating illness and affects an estimated 700 000 children under 16 years of age, with a significant morbidity associated with lost schooling (DoH, 1991). The prevalence of asthma tends to be higher in the south of Britain than in the north but shows little urban–rural difference (Anderson, 1992).

There is a great deal of continuing research into the cause of asthma, particularly extrinsic asthma which occurs in childhood and is triggered by certain external factors or allergens. Studies such as that by Read (1991) demonstrate a link between air pollutants and asthma. Children are especially vulnerable in this context because they spend more time playing outdoors. In addition, asthma can influence the psychological and social development of the child, particularly if the child is treated as frail and excluded from certain activities at school. The child may develop a lack of self-confidence and low self-image which can continue into adulthood (Taylor and Newacheck, 1992).

As the number of hospital admissions among children is escalating (Strachen and Anderson, 1992), it becomes increasingly important for community health care nurses to develop effective working relationships with the asthmatic children, their parents, teachers and colleagues in order to minimize the debilitating effects of the illness. Adopting a school policy, raising awareness among school staff and developing closer liaisons between the teacher, the child, the parents and the PHCT are ways in which community health care nurses may improve communications about asthma (McLean, 1992). This, alongside the 'Health of the Nation' aims for reducing the incidence of asthma (DoH, 1992a), could diminish the impact of this illness on the developmental progress of the child and prevent dysfunction in the long term.

Eczema, sometimes associated with asthma, may affect any part or almost the whole skin. Damage to the psychological development of the child can be lasting, as the appearance of the skin can frighten other children and teachers into believing the condition is infectious. This results in the child being isolated and possibly emotionally scarred for life through being treated differently (National Eczema Society, 1992).

Diabetes can also affect the lifecourse of the child. This is of particular concern as the incidence of diabetes mellitus in children and adolescents (0–19 years of age) appears to be increasing at 10–15 new cases per 100 000 population each year (DoH, 1991), and the prevalence in Asian groups is reported to be three to four times higher than the national average of 1% and 2% of the general population (Mather and Keen, 1985). Controlled by diet and insulin, the key to caring for the diabetic child revolves around education and support provided by the PHCT (Walker, 1993). It is essential that all community health care nurses have up-to-date knowledge about the condition, treatments and acceptable levels of control. In this way the child can achieve the right balance between quality of life and control of the diabetes. Adapting to the diabetes involves a total reassessment of lifestyle for the child and it is therefore important that attitudes of teaching at school do not encourage overprotection. In addition, disassociation or exclusion of the child from certain curricular activities may lead to resentment and anger by the child. The child needs empathetic understanding and to be empowered with the knowledge of how to make appropriate life choices in relation to diet and lifestyle, as this will limit the complications that can arise in later life. Through understanding the nature of the problems the child might face and developing effective, appropriate interventions it is possible to help facilitate a healthy passage into adolescence.

● **The management of health**

All children should be treated as individuals within a society's health care system. Emphasizing the role and responsibility of parents for the moral as well as the physical development of their children enables a society to develop a number of ways of working with children. Within the

UK, the community health care nurse can enable the child and the parents to make healthier choices through providing information as part of health education programmes, as part of outreach services and being involved in opportunistic screening programmes. By being accessible and responsive to the needs of the child, the community health care nurse can try to ensure that effective treatment, care and rehabilitation are offered at the first sign of any deviation from the normal lifecourse. The principles of good practice for all community health care nurses in the UK are clearly outlined by the Department of Health (DoH, 1993c) and are based on evidence of 'good practice'. The scope of good practice involves a full range of nursing activities that contribute to improving the health of the child through influencing individual behaviour by participating in health promotion and developing activities to challenge policies and practices affecting the environment in which children live. Within this context, the development of a workforce that reflects the ethnic composition of a neighbourhood enables language and cultural barriers to be overcome so that the service all children receive is appropriate to their needs (Potrykus, 1994). Health improvements can be made by supporting and promoting healthy environments where children live and play and through forming healthy alliances with a wide range of organizations (DoH, 1993c). In England, the Court Committee recommended an integrated child health service to facilitate the abilities of parents to care for their children, with prevention as the main thrust and close links between the preventive and curative elements of the child care service (Court, 1976). In concluding this section, three initiatives in child health will be looked at in relation to the sick child, the well child and finally the development of an information system to monitor development.

The sick child

The development of family-centred care identifies a holistic approach to the care of the sick child and, as Campbell and Summersgill (1993) point out: 'The role of the nurse as patient and family advocate has become well established.' Within the framework of family-centred care the nurse must understand and incorporate the developmental and emotional needs of children and their families into the health care system (Shelton *et al.*, 1987, cited in Campbell and Summersgill, 1993). Family nursing can be seen as the logical extension of the paediatric nursing role, particularly with the current emphasis on care in the community. Whyte (1992) explores the paediatric nursing contribution to the support of the family caring for a child with a chronic illness and concludes that nursing support involves

a complex blend of information giving, befriending, family counsel-
ling and advocacy as the nurse moves in and out of the family system
and links the family with support networks in the social system.

Perhaps the main point made by Whyte (1992) is that in reality there is a shift in focus of 'paediatric nursing from the ill child to the whole family as a unit of care'.

The well child

Although preventive child health services and the criteria for the delivery of surveillance services remain an issue for debate, innovations in community health care nursing are developing where parents are acknowledged as partners in the care and development of the child health. One such innovation is 'Family Health Matters', developed by health visitors in York, in an assessment tool which empowers families to assess their own health status and encourages them to work with the community health care nurse to plan improvements or maintain their health status (York Health Visitors, 1988). This in turn offers the nurse a clearer picture of the family's health, enabling them to target their input more effectively. Authors such as Bellman (1989) argue that it is only through a team approach to child development that success can be achieved.

Directives from the European Union provide a framework for many areas of child health which national legislation then converts into regulatory form. An international approach such as this allows for the transfer of experience from one country to another and should enable easier co-ordination of regulations. Child health and development policies must be flexible enough to respond to the individual needs of both a disadvantaged population and those that are more affluent. Similarly, a target nurse-led school nursing service allows for health interviews to be carried out with children and parents who have the greatest need of the service (HVA, 1991). This can be done through identifying health education topics linked to specific age groups and local health issues. Through discussing problems openly, children and parents play an active role in the decision-making process – a process which alongside parent-held child records allows the parent and/or child to take responsibility for their own health and development.

Monitoring development

The use of information systems to provide essential information for caseload management is another important innovation. The National Child Health System in the United Kingdom (Durbin, 1993) is a computer software system designed for monitoring child health and development. It aims to promote and maintain the health of children through providing essential information for health professionals. This computerized framework allows for organizing, planning of appointments, monitoring and managing the developmental health of children. It provides the means for pre-school children receiving regular developmental examinations and screening, with results and special needs recorded so that the intervention is offered at the appropriate point in the child's development. This system focuses on the needs of the child, and enables the community health care nurse to evaluate practice and improve the efficiency and effectiveness of the service offered.

● **Conclusion**

Developments in the delivery of services for children should enhance co-operation between all professionals involved in child care throughout the world. Enabling the sharing of expertise in the field of child development provides a more effective response to the needs of children and acts 'as a process of adaption to the changing demands of living and the changing meanings we give to life' (Dubros, 1960, cited in Parmer, 1985).

References

Adams, C. (1993) Getting the message across on safety. *Health Visitor*, **66**(2), 63–64

Anderson, H.R. (1992) Epidemiology of asthma. *British Journal of Hospital Medicine*, **47**, 99–105

Armstrong, N. (1993) Promoting physical activity in schools. *Health Visitor*, **66**(10), 362–364

Balding, J. (1989) *Young People in 1988*, Health Education Authority, Schools Health Education Unit, University of Exeter

Barker, D.J.P. (ed.) (1992) Relation of fetal and infant growth to plasma fibrinogen and factor VII concentration in adult life. *British Medical Journal*, **304**, 148–152

Barker, W. (1988) The value of developmental tests. *Health Visitor*, **61**(12), 373–374

Barker, W. and Anderson, R. (1988) *The Child Development Programme: An Evaluation of Process and Outcomes*, Early Childhood Development Unit, University of Bristol

Batchelor, J. (1990) *Failure to Find*, Whiting and Birch, London

Bellman, M. (1989) A team approach to child development. *Midwife, Health Visitor and Community Nurse*, **5**, 180–184

Bhatt, A. and Dickinson, R. (1992) An analysis of health education materials for minority communities by cultural and linguistic group. *Health Education Journal*, **51**/2, 72–77

Billingham, K. (1989) 45 Cope Street: working in partnership with parents. *Health Visitor*, **62**(5), 156–157

Bittles, A.H. and Roberts, D.F. (1990) *Minority Populations: Genetics, Demography and Health*, Galton Institute, London

Boyle, G. and Gillam, S. (1993) Parents' views of child health surveillance. *Health Education Journal*, **51**/1, 42–44

Bradshaw, J. and Morgan, J. (1987) *Budgeting Benefit*, Family Policy Study Centre, London

Campbell, S. and Summersgill, P. (1993) Keeping it in the family. *Child Health*, June/July, 17–20

CAPT (1989) *Basic Principles of Child Prevention, a Guide to Action*, Child Accident Prevention Trust, London

Child Growth Foundation (1993) *Disorders of Growth – A Guide*, Series 1, Child Growth Foundation, London

COMA (1989) *The Diets of British School Children*, Final Report from the Chief Medical Officer's Committee on Medical Aspects of Food Policy, HMSO, London

Court, S.D.H. (1976) *Fit for the Future*, Report of the Committee on Child Health Services, HMSO, London

DoH (1991) *The Health of the Nation: A Consultation Paper*, HMSO, London

DoH (1992a) *The Health of the Nation: A Strategy for Health in England*, HMSO, London

DoH (1992b) *Immunisation Against Infectious Diseases*, HMSO, London

DoH (1993a) *Targeting Practice: The Contribution of Nurses, Midwives and Health Visitors*, HMSO, London

DoH (1993b) *The Health of the Nation: A Strategy for Health in England. Key Area Handbook*, HMSO, London

DoH (1993c) *Working Together for Better Health*, HMSO, London

Drennan, V. and Stern, J. (1986) Health visitors and homeless families. *Health Visitor*, **59**, 340–343

Drillien, C. and Drummond, H. (1983) *Developmental Screening and the Child with Special Needs*, Heinemann, London

Durbin, J. (ed.) (1993) Child health system. *Child Health Matters*, newsletter no. 9, summer

Forfar, J. (1988) *Child Health in a Changing Society*, Oxford University Press, Oxford

Graham, H. (1993) *Hardship and Health in Women's Lives*, Harvester Wheatsheaf, UK

Hall, D. (1991) *Health for all Children*, 2nd edn, Oxford Medical Publications, Oxford

Hall, D.M.B., Hill, P. and Ellman, D. (1990) *The Child Surveillance Handbook*, Radcliffe Medical Press, Oxford

HASS (1991) *Home Leisure Accident Research*, Consumer Safety Unit, Department for Enterprise, UK

HEA (1991) *A Handbook of Dental Health for Health Visitors*, Health Education Authority, London

HEA (1992) *Allied Dunbar National Fitness Survey*, Sports Council and Health Education Authority, London

HEA (1993) *Nutrition Interventions in Primary Health Care*, A literature review, Health Education Authority, London

House of Commons (1989) *The Children Act*, HMSO, London

HVA (1991) *Project Health*, Health Visitors' Association, London

Johnson, J. (1991) Classroom health promotion. *Health Visitor*, **64**(5), 152–153

Law, J. (1990) Identifying language impairment. *Health Visitor*, **63**(9) 297

Levene, S. (1990) Approaches to child accident prevention. *Midwife, Health Nurse*, **26**, 211–215

McCarthy, N. (1990) Children with restricted growth: *Nursery World*, 11–14 Oct., 11

McLean, F. (1992) Asthma in school: why nurses must campaign. *Professional Care of Mother and Child*, February, 37–38

Mares, P., Henley, A. and Baxter, C. (1985) *Health Care in Multiracial Britain*. Health Education Authority/National Extension College, London

Mason, P. (1992) A load of junk. *Nursing Times*, **88**(9), 20

Mather, H.M. and Keen, H. (1985) Southall diabetes survey: prevalence of known diabetes. *British Medical Journal*, **291**, 1081–1084

Moon, A. (1985) Children's perceptions of health and illness. MA Dissertation, University of Southampton

National Eczema Society (1992) Managing child eczema. *Primary Health Care*, **12**(5), 10–14

NHSME (1993) *Nursing in Primary Health Care, New World New Opportunities*, HMSO, London

Parmer, M.D. (1985) Family care and ethnic minorities communication. *Nursing*, 2nd Series, 1068–1071, Baillière Tindall, London

Paton, D. and Brown, R. (1991) *Lifespan Health Psychology. Nursing Problems and Interventions*, Harper Collins, London

Polnay, L. and Hall, D. (1985) *Community Paediatrics*, Churchill Livingstone, Edinburgh

Potrykus, C. (1994) Government tackles NHS barriers. *Health Visitor*, **67**(2), 45

Quine, P., Wade, K. and Hargreaves, R. (1991) Learning to sleep. *Nursing Times*, **87**(48), 41–43

Read, C. (1991) *Pollution and Child Health*, Greenpeace, London

Reid, J.A. (1991) Developing the role of the school nurse in public health. *Health Education Journal*, **50**(3), 112–118

Riley, I. (1987) Childhood as a period of change and development. *The Add-on Journal of Clinical Nursing*, **3**(23), 858–861

Roberts, H. (1991) Accident prevention: a community approach. *Health Visitor*, **64**(7), 219–220

Rousseau, N. (1983) Give us a play piece, please not lectures. *Journal of Royal Society of Health*, **103**, 104–111

Saffin, K. (1992) School nurses immunising without a doctor present. *Health Visitor*, **65**(11), 394–396

Sefi, S. and Macfarlane, A. (1989) *Immunising Children*, Oxford Medical Publications, Oxford

Smith, S. (1993) Immunisations – fact pack. *Community Outlook*, March, 16–17

Stallard, P. (1993) Routine assessment of children at three years. *Health Visitor*, **66**(11), 397–398

Strachen, D. and Anderson, H.R. (1992) Trends in hospital admission rates for asthma in children. *British Medical Journal*, **304**, 819–890

Suppiah, C. (1994) Working in partnership with community mothers. *Health Visitor*, **67**(2), 51–53

Tanner, J., Moss, J. and Silver, L. (1985) Child growth, catching them early. *Community Outlook*, April, 19–24

Taylor, W. and Newacheck, P. (1992) Impact of childhood asthma on health. *Paediatrics*, **90**(5), 657–662

Todd, J.E. and Dodd, T. (1985) *Children's Dental Health in the UK in 1983*, HMSO, London

Turner, M. (1993) *Nutrition and Children Aged One–Five*, National Council, London

Walker, R. (1993) Care and control of diabetes: finding the right balance. *Primary Health Care*, **3**(10), 16–20

Whitehead, M. (1988) *Inequalities in Health*, Penguin Books, London

Whyte, D.A. (1992) A family nursing approach to the care of the child with a chronic illness. *Journal of Advanced Nursing*, **17**, 326–327

Williams, T. and Wetton, N. (1990) *Promoting Our Children's Health in Schools, A Working Partnership*, Health Education Authority, London

Wolfendale, S. (1989) All about me: a parent completed development profile. *Health Visitor*, **62**, 334

York Health Visitors (1988) *Family Health Matters*, York Health Services Trust, England

20

The adult

Denise Knight

● **Introduction**

The adult clients of community health care nurses are an extremely variable group in terms of their roles, personal relationships, work and leisure patterns and family structure. The health needs of this client group also reflect this heterogeneity and are often determined by the particular phase of the lifecourse which the individual is experiencing at that moment. For instance, many young adults are beginning a family and must therefore adapt to the physical, emotional and other stresses associated with bearing and raising children. Similarly, many adults in their fifties are beginning to think about and hopefully plan for retirement which represents a major change in their social, economic and personal circumstances.

Pickin and St. Leger (1993) suggest a lifecycle framework is a useful tool in the assessment of health need. They point out that during each period in the lifecycle, factors characteristic of that stage tend to be dominant in determining the health experience of individuals and are thus associated with 'particular opportunities to promote health and with particular risk of ill health'.

This chapter seeks to inform the community health care nurse of the characteristic developmental changes occurring during the adult phase of the lifecourse. It will explore the complex interrelationship of biological, social and psychological factors which determine the nature of developmental change. The chapter will also introduce the community health care nurse to some of the main theoretical issues which are found within the study of development in the adult. In this way the nurse will be able to hold an informed, critical perspective of adult development, allowing a more complete understanding of her or his adult clients and their health needs.

The lifespan approach of human development outlined within this chapter suggests that there is considerable flexibility and potential for change within individual development (Baltes and Baltes, 1990). This offers the community health care nurse opportunities to effect changes which will enable the individual to adapt successfully to the stage of development they have reached. Possible ways in which nursing intervention can facilitate optimal development in the adult are explored.

● Development and the adult phase of the lifecourse

Definitions and related concepts

Development and ageing processes are characteristic of all living organisms. Development involves both qualitative and quantitative changes in a particular skill, ability of function which is organized and adaptive. Hayslip and Panek (1993) state that the development of an individual is influenced by a complex interrelationship of moderating factors including inner biological influences such as health or illness, maturation, genetic endowment, physical or cultural aspects of the environment and individual psychological factors. Baltes *et al.* (1980) suggest that a consideration of three types of influence is essential in understanding change in adulthood.

- **Normative age-graded factors** affect all individuals of a given age and may be physiological such as the onset of puberty and the menopause, or environmental factors such as culturally defined age norms for retirement or marriage. Age-graded influences tend to be greater during childhood and the later years of life.
- **Normative history-graded factors** or cohort influences are shared by most members of a society at a particular time, characteristics of which may exert a powerful influence on development, particularly that of adolescents and young adults. Examples of history-graded factors include the swinging sixties, the roaring twenties and periods of war.
- **Non-normative factors** are those which are not related to age or history but which will have an impact on the individual experiencing them, such as being sacked from a job or having an accident. These influences tend to increase in significance with increasing age.

The continuing and complex interrelationship of normative and non-normative influences on development have implications for the reliability and validity of developmental research. Most developmental research examines the effect of age on one or more variables such as personality or intelligence. However, other influences on development such as history-graded factors or non-normative factors may be contributing to the observed relationship as well as to age-related factors. Neither cross-sectional nor longitudinal research designs, which are commonly used in developmental research, are able to account adequately for the myriad influences, as well as age, which influence development (Schaie, 1965; Baltes, 1968).

● The lifecourse/lifecycle

The terms lifecycle and lifecourse are often used interchangeably to refer to the pattern and structure of a life from its beginning to its end. Levinson (1986), however, suggests that the two terms are not synonymous. Lifecourse is a descriptive term related to the sequence and temporal flow of a life, together with all its main aspects such as family, work and other social systems, bodily changes and love relationships, whereas lifecycle is a metaphorical term denoting the underlying order in the human lifecourse where each individual follows the same basic sequence although each life is unique.

The lifecycle is often viewed as a number of qualitatively different phases and many metaphors are used to describe the sequence of phases which constitute a lifecycle. Jung (1972), for example, uses the analogy of the daily passage of the sun through the heavens, with childhood viewed as the morning of life and decline into old age commencing at the noon of an individual's life. Hockey and James (1993) point out the common use of negative metaphors to describe the later phases of the lifecycle, with the adult viewed as moving towards the twilight, or winter, of life with a resulting disengagement from society (Cumming, 1963). Thus, use of negative analogies is both caused by, and contributes towards, the ageist attitudes prevalent in society (Hockey and James, 1993).

Empirical study of the adult phase of lifecourse has only become established over the past two decades (Baltes, 1987). Major developmental theorists such as Freud (1924) and Piaget (1970) originally suggested that development is largely completed by the end of adolescence with little change occurring in the adult.

Defining adulthood

The adult phase is the longest period within the lifecourse and is generally viewed as the period between 21 years and 70 years encompassing the time between the end of adolescence and the onset of senescence and the advanced ageing process (Dewald, 1980). The upper and lower limits to adulthood are, however, arbitrary and are often defined by the society in which the individual lives. Thus, in the UK the age of majority was changed from 21 years to 18 years, yet individuals aged between 18 and 21 years change little in terms of their physical, social or psychological functioning at this time.

Other definitions of adulthood face similar difficulties; for example, adulthood may be defined in terms of the assumption of age-appropriate roles and responsibilities such as marriage and the establishment of a family. However, many adults do not choose to marry or establish a family (Sugarman, 1986). Whitbourne and Weinstock (1979) suggest that psychological maturity distinguishes the adult from the non-adult. This involves the ability to shoulder responsibilities, make logical decisions and accept one's social role. Again this definition is limiting, since many adults are not able to fulfil all of these criteria or may fulfil some of them only partially.

Chronological age as a marker of adult development

Chronological age has been criticized as indicating very little about adult development (Birren, 1969). It is suggested that the following age indices allow a more complete understanding of the adult individual:

Biological age refers to the relative age or condition of the systems and organs within the body and is usually, although not always, related to chronological age (Birren, 1969). Thus a 50-year-old male marathon runner may have a biological age similar to that of a 25 year old who avoids exertion wherever possible.

Psychological age denotes the adaptive capacities of the individual in terms of her or his intelligence, coping ability and problem-solving skills. Many older adults may possess good adaptive skills and be able to respond to change more positively than young adults.

Social age refers to the individual's behaviour, habits and activities relative to the expectations of society in terms of age norms or age-appropriate behaviours, that is described by Neugarten (1977) as the 'social clock'.

Functional age is closely related to the concept of biological age and is determined by the individual's capacity to carry out the functions expected of her or him (Birren, 1969). Once again this may have only a limited relationship with chronological age.

Chronological age alone is therefore extremely limited as a marker of adult development. The community heath care nurse should therefore consider the use of other age indices when assessing the adult client.

● **The nature of adult development**

All theories of adult development adopt a particular perspective or view of change in the adult. Authors such as Erikson (1963) and Levinson *et al.* (1978) suggest that development occcurs in a series of qualitative different stages and describe the nature of psychodynamic and socio-cultural change across the lifecourse. Other writers examine specific areas of adult development such as personal–social components or cognitive–intellectual components (McCandless and Evans, 1973). It is important for practitioners to have knowledge of each of these approaches since, in this way, a broad knowledge base is acquired which is essential for an informed understanding of adult clients. An eclectic approach is adopted in this chapter in which the major stage theories are presented followed by discussion of the key areas of development in the adult individual. It is, however, important to emphasize that the material presented here is a summmary of the findings related to adult development. The reader is also advised to consult developmental tests such as Hayslip and Panek (1993) which offer a comprehensive and critical discussion of adult development.

Stage theories of adult development

Stage theories of development focus on the individual's achieve-ment of certain development tasks which are characteristic of each stage of the lifecourse. A developmental task has been defined by Havighurst (1972) as

a task which arises at, or about, a certain period in the life of the individual, successful achievement of which leads to his happiness

*and to success with later tasks, while failure leads to unhappiness in
the individual, disapproval by society and difficulty of later tasks.*

A summary of the major stage theories of adult development is
presented in Tables 20.1–20.4, which the following text discuss.

Table 20.1   Psychosocial crises in adult life (After Erikson, 1963)

Chronological age	*Psychological conflict*	
20–35 yrs Early adulthood	Intimacy vs. isolation	Need to form a close relationship with another. May risk newly developed sense of identity and thus may be avoided by same. May be used as a means of resolving identity crisis but leads to unequal relationship

35–65 yrs
Mid and late
  adulthood
	Generativity vs.
	  stagnation
		Concern with establishing and guiding the next generation. May be concerned with parenthood or other creative activities

Table 20.2   Developmental stages in adult life (After Levinson *et al.*, 1978; Levinson, 1986)

Developmental stage	
Pre-adulthood	Growth from highly dependent undifferentiated childhood to beginnings of responsible adult life
17–22 yrs Early adulthood transition	Less dependent on support and authority from parents – modifies relationship with parents and others
22–28 yrs Entering the adult world	'Novice phase' formation and living out of the 'dream', i.e. vision of role in adult world may be helped by mentor relationship with older adult. Forming an occupation. Forming a love relationship, marriage and family
28–33 yrs Age thirty transition	Modifying the first life structure above to remedy flaws and limitations. Choices regarding family career, etc., become more permanent
33–40 yrs Settling down period	Continuation of above. Sense of 'Becoming one's own man'. Strong commitment to personal, familial and occupational future
40–45 yrs Mid-life transition	Shift from an acquisition orientation to more evaluative one – period of soul-searching and examination of life, i.e. mid-life crisis which, for some, may involve a new start (crisis may occur at around age 30 for women (Reinke *et al.*, 1985))
45–50 yrs Entering middle adulthood	Formation of new life structure – may be influenced by 'marker' events, e.g. illness, divorce, job change, bereavement
50–55 yrs Age 50 transition	Opportunity to change and/or further solidify life structure above. For some, mid-life crisis may be experienced here
55–60 yrs Culmination of middle adulthood	Relatively stable
60–65 yrs Late adult transition	Beginning of, and preparation for, late adulthood

Table 20.3   Transformations in adult life (After Gould, 1978)

Adult stages	
20–25 yrs Struggle to leave parents' world	Challenge and resolution of false assumptions from childhood consciousness, e.g. 'I can see the world only through my parents'. My parents must be my only family
25–30 yrs I'm nobody's baby now	Challenge and resolution of new false assumptions, e.g. 'rewards will always follow if we do what we are supposed to do'. There is only one right way to do things
30–40 yrs Challenging the illusion of absolute safety	Need to confront loss of power in parents. Shift in time orientation to more limited future. Questioning of life's directions
40–50 yrs	Concerns with adolescent children – struggle for power. Turning inward to face own needs
50+ yrs 'I own myself'	Childhood illusions of control given up. Acceptance of what one has

Table 20.4   Developmental tasks in adulthood (After Havighurst, 1972)

Stage	Developmental task
Early adulthood	Selecting a mate Learning to live with marriage partner Starting a family Rearing children and managing a home Getting started in an occupation Taking on civic responsibility and finding a congenial social group
Middle age	Assisting teenage children to become responsible and happy adults Achieving civic and social responsibility Reaching and maintaining satisfactory career performance Relating to one's spouse as a person Accepting and adjusting to physiological changes Adjusting to ageing parents

Psychosocial crises in adult life

This theory suggests that the individual attempts to resolve psychosocial conflicts brought about by biological maturation and cultural demands, the resolution of the conflicts being influenced by social and cultural factors. According to Erikson (1963), eight conflicts confront the individual throughout the lifespan, with one conflict predominating at each stage. Each conflict does, however, exist throughout life and may therefore be addressed and resolved at times other than the peak time for this conflict. Within this, Erikson (1963, 1980) suggests that the adult faces two psychological conflicts – intimacy vs. isolation and generativity vs. stagnation – which are shown in Table 20.1.

Developmental stages in adult life

Levinson, following an in-depth study of a small group of men, suggested that an individual's life follows a sequence of seasons or 'eras' (Levinson *et al.*, 1978). Each era represents a change in the nature of life. A transitional, or structure-changing, period lasting about 5 years marks the end of one era and the beginning of another when the next structure is built upon. Personality, culture, social roles, major life events and biological changes all interact to exert an influence on the active nature of an individual life. Levinson (1986), however, argues that life structure has a basic nature and time pattern which is common to all.

Transformation in adult life

Gould (1978) describes the evolution of adult consciousness. Development takes place against a shifting time perspective in the adult. As a child, time holds no meaning for the individual in her or his sheltered environment protected by parents or other adults. Adults must develop a belief in their ability to create and control their own destiny. This must be achieved against a sense that time is running out and leads to the evolution of adult consciousness. Each adult stage is concerned with the challenging of a particular false assumption.

Developmental tasks in adulthood

Havighurst (1972) suggests that developmental tasks arise through the interaction of the physical maturation processes, individual values and cultural expectations. He discusses a number of developmental tasks for each of six stages throughout the lifecourse. The developmental tasks were defined through empirical methods such as observation and interviewing.

The role of the community health care nurse

The stage theories of adult development described above share many common themes. For example, each of the theories describes the establishment of a sexual and occupational identity and the need to cope with the recurring themes of love, marriage and family and physical peaks and declines (Sugarman, 1986). They highlight the importance of these themes for the developing adult and suggest that conflict may occur for some individuals as they try to work through each era or task. This would suggest that the community health care nurse should be aware of challenges faced by clients which arise from their individual phase of development, offering help where appropriate. It is, however, important to remember that most individuals are able to work through each developmental stage without assistance.

Many of the stage theories of adult development have, however, been derived from work on small samples of individuals. The theories also suggest a generally benign view of society, always working towards positive development of the individual and not acting in a coercive or repressive way (Buss, 1979). Optimal development also occurs only when the individual fulfils society's expectations of age-appropriate roles and behaviours. Many clients may choose to ignore societal and cultural norms in the way they behave and readers might like to consider their role with these clients as advised by the *Code of Professional Conduct* (UKCC, 1992).

Changing health patterns in the adult

Pickin and St Leger (1993) discuss the ways in which the health needs of adults change across the lifecourse. The major health needs proposed are presented in Table 20.5. The health needs of men and women are presented separately since, for women in the early years of adult life, health services used are often associated with fertility, pregnancy and childbirth.

The health needs highlighted demonstrate an emphasis on physical health needs but can suggest areas in which the skills of the community health care nurse at primary, secondary and tertiary levels of prevention are required (Caplan, 1964) (see Chapter 10). Thus the levels of ischaemic heart disease rise in mid and late adulthood, suggesting that secondary prevention in the form of screening programmes is appropriate for this age group. Primary prevention through health education is required prior to the development of disease process and is required in earlier phases of the lifecourse.

● **Physical change and adulthood**

It is frequently assumed that all the physical changes occurring during adulthood are negative. Bee and Mitchell (1984) reflect this assumption when they suggest that all the associated bodily changes may be summarized as smaller, slower, weaker, lesser and fewer. It is, however, important to remember that functional age need not reflect chronological age; for example, an individual who engages in good health behaviours may have a young functional age. Changes associated with normal ageing should also be differentiated from those associated with pathological ageing where coexisting disease also contributes to physical deterioration. Between the ages of 20 and 30 years most individuals are at their physical peak. Muscle strength reaches its highest level at about 30 and brain cell development is completed during the 20s.

A gradual deterioration in many body systems may be detected from the age of 30 onwards, although the degree to which this hampers individual functioning is difficult to predict for reasons already discussed. Bones begin to lose mass and density and there is degeneration of the intervertebral cartilage in the spine. This leads to compression of the spinal column, with a resultant loss in height. On average, adults may decrease in height by one-eighth of an inch (3 mm) between the ages of 20 and 40 years (Batten, 1984). Muscles begin to decline in size and strength, with regular exercise slowing this change. The heart and lungs and circulatory system may also show degenerative changes, with a resultant decrease in pulmonary and cardiac function. Problems with hypertension become more common during this time, particularly in males (Pickin and St Leger, 1993).

Degenerative changes also occur within the endocrine system – a gradual reduction in basal metabolic rate (BMR) linked to the loss of muscle tissue. The secretion of thyroid hormones decreases to compensate for their reduced blood clearance (Ingbar and Woeber, 1981). Sex

Table 20.5 Adult stages of lifecycle and major health needs (After Pickin and St. Leger, 1993)

Life stage	Main cause of mortality		Main reasons for GP consultations	
	Male	*Female*	*Male*	*Female*
15–24 yrs Early adulthood	Accidents* and violence, suicide and self-inflicted injury Cancers	Accidents and violence Cancers Suicide and self-inflicted injury	Respiratory disease Accidents and violence Skin disease	Family planning Respiratory diseases Pregnancy care
25–44 yrs Middle adulthood	Cancers (leukaemia, lung, brain) Accidents Ischaemic heart disease	Cancers* (breast, cervix, leukaemia) Accidents Suicides	Respiratory diseases Musculoskeletal problems Accidents and violence	Respiratory diseases Genitourinary disease Family planning
45–64 yrs Late adulthood	Ischaemic heart disease Cancers (lung, bowel, stomach) Respiratory diseases	Cancers* (breast, lung, large bowel) Ischaemic heart disease Cerebrovascular disease	Respiratory diseases Musculoskeletal problems Diseases of circulation	Musculoskeletal problems Respiratory diseases Ill-defined conditions

*Cause nearly 50% of all deaths.

hormone production decreases, particularly in the female where falling levels of oestrogen in women aged over 30 years may contribute to the increasing incidence of pre-menstrual tension in the older woman (Gregerman and Bierman, 1981). Changes in the menstrual cycle may also occur, with time between menses becoming usually shorter but occasionally longer and more irregular (Whitbourne, 1985). The end of the female reproductive cycle occurs at the menopause, on average at age 50 years (Gregerman and Bierman, 1981).

The menopause may be associated with a number of physical and/or psychological symptoms, e.g. hot flushes, palpitations, tingling in fingers and toes, forgetfulness, depression, anxiety, etc., but these negative symptoms affect only a minority of women and may be associated with other events happening in the woman's life at the same time. Woods (1982), for example, found that women who were satisfied with their lives were less likely to report symptoms associated with the menopause. For many women the end of their reproductive years means an end to their fear of pregnancy which, when coupled with declining family and domestic responsibilities, can lead to an increased sexual drive (Masters and Johnson, 1966).

In men, androgen levels decline much more slowly and changes such as delayed erection time and reduced ejaculatory time may not be noted until their 70s or 80s. For some men, increased age can be associated with a decrease in sexual activity. This is, however, influenced by several factors, such as level of sexual activity in earlier years, strength of relationship with partner and preoccupation with concerns regarding career or finances (Masters and Johnson, 1966). For many individuals, later adulthood represents a sexually positive phase of life (Idiculla and Goldberg, 1987).

Degenerative changes may occur in the sensory processes. Hearing loss due to the thickening of the ear drum, hardening of the ossicles and inner ear degeneration begins at about age 30 in men and in the late 30s for women (Welford, 1980) with, in particular, a reduced ability to discriminate high-pitched sounds. Visual acuity and accommodation declines from about age 40 (Corso, 1971). There is also a decreased ability to adapt to dark conditions and less tolerance for glare. There may appear to be minor changes in preference for certain tastes and smells, although Engen (1977) suggests that these may occur through the effects of smoking, disease and the effects of sex hormones.

Physical appearance also changes with age and it is often these changes that cause the greatest concern to individuals. This worry is linked perhaps to the high value placed on youth and physical attractiveness by Western society (Sugarman, 1986). The hair becomes grey and may be lost, particularly in the male. Loss of elasticity in the skin leads to wrinkles (Rossman, 1977). Changes in the basal metabolic rate and decreased exercise patterns may lead to a gain in weight. Many of the degenerative changes described above could be avoided, or minimized, through regular exercise and a sensible, well-balanced diet. The community health care nurse should work in co-operation with clients so that these simple health-promoting measures are adopted.

● **Cognitive and personality changes in adulthood**

It is generally accepted that performance in tests of memory and intelligence are adversely affected by age (Willis and Baltes, 1980; Schaie, 1980). However, many factors contribute to this decline other than age alone, such as a more cautious approach by the individual and the release from formal schooling. Since many studies of the effects of ageing on memory involve reaction-time measures, slower psychomotor skills in many older adults may contribute to the differences found. Schaie (1980) suggests that changes in intellectual functioning occurring before the age of 60 are likely to be due to underlying pathology such as disease or due to poor socio-economic conditions rather than ageing alone.

There is a complex interrelationship between personality and increasing age. An individual's experience of ageing may thus affect her or his personality type and in turn may affect the individual's experience of ageing (Neugarten, 1977). Several studies have shown the relative stability of personality traits with increasing age (Costa and McRae, 1978; Schaie and Parham, 1976), although traits such as general activity, thoughtfulness, tolerance for others and willingness to take risks have been shown to decrease with advanced age (Douglas and Arenberg, 1978). Elder (1979) discusses the important influence that personality effects have in determining the manner of adaptation to ageing. Mussen et al. (1982), for example, found that women who had a buoyant responsive attitude towards life, and men with good emotional and physical health, at age 30, were more likely to report high levels of life satisfaction 40 years later.

Social relationships in the adult

Social relationships play an important role in adult life. Kahn and Antonucci (1980) suggest that adult relationships with individuals such as friends, family and work colleagues form a social support system or convoy which enables the individual to cope with life changes. Relationships with friends assume a greater significance in later life and may even be rated more positively than relationships with family members. Good social support convoys, as perceived by the individual, have been linked with positive health outcomes (LaRocco et al., 1980). Perceptions of social support could therefore be usefully explored during client assessment.

The family and the adult

The adult's family will consist of relationships with siblings and ageing parents and with the adult's partner and children. Earlier conceptions of the family described a nuclear family which evolved through a series of developmental stages, for example, birth of first child, preparing adolescent children for independence and the 'empty nest' period. More recent views of the family, however, suggest a dynamic changing system with reciprocal influence between family members and the wider society (Featherman, 1983; Weeks and Wright, 1985; Parke, 1988). This theoretical perspective is able to deal successfully with the changing nature of family life today such as single parenthood and step-families (Hayslip and Panek, 1993).

Within the family, relationships with siblings continue to play an important role in adulthood, particularly if they had been positive in nature (Mosatche *et al.*, 1983). Matthews *et al.* (1990) and Cicirelli (1989) have shown that a close relationship with siblings leads to increased personal support in times of stress and fewer reports of depression. This again demonstrates the importance of exploring clients' perceptions of their relationships with others as part of the assessment process, particularly since relationships between family members of different generations are assuming a greater significance now with the 'greying' of the population (Victor, 1991). Four- and even five-generation families are now possible. Older members of the family group generally give, and receive, help within the family, although as Sussman (1985) suggests, the exact pattern of inter-generational relationships varies with ethnicity and race. Generally, in all societies, close emotional ties exist between parent and child (Rossi and Rossi, 1990). As parents age, adult children are generally expected to assume filial responsibility for their elderly parents by providing, for example, support and assistance. This expectation, which varies greatly between different cultures, often engenders stress in the adult providing care (Finley *et al.*, 1988). It is now important to acknowledge that it can be alleviated by appropriate intervention and support from the community health care nurse.

Work and the adult

Work is an important feature of the adult's development, as suggested by most of the stage theories. It may serve to define self-esteem, self-concept and perhaps, identity (Chown, 1977; Coleman and Antonucci, 1983). Work often produces intrinsic satisfaction greater than that derived from earnings alone, and can influence our beliefs about our intellectual adequacy (Cohn, 1979; Rebok *et al.*, 1986). For both women and men, being in work leads to greater self-esteem and wellbeing than unemployment (Stein *et al.*, 1990). Job loss can lead to declines in physical health and self-esteem, depression, anxiety and even suicide (DeFrank and Ivanevich, 1986).

Job loss also affects the psychological, sociological and economic functioning of all the family. In today's economic climate, the community health care nurse will be increasingly involved with individuals and families affected by unemployment. Although this may not be the main reason for professional involvement with the client, the practitioner must be aware of the immense pressures which may be caused by unemployment and should seek to ameliorate them through careful assessment and appropriate intervention.

● **Lifespan development: opportunities for practice?**

Neither the stage theories of adult development nor examination of the more specific changes found in adulthood account adequately for the considerable variability which is found between individuals. There is a failure also to explain and describe the interaction of diverse influences on adult development. Very little systematic study has, for example, taken place into the influence of ethnicity and race on adult development. The lifespan developmental perspective as described, for example, by Baltes (1987) attempts to overcome such difficulties. This emphasizes the importance of the many contextual factors which influence development and the reciprocal nature of the relationship between the individual and the environment. According to a lifespan perspective, development occurs throughout the lifecourse with no assumption of automatic decline in the later stages of life. Development is, instead, a process, involving both gain (growth) and loss (decline). As the individual ages there is a shift in the gain/loss proportion towards loss. The individual may, however, use related skills to compensate for loss in a particular area. In addition, the considerable plasticity or potential for change in human development, proposed by the lifespan perspective, means that many functions can be maximized by appropriate rehearsal and activity schedules. A lifespan approach can thus explain the considerable hetero-geneity between adults and, furthermore, allows a more optimistic view of advancing age. It also suggests that a number of interventions may be possible to maximize developmental gains and foster successful ageing (Baltes and Baltes, 1990).

Baltes and Baltes (1990) agree that the association of ageing with success might appear contradictory. The term is, however, to be encouraged, they suggest, since it leads to the creation of late adulthood as a positive phase of life. A critical analysis of the concept may, they suggest, develop the idea that the constituents of 'success' in later life may be different from those in earlier phases of the lifecycle. Factors such as biological health, mental health, cognitive competence, adaptability, personal control and life satisfaction contribute toward the definition of success.

Adaptation to life changes is essential for human development. Baltes and Baltes (1990) suggest that successful adaptation together with a minimization of developmental loss occurs through three processes: *selection*, *optimization* and *compensation*. Faced with losses in some areas of life, the ageing adult must select those aspects of life which are important to them and should concentrate motivation and skills on these high-priority life domains. Such selection may mean the individual is involved in fewer life activities, but because these are carried out more efficiently, greater satisfaction and sense of control is achieved. Optimiza-tion and compensation in development occurs through the use of related skills and knowledge. Thus the older car driver whose reaction times are becoming slower may adapt to this by optimizing her or his skills in 'reading' the road ahead to compensate for this loss. Clients should be helped to recognize ways in which they can optimize their behaviour through selection and compensation.

Physical health is an important factor in optimal adult develop-ment. Fries (1990) suggests that chronic disease is a major obstacle to successful ageing. The avoidance of this can be facilitated by the community health care nurse through successful primary and secondary health intervention programmes. Baltes and Baltes (1990) suggest further that plasticity in development offers the potential of sizeable reserves in social, mental and physical capacities which may be exploited via appropriate education, exercise and training. Again, the practitioner can help to achieve these successful outcomes through appropriate health education. A lifespan approach to adult development thus suggests many areas in which the community health care nurse can seek to effect changes that will enable the individual to adapt successfully to age.

Lerner and Ryff (1978) and Sugarman (1986) suggest that adequate education about the nature of ageing in adulthood and the successful management of change would challenge the association of change with decline and would enhance the ability to cope with increasing age. This form of education could be usefully incorporated by the community health care nurse within health education programmes such as pre-retirement programmes. Lerner and Ryff (1978) further point out that the emphasis on the variability in human development and wide range of possible supportive measures means that any help must be planned on an individual basis and in co-operation with that individual. This assertion bears interesting parallels to the concepts of individualized care and negotiated care-planning found within nursing and should, therefore, be easily incorporated within nursing interventions.

● **Conclusion**

This chapter has reviewed the key health needs and major developmental features and has examined some of the theoretical issues associated with this field. These issues involve the complex interrelationship of biological, social and psychological factors. It has also pointed out where developmental consideration might offer opportunities for the community health care nurse to promote health and successful ageing during the adult years. Readers will hopefully be encouraged to consider ways in which these opportunities might be exploited with the clients with whom they have contact.

References

Baltes, P.B. (1968) Longitudinal and cross-sectional sequences in the study of age generation effect. *Human Development*, **11**,145–171

Baltes, P.B. (1987) Theoretical propositions of life-span developmental psychology: on the dynamics between growth and decline. *Developmental Psychology*, **23**(5), 611–626

Baltes, P.B. and Baltes, M.M. (1990) *Successful Ageing, Perspectives from the Behavioural Sciences*, Press Syndicate of the University of Cambridge, Cambridge

Baltes, P.B., Reese, H.W. and Lippit, L.P. (1980) Life span developmental psychology. *Annual Review of Psychology*, **31**, 65–110

Batten, M. (1984) Life spans. *Science Digest*, **98**, 46–51

Bee, H. and Mitchell, S.K. (1984) *The Developing Person: A Life Span Approach*, 2nd edn, Harper and Row, San Francisco

Birren, J.E. (1969) The concept of functional age; theoretical background. *Human Development*, **12**, 214–215

Buss, A.R. (1979) Dialectics, history and development. The historical roots of the individual – society dialectic. In *Life-Span Development and Behaviour*, Vol. 2 (eds P.B. Baltes and O.G. Brim), Academic Press, New York

Caplan, G. (1964) *Principles of Preventative Psychiatry*, Basic Books, New York

Chown, S.M. (1977) Morale, careers and personal potentials. In *Handbook of the Psychology of Aging* (eds J.E. Birren and K.W. Shaie), Van Nostrand Reinhold, New York

Cicirelli, V.G. (1989) Feelings of attachment to siblings and well-being in later life. *Psychology and Ageing*, **4**, 211–216

Cohn, R.M. (1979) Age and satisfaction from work. *Journal of Gerontology*, **34**, 264–272

Coleman, L.M. and Antonucci, T.C. (1983) Impact of work on women at mid-life. *Developmental Psychology*, **19**, 290–294

Corso, J.F. (1971) Sensory processes and age effects in normal adults. *Journal of Gerontology*, **26**, 90–105

Costa, P.T. and McRae, R. (1978) Objective personality assessment. In *The Clinical Psychology of Aging* (eds M. Sterandt, I. Siegler and M. Elias), Plenum, New York

Cumming, E. (1963) Further thoughts on the theory of disengagement. *International Social Science Journal*, **15**, 377–393

DeFrank, R.S. and Ivanevich, J.M. (1986) Job loss: an individual-level review and model. *Journal of Vocational Behaviour*, **28**, 1–20

Dewald, P.A. (1980) Adult phases of the life cycle. In *Psycholanalytic Contributions Towards Understanding Personality Development: Adulthood and the Ageing Process*, Vol. 3 (eds S.I. Greenspand and C.H. Pollock), NIMH, Washington D.C.

Douglas, K. and Arenberg, P. (1978) Age changes, age differences and cultural change on the Guilford-Zimmerman Temperament Survey. *Journal of Gerontology*, **33**, 737–747

Elder, G.H. (1979) Historical changes in life patterns and personality. In *Lifespan Development and Behaviour* (eds P.B. Baltes and O.G. Brim), Academic Press, New York

Engen, T. (1977) Taste and smell. In *Handbook of the Psychology of Aging* (eds J.E.Birren and K.W. Schaie), Van Nostrand Reinhold, New York

Erikson, E.H. (1963) *Childhood and Society*, W.W.Norton, New York

Erikson, E.H. (1980) *Identity and the Life Cycle: A Reissue*, W.W. Norton, New York

Featherman, D.L. (1983) Lifespan perspectives in social science research. In *Lifespan Development and Behaviour*, Vol. 5 (eds P.B. Baltes and O.G. Brim), Academic Press, New York

Finley, N.J., Roberts, M.D. and Banahan, B.F. (1988) Motivators and inhibitors of attitudes of filial obligation toward ageing parents. *Gerontologist*, **28**, 73–78

Freud, S. (1924) On psychotherapy. In *Collected papers of Sigmund Freud*, Vol. 1, Hogarth Press, London

Fries, J.M. (1990) Medical perspectives on successful aging. In *Successful Aging: Perspectives from the Behavioural Sciences* (eds P.B. Baltes and M.M. Baltes), Press Syndicate of the University of Cambridge, Cambridge

Gould, R.L. (1978) *Transformations: Growth and Change in Adult Life*, Simon and Schuster, New York

Gregerman, R.I. and Bierman, E.L. (1981) Ageing and hormones. In *Textbook of Endocrinology*, 6th edn (ed. R.H. Williams), Saunders, Philadelphia

Havighurst, R.J. (1972) *Developmental Tasks and Education*, 3rd edn, David McKay, New York

Hayslip, B. Jnr and Panek, P.E. (1993) *Adult Development and Aging*, 2nd edn, Harper Collins, New York

Hockey, J. and James, A. (1993) *Growing Up and Growing Old: Ageing and Dependency in The Life Course*, Sage, London

Idiculla, A.A. and Goldberg, G. (1987) Physical fitness for the mature woman. In *Medical Clinics of North America: The Post Menopausal Woman*, Vol. 71/1 (ed. D.M. Barbo), W.B. Saunders, Philadelphia

Ingbar, S.H. and Woeber, K.A. (1981) The thyroid gland. In *Textbook of Endocrinology*, 6th edn (ed. R.H. Williams), Saunders, Philadelphia

Jung, C.G. (1972) The transcendent function. In *The Structure and Dynamics of the Psyche*, 2nd edn, Vol. 8 of *The Collected Works of C.G. Jung* (eds H. Read, M. Fordham, G. Adler and W. McGuire), Routledge and Kegan Paul, London

Kahn, R. and Antonucci, T. (1980) Convoys over the life-course: attachment, roles and social support. In *Life-span Development and Behaviour*, Vol. 3 (eds P.B. Baltes and O.G. Brim), Academic Press, New York

LaRocco, J.M., House, J.S. and French, J.R. (1980) Social support, occupational stress and health. *Journal of Health and Social Behaviour*, **21**, 202–218

Lerner, R.M. and Ryff, C.D. (1978) Implementation of the life-span view of human development: the sample case of attachment. In *Life Span Development and Behaviour*, Vol. 1 (eds P.B. Baltes and O.G. Brim Jnr), Academic Press, New York

Levinson, D.J. (1986) A conception of adult development. *American Psychologist*, **41**(1), 3–13

Levinson, D.J., Darrow, D.N., Klein, E.B., Levinson, M.H. and McKee, B. (1978) *The Seasons of a Man's Life*, A.A.Knopf, New York

McCandless, B.R. and Evans, E.D. (1973) *Children and Youth: Psychosocial Development*, Illinois Dryden Press, Hinsdale, Ill.

Masters, W.H. and Johnson, V.E. (1966) *Human Sexual Response*, Little Brown, Boston

Matthews, S.H., Werkner, J.E. and Delaney, P.J. (1990) Relative contributions of help by employed and non-employed sisters to their elderly parents. *Journal of Gerontology: Social Sciences*, **49**, S36–44

Mosatche, H.S., Brady, E.M. and Noberini, M.R. (1983) A retrospective life span study of the closest sibling relationship. *Journal of Psychology*, **113**, 237–243

Mussen, P., Honzik, M.P. and Eichorn, D.H. (1982) Early adult antecedents of life satisfaction at age 70. *Journal of Gerontology*, **37**, 316–322

Neugarten, B.L. (1977) Adaptation and the life-cycle. In *Counselling Adults* (eds N.K. Schlessberg and A.D. Entine), Monterey, California

Parke, R.D. (1988) Families in life span perspective. A multilevel developmental approach. In *Child Development in Life-Span Perspective* (eds E.M. Hetherington, R.M. Lerner and P.B. Baltes), Erlbaum, Hillsdale, N.J.

Piaget, J. (1970) Piaget's theory. In *Carmichael's Manual of Child Psychology*, Vol. 1, 2nd edn (ed. P. Mussen), Wiley, New York

Pickin, C. and St Leger, S. (1993) *Assessing Health Need Using the Life Cycle Framework*, Open University Press, Buckingham

Rebok, G., Offerman, L.R., Wirtz, G. and Montaglione, C.J. (1986) Work and intellectual aging: the psychological concomitants of social-organisational conditions. *Educational Gerontology*, **12**, 359–374

Reinke, B.J., Holmes, D.S. and Harris, R.L. (1985) The timing of psychosocial changes in women's lives: the years 25–45. *Journal of Personality and Social Psychology*, **48**, 1353–1364

Rossi, A.F. and Rossi, P.H. (1990) *Of Human Bonding: Parent–Child Relationships Across the Life Course*, Aldine, New York

Rossman, I. (1977) Anatomic and body composition changes with ageing. In *Handbook of the Biology of Ageing* (eds C.E. Finch and L. Hayflick), Van Nostrand Reinhold, New York

Schaie, K.W. (1965) A general model for the study of developmental problems. *Pyschological Bulletin*, **64**, 92–107

Schaie, K.W. (1980) Intelligence and problem solving. In *Handbook of Mental Health and Ageing* (eds J.E. Birren and R.B. Sloane), Prentice-Hall, Englewood Cliffs, N.J.

Schaie, K.W. and Parham, I.A. (1976) Stability of adult personality traits: fact or fable? *Journal of Personality and Social Psychology*, **34**, 146–158

Stein, J.A., Newcomb, M.D. and Bentler, P.M. (1990) The relative influence of vocational behaviour and family involvement on self-esteem: longitudinal analyses of young adult women and men. *Journal of Vocational Behaviour*, **36**, 196–212

Sugarman, L. (1986) *Life-Span Development: Concepts Theories and Interventions*, Methuen, London

Sussman, M.B. (1985) The family of old people. In *Handbook of Ageing and the Social Sciences* (eds R. Binstock and E. Shanas), Van Nostrand Reinhold, New York

UKCC (1992) *Code of Professional Conduct*, UKCC, London

Victor, C.R. (1991) *Health and Health Care in Later Life*, Open University Press, Buckingham

Weeks, G.R. and Wright, L. (1985) Dialectics of the family life cycle. *American Journal of Family Therapy*, **27**, 85–91

Welford, A.T. (1980) Sensory, perceptual and motor processes in older adults. In *Handbook of Mental Health and Ageing* (eds J.E. Birren and R.B. Sloan), Prentice-Hall, Englewood Cliffs, N.J.

Whitbourne, S.K. (1985) *The Ageing Body: Physiological Changes and Psychological Consequences*, Springer Verlag, New York

Whitbourne, S.K. and Weinstock, L.S. (1979) *Adult Development; The Differentiation of Experience*, Holt, Rinehart and Winston, New York

Willis, S.L. and Baltes, P.B. (1980) Intelligence in adulthood and ageing: contemporary issues. In *Ageing in the 1980s: Psychological Issues* (ed. L.W. Poon), APA, Washington D.C.

Woods, N.F. (1982) Menopausal distress: a model for epidemiologic investigation. In *Changing Perspectives on Menopause* (eds A.M. Voda, M. Dinnerstein and S.R. O'Donnell), Unversity of Texas Press, Austin

21

Ageing

Liz Day

● **Introduction**

Although the ageing process is often associated with disease and ill-health, as identified by Scrutton (1992), chronological age is a poor indicator of health and ability. However, it is a major determinant of social expectations and social roles, so it is important to look beyond the assumptions associated with age and ageing and to challenge simple explanations which associate disease with age. *The Health of the Nation* (DoH, 1992) provides an opportunity for promoting health throughout the lifespan. Indeed, this chapter uses the targets for health promotion set out in this document as a framework for debate on health issues relating to older people. The strengths and weaknesses of the targets are explored, and application to practice and areas for further research are highlighted. Within this framework an important focus in this chapter is that older people are people who have aged and who have similar needs to the rest of the population. As Comfort (1982) suggests, old people need what people need.

● **The ageing process**

It is difficult to define when or if development ceases and when ageing starts. As Whitbourne (1985) states, ageing is a normal and gradual alteration in the ability to adjust to changing circumstances through homeostatic mechanisms. The Medical Research Council argue that the way in which people experience the ageing process is a consequence of the interaction between internal and biological processes and extrinsic or environmental factors (MRC, 1994). The environment may be adapted to meet the changing needs of the older person, but eventually the individual will be unable to adapt and these changes will ultimately lead to death. Adapting the environment and promoting independence may lead to a shorter period of dependency, suggesting that prevention and health promotion is crucial to the wellbeing of older people.

● An ageing society

One of the major successes of public health measures is an increase in life expectancy at all stages throughout the lifespan. Such measures include good housing, sanitation, clean water supply, maternal and child care, improvements in occupational health and the elimination of life-threatening infectious diseases in childhood, such as diphtheria. Not only are people living longer, but more people are achieving old age than at any other time in history (Victor, 1991a,b). It is difficult to predict whether or not this trend will continue as new problems and health issues emerge, such as HIV/AIDS and environmental pollution, which need to be addressed.

Coupled with the increase in life expectancy is the decline in the birth rate, which has led to Britain, Sweden, Japan, Greece and the USA becoming 'ageing societies' (Kosberg, 1992). This means that the number of people achieving old age in the population is growing at the same time as the mortality rate falls below the birth rate. This leads to a population which consists of more than 15% over retirement age and a birth rate of about 13% (WHO, 1989; Kosberg, 1992). Health promotion throughout the lifespan may contribute to longevity and a reduction in mortality and morbidity which are the main aims of the government's 'Health of the Nation' initiative.

● The health of the nation

The government's welcome attempt to bring health promotion to the forefront of health care, rather than it being an optional extra, culminated in the publication of the White Paper *The Health of the Nation* (DoH, 1992), containing health targets for England. The purpose of the document was to raise awareness of the need to reduce the incidence of avoidable ill-health and put health promotion firmly on the health care agenda. Grimley Evans (1991), in a debate during the consultation stage of the document, argued that the proposals emphasized preventive strategies for people *prior to* retirement. He argued that if health promotion is to be successful it should continue throughout the lifespan and into old age. Victor (1991b) suggests that premature mortality is not the main health concern for older people, but rather that of not being able to cope with the changes which occur with ageing and chronic health problems which may or may not restrict daily living.

● Health promotion

Kalache (1988) says that there are four key requisites needed for health promotion. These four key requisites, which are important for everyone including older people, are:

- **information/knowledge** about factors affecting health
- **appropriate skills** to promote health, including negotiating and

lobbying skills to improve the socio-economic factors influencing health
- **supportive environments** which enhance health and do not 'blame the victim' and therefore acknowledging that there are wider issues than simply lifestyles which affect health
- **opportunities for healthier choices** which include an adequate income, appropriate attitudes and opportunities for rehabilitation, exercise and recreation.

Armed with the necessary information, older people and professionals with whom they are in contact are in a good position to act as advocates for each other and for other groups in society who share their concerns and their issues. Taking account of the four key requisites highlighted above, as well as the reservations expressed by Victor (1991a) and Grimley Evans (1991) of the relevance of the targets to the health concerns of older people, the targets set out in the 'Health of the Nation' initiative will be explored. In discussing these targets, issues will emerge which demonstrate that a non-ageist approach to health promotion has direct relevance to older people. The document identifies five key areas in which substantial improvements in health status can be achieved, and for each of these areas identifies national targets. These areas are:

- coronary heart disease and stroke
- cancers
- mental illness
- HIV/AIDS and sexual health
- accidents.

When considering these topics, some of the physiological, psychological and socio-economic changes that may occur with ageing are raised.

Heart disease and stroke
There have been a number of recommendations made in the health promotion literature for the prevention of heart disease and stroke in recent years, particularly in the light of the high mortality from circulatory disease in old age. One of the recommendations includes helping people to quit smoking, although the Medical Research Council suggests that this issue is not so well addressed with older people (MRC, 1994). The General Household Survey (1988), cited by Askham *et al.* (1992), demonstrated that 51% of respondents over the age of 60 years who smoked reported poor health. It has been shown that older people benefit from giving up cigarette smoking, in particular when they experience high levels of serum cholesterol, according to Grimley Evans (1992).

Tilston and Williams (1992) suggest that health promotion strategies which include exploring ways in which the daily diet can be changed to reduce the intake of cholesterol have proved to be well received by older people and may also be effective in reducing serum lipids (Grimley Evans, 1992; MRC, 1994), thus reducing the risk of coronary heart disease.

Exercise may also contribute to the physical, mental and functional ability and wellbeing of people of all ages. The MRC (1994) demonstrated strong correlation between physical fitness and the retardation of cognitive changes in old age. Hardman (1992) highlights the benefits of exercise to older women in terms of improvements in functional capacities, increased muscle strength, decreased rate of loss in bone density after the menopause and increased stamina. Despite the positive benefits of some daily exercise, older people tend to undertake less physical activity with age (Askham *et al.*, 1992). In a recent study, Ashworth *et al.* (1994) also found that in comparison with people whose mean age was 27 years, people with a mean age of 70 years undertook lower levels of basic daily living activities. The Health Education Authority has been involved in the training of people to lead 'Look After Your Heart' groups, and it is important that these and other health promotion strategies are targeted at older people, who should be encouraged to pursue a planned programme of exercise of two or three sessions a week including brisk walking, swimming, cycling and dancing (Hardman, 1992). However, MRC (1994) highlights the need for further research into optimum levels of exercise for older people as well as reasons why exercise levels are low.

In terms of secondary prevention, the MRC (1994) also argue that screening for hypertension and the management of high blood pressure in people up to the age of 80 years can have beneficial effects, although it is suggested that there is a need for more research in this area too. Indeed, screening or case-finding is a controversial issue, not least because there may be some unwanted side-effects such as identifying a problem not previously recognized, or false-positive and false-negative results creating undue anxiety. However, Tilston and Williams (1992) suggest that there are some positive non-medical benefits of screening and case-finding, including an increased uptake of health and social services, shorter stays in hospital and the benefit of positive attention being paid by individuals to health.

Cancers

Despite some of the benefits of screening and the higher incidence of cancer in older people, Zabalegui (1994) demonstrates a lower uptake of screening in this age group. Kemppainen *et al.* (1993) also found, in their study of patients with colorectal cancer, that elderly people may also delay seeking medical advice. Delays from the first symptom being experienced to the first consultation may be between 12 and over 16 weeks. However, Curless *et al.* (1994) found that there was no difference in the delay between younger and older patients, although they did find that older patients had different symptom presentations, including anorexia, which could obscure the seriousness of the condition.

Fletcher (1992) argues that the outcomes of screening programmes are mixed and inconclusive and generally based on studies of younger people. However, when older people are included in studies, their uptake of the service remains low. The reason for this warrants some discussion. The MRC (1994) identified possible explanations for the poor uptake of screening or delays in seeking treatment or advice, which included lower expectations of health, previous experience and socio-economic differences. Older people may also have experienced a time when the outcome of treatment for some conditions was unsuccessful. However, in terms of some diagnoses and the subsequent response to treatment, evidence suggests that older people do as well as younger people (Kelly *et al.*, 1991; Fletcher, 1992). Kelly and colleagues undertook a retrospective study of survival of young patients and older patients with small-cell lung cancer who received a combination of treatments. They concluded that there was no difference between the survival curve of young and older patients or between men and women. The outcome of screening and the results of interventions need to be examined and older people made aware of the information so that they can make informed choices about screening and about the potential outcome of treatments.

Many of the studies on the benefits of screening and the outcomes of treatments have excluded elderly people despite the evidence that half of all the new malignancies occur in people over the age of 70 years, according to Henwood (1990). Although elderly people may request breast and cervical screening, the age group targeted is 50–65 and the evidence demonstrates that older people may not come forward and make such requests. It is also clear that further studies need to be undertaken to investigate the benefits of screening procedures for older people as well as their response to treatment.

Mental health and mental illness

Retirement and old age is a very positive experience for many people, offering new challenges and opportunities. Many older people report that they do not feel their age and that they are enjoying their lives, wondering how they had time to work (Thompson *et al.*, 1990). Although mental health promotion is of importance to people whatever their age, ageing may bring adverse life events which are concentrated in a relatively short time span. Bereavement and the onset of health problems are examples of such events which require new coping strategies and ongoing support. Indeed, the government initiative identifies important areas for primary, secondary and tertiary prevention which are relevant to all age groups (see Chapter 10). These include counselling and advice for people experiencing redundancy and unemployment, family circumstances such as bereavement and social isolation, sensory and physical impairment and coping with stress.

Depression is under-reported in people with common health problems such as respiratory and cardiovascular disease requiring hospital admission (Baldwin and Jackson, 1993). This study was undertaken in hospital and included the use of a self-complete 30-item Geriatric Depression Scale together with the Geriatric Mental Status Schedule completed by the psychogeriatrician. Nurses in the general medical ward were also asked to undertake a simple observation scale for the detection of depression which proved not to be sensitive to detecting depression. It was suggested that nurses should undertake training to improve their skills in detecting depression in older people and that the Geriatric

Depression Scale should be incorporated into routine practice. This could contribute to the assessment of older people in the community

Support networks

Although Scrutton (1992) argues that social isolation contributes to mental ill-health, other authors state that though effective social support networks can buffer the effects of stress, decrease psychological stress and contribute to the physical and mental wellbeing of older people, there is little agreement as to the features of social networks which make them supportive (Grant *et al.*, 1988).

In a longitudinal study of older people, Grant *et al.* (1988) identified four different types of support and related them to the number of supportive people available (network size), satisfaction with the support received and the consistency of the support available to older people without dementia who were living in the community, over a span of two years. The four types of support were 'thing giving', 'help giving', 'advice giving' and 'emotional support giving'. Thing giving was associated with being able to borrow money or resources. Help giving was being looked after while ill or following an accident. Advice giving referred to information, guidance and problem-solving, while emotional support giving was having someone to confide in. It was found that there were more self-reports of depression in subjects who had fewer 'emotional supports' from relatives. Although consistent with earlier research, the difference between this and the earlier research was that it identified the importance of family 'emotional support' rather than simply 'help giving' or 'advice giving' support in maintaining the mental health of older people. The researchers, however, did not indicate how this emotional support was given. The method of giving the support, whether through direct contact, letters or telephone contact, may be quite important, given the mobility of the working population.

In addition to poor social support, physical changes such as alterations in sleep patterns have been linked with the incidence of depression. Livingston *et al.* (1993), in a longitudinal study of the prevalence of sleep disturbances and its relationship with other health indices, which included depression, disability and social circumstances, found that people who were depressed were more likely to experience sleep disturbance. It was suggested that reports of insomnia may be an effective predictor of new depression and that sleep disturbances may lead to depression. Farquhar *et al.* (1993), in a study of the use of services by elderly people living in East London and Mid Essex, found that the second highest self-reported health problem was sleeplessness in the East London sample and the fourth in Mid Essex sample. The highest problem in both samples was that of aches, pains and stiffness in muscles and joints. In this study the researchers used the Goldberg General Health Questionnaire which they suggested correlated well with independent psychiatric diagnosis of depression, finding that the East London group had a higher incidence of depression. However, they did not make the connection between reports of sleeplessness and the incidence of depression, which suggests the need for further research. It is important to note that the studies by Livingston and Farquhar and colleagues did not focus on the quality of family emotional support in the way in which Grant and co-workers did. There may be a need for detailed multidisciplinary research which pulls together the various strands which have emerged from earlier studies.

In terms of the 'Health of the Nation' target of promoting mental health, health checks offered to older people could incorporate screening for insomnia and an assessment of the social support networks, in order to detect and effectively treat depression. Failure to diagnose depression and associated insomnia, is leading to the inappropriate prescribing of benzodiazepines which not only do not tackle the cause of the depression but may lead to falls and fractures due to the continuing sedating effects when the patient is mobile the following day (Nutt, 1993).

Nutt points out that the depressed people experience disturbances in their sleep waves, causing the dreaming phase to be brought forward and reducing the available time for restorative sleep. He suggests that fluvoxamine is a more appropriate medication as it lacks the sedative effects of benzodiazepines. The treatment of depression and the subsequent follow-up of people in the community is important in tertiary prevention. Community health care nurses are in a prime position to follow up and monitor clients who are being treated for depression. They may also be in a good position to share stress-relieving strategies such as relaxation techniques which may contribute to the overall wellbeing of older people.

In relation to suicide, Bowles (1993) highlights risk factors based on the work of earlier authors. These risks factors include bereavement without adequate support, caring for a dependent person, especially one who is cognitively impaired, has chronic health problems such as Parkinson's disease or following a cerebrovascular accident, a history of depression or alcoholism, and a recent visit to the doctor. Bowles suggests that nurses may feel sympathetic to older people who have experienced losses of partners, health and home and who express suicidal wishes. She points out, though, that suicide is a maladaptive response and the underlying depression and unresolved grief need to be addressed. Counselling and the appropriate use of medication may contribute to the older person's recovery. She too recommends training in assessing older people and in supporting them to improve their self-esteem and wellbeing.

Dementia

Dementia implies an irreversible global impairment of cognitive functioning, although people are affected differently depending upon the level of involvement of memory, perception, attention and reasoning (Grimley Evans, 1991). The commonest type of dementia is that of Alzheimer's disease, but this diagnosis should only be reached after other potentially reversible or treatable conditions have been excluded. Older people may react differently to infections, drugs, HIV/AIDS and other conditions. Appropriate diagnostic investigations should always be undertaken when disabling memory loss and confusion are present (Smith and Leigh, 1986).

Different approaches have been adopted to develop the mental wellbeing of people with dementia. Some of these approaches, including reminiscence therapy, have achieved mixed results (Redfern, 1991). Budge (1990) describes a range of approaches for creating recreational activities such as educational and social activities with older people, including those with dementia. However, Feill (1993) suggests that people with dementia may need special considerations such as validation therapy as a way of valuing, respecting and empathizing with them. Validation therapy is based on underlying principles and values which acknowledge that each person is unique in their history, their needs and their aspirations. Feill also recognizes that people may have unresolved issues which they need to explore whether they have dementia or not. She describes the use of validation in the community and highlights ways of introducing it in a group setting. This approach may have some benefits for promoting the mental health of people with dementia. The evaluation of validation therapy in this country and in the community should be a priority, if mental health promotion with people with dementia is to move forward. Another important point is to acknowledge that people with dementia, living in the community, are often supported by relatives, friends and neighbours, and the needs of these carers must be considered if community care is to be successful.

Carers and community care

The majority of older people with chronic health problems live in their own homes supported by relatives and friends. Community care frequently means that carers undertake a range of caring tasks from shopping to bathing, lifting, moving and feeding the dependent person. These carers may themselves be older and may find it difficult to cope with some of the aspects of caring. Carers may be of either gender, from different ethnic groups, of different ages, and from different social classes (Bornat *et al.*, 1993). Lynch and Perry (1992) describe a range of innovative approaches for working with carers. These include the provision of community gardens, day centres for ethnic minority groups, community projects and projects for people with Alzheimer's disease, all of which offer some respite from the stresses of caring (see section on carers in Chapter 13).

Sexual health and HIV/AIDS

Another key area in the initiative is the promotion of sexual health and the prevention of sexually transmitted diseases including HIV and AIDS. The target groups are women and men in the general population as well as defined groups of people such as gay and bisexual men, drug and substance misusers and prostitutes and their clients. The aim of health promotion in the context of sexual health is to improve levels of knowledge and encourage people to adopt healthy and safer patterns of sexual behaviour. Although the groups defined in the *Key Area Handbook* produced on HIV/AIDS and sexual health (DoH, 1993) does not directly exclude older people as part of the general population, the words 'young' and 'family planning' frequently appear in the document. This raises the question of whether education about sexual health will feature in future health promotion strategies with older people. However, Gibson (1992) identifies some important issues for sexual health promotion with older people. He suggests that older people may have been socialized not to discuss sexual matters openly, either with each other or with people including professionals. They may have been brought up to believe that masturbation could cause physical or mental ill-health, and Gibson (1992) suggests that there are many areas which could be the focus of health education including correcting past misinformation.

Sexuality and older people

According to Davies (1986), sexual desire continues into very old age and the physical expression of this desire may be through touching, stroking and caressing as well as sexual intercourse. Men and women may have different ways of expressing sexuality, depending upon their past experiences and expectations. Gibson (1992) points out that older men see penetration as evidence of manhood, whereas older women may enjoy the physical contact of touching and stroking which is often referred to as foreplay. These different expectations may lead to problems in a relationship, and sexual health education may provide opportunities for open discussion about such issues and contribute to a greater appreciation and understanding of sexuality. Jerrome (1993), on the other hand, cautions health practitioners to avoid overrating sexual activity in old age and putting new pressures on older people who may be quite happy with minimal sexual activity.

One of the social reasons why people may be denied the opportunities to express sexuality in later life is through the death of a partner. Older lesbian women appear to have wider possibilities of making new relationships in old age than heterosexual women (Jerrome, 1993). The changing nature of relationships in society needs to be recognized when undertaking assessments. It may no longer be appropriate to enquire as to 'next of kin', but to ascertain the 'significant other' person who needs to be informed of care decisions.

Physical changes

As well as social reasons for the limiting of opportunities for sexual relationships, there are also physical reasons. One of the physical changes which takes place in older women during the menopause is the reduction in vaginal secretions (Dickson and Henriques, 1992). This may, according to Leroy (1993), make sexual intercourse painful, but this pain may be alleviated by the use of specific lubricants and also exploring new and different ways of sexual intercourse. This may be particularly useful where individuals have undergone surgery such as joint replacements or if they have a limiting condition such as arthritis. The onset of a limiting health condition may have an impact on an individual's perception of themselves, as it may change their body image. It may also cause pain, limitation of movement or decreased sensitivity.

Interventions and advice

Certain interventions and medications may cause impotence or other sexual difficulties. It is important for professionals to be aware of the effects of physical conditions on an individual's sexuality and to be competent to undertake a sensitive assessment, seeking to modify or address the problem. Advice on the timing of medication may reduce pain and enable people to undertake sexual activity. Some medication, such as hypotensive drugs, may induce impotence in men and women. These drugs could be changed, provided that the practitioner is aware and able to advocate on behalf of the client.

Sexual health promotion

Kaufman (1993) argues that because sexuality in older people is often ignored, lifestyles are often assumed and are rarely questioned, so HIV/AIDS is rarely discussed. She points out that some heterosexual men may also have had homosexual relationships. Widows and widowers may seek partners and may also travel abroad, yet the information regarding HIV/AIDS is not usually targeted at this group (Gibson, 1992). Kaufman points out that HIV/AIDS should be considered when older people are admitted to hospital. Recurrent infections, dementia and other symptoms should be thoroughly investigated if the correct diagnosis is to be made and the appropriate treatment and interventions initiated.

The care of older people with HIV/AIDS needs the same considerations and attention as the care of younger people, but the needs of older people require special attention as resistance to infection, response to treatments, recovery rates and adaptation to physical changes may all be adversely affected by the ageing process (Kaufman, 1993). There are other ways in which HIV/AIDS touches the lives of older people, which include their families and friendships. Older people may be parents, grandparents, carers and partners of people with HIV/AIDS. They too will experience the bereavements which have come to be associated with younger people but, with a diminishing circle of friends and family, such losses may be compounded by the increase in the experience of bereavement in ageing friends and family.

The important message in relation to sexuality and health promotion with older people is to see older people as simply people who have aged. They are as diverse as the rest of the population.

Accidents

The aim of the key target relating to accidents in older people is to reduce mortality and morbidity rates, particularly those from falls and road traffic accidents. According to data published by OPCS (1993), 3% of people over 60 years reported some kind of accident in the preceding 3 months which required seeing the doctor or attending hospital. The reported incidence of accidents is higher among women than men and higher among people over 80 years who rated their health as 'not so good'. In 75 year olds in 1991, falls were responsible for 67% of female and 52% of male accidental deaths. Half a million people over 65 years require hospital attention and 65% of these are falls and there are many road traffic accidents among pedestrians (DoH, 1993).

Accidents and falls may result from either internal factors related to the older person's health, or from external factors in the environment. These external factors may occur in the immediate environment of the home, or in the wider environment of the local community. In relation to internal factors, it is important to recognize that the ageing process creates changes in physical functioning. An awareness of the physiology of ageing, as a basis for providing realistic health promotion, will enable older people to make changes in their lifestyle and their environment which could accommodate their changing physiological processes.

Visual changes

Visual changes occur which make it difficult for the older person to adjust quickly to changes in lighting levels; moving from a light to a dark environment causing temporary blindness provides an example. It is important to ensure that throughout the house the lighting level is adequate and even. Regular vision testing is important for the early detection of visual changes. One strategy adopted in an outpatient department involved the opportunistic screening of the vision of older people using a Snellen chart. Long (1991) recommended that the Snellen chart was used as a quick and objective way of detecting changes and obtaining early treatment. Although authors such as Thompson *et al.* (1989) and Long (1991) recognize the limitations of the Snellen chart, they suggest that screening vision in this way might identify people who are at risk of falls. Screening for glaucoma is another important area in which health promotion could be adopted on a wide scale. A glaucoma chart for the purpose of oculokinetic perimetry has been developed for use by non-specialists in the community to test for glaucomatous visual field loss (Mutlukan *et al.*, 1993). This screening should preferably be undertaken as part of a combined strategy with ophthalmological services.

Opportunistic screening, planned screening and self-examination of vision has not been universally adopted by community health care nurses either in the clinics or in the home. Indeed, this is an area for future research, evaluation and recommendations, since it is largely left to the self-reporting of problems. Community health care nurses are in a good position to undertake research in these important preventive measures and to provide guidance to future practice. Indeed, in terms of secondary and tertiary prevention, older people need help, guidance, support and counselling in the event of sight loss. Conyers (1992), in a survey of 122 outpatients who had been diagnosed and registered as blind or partially sighted, found that the most commonly reported feeling was one of depression. Fifty-eight people said that they did not receive enough help to prepare them for the loss of their sight, and 48 said they felt the ophthalmic consultant did not have enough time for them to discuss the implications.

The study recommended that there should be greater liaison

between ophthalmic staff and social workers, with more collaboration between all professionals to ensure that counselling and support is available. This is particularly important with people from minority ethnic groups where unrealistic assumptions are frequently made about the amount of support which families can offer (Atkin *et al.*, 1988; Glendenning and Pearson, 1988). Help through short-term crisis intervention to assist the client over the acute psychosocial distress they may experience could play an important part in adjustment to visual problems. It is important to help people cope with the activities of living, preventing accidents and improving overall confidence.

Hearing impairment

Although hearing impairment is common in older people, Bennett and Ebrahim (1992) argue it is difficult to attribute this solely to the ageing process. The most common cause of hearing impairment is due to obstruction in the external auditory meatus, owing to a reduction in skin moisture leading to drier cerumen being secreted, an increase in irritation, cracking, crusting and bleeding and a build up of debris. Bennett and Ebrahim (1992) suggest that the removal of this debris remedies this simple form of conductive deafness. The second type of hearing loss, known as presbycusis, is a sensorineural loss, due to the damage to the cochlea or to the auditory nerve fibres leading to decreased sensitivity to high-frequency sounds (Gillick *et al.*, 1989). Because speech and other sounds are made up of a combination of frequencies and the individual with presbycusis can only distinguish low frequencies, it means that speech may be distorted and misinterpreted, leading to misunderstandings, impatience and feelings of isolation. This type of hearing loss is very gradual and the individual may be unaware of it and therefore fail to seek help.

MacPhee *et al.* (1988) developed a simple screening test using free-field voice testing of a whisper at 2 feet (0.6 m) from the ear. They found that once certain conditions such as dysphasia, terminal illness and acute conditions had been accounted for, this test was sensitive and predictive of hearing impairment. Since this study was undertaken in hospital, it would be a study to replicate in the community. In another study undertaken by Counsel and Care (1993) of elderly people in residential and nursing homes, it was found that frequently hearing problems were undetected and where a hearing aid had been provided this could not be used because of the lack of maintenance. This study may represent 'the tip of the iceberg' in the community and identifies the need for practitioners to adopt MacPhee's hearing assessment as well as training, so that they are familiar with hearing aids and equipment such as induction loops. Practitioners should also liaise with voluntary bodies which specialize in hearing impairment and should be trained in communication skills.

Hearing is not simply a sense which allows people to hear and interpret language, it also has a protective function which enables people to hear traffic, hear audible bleeps on pedestrian crossings and hear people approaching. Without this important sense, older people may be more vulnerable to accidents. It is therefore important that measures are implemented which will reduce this vulnerability and improve the quality of life.

Physical factors and falls

Other internal factors related to the incidence of accidents and falls include physical health and strength, activity levels, speed of walking, medication and alcohol consumption. Askham *et al*. (1992) and Thompson *et al*. (1990) suggest that people who report accidents generally have some medical condition. The most frequent conditions cited by men aged between 60 and 64 years were arthritis/rheumatism, hypertension, heart attack, and other bone/joint problems. These were different for men over 80 years who cited arthritis/rheumatism first, followed by hearing problems, visual problems and heart attack. Women aged 60–64 years reported arthritis/rheumatism, hypertension, back problems and heart attack. This changed to arthritis/rheumatism followed by visual problems, other bone/joint and muscle problems, heart and hearing problems, with older women. This evidence suggests that chronic health problems require further investigation if the target of reduced morbidity and mortality from falls is to be achieved.

In a survey of 1042 people over the age of 65 years, Blake *et al*. (1988) found that of the 34% (356) people reporting falls, 53% reported tripping (environmental factors) while 6% reported blackouts and 19% reported no reason. The researchers found that there was a significant association between falls and the use of hypnotics and antidepressants. There was also an association between handgrip strength, giddiness and foot difficulties reported. Physical restrictions including those imposed by arthritis and rheumatism may lead to inactivity and falls. Pain-relieving strategies may help an older person undertake increased physical activity, which is particularly important since Boyce and Vessey (1988) suggest that physical inertia is implicated in the risk of falls and fractures. In their study of 139 selected patients with confirmed fractured femur matched by age and sex with a control group in the community, they carried out an interviewer-administered questionnaire survey which demonstrated that where people were less active in the mid-life, there was an increase in the risk of fracture. They also cite studies which indicate the importance of activity in maintaining bone mass and suggest that this increased bone mass reduced the risk of fractures. However, other authors such as Lehmann (1992) suggest that under-nutrition may be responsible for hip fractures and cardiovascular events in older people, especially in winter.

It is clear from the 'Health of the Nation' key targets that accidents, particularly falls, are of concern to policy-makers as well as older people, not only because of their frequency in old age but also because the outcome of a fall may have serious consequences for the individual. Falls and accidents may be symptoms of disease or other problems which may alert practitioners to consider the possibility of elder abuse.

Elder abuse

The definition of elder abuse has been debated recently in journals and in research articles (Steinmetz, 1988; Pritchard, 1992; Bennett and Kingston, 1993). The different types of abuse which have been identified are as follows:

- Physical abuse – violence and assaults:
  misuse of medications and treatments
  physical constraints, e.g. confining to room or tying to chair
  sexual abuse
  withholding treatments, aids and appliances
  inadequate care and neglect
- Psychological abuse – humiliation:
  harassment
  name calling
  threats
- Financial abuse – theft of money or property:
  exploitation of money or property

However, these categories of abuse are by no means clear and remain open to debate. Although some local authorities have developed guidelines and policies for their staff, these are not as well developed as those for child abuse (Bennett and Kingston 1993).

It is essential for community health care nurses to be aware of the possibilities that abuse might occur. Local guidelines and local discussions will help to clarify the assessment tools and need for action in the event of abuse being identified. Eastman (1984) identified concerns for both the carer and the client, as he suggested that there are two victims of abuse – the abused and the perpetrator. This view is also supported by Steinmetz (1988), who highlighted in her research how carers tend to drift into the caring situation, often with the expectation that it would be for a limited period of time and that they could cope. Although their intention was to provide care, they failed to recognize the demands and the stress which could be created in the dependency situation.

Therefore, when practitioners are carrying out assessment, recognition should be given to the individual needs of both parties, independent and confidential from each other. Consideration should be given not only to whether the home environment is the most appropriate place for interviewing both carer and client, but also whether one worker can advocate for both individuals in the event of action being required. It is also important for both the carer and the client to be aware of the implications of divulging information to health care professionals. The outcomes may be positive, in that the carer may be relieved of some of the caring responsibilities by modifications and expansion of the 'care package', or the outcome could be negative, in that the older person is removed from their home. Steinmetz found that some older people, despite the physical threat to their wellbeing, preferred to remain in the abusing situation rather than be removed to a new and alien environment. A new organization 'Action on Elder Abuse' was launched in the UK in 1993, and is seeking charitable status and funding from government and from Age Concern, England. The organization is hoping to raise the profile on elder abuse, educate professionals and carers and undertake research in order to prevent abuse taking place.

Accidents and falls are complex and it would be inappropriate to suggest that one assessment of an older person, followed by changes in lifestyle and environment, would dramatically change the present situation. Although it may contribute to the wellbeing of older people, further research is needed if accidents and falls are to be fully understood.

However, accidents and falls are symptoms of physical and environmental problems as well as possible indications of elder abuse. It is important therefore that community health care nurses are aware of the complexity of assessing the health promotional needs of older people, and recognize the significant contribution of all agencies involved in providing services to older people.

● Conclusion

In exploring the relevance of the 'Health of the Nation' targets to older people, this chapter has highlighted the significance of practitioners looking beyond simple biological explanations for health problems in old age. Other people's lives could be adversely affected by negative attitudes and assumptions, but positive attitudes will enhance and promote the health of older people, whatever their age and their abilities. Although there is considerable research available to practitioners indicating the potential for health promotion with older people, there is clearly a need for further research. Indeed, changes in the delivery of health and community care for older people, the health targets identified in *The Health of the Nation* and *The Patient's Charter* and the new consumerism in the public sector all present challenges and opportunities for practitioners in caring for older people.

References

Ashworth, J., Reuben, D. and Benton, L. (1994) Functional profiles of health in older persons. *Age and Ageing*, **23**, 34–39

Askham, J., Barry, C., Grundy, E., Hancock, R. and Tinker, A. (1992) *Life After 60. A Profile of Britain's Older Population*, Age Concern/Institute of Gerontology, King's College, London

Atkin, K., Badger, F., Cameron, E. and Evers, H. (1988) *The Community Care Project: Why don't GPs Refer Black Disabled Patients to District Nurses?* Community Care Project, Working Paper 23, Central Birmingham Health Authority

Baldwin, R. and Jackson, R. (1993) Detecting depression in elderly medically ill patients: the use of geriatric depression scale compared with medical and nursing observations. *Age and Ageing*, **22**(5), 349–353

Bennett, G.J. and Ebrahim, S. (1992) *The Essentials of Health Care of the Elderly*, Edward Arnold, London

Bennett, G. and Kingston, P. (1993) *Elder Abuse: Concepts, Theories and Interventions*, Chapman and Hall, London

Blake, A.J., Morgan, K., Bendall, M.J. *et al*. (1988) Falls by elderly people at home: prevalence and associated factors. *Age and Ageing*, **17**, 365–372

Bornat, J., Pereira, C., Pilgrim, D. and Williams, F. (1993) *Community Care: A Reader*. Open University Press, Buckingham

Bowles, L. (1993) Logical conclusion. *Nursing Times*, **89**(31), 32–34

Boyce, W.J. and Vessey, M.P. (1988) Habitual physical inertia and other factors in relation to risk of fracture of the proximal femur. *Age and Ageing*, **17**, 319–327

Budge, M. (1990) *A Wealth of Experience. A Guide to Activities for Older People*. MacLennan and Petty, Sydney

Comfort, A. (1982) Old people need what people need. *New Internationalist*, June, 12

Conyers, M. (1992) *Vision for the Future. Meeting the Challenge of Sight Loss*. Jessica Kingsley Publications, London

Counsel and Care (1993) *Sound Barriers. A Study of the Needs of Older People Living in Residential Care and Nursing Homes*, Counsel and Care, London

Curless, R., French, J., Williams, G. and James, O. (1994) Colorectal carcinoma: do elderly patients present differently? *Age and Ageing*, **23**, 102–107

Davies, M. (1986) Sexuality and elderly people. In *Sexuality in Later Life* (ed. C. Wild), Working Papers on the Health of Older People No. 4, HEC in association with the Department of Adult and Continuing Education, University of Keele

Dickson, A. and Henriques, N. (1992) *Menopause. The Women's View,* Quartet Books, London

DoH (1992) *The Health of the Nation*, HMSO, London

DoH (1993) *The Health of the Nation. Key Area Handbook*, HMSO, London

Eastman, M. (1984) *Old Age Abuse*, Age Concern England, London

Farquhar, M., Bowling, A., Grundy, E. and Formby, J. (1993) Elderly people's use of services: a survey. *Nursing Standard*, **7**(47), 31–36

Feill, N. (1993) *The Validation Breakthrough. Simple Techniques for Communicating with People with Alzheimer's-type Dementia*. Health Professions Press, London

Fletcher, A. (1992) Controversies in screening for breast and cervical cancer. In *Health Care for Older Women* (eds J. George and S. Ebrahim), Oxford Medical Publications, Oxford

Gibson, H.B. (1992) *The Emotional and Sexual Lives of Older People. A Manual for Professionals*, Chapman and Hall, London

Gillick, W.L., Gescheider, G.A. and Frisina, R.D. (1989) *Hearing: Physiological Acoustics, Neural Coding and Psychoacoustics*, Oxford University Press, Oxford

Glendenning, F. and Pearson, M. (1988) *The Black and Ethnic Minority Elders in Britain: Health Needs and Access to Services*, HEA in association with the University of Keele

Grant, I., Patterson, T.L. and Yager, J. (1988) Social support in relation to physical health and symptoms of depression in the elderly. *American Journal of Psychiatry*, **145**(10), 1254–1258

Grimley Evans, J. (1991) Challenge of ageing. In *The Health of the Nation: The BMJ View* (ed. R. Smith), BMJ, London

Hardman, A. (1992) Exercises and older women. In *Health Care for Older Women* (eds. J. George and S. Ebrahim), Oxford Medical Publications, Oxford

Henderson, P. and Armstrong, J. (1993) Community development and community care: a strategic approach. In *Community Care: A Reader* (eds J. Bornat *et al.*), Oxford University Press, Oxford

Henwood, M. (1990) No sense of urgency. In *Age. The Unrecognised Discrimination. Views to Provoke Debate* (ed. E. McEwen), Age Concern England, London

Jerrome, D. (1993) Intimacy and sexuality amongst older women. In *Women Come of Age* (eds M. Bernard and K. Meade), Edward Arnold, London

Kalache, A. (1988) *Promoting Health Among Elderly People*, King's Fund Publishing, London

Katz, A. (1986) Self-care and self-help programmes for elders In *Self-Care and Health in Old Age* (eds K. Dean, T. Hickey and B. Holstein), Croom Helm, London

Kaufman, T. (1993) *A Crisis of Silence: HIV, AIDS and Older People*, Age Concern Greater London, London

Kelly, P., O'Brien, A., Daly, P. and Clancy, L. (1991) Small-cell lung cancer in elderly patients: the case for chemotherapy. *Age and Ageing*, **20**, 19–22

Kemppainen, M., Raiha, I., Rajala, T. and Sourander, L. (1993) Delay in diagnosis of colorectal cancer in elderly patients. *Age and Ageing*, **22**, 260–264

Kosberg, J.I. (1992) *Family Care of the Elderly. Social and Cultural Changes*, Sage Publications, London

Lehmann, A. (1992) Measuring the nutritional status of old people. In *Gerontology. Responding to an Ageing Society* (ed. K. Morgan), Jessica Kingsley Publications, London

Leroy, M. (1993) *Pleasure. The Truth About Female Sexuality*, Harper Collins, London

Livingston, G., Blizard, B. and Mann, A. (1993) Does sleep disturbance predict depression in elderly people? *British Journal of General Practice*, **43**, 445–448

Long, C.A. (1991) Opportunistic screening of visual acuity of the elderly. *Ageing and Society*, July, 233–235

Lynch, B. and Perry, R. (1992) *Experiences of Community Care. Case Studies of UK Practice*, Longman, Harlow

MacPhee, G.J.A., Crowther, J.A. and MacAlpine, G.H. (1988) A simple screening test for hearing impairment in elderly patients. *Age and Ageing*, **17**, 347–351

MRC (1994) *The Health of the UK's Elderly People*, MRC Topic Review, Medical Research Council, London

Mutlukan, E., Domato, B.E. and Jay, J. (1993) Clinical evaluation of a multi-fixation campimeter for the detection of glaucomatous visual field loss. *Journal of Ophthalmology*, **77**, 332–338

Nutt, D. (1993) Drug warning for elderly sufferers from insomnia. *Nursing Standard*, **8**(2), 16

OPCS (1993) Monitor. PP2 93/1, HMSO, London

Pritchard, J. (1992) *The Abuse of Elderly People. A Handbook for Professionals*, Jessica Kingsley Publications, London

Redfern, S. (1991) *Nursing Elderly People*, 2nd edn, Churchill Livingstone, London

Scrutton, S. (1992) *Ageing, Healthy and in Control: An Alternative Approach to Maintaining the Health of Older People*, Chapman and Hall, London

Secretary of State for Health (1991) *The NHS and Community Care Act*, HMSO, London

Smith, L.A. and Leigh, N. (1986) The biology of ageing. The ageing brain. *Geriatric Nursing and Home Care*, November/December, 21–25

Steinmetz, S. (1988) *Duty Bound. Elder Abuse and Family Care*, Sage Publications, London

Thompson, J.R., Gibson, J.M. and Jagger, C. (1989) The association between visual impairment and mortality in elderly people. *Age and Ageing*, **18**, 83–88

Thompson, P., Itzin, C. and Abendstern, M. (1990) *I Don't Feel Old. The Experience of Later Life*, Oxford University Press, London

Tilston, J. and Williams, J. (1992) Everyone wants to go to heaven, but no one wants to die. Screening women over 75—a health promotion approach. In *Health Care for Older Women* (eds J. George and S. Ebrahim), Oxford Medical Publications, Oxford

Victor, C. (1991a) Continuity or change: inequalities in health in later life. *Ageing and Society*, **11**, 23–39

Victor, C. (1991b) *Health and Health Care in Later Life*, Open University Press, Buckingham

Whitbourne, S.K. (1985) *The Aging Body. Physiological Changes and Psychological Consequences*, Springer Verlag, New York

WHO (1989) *Health of the Elderly* (Technical Series Report 779), WHO, Geneva

Zabalegui, A. (1994) Barriers to health. Cancer screening. Older people. *Nursing Times*, **90**(1), 59–61

22

Death and dying

Virginia Dunn

● **Introduction**

To modify a well-known saying: 'The dying we will have always with us.' Indeed, the dying have always been with us, but in the 1950s it became clear that death had become increasingly unfamiliar and marginalized. While there is debate in the literature about whether in fact death is denied (Kellehear, 1984), it is clear that most people are personally unfamiliar with the experience of dying and death. One reason is that the pattern of death has changed. In common with other advanced industrial societies, the UK has an ageing population. Infant mortality has decreased and life expectancy increased to the extent that in 1991 life expectancy was 73.2 years for males and 78.2 years for women (Field and James, 1993). Acute diseases now rarely have fatal outcomes and the main causes of death are chronic degenerative disease of the circulatory and pulmonary systems and cancers. Blauner (1966) notes:

as death . . . becomes increasingly a phenomenon of the old, who are usually retired from work and finished with their parental responsibilities, mortality in modern society rarely interrupts the business of life.

Another reason for the discomfort is the shift in the place of care. The majority of deaths before this century occurred at home, but within the life of the NHS the proportion of people dying in institutions for the sick increased to the extent that, by the mid-1960s, two-thirds of all deaths in the UK took place in hospitals or other places. But Cartwright (1991) noted that while it is highly likely that dying people will die in a hospital or hospice, recent improvements in medical techniques and the political emphasis and developments in community care have resulted in dying patients spending a shorter time in hospital. In the last year of life, most care is given in their own homes, with that care provided mainly by unpaid, untrained lay carers.

Definition of palliative care

The World Health Organisation (WHO, 1990) defines specialist palliative care as the *active total care of patients whose disease is not responsive to curative treatment. Control of pain and other symptoms, and of psychological, social and spiritual problems is paramount. The goal of palliative care is achievement of the best quality of life for patients and their families.*

It encompasses the following dimensions:

- to affirm life and to regard death as a normal process, neither hastening or postponing it
- to integrate the physical, psychological and spiritual aspects of care so that patients may come to terms with their own death as fully and constructively as possible
- to support patients to live as actively and creatively as possible until death
- to offer support to families during the patient's dying and in bereavement.

Death is the most certain event of human life and has always been understood to be more than a mere physiological act. It shapes and is shaped by the whole of an individual's being. And while this last statement implies the unique and personal nature of dying, death is also most unquestionably a social and cultural event as well. So the expectations and experiences around dying and death are formed by many factors. While the physical symptoms may establish one area of focus, the individual's own personality and history will also contribute to the emotional and psychological responses. The wider canvas of cultural background and religious beliefs define expectations for the individual within a larger social context. There may be specific roles to play and duties to perform related to the ending of life (Neuberger, 1987). The individual, the family and the wider sociocultural network hold beliefs and values that will also govern the content and the manner of support which the health professional can offer to meet expectations and needs of this event.

● Dying at home

There are many reasons why a dying person will want to be at home (Billings, 1985; Spilling, 1986; Dunlop *et al.*, 1989; Townsend *et al.*, 1990; Hinton, 1994). First, when palliative care occurs in the home, the control of the process of dying shifts back to the dying person and the family (Field, 1980). Decisions about such questions as Who is around?, What is the focus of care?, Who provides the care? and How is care provided? are really made by the patient and family and not the health care professional, who is intermittently present. This is contrasted with care in hospital where often the focus is on physical aspects of care, the use of powerful and sophisticated interventions and the involvement of multiple teams of people (James and Field, 1992). In the acute hospital, the dying may not experience a clearly acknowledged transition from the state of being sick, and thus treatable, to one of knowing that dying is taking place (Williams, 1982). The failure to acknowledge death prevents the individual, family and the wider sociocultural group from engaging in activities that make this a significant life event.

Secondly, death is the ultimate separation from the living for the one who is dying. Being in an institution, regardless of how good the care, the dying are separated from important connections – personal, social and cultural. The trappings of life are absent. The patient (not John or Dad) has one major role – to co-operate with the medical plan and get better. Some writers use the term 'social death' to describe the cessation of the individual person as an active agent in others' lives. While hospitalization does not always result in this separation from usual life, it is difficult to sustain involvement in family and community life. Being at home as long as possible is one major attempt to maintain that involvement and to live until death.

Thirdly, freedom to live as one chooses is an important part of one's individuality. The previous point raises the issue of the loss of a meaningful contribution by the person who is dying to the lives of those who are important. This point now identifies another loss brought about by hospitalization, that of the loss of control over the ordinariness of life. This ordinariness is seen in the privacy, familiarity and continuity with normal life. It is a manifestation of personal autonomy. As one patient said, 'Home is your own turf. Here, I can call the shots' (Billings, 1985).

It is therefore not surprising that when asked for their preference about where care should occur, most patients identify home (Dunlop et al., 1989; Townsend et al., 1990). Having said the above in support of care at home, there are crucial factors besides patient preference that need to be taken into account when making decisions about the place of care; these include the availability, ability and commitment of carers to provide continuous and sustained care (Hinton, 1994). Thus, addressing family needs constitutes a major activity when supporting the dying person in the community. The ability to manage distressing symptoms also influences whether care can occur at home. Spilling (1986) notes that one of the factors that may make death difficult at home is that family's direct confrontation with the distress of dying. Therefore, the right of carers *not* to be primary providers of care should be acknowledged and supported. So while there is a philosophical commitment within palliative care to provide, where possible, care where patients choose, in actuality patients may require intermittent care in in-patient settings, either hospice or hospital, for limited periods of time, including the acute terminal period.

● **The contribution of research to palliative care**

Much of the literature and research about dying originates from North America and focuses on dying from cancer. Thus questions arise about the applicability of this base as a foundation for practice in the UK. In addressing the first concern about using material from another culture, one must assess what critical aspects do North American and contemporary British societies share that will legitimate generalizing from the one to the other.

Both are modern industrialized societies where death is peripheral and rarely interrupts the 'business of life' (Blauner, 1966). As mentioned earlier, an unfamiliarity with death occurs and this unfamiliarity is present in both cultures, resulting in the discomfort with direct communication about death and uncertainty about how to act for all participants – the patient, family and professional carers. In both societies, the hospice movement challenges the predominantly physical and medical manner of institutional dying and places an emphasis on (w)holistic care.

Both societies are organized in smaller nuclear families, with the extended family often living in other parts of the country. Also, in the past, informal care of the kind needed in situations of prolonged dying from chronic diseases was largely determined by demography and kinship. The extended family is committed to help, but for the most part do not live geographically close enough to provide the day-to-day support in prolonged chronic situations (Neale, 1991). Patterns of employment and a shift in traditional gender roles, particularly for the unmarried woman, means that while modern families want to fulfil their familial responsibilities of care, there may be a lack of a family member who can provide the continuous sustained care needed. Thus there is a common dependence in both cultures on the support of professional carers to provide guidance, support and actual care at home.

Some differences are found in the ethnic make-up of the two countries, but while the particular multi-cultural make-up may differ, both societies are multi-cultural and pluralistic in orientation. The general organizational differences in health care are rapidly diminishing with the NHS reforms in this country (Roemer, 1986; Leathard, 1990). However, in the USA, there is not an extensively developed primary care network. Therefore, the literature from North America identifies the use of specialized services almost exclusively for palliative support in the community instead of the negotiated partnership of specialist nurses with community health care nurses.

The second issue is that the disease focus of much of the research and literature about the care of people from anticipated death and their carers has evolved in the context of cancer care (James and Field, 1992). Cancer may produce a different array of physical symptoms than is experienced in other chronic diseases, but many are similar, for example fatigue, breathlessness, nutritional difficulties as well as pain. Cancer also provokes an intense emotional response that has been extensively written about in the literature, but the author would suggest that dying from any cause provokes similar anxieties and concerns which need to be addressed.

So despite some differences, it is reasonable to agree with Field (1989) when he concludes in *Nursing the Dying*, that

> *it does seem that the problems experienced by British and North American nurses in nursing people who are dying are very similar, and that each can learn from the research and attempted solutions found in the other.*

● Patient needs

Introduction

This section will explore the major areas of physical deterioration and some spiritual issues that frequently arise for patients. However, before these specific areas are examined, there are some general points that apply to all these areas and will influence the provision of nursing care.

First, dying is not a static event but a dynamic process, changing over time. Research has identified these changes which include not only physical deterioration but also changes in other important areas. For example, Abrams (1966), in an early paper, reported the way communication patterns changed between patients, health care professionals and family members as patients travelled their course with cancer. Herth (1990) found that patients defined hope differently as they neared death. So although there may be periods of relative stability, practitioners should anticipate that change will occur, and be open to new patient issues or perspectives. Patient priorities change over time and what was crucial at one point in time may fade to insignificance at another time. It is not unusual for a patient at one time to desperately want any treatment that is available regardless of the side-effects and efforts, and at a later stage feel that some treatments are not worth the cost. So, as mentioned earlier, when assessing patient symptoms, it is important to understand that *what has been* may not be *what is now* and assessment is a continuous re-evaluative process.

Secondly, many areas of patient concern are subjective, that is, they are known only to the person experiencing it and known only to others if shared with them. Even with physical deterioration, only hints may be available to the observer to indicate a problem or concern exists. Assessment becomes especially difficult if the individual is unknown, because the hint may only be a change from the usual behaviour or demeanour, as is seen in pain of long-standing duration, anorexia with nausea, sleeplessness, or guilt. The practitioner cannot assume that if the person does not take the initiative and raise a concern, there is no problem. Patients should be offered opportunities to share their concerns.

Thirdly, all aspects of the person are affected by dying, thus raising potential patient concern in any and all areas of their being. Some of these areas are extremely important because when there are problems, much distress results, for example, with issues of spirituality and family relationships. But these same areas can also be major sources of strength. Most practitioners are comfortable with assessing and working with physical changes, but there is less comfort when addressing some of the other areas. There are understandable reasons why this discomfort exists.

These are areas which the predominant culture in the UK considers 'private' and this label highlights several issues. The patient may not feel that they can raise it for discussion. They may wonder, 'Is the nurse a person who is interested in this area of my experience?'. Community health care nurses are committed to holistic care and therefore can provide a consistent and available resource who has regular and frequent contact with patients and their families. Therefore, it is reasonable for a community health care nurse to become a keyworker for the patient, not just in liaison work but in assessing and monitoring the experiences for the dying person and the family. A second patient question may also arise, 'If the community health care nurse is interested and available, can she do anything about it?'. Many practitioners have concerns about their knowledge and skills in supporting patients in these areas. Yet there are generic nursing skills that provide a starting point to address these areas. Nurses already possess the communication skills to respond to cues from the patient. They can also establish a non-judgemental emotionally supportive environment where uncomfortable issues can be exposed and explored to identify the important issue behind the initial cue. With most of these areas, often clarifying the issue through therapeutic listening allows the patient to work through to their own understanding and solution. If the patient does require more specialized help, there are resources available, such as a specialist nurse, the chaplain/religious leader, clinical psychologist, social worker or counsellor.

It is against this backdrop that it is important to consider some of the needs of patients: the distressing symptoms of progressive physical deterioration (using pain as an example) and spiritual issues raised by dying.

Progressive physical deterioration

In considering the distressing physical symptoms that are present for many dying patients, there are some general issues that need to be raised and, to explore these, pain is used as an example. First, assessment of a symptom does not mean only noting its presence or its intensity, important though these are. Assessment is a process by which practitioners come to some conclusion about a particular problem (Fordham and Dunn, 1994): What is the problem? What is it like? How is it experienced? What does it mean to the patient? How important is it to the patient? What influences it? What resources and strategies can be brought to the situation to address it? These questions all need to be addressed, on the one hand, to identify the significant problem for the patient and, on the other, to develop an effective plan that is likely to work. For example, pain for one individual may mean that life, though difficult, is still present and attempts to eradicate it may be met with resistance. For another, any pain, even a pain unrelated to the underlying disease, is interpreted as further progression of disease and any experience of pain carries with it increased anxiety about the process of dying. Therefore, just noting that pain is present at a moderate level does not provide enough information to know where to focus the resources the nurse brings.

Secondly, palliative treatment means an *active* engagement with these symptoms. While it is recognized that interventions may not change the course of the underlying disease, there are still ways in which the underlying disease can and should be addressed. In the case of unrelenting pain from metastatic bone disease that limits mobility and demands almost all the energy of the person experiencing it, limited radiotherapy may provide relief or bring the pain within manageable bounds for the patient. It is therefore important to recognize that active involvement rather than therapeutic passivity may be entirely appropriate, even in the context of terminal disease. Decisions need to be made by a multi-professional team where a variety of expertise is brought together and therapeutic options weighed in the context of the patient's unique beliefs and priorities.

Another aspect of active involvement attempts to counter the isolation that many patients feel when their symptoms are difficult to relieve. Unrelieved patient symptoms can be a reminder of professional impotence. One hospice nurse noted:

> *J.'s pain caused me anxiety, anger and feelings of guilt. I felt inept, awkward, inadequate and almost fearful to answer her call bell. My anger came from frustration at the inability to make J. comfortable.*

The patient is often aware of the distancing that occurs in this situation and will experience feelings of abandonment. It is therefore important, despite professional distress and feelings of helplessness, to acknowledge the patient's pain and continue to address it using all the skill and knowledge available, including referral to a specialist if needed.

Specific areas for nurse involvement include the following activities (Fordham and Dunn, 1994):

- influencing prescribing decisions when a regimen is established
- individualizing the regimen
- enhancing the action of prescribed drugs
- preventing or minimizing complications
- monitoring the therapeutic and toxic effects

Influencing prescribing decisions

While the physician prescribes drugs to manage pain, the decision-making is guided not only by medical assessment of the patient and knowledge of pharmacology, but by the different assessment information provided by the nurse. Using the established relationship with the patient and direct observations of the person, the practitioner can provide helpful information which can shape a regimen more effectively. Particular patient concerns need to be clearly communicated when decisions are made.

Individualizing the regimen

Therapeutic regimens are shaped or individualized for a particular patient. The process of individualization works through three questions: What is desirable? What is possible? What is acceptable? Depending on who answers these questions – the patient, health care professional or the family – there will be different answers. While it would be easy if everyone had the same answer, more often priorities are negotiated to establish the most effective (desirable and effective) and satisfying (acceptable) plan. Usually there is agreement about what is desirable.

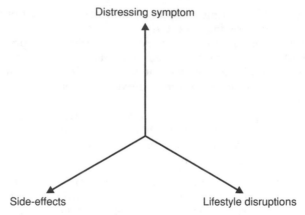

Figure 22.1 Individualizing a regimen (From Fordham and Dunn, 1994, by permission)

However, the ideal is not always possible, often due to side-effects and impact on lifestyle. So, in reality, individualizing a therapeutic regimen is a balancing act among three components: the distressing symptom; the side-effects of treatment; and the degree lifestyle disruption. This balance is illustrated in Figure 22.1. In the last analysis, it is the patient who sifts and weighs the range of possibilities and who answers the last question about acceptability.

Using pain as an example, it is ideal to eliminate the cause of the pain. When this is not possible, as in a palliative context, analgesics are prescribed. Pain can be eradicated using high doses of analgesics, but there are some unwanted side-effects such as sedation which has an important impact on lifestyle. Some patients, when weighing up the balance between no pain and drowsiness, may choose to experience some pain because they want to be alert to be with family. Helping patients articulate and express their priorities and values and finding creative ways to honour these considerations is one of the satisfying aspects of nursing with this group of patients (Fordham and Dunn, 1994).

Enhancing drug action
Pain, like many other physical symptoms such as breathlessness and nausea, is multidimensional, with many factors that influence it. Enhancing a pharmacological regimen may focus on ensuring that medication is taken as prescribed. Many people have deeply held fears about analgesia which need to be explored. These fears may include becoming addicted, or taking potent drugs too early and not having them available for effective use later when really needed. Neither is true and both the patient and the family need to be reassured about this. In the community, this issue is crucial since the patient and family take over the administration of medication and these fears can influence the family giving the drugs and the patient taking them. For example, they need to know that in the context of continuous pain, regular administration

results in sustained pain relief and smaller amounts of drug being needed than when the pain is allowed to increase to severe levels before taking anything.

Another strategy to enhance the action of prescribed drugs involves using techniques such as relaxation to address the anxiety that exaggerates many physical symptoms. Many of these strategies act synergistically with the drugs, reducing the dose required to treat the symptom. These techniques also offer the patient and family a more 'natural' way to address their physical problems, and provide a way to contribute to care.

Preventing or minimizing complications

All medications have desired and undesired effects. The issue is about how to manage the undesired effects that for some patients can be worse than the symptom itself. Nursing involvement may be anticipatory, vigilant or reactive. To make decisions about the nature of the activity, the practitioner needs to know the incidence of a particular side-effect. If a side-effect is certain to occur, such as constipation when opioids are used, it is important to prepare the patient and family for its occurrence and a concurrent plan developed to prevent or manage it. Thus, patients who begin opioids should also have their usual bowel pattern assessed and a bowel regimen of stool softeners and peristaltic simulants initiated at the same time.

However, some side-effects occur with less frequency or decrease after an initial period. Nausea and vomiting, for example, normally follow this pattern. The nurse may take an anticipatory or preventive approach and ensure that an anti-emetic is available and given on a regular basis when the opioid is begun. Another approach could be, 'Be prepared for the worst, but hope for the best!' An anti-emetic could be available, that is, ordered by the General Practitioner and on hand for administration if necessary. The patient is monitored vigilantly during the first couple of doses for the appearance of these effects and treated immediately, thus minimizing patient distress. Either approach is appropriate and which one is chosen depends on the patient's anxieties, GP preference and nursing style.

Monitoring effects

Effective symptom management needs fine tuning, with the desired effect being compared with the patient's experience. The assessment data is used as a baseline to measure the effectiveness of the prescribed regimen. Consideration in pain management might include:

- How much pain is the person experiencing?
- Does the medication ever take the pain away completely? (Are the drug and the dose adequate for the pain that the patient is experiencing?)
- Does the patient's pain return before it is time for the next dose of medication? (Is the interval of administration adequate?)

- What undesired effects does the patient experience?
- In what activities is the patient able to engage? (Pain-free at rest, pain-free on movement?)

Spiritual needs

The spiritual dimension is the integrating and unique aspect of the individual. While it is distinct from other aspects of the individual such as physical and social aspects, it is interrelated with them, both influencing them and being influenced by them. It is often perceived as being concerned with meaning and purpose as well as 'right-relatedness' (Mud & Stars, 1991).

Questions of meaning

Spirituality becomes important at times of great change or distress when questions of meaning arise. These questions often focus on 'why': Why is *this* happening? Why is this happening *to me*? Why is this happening to me *now*?

Working with these questions forces the person to look for a way to interpret the present experiences in the context of some deeper positive meanings (Frankl, 1987). Sometimes there is a bewildered response by the dying person if they have never had to confront these profound issues. The way the world works and their understanding of it have never been questioned. It is assumed that, 'If I'm good, everything will be OK'. Some people are brought up short and have to begin to think through these assumptions.

There may be other responses. Kushner (1982) raises the question, 'Why do bad things happen to good people?', which begins the struggle to reconcile previously held beliefs with current experience. The struggle can be profound, shaking people to the very roots of their understanding and being. Spiritual distress occurs as a person experiences or is at risk of experiencing a disturbance in the personal belief or value systems that are the source of strength and hope (Carpenito, 1983). This is powerfully illustrated in David Watson's autobiography, *Fear No Evil* (Watson, 1984). As an Anglican priest actively engaged in a healing ministry, he and friends prayed for healing when he was diagnosed with bowel cancer. When it became clear that he had not been healed, he struggled with trying to bring together his previously held beliefs about a powerful God who longs to heal, and his current experience of not being healed. Watson asks, 'Can God heal?' and 'If He can heal, why didn't He heal me?' He finally decided that there was no way to reconcile them and that he must live holding them together because they both seemed true.

Although Watson accepted the tension of holding together seeming irreconcilable beliefs, others get angry, metaphorically and sometimes actually, crying out at the injustice of what is happening to them. This anger sometimes is focused on to the GP who did not diagnose the cancer when it first appeared, or at the hospital for the delay in starting treatment. But many finally realize that they are basically angry that they have to die. It is even more distressing when death is untimely and there are outstanding responsibilities or unfinished business. There may be no answers.

In fact, the role of helper in these situations is to give permission for people to explore the depths of these questions of meaning, acknowledging the distress and anger. Sheila Cassidy powerfully speaks of this activity in her book, *Sharing the Darkness*, when she acknowledges that people may *only* (present author's emphasis) be able 'to be with' the patient (Cassidy, 1988). But it is in 'witnessing' the person's pain and distress that their pain and distress are acknowledged as real and they are not left to experience it alone.

Right-relatedness

Harmony forms the content of the concept of right-relatedness and issues are raised at several levels: the personal level with oneself; the social level with others; and if one believes in a higher being, at a religous level. These issues often arise during the life review that naturally occurs as people face this ending and is commonly associated with a need for forgiveness, reconciliation and affirmation of worth (Clark, 1990). At a personal level, it may encompass coming to terms with life choices that did not work out as expected or the need to feel that one's life has been worth while. At a social level, mending broken relationships may be required. Religiously, there may be rituals and activities that need to be done. Working toward right-relatedness constitutes one aspect of dealing with 'unfinished business'. Garrison Keillor, the American humorist and writer, when asked 'How would you like to die?' answered, 'Slowly and gently', . . . with time enough to clean up my mess'.

The community health care nurse can again listen as the dying person identifies the relationships that need to be confronted and explored and what they want to do about them. It may entail helping in concrete ways — telephoning long-estranged relatives and friends or contacting the priest or religious leader. In *Final Gifts* (Callanan and Kelley, 1992), the authors identify that there are important things that need to be done or said before a person dies and these things are often communicated in coded or symbolic language, especially as people near death. Taking care to understand and act on the coded message can bring a sense of resolution and peace to everyone in the face of death.

● Family needs

Since the beginning of the hospice movement, it has been recognized that the family as well as the dying person comprise the focus of care. What is meant by family is quite broad and includes those who are important to the dying person. Most often it is a kin relationship, but work with patients with AIDS has highlighted the larger range of people who significantly participate in the dying process.

In a recent UK study exploring the experience of 232 adult cancer patients who were dying, Hinton (1994) underscored the important family contribution to care at home by noting that few patients living alone or with unfit relatives were able to stay at home. Another observation was that patients were increasingly admitted for in-patient care as the time of dying lengthened, hinting at the wearing aspect of providing long-term care in the community. The community health care nurse's involvement with the family is to prepare and support them to adapt to the changes that happen because one of them is dying (RCN, 1993). In the following section, the family experiences and what support they may need to deal with the changes that are an expected part of dying, particularly at home, are explored.

Family experiences

Each family has its own unique history, traditions, values, communication patterns and characteristic ways of managing the everyday details of life (Ferszt and Houck, 1986). When a member of the family requires palliative care, the family's usual way of living is disrupted, forcing change in areas such as relationships (Ferrell et al., 1991), roles (Pederson and Valanis, 1988) and tasks (Giaquinta, 1977; Mahon, 1991). These changes develop and alter through the course of dying (Chekryn et al., 1991), and one writer notes that the disruption may be greatest during a transition from one developmental stage to another (Gray-Price and Szczesny, 1985).

One group of researchers used a conceptual framework of transition to understand what families experience (Chekryn et al., 1991). They used the definition by Parkes (1971) of psychological transition as a change that necessitates the abandonment of one set of assumptions and the development of a new set to enable the individual to cope with a newly altered life space. Interviewing 24 family members, including the dying person and adult children who belonged to eight families, they identified three phases to the transition. The first was an ending of the old way of life, followed by a neutral period and finally a period of beginning. These phases are identified in Figure 22.2.

Ending

The ending was signalled for the family by the decline in the dying person's physical condition and resulted in the perception that, undeniably, the person was 'fading away'. Unrecoverable weakness, inability to get around, loss of independence in personal care and loss of mental clarity were visible signs of the person's impending death. During this time, the family had to redefine themselves as family, identifying and acknowledging the losses that had already occurred, were now incurring and those they anticipated. Also, there were the extra demands that occur when families care for a terminally ill member and need to carry on the usual business of living.

The physical aspects of caring may be the most easily seen of the family's demands. Twigg and Atkin (1994) suggest that physical care can be divided into broad categories: 'personal care'; management of incontinence; medical and nursing care; and household management.

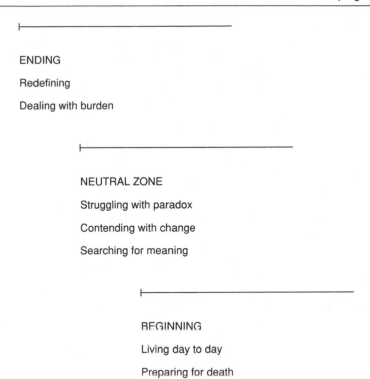

Figure 22.2 Phases and tasks of the transition of 'fading away' (After Chekryn Reimer *et al.*, 1991, by permission)

There must be an assumption that the family can deal with all the 'unskilled' elements of physical care including bathing, dressing and dealing with incontinence. Incontinence, one of the most stressful aspects of caring for both the family and the dying person, is often hidden or underplayed because of embarrassment or a wish to protect the dying person (Charles-Edwards, 1986). Incontinence, like bathing, are areas of care that are intimate in nature and Ungerson (1987) argues that it involves taboo subjects that can cause problems in caring kinship relationships. There can be difficulties, especially when the caring is by someone of the opposite gender, since intimate physical care is more culturally acceptable for women to do and difficulties may occur when a male is caring for a woman (Twigg and Atkin, 1994).

Another area of demand concerns the financial costs of caring which can be considerable and have been documented recently by Glendinning (1992). Loss of earning is one financial aspect of caring, but care at home may result in higher day-to-day living expenses due to expenditures like laundry, heating, transport, housing adaptations and special foods. Graham (1983) highlighted that a lack of information was the main factor preventing family members claiming the financial support that would help.

Neutral zone

The ending cut the connections with old ways of living and, as a result, the families moved into a kind of limbo between their previous, familiar way of life and an unknown new way. Chekryn and colleagues talk about the confusing reality that families experience and call it a 'neutral zone' – neither the old but not yet the new. It is during this time that families struggle with the paradox of living and dying at the same time. Also they have to contend with change which is occurring at both a family and individual level. Finally they, like the dying person, struggle to make sense of what is happening and search for meaning that will place the events into a deeper, more positive context.

One problem reported by Spinetta (1982), in studying childhood dying, was balancing the needs of the other family members and the dying person. Pederson and Valanis (1988) concluded that reassignment of housework, child care and other duties to other family members may create difficulties in relations as individual goals and needs are put aside. When the dying person is the family co-ordinator and determines interactions, the family is more extensively affected (Welch-McCaffrey, 1988). Another dimension of the role change reported by families was the adjustments required because of a lack of constancy in the patient's ability to carry out their usual roles (Matocchio, 1982; Loomis and Williams, 1983). On the one hand, the dying may have a steady downward progression resulting in a gradual decrease in the patient's abilities. The family must then respond to subtle changes in the individual's condition and gradually assume more tasks. In contrast, the process may also be marked by periods of remission and exacerbations, necessitating sudden changes in family responsibilities.

Matocchio (1982) documented the problems that occur with different patterns of dying. Family exhaustion, conflict and guilt occurred when there were differences between what the family expected to happen and what actually occurred. In situations where the course was sudden with rapid deterioration, interactions were intense and crisis-like, with less information provided by health professionals and less time to prepare for the patient's death. In instances when the patient did not 'die on time', the lingering, prolonged vigil and guilt associated with waiting for death and desiring it for everyone's relief, as well as the physical exhaustion, were additional stressors for the family.

Beginning

At some point, usually difficult to pinpoint, the family reorients to life 'as it is now' and develops a perspective of living day to day. While living day to day, they also were preparing for the death. One particular difficulty that family members identify is 'juggling' the demands of managing household task and the strain of 'standing by' and being continuously on duty (Stetz, 1987; Oberst *et al.*, 1989). Twigg and Atkin (1994) use 'restrictedness' to describe an experience which is central to the lives of most carers, that of feeling, or actually being, unable to leave the dying person and includes broader ways that care at home can limit the carer's life. Feelings of frustration, boredom and claustrophobia have all been identified by family members, and it is not only the concrete tasks of caring that restrict them, but an anxiety about what might occur in their absence, resulting in increased stress (Twigg and Atkin, 1994)

Support

The family's needs have been explored to understand what they perceive they require from health professionals in order to cope with the situation. Informal care in the home increasingly becomes nursing care of the bedbound patient and Grobe et al. (1982) found that families reported dissatisfaction with the trial-and-error method they used to learn the skills necessary to care for the dying person. Ferrell et al. (1988, 1991) reported the importance of patient comfort as a priority for families. Caring for a loved one in pain which was often not effectively managed at home posed many physical and psychological burdens for the family, including mood disturbance and disrupted relationships.

The flexibility of family members, and their tolerance to change, require clear communication and much negotiation (Lloyd and Coggles, 1990). As Benoliel (1979) noted, communication, when the future is ambiguous and uncertain, is difficult and there are no rules to govern it. One area of support for families is to provide opportunities to talk about what they are experiencing and what those changes mean to them as individuals and as a family. Family members will vary in their ability to acknowledge and adapt to the changes and will have different ways of coping with them.

Another important area is preparing and supporting children who are facing the death of an important adult. It requires special attention, since they are often overlooked and one must have information about the particular issues related to their development. The understanding of death is a gradual developmental process, partly occurring naturally as children see, interpret and understand the events in the world around them while other aspects are taught. There are four basic concepts about death that will affect the child's response (Wass, 1984). These are:

Irreversibility. Death is a permanent phenomenon from which there is no return or recovery.

Finality. Death is a state in which all life functions cease completely.

Universality. Death is a natural phenomenon that no living being can escape indefinitely.

Causality. The child develops a realistic understanding of the causes of death.

Children under 5 years of age are aware of death and at this age they perceive death as a departure or a sleep associated with a lack of movement. They may believe that death is reversible (i.e. a temporary phenomenon) like cartoon or television characters that die and return to life next week. At this stage of development, the pre-school child views death as caused externally either by accident or by acts of violence. In mid-childhood (between 5 and 9 years of age), children are gradually accumulating the components for a full concept of death. By the age of 9, the child's understanding of death is equivalent to that of an adult.

There are two major features of children's development of the concept of death which may cause misunderstandings. The first feature is the notion of causality. McCown (1988) suggests that children younger than 7–8 cannot consider events happening by chance, their understanding being influenced by justice, a belief in which goodness is rewarded and badness punished. Thus children at this stage of development have a tendency to view illness as a form of punishment for wrongdoing. In addition to the development of the concept of causality there is, at this stage, the development of the child's conscience and the sense of right and wrong. The child may readily associate their parent's illness with their own wishes or behaviour (Raphael, 1992).

The second feature is their incomplete understanding of irreversibility. Misunderstanding may be recognized by the belief that the child or their family are immortal. In addition, if death is not considered inevitable, the child between 5 and 9 years may consider the death to be a punishment for bad behaviour of either the dying person or the child. The child who does not have a realistic knowledge and understanding of the causes of death may, through magical thinking, assume responsibility for the death of a parent; for example, that the death is caused by the child's bad thought or other (unrelated) actions.

Stedeford (1994) investigated the variables that influenced the way children were prepared for the death of a parent. In a study of 19 couples who had children under 18 years of age, she identified three main factors: parental attitude to death; openness with children in general and the family communication style; available support from extended family. The importance of this research is highlighted when attempting to prepare children to deal with an anticipated death of a significant adult. The most frequent advice concerns 'honesty is the best policy' (Stokes, 1994). Over time, children can gradually begin to acknowledge the obvious deterioration in health. In doing so, they continue to assimilate information which enables them to face the reality of their impending loss. They will need the context of loving, honest and trusting relationships in order to cope with the unpredictable future.

Parents may feel it is difficult to be honest in this particular situation. The perceived need for secrecy often rests on good intentions. These include not having a clear predictable picture of what the course of the dying will be and feeling there is a need to have the complete answer before the issue is opened up. Another reason focuses on what to say, how to say it and how to deal with the child's response. For the parent, having to tell children entails acknowledging the loss of life and the pain of feeling that they are abandoning their child. Children are intuitive and are often aware that something is not right and their guilty misconceptions are more harmful than the pain of sharing the loss together. Finally, parents are also understandably sensitive to the number of losses their child may have already experienced and they feel they are protecting them by not confronting the issue of disclosure.

Disclosure should not be perceived as a single act, but rather as an ongoing process which allows trust to be maintained and anxiety to be contained. Tasker (1992) identifies four general phases which provide a useful clinical framework for supporting parents as they confront the task of disclosing an impending death to children. These include:

Secrecy phase → Exploratory phase →

Readiness phase → Disclosure phase

Practitioners should acknowledge the parent's desire for secrecy and explore what fears are present. Also, it is important for parents to understand that talking about dying is not an easy task. The decision to exclude children from the dying process through secrecy joins the family in a conspiracy of silence that deprives children of the opportunity to confront, question and resolve their own feelings. The literature consistently reports that a child's ability to cope, especially in bereavement, will be enhanced by being informed by a trusted adult addressing their particular concerns about the impact on their care and taking account of their particular understanding of the concepts of death (Silverman and Worden, 1993).

There is some debate within the literature as to when children grasp the different concepts and whether a child's own experience will affect the rate of development. The important consideration in dealing with children facing the death of a parent or other significant adult, is not their chronological age, but what they understand of the four principal concepts of death. The exploratory phase then gathers information on what the child understands about death and what are their particular concerns.

Assessing readiness primarily identifies the concerns that the child has, and frequently includes why is this happening, did they cause it, and who will look after them? It is important to gain a sense of what the child understands about dying in general and specifically in their situation. Preparing the parent about common questions that children ask allows the parent to resolve some of their own fears and thinking through ways to answer the concerns prior to facing the children. It also allows the parent to confront some of their own fears.

In talking with children, parents should use clear and simple information, in language that is comfortable. The use of books has been explored as a means of addressing some of the issues of death in a gentler way, allowing death to be shared side by side rather than confronted directly. Books can be chosen to match the child's cognitive development and the family's beliefs and values. Seibert and Drolet (1993) identify four ways to use children's books:

- to share and explore feelings about death
- to gain knowledge about death
- to discuss beliefs and values related to death
- to identify skills for dealing with death

Barbara Greenall, the then librarian at St Christopher's Hospice, compiled a review of books available in Britain which may be helpful (Greenall, 1988).

● **The nurse's needs**

Working with the dying person and their family can be extremely satisfying. However, it can also be stressful. Saunders and Valente (1994), surveying 300 oncology and hospice nurses, articulated several characteristics that contributed to a distressing death for them. These included:

- untimely death or an unjust death
- person unable to complete important tasks
- nurse did not deliver best quality of care possible
- person's distress or symptoms not relieved by current knowledge and technology.

In the first situation, a patient's death may raise deep and profound spiritual questions of justice and meaning for the nurse as well as the patient and family. The practitioner must confront these questions and find a way to live with them that enables her or him to continue working with the patients who may die.

In the next situation, there may be many reasons why the person was not able to tie up the 'loose ends of life'. Sometimes death comes so quickly that no one has time for anything except living the experience. However, from the previous discussion about an anticipated death, it is clear that a major reason for inadequate time may be that not everyone was aware that death was imminent. A clear transition from battling for a cure or sustained life to one of support and palliation may not occur (Dunn, 1992). Members of the health care team, as well as the patient and family, may not understand – intellectually and emotionally – that this shift has occurred. Mixed messages may sustain an unrealistic hope and prevent engagement with important tasks. So the underlying problem is not so much a lack of time as a lack of agreement.

This lack of agreement or shared vision may underlie the next characteristic of a distressing death, that of not delivering the best quality of care. Care of the dying is a shared activity, as noted in the earlier discussion. The nurse's ability to shape or control the entire process does not exist. Vachon (1987) noted that a major source of stress for professional carers arose in relation to organizational and interprofessional aspects of care. Another source of poor quality care may be the nurse's lack of up-to-date knowledge and skills.

Finally, there is the reality of being unable to eliminate all suffering and to guarantee a peaceful death. Although there is much that practitioners can do to ameliorate the wretchedness of physical deterioration and separation, in the end both happen. Patients and families need to have those who can stay with them (Cassidy, 1988; Fordham and Dunn, 1994) and share the pain. Davies and Oberle (1990), when discussing the core dimension of preserving the nurse's integrity, noted that to work with the dying, the practitioners must have a way of understanding and valuing what is possible and can be achieved in a specific situation, and coming to terms with the limitations that are inescapable in this area of care.

Each of these causes of distress will point to a different approach for support. Some approaches involve focused educational and clinical development. Others are more philosophical and spiritual, while others will be problem-solving about team relationships. It is important to acknowledge that this kind of work is distressing and far from being a sign of personal inadequacy; rather, it opens the way for personal and professional growth.

References

Abrams, R. (1966) The patient with cancer: his changing pattern of communication. *New England Journal of Medicine*, **274**(6), 317–322

Benoliel, J.Q. (1979) Dying is a family affair. In *Home Care: Living with Dying* (eds E.R. Pritchard, J. Vollard, J. Starr, J. Lockwood and A. Kutscher), Columbia University Press, New York

Billings, J.A. (ed.) (1985) Why dying people and their families seek home care. In *Outpatient Management of Advanced Cancer: Symptom Control, Support and Hospice-in-the-Home*. J.B. Lippincott, Philadelphia

Blauner, R. (1966) Death and social structure. *Psychiatry*, **29**, 378–394

Callanan, M. and Kelley, P. (1992) *Final Gifts: Understanding and Helping the Dying*, Hodder and Stoughton, London

Carpenito, L.J. (1983) *Nursing Diagnosis: Application to Cinical Practice*, J.B. Lippincott, Philadelphia

Cartwright, A. (1991) The role of hospitals in the last year of people's lives. *Age and Ageing*, **20**, 271–274

Cassidy, S. (1986) Emotional distress in terminal cancer. *Journal of the Royal Society of Medicine*, **79**, 717–720

Cassidy, S. (1988) *Sharing the Darkness*, Darton, Longman and Todd, London

Charles-Edwards, A. (1986) Nursing care at home. In *Terminal Care at Home* (ed. R. Spilling), Oxford Medical Publications, Oxford

Chekryn Reimer, J., Davies, B. and Martens, N. (1991) Palliative care: the nurse's role in helping families through the transition of 'fading away'. *Cancer Nursing*, **14**(6), 321–327

Clark, R. (1990) Forgiveness in the hospice setting. *Palliative Medicine*, **4**, 305–310

Davies, B. and Oberle, K. (1990) Dimensions of the supportive role of the nurse in palliative care. *Oncology Nursing Forum*, **17**(1), 87–94

Dunlop, R.J., Davies, R.J. and Hockley, J.M. (1989) Preferred versus actual place of death: a hospital palliative care support team experience. *Palliative Medicine*, **3**, 197–210

Dunn, V. (1992) Palliative care: problems addressed and problems created. In *Changing Frontiers in Palliative Care*, Proceedings of the 7th International Conference on Cancer Nursing. International Society of Nurses in Cancer Care by Scutari Projects Ltd, London

Ferrell, B.R., Berrell, B.A., Rhiner, M. and Grant, M. (1991) Family factors influencing cancer pain management. *Postgraduate Medical Journal*, **67**(Suppl.), 64–69

Ferrell, B.R. and Schneider, C. (1988) Experience and management of cancer pain at home. *Cancer Nursing*, **11**, 84–90

Ferszt, G.G. and Houck, P.D. (1986) The Family. In *Nursing Care of the Terminally Ill* (eds M.O. Amenta and N.L. Bohnet), Little Brown, Boston

Field, D. (1989) *Nursing the Dying*. Tavistock/Routledge, London

Field, D. and James, N. (1993) Where and how people die. In *The Future for Palliative Care: Issues of Policy and Practice* (ed. D. Clark), Open University Press, Buckingham

Firth, S. (1993) Cultural issues in terminal care. In *The Future for Palliative Care: Issues of Policy and Practice* (ed. D. Clark), Open University Press, Buckingham

Fordham, M. and Dunn, V. (1994) *Alongside the Person in Pain: Holistic Care and Nursing Practice*, Baillière Tindall, London

Frankl, V. (1987) *Man's Search for Meaning*, Hodder and Stoughton, London

Giaquinta, B. (1977) Helping families face the crisis of cancer. *American Journal of Nursing*, **77**, 1585–1588

Glendinning, D. (1992) *The Costs of Informal Care: Looking Inside the Household*, HMSO, London

Graham, H. (1983) Caring: labour of love. In *A Labour of Love: Women, Work and Caring* (eds J. Finch and D. Groves), Routledge and Kegan Paul, London

Gray-Price, H. and Szczesny, S. (1985) Crisis intervention with families of cancer patients: a developmental approach. *Topics in Clinical Nursing*, **7**, 58–70

Greenall, B. (1988) Books for bereaved children. *Health Libraries Review*, **5**, 1–6

Grobe, M.E., Ahmann, D.L. and Ilstrup, D.M. (1982) Needs assessment for advanced cancer patients and their families. *Oncology Nursing Forum*, **9**(4), 26–30

Herth, K. (1990) Fostering hope in terminally-ill people. *Journal of Advanced Nursing*, **15**, 1250–1259

Hinton, J. (1994) Which patients with terminal cancer are admitted from home care? *Palliative Medicine*, **8**, 197–210

James, N. and Field, D. (1992) The routinization of hospice: charisma and bureaucratization. *Social Science and Medicine*, **34**(12), 1363–1375

Kellehear, A. (1984) Are we a 'death-denying' society? A sociology review. *Social Science and Medicine*, **18**(9), 713–723

Kristjanson, L.J. and Ashcroft, T. (1994) The family's cancer journey: a literature review. *Cancer Nursing*, **17**(1), 1–17

Kushner, H.S. (1982) *When Bad Things Happen to Good People*, Pan Books, London

Leathard, A. (1990) *Health Care Provision: Past, Present and Future*, Chapman and Hall, London

Lloyd, C. and Coggles, L. (1990) Psychological issues for people with cancer and their families. *Canadian Journal of Occupational Therapy*, **57**, 211–215

Loomis, M.T. and Williams, T.F. (1983) Evaluation of care provided to terminally ill patients. *Gerontologist*, **23**, 493–499

McCown, D. (1988) When children face death in the family. *Journal of Paediatric Health Care*, **2**, 14–19

Mahon, S.M. (1991) Managing the psychosocial consequences of cancer recurrence. Implications for nurses. *Oncology Nursing Forum*, **18**(3), 557–583

Matocchio, B.C. (1982) *Living while Dying*, Robert J. Brady Co., Bowie, Maryland

Mud & Stars (1991) The Report of a Working Party on the Impact of Hospice Experience on the Church's Ministry of Healing, Sobell Publications, Oxford

Neale, B. (1991) *Informal palliative care: a review of research on needs, standards and service evaluation*. Occasional Paper No. 3, Trent Palliative Care Centre, Sheffield

Neuberger, J. (1987) *Caring for Dying People of Different Faiths*, Austin Cornish/The Lisa Sainsbury Foundation, London

Oberst, M.T., Thomas, S.E., Gass, K.A. and Ward, S.E. (1989) Caregiving demands and appraisal of stress among family caregivers. *Cancer Nursing*, **12**, 209–215

Parkes, C.M. (1971) Psycho-social transitions: a field for study. *Social Science and Medicine*, **5**, 101–115

Pederson, L.M. and Valanis, B.G. (1988) The effects of breast cancer on the family: a review of the literature. *Journal of Psychosocial Oncology*, **6**, 95–119

Raphael, B. (1992) *The Anatomy of Bereavement*. Routledge, London

RCN (1993) *Standards of Care: Palliative Nursing*, Royal College of Nursing, London

Roemer, M. (1986) *An Introduction to the US Health Care System*, 2nd edn, Springer, New York

Saunders, J.M. and Valente, S.M. (1994) Nurses' grief. *Cancer Nursing*, **17**(4), 318–325

Seale, C. (1991) Communication and awareness about death: a study of a random sample of dying people. *Social Science and Medicine*, **32**(8), 943–952

Seibert, D. and Drolet, J. (1993) Death themes in literature for children ages 3–8. *Journal of School Health*, **63**(2), 86–90

Silverman, P. and Worden, J.W. (1993) Children's reactions to the death of a parent. In *Handbook of Bereavement: Theory, Research and Intervention* (eds M. Stroebe, W. Stroebe and R.O. Hansson), Cambridge University Press, Cambridge

Spilling, R. (ed) (1986) *Terminal Care at Home*, Oxford University Press, Oxford

Spinetta, J.J. (1982) Behavioral and psychological research in childhood cancer. *Cancer*, **50**, 1939–1943

Stedeford, A. (1994) *Facing Death: Patients, Families and Professionals*, 2nd edn, Sobell Publications, Oxford

Stetz, K.M. (1987) Caregiving demands during advanced cancer: the spouse's needs. *Cancer Nursing*, **10**, 260–268

Stokes, J. (1994) Anticipatory grief in families affected by HIV/AIDS. *Progress in Palliative Care*, **2**(2), 13–18

Tasker, M. (1992) *How Can I Tell You?* Association for the Care of Children's Health, Bethesda, Maryland

Townsend, J., Frank, A.O., Fermont, D., Dyer, S., Karran, O., Walgrove, A. and Piper, M. (1990) Terminal cancer care and patients' preference for place of death: a prospective study. *British Journal of Medicine*, **301**, 415–417

Twigg, J. and Atkin, K. (1994) *Carers Perceived: Policy and Practice in Informal Care*, Open University Press, Buckingham

Ungerson, C. (1987) *Policy is Personal: Sex, Gender and Informal Care*, Tavistock, London

Vachon, M. (1987) *Occupational Stress in the Care of the Critically Ill, the Dying and the Bereaved*, Hemisphere, Washington D.C.

Wass, N. (1984) Concepts of death: a developmental perspective. In *Childhood and Death* (ed. H. Wass), Hemisphere, Washington D.C.

Watson, D. (1984) *Fear No Evil: A Personal Struggle with Cancer*, Hodder and Stoughton, London

Welch-McCaffrey, D. (1988) Family issues in cancer care: current dilemmas and future directions. *Journal of Psychosocial Oncology*, **6**, 199–211

WHO (1990) *Cancer Pain Relief and Palliative Care*, Report of a World Health Organisation Expert Committee, WHO Technical Report Series 804, World Health Organisation, Geneva

Williams, C.A. (1982) Role considerations in care of the dying. *IMAGE: Journal of Nursing Scholarship*, **14**(1), 8–11

Part VI

Interventions and skills for practice: needs and priorities

The previous parts of this book have attempted to consider some of the major factors which have implications for practice in community health care nursing. This has included not only the philosophy of care of the practitioner, but also the contextual setting in which practice takes place, of which obviously the changing structure of health care in the UK has enormous implications. In addition, some more general issues have been included such as the contribution of research to the provision of high-quality care. Indeed, frequently in a community setting practitioners work in relative isolation from each other, making the implementation of research findings and the consequent development and change in practice a more difficult process than in the institutional setting.

This part of the book considers specific strategies in practice, in particular the interventions and skills of practitioners and how they contribute to patient and client care. The selection of appropriate interventions and skills was not an easy task, since practice takes place in dynamic settings where priorities and trends continually change. However, as identified within documents such as the Heathrow Debate (DoH, 1994), there are issues and strategies in practice which will continue to play a central role in the delivery of patient and client care into the next century.

In order to select interventions and skills for practice for discussion the editors have drawn not only upon policy documents but also recent legislation and research directly affecting community health care nursing, all of which have implications for the delivery of care. Once again to reflect the purpose of the book, the interventions focus on principles for practice. Therefore this part not only includes interventions such as advocacy, partnership in care and community development work, but also the promotion of health and assessment of health need. In addition, key topic areas such as change and case management, and the role of the clinical nurse specialist, are covered.

As readers may observe, there are interventions which have not been included, of which perhaps standard setting provides an illustration. The question of interventions such as standard setting raised an interesting point of discussion for the editors as to whether or not this process should be described as a practice intervention, directly contributing to the delivery of care. The outcome was that these interventions need to be considered in a wider context – in the example of standard setting, this would need to be assessed within the context of quality assurance, which suggested that it was more appropriate for readers to access specific texts of the topic. Although readers may identify other interventions which they feel should have been included, the editors believe that the interventions which have been presented here provide a platform for lively and informed debate. They will not only allow practitioners to reassess their own practice, but also contribute to the continuing development and improvement of health care.

Reference

DoH (1994) *The Challenges for Nursing and Midwifery in the 21st Century*, Chief Nursing Officers for England, Scotland, Wales and Northern Ireland, Department of Health, London.

23

Assessing health needs

Jennifer Billings

● **Introduction**

The aim of this chapter is to provide practitioners with a critical understanding and working knowledge of the various approaches to needs assessment, with particular reference to health profiling. First, the complex nature of needs assessment will be discussed, attempting to define it from the differing perspectives of three dominant approaches, namely sociology, epidemiology and health economics. The chapter continues by discussing what is meant by 'community health profile', highlighting its use in the literature and in particular strengths and weaknesses in relation to practical compilation and validity and reliability of data sources. The importance of including a 'positive health' perspective in needs assessment is also considered. Following this, the consumer perspective is reviewed, as well as issues surrounding the ethics of data collection. Throughout the chapter, issues are discussed with reference to the community nursing perspective and current changes within the health service.

Although needs assessment has always been a priority issue for those concerned with community health, the publication of the Acheson Report led to renewed interest, proposing as it did that directors of public health should be responsible for assessing the needs of their local populations (DHSS, 1988). Since this proposal, successive Department of Health papers (DoH, 1989a, 1989b, 1990, 1992, 1993) have broadened the professional scope and application of needs assessment by reaffirming its importance as a means of determining the provision and extent of health care. As a result, this so-called 'needs-led' style of planning signals a departure from previous approaches, which were predominantly service led (Stalker, 1993). Needs assessment has been defined simply as 'a description of those factors which must be addressed in order to improve the health of the population' (Harvey, 1994).

Even though needs assessment was initially seen as the primary responsibility of potential purchasing and commissioning authorities, necessary to inform the contracting process (DoH, 1989c), community provider units are now recognizing the important contribution they can make towards the identification of local population needs, particularly through the work of community health care nurses (Day, 1992; Goodwin,

1994). The ability to carry out a full assessment of the needs of individuals, families and communities has always been a central feature of nursing in the community, as an assessment of individual client needs is fundamental to ensuring suitable service provision (Goodwin, 1988). Indeed, the Council for the Training of Health Visitors specified in 1977 that the search for health needs and a stimulation of their awareness were the principal objectives within health visiting practice. Considering the challenges of today's practitioners, such as increasing social deprivation and poverty (Blaxter, 1990), inequalities in health (Phillimore et al., 1994) and the growing morbidity and mortality from heart disease and AIDS (DoH, 1992), these principles are as relevant today for all practitioners as they were for health visitors in the 1970s (Twinn and Cowley, 1992).

● Approaches to definitions of needs assessment

Assessment of health needs has been the subject of much inquiry over the past two decades, escalating in recent years due to the pressure of government legislation (Buchan and Gray, 1990). The complex, multi-dimensional nature of needs assessment has been revealed, and those health care managers and practitioners working in this field have recognized that the task is far from straightforward. Defining what is meant by 'needs' is one example. Orr (1992a) provides an initial interpretation that reveals the multiple meanings attached to the concept, defining need as 'social, relative and evaluative'; social being defined according to standards of communal life, relative since its meaning will vary between people and societies, and evaluative in that it is based upon value judgements. The difficulties of operationalizing these notions for assessment purposes becomes apparent. In a broader perspective, sociologists, epidemiologists and health economists have each defined needs from their own standpoint.

Sociological perspective

Generally, the sociological view is exemplified by Bradshaw (1972), whose taxonomy of normative need, felt need, expressed need and comparative need remains relevant to health care, distinguishing as it does the important differences between needs as identified by professionals (normative) and those 'felt' by the individual. The influence of Bradshaw is also evident in community health care nursing, where the concept of need is perceived as personal, subjective and variable (Twinn and Cowley, 1992). The perspective does, however, raise issues concerning the difficulty of forming clear and comparable criteria for needs assessment. Buchan and Gray (1990) argue that qualitative definitions of need tend to be nebulous and of little help in determining appropriate levels of care delivery. In a study of social welfare provision, for example, Thayer (1973) concluded that the taxonomy of need was a useful way to identify different approaches to assessment, but there was little methodological evidence to suggest that the concepts could be operationalized in a meaningful way. In general terms, however, health is such a broad concept, as demonstrated by Seedhouse (1986), that there would appear to be unlimited scope for people to consider themselves unwell.

Epidemiological perspective

The traditional epidemiological approach to needs assessment has been to use morbidity and mortality data to measure the total amount of ill-health in the community. This information is then used to set priorities for allocating resources between different diseases (Ashley and McLachlan, 1985). Need is thus defined in terms of lives lost, life years lost, morbidity, or loss of social functioning. Indicators of deprivation are used in a similar fashion, based upon census data. Variables such as numbers of single parents, elderly living alone, families with pre-school children and ethnicity are measured, combining social and material deprivation into a composite index. This ultimately provides a means of scoring and ranking areas according to their degree of relative disadvantage or affluence (Jarman, 1984; Townsend et al., 1988).

These approaches have the potential to provide valuable information about the need for health. However, by focusing upon 'normative' or professionally defined need, there is the assumption that, once categorized, population groups are automatically in need of services which may not be the case (Orr, 1992a). This lack of specificity regarding the identification of the need for health care has also been highlighted by Stevens and Gabby (1991), who argue that the need for health care must be the focus of community needs assessment if service provision is to be effective.

Health economist perspective

The health economists' contribution has been in contrast to previous perspectives, defining need within the context of cost-effectiveness and supply and demand. The main thrust of the argument is to emphasize that areas of needs are relative and can be 'traded off' against each other, given limited resources (Culyer, 1976; Donaldson and Mooney, 1991). With the assumption that the objective of health care policy is to maximize that contribution of health care resources to the health of the community (defined in terms of Quality Adjusted Life Years, QALYs), some authors argue that more resources within the health care budget should be allocated to treatments with a low marginal cost per QALY and less to those with a high marginal cost per QALY gained. Bryan et al. (1991) give the example of expanding a community chiropody service while contracting home dialysis, as more QALYs would be produced without any increase in expenditure.

Supporters of this approach state that it does not require any assessment of total needs, and that the key concept is getting the greatest benefit for each pound spent (Williams, 1987). Although the economic viewpoint may rationalize service provision in a 'cut and dried' fashion, it is not difficult to imagine that the perspective has been strongly criticized for its unethical stance; in particular as it neglects consumer views and issues relating to maintenance of quality of life in illness (Loomes and McKenzie, 1989). In addition to this, the economist viewpoint is frequently difficult to grasp, as demonstrated in the paper by Bryan *et al*. (1991). For this reason, those health care professionals unfamiliar with the language may be too critical or dismissive of the approach.

Notwithstanding the ambiguities surrounding differing interpretations of need, defining what is meant by 'community' and 'population' within this context also highlights inconsistencies and lack of clarity when undertaking an assessment procedure. Briefly, with reference to community, Orr (1992b) states that the various meanings and confusion surrounding the concept of community occurs because it is used in a descriptive, evaluative and emotive manner, which makes a precise definition difficult, a view shared by Benson (1976). In addition, community agencies are expected to set out the needs of the population they serve (DoH, 1990). Stalker (1993) questions whether the term refers to existing service users, potential service users, or the totality of residents in a region. Thus, attempting to identify community needs within a population against this complex and multi-faceted backdrop is an enormous task for professionals.

● **Community health profile**

An approach that is gaining interest and application in determining community need is the development of an area or community profile, which incorporates some of the elements of the perspectives described above. For community health care nurses in particular, the advent of fundholding GP practices has necessitated that they consider more closely their marketable properties in order to demonstrate to purchasers their value in the community health arena, and profiling is becoming a central 'selling' point (RCN, 1993; Goodwin, 1994; NHSE, 1994). A profile is believed to emphasize the important and unique contribution that practitioners can make to community health knowledge, not only in searching for health needs (Hawtin *et al*., 1994), but also by their acquisition of 'soft' data relating to families, augmenting empirical information.

The concept is not new, and has been a requirement of health visitor training since the 1970s (Hunt, 1982). The approach is appealing in that it combines quantitative data such as demographic information, epidemiological data and indicators of deprivation with qualitative data, such as information from health care professional caseloads and individual assessments (Richards, 1991). In order to understand fully what is meant by community profile, the term will be discussed, exploring its uses in the literature and summarizing predominant characteristics in a structure, process and outcome model (Donebedian, 1977). Outcomes of profiling will be explored more fully, looking at both positive and negative consequences. The practicalities of obtaining information will be discussed, and a research method for analysing the multiple data sources will be put forward. To end the section on profiling, some of the more established and empirical data sources will be considered in relation to issues of reliability and validity.

Uses in the literature

Health-related literature identifies three main levels of profiling that can be undertaken, all involving the accumulation of a range of health data and identifying differing populations:

- community health profile
- caseload profile, which also includes information relating to individual health profiles
- practice profile.

Community health profile

First, a community health profile as defined by Hubley (1982) is that process by which there is an attempt by the community worker to understand and describe the locality in which she or he may be working, in order to prioritize need. Orr (1992a) describes its importance in the identification of 'at risk' groups using socio-economic indicators, and data illustrating the experiences of clients. The community profile can include information from caseload and practice profiles.

Cernik and Wearne (1992) elaborate more fully by defining the community health profile as a 'snapshot' of the population, which provides a systematic approach to assessing community health needs and resources. This process provides purchasers, trusts and workers with information upon which to make informed choices about the care provided, as well as helping to set targets for health prevention and promotion. Kennedy (1992) offers a similar explanation, but emphasizes that 'health' should be interpreted positively, and not be taken to mean purely the absence of disease. A multi-agency approach is advocated, and thought to have considerable benefits. Indeed, Peckham and Spanton (1994) state that community health care nurses can build local networks and alliances with groups and individuals, increasing their understanding and awareness of local issues, and adapting work priorities accordingly. Both Cernik and Wearne (1992) and Kennedy (1992) state that a profile should be compiled annually to provide information relating to trends, and to facilitate evaluation of health promotion activity.

Further interpretations are offered by Twinn et al. (1990), who although discarding the term community, owing to its perceived ambiguity previously outlined, describe the health profile as a systematic collection of data for needs identification, and the analysis of that data to assess and prioritize strategies in health promotion. Although they state the process as being essential to directing and targeting health visiting, it is also essential to other practitioners in the community. Cernik and Wearne (1992) suggest either practitioner working parties or specialist researchers with community experience should be considered for the task.

Goodwin's use of the term (Goodwin, 1994) urges their application by practitioners to assess the effectiveness of their current practice of health promotion among the well population. From a community nurse management viewpoint, Hull (1989) explores the use of information technology in the process and analysis of health profiling, concentrating on empirical data.

Caseload profile

Caseload profiles concentrate more upon the clientele of the community nurse, and were first advocated by Hunt (1982). The caseload profile is described as the analysis of all individual records held by each community health care nurse according to certain health dimensions to identify characteristics and trends, highlighting individual and family need, facilitating prioritization and the targeting of health promotion work (Hunt, 1982; Drennan, 1990).

Much of the caseload profile will incorporate information which has been amassed during health profiles. Bell (1993) refers to the health profile in terms of individual assessment, necessary to determine individual or group needs, problems and resources, and their referral to other agencies if necessary. This level of profiling is most familiar to practitioners, being an integral part of everyday practice.

Practice profile

Following the National Health Service Management Executive document (NHSME, 1992) stating that fundholding practices must profile their practice population twice a year, the use of the term practice profile has been adopted. A recent Royal College of Nursing publication (RCN, 1993) urges all members of the primary health care team to be involved in the process. The RCN defines the practice profile as incorporating elements of health needs assessment and community profiling, the purpose of which is to provide information to determine priorities for pro-active and reactive care. Hugman and McCready (1993) describe its use in defining the detail of the service, acting as a tool to set aims and objectives for the practice, and to define the state of nursing within the practice.

Therefore, this review of the use of the term profile, although demonstrating different levels of operations, has common themes. A combination of approaches is becoming an accepted way of profiling for health needs, providing as it does a more comprehensive approach (Yorkshire Health, 1990; Billingham, 1991).

In order to clarify fully the major features of the multi-dimensional interpretation of the term profile, the model developed by Donebedian (1977) will be used to explore its uses in the literature, as demonstrated in Table 23.1. This model allows a summary to be made of the *structure* (what must be in place before profiling can be undertaken), *process* and *outcome* components.

Table 23.1 Structure, process and outcome components of profiling

STRUCTURE

Before a profile can be undertaken, the literature suggests that the following need to be in place:

- collaboration between and among professional groups and agencies in the community
- adequate time for practitioner(s) or an experienced non-practitioner/researcher
- access to client information and consumer opinion
- information technology.

PROCESS

Central to the process of compiling a profile is the annual collection of data relating to:

- the population within the community, caseload and/or practice, and individual assessment
- empirical health data and/or 'soft' data illustrating the experiences of clients
- resources within the community and individuals
- states of positive health, as well as morbidity and mortality.

The process of the profile also includes its analysis combining quantitative with qualitative data, and using descriptive statistics where appropriate to facilitate cross-comparison between groups.

OUTCOME

Intended outcomes and uses for the analysed data include:

- the identification and prioritization of community, group, family and individual need
- the provision of information to purchasers, trusts, workers and users of the services upon which to make informed choices about health
- the setting of targets for health prevention and promotion
- determining the direction for the provision of community nursing and setting aims and objectives
- assessing and evaluating the effectiveness of health promotion activity
- the identification of population, group and individual characteristics and trends.

Outcomes of profiling

Positive outcomes

Elaborating upon those outlined, supporters of profiling offer a range of potentially positive outcomes or consequences. Hubley (1982) states that information from a community profile will facilitate the planning of community-based health education programmes and initiatives, and justify additional funding to concentrate activity in a locality. This may also allow a more even distribution of scarce resources (Klein and Thomlinson, 1987).

From a health visiting perspective, authors emphasize its value in demonstrating effectiveness, linking profiling with quality assurance and audit and in the identification and correction of mismatches between needs and service delivery (Dobby, 1986; Drennan, 1990). Issues relating to practice that may evolve from the profile include the identification of areas for research and development and staff training needs (Drennan, 1990; Twinn *et al.*, 1990). Hunt (1982) focuses upon the consumer, stating that caseload analysis may bring together individuals who share common problems and needs. She also highlights the benefits to the practitioner, who may identify issues such as low breastfeeding incidence or high rates of unsupported carers. This information will enable the practitioner to justify health promotion activity in a specific area. On a broader note,

Cernik and Wearne (1992) describe their vision of how data from the profile should not only act as resource for the Primary Health Care Team, but be given to local people, encouraging them to become involved in planning and policy formation.

Some studies give an indication of actual outcomes from the formation of a profile. Drennan (1990) describes how caseload profiles were used to develop a weighting system for district nurse caseloads. Colin-Thome (1993) describes how the findings of the practice profile formed by a collaborative team of staff and patients were used to construct a practice health strategy – identifying the scope for health improvement through a range of initiatives. In Milton Keynes, practice profiles have been used to change the level and type of nursing it purchases, determined by identified need (Hugman and McCready, 1993). Others have looked specifically at the development of a health visiting strategy from community profile data (Jackson, 1989) and 'goodness of fit' between existing primary health care and population needs (Cernik and Wearne, 1991).

Negative outcomes

However, despite the advantages of profiling for practice it is important that practitioners should be aware of its limitations. Goodwin (1992) questions its ultimate usefulness when limited budgets may be unable to meet the cost of outcome implementation. There is also the possibility of revealing social needs that the caring professions are unable to act upon (Twinn *et al.*, 1990). This may result in frustrations and disillusionment for both provider and recipient and raise serious professional issues related to accountability. A similar concern is that resulting strategies from profile information may not be compatible with purchaser, Trust or Department of Health priorities (Rodrigues, 1989). Equally important, completing a profile may be a waste of time and resources if health care professionals are not willing to radically alter their attitudes to practice, or are not supported during the necessary change in practice. Cernik and Warne (1992) argue that with no standardized tool from which to record the type and amount of data, results may be fragmented and uncoordinated. Also, if components for measurement do not reflect the consumer perspective, data may result that is not relevant to the felt needs of the population (Knights and Hayes, 1981). In a similar fashion, a caseload analysis focus may provide data that is professionally owned and therefore not automatically available for use by other community workers or agencies (Jackson, 1989). Also, the multidisciplinary-collaborative approach advocated by Drennan (1990) may in reality be difficult to achieve, given the increasing workloads of practitioners and limited time available (HVA, 1994). A more threatening consequence may be that information from a profile may be used for staff cost-cutting exercises, by reducing or diluting nursing roles through inappropriate grade or skill mix.

An additional concern is that profiles are seen by some authors as instrumental in the survival of some community professionals, particularly the health visiting service. A somewhat 'profile or perish' approach is detected in the literature (Denny, 1989; Day, 1992), with not only token recognition of the skills needed to undertake this task, but also the time constraints of practitioners. Gooch (1989) extends this approach by stating that the profile will provide those sceptical of the value of practitioners in the community with measurable evidence of what the profession can accomplish. While this may be a reasonable supposition, profiling should be placed in perspective, and is indeed only one feature of the complexity of nursing practice in the community.

●   **The practicalities of profile compilation – approaches to data collection**

The identification of factors that assist practitioners to profile their practice or caseloads appears to vary tremendously within the literature. Most authors appear to agree that the data required will depend upon the particular focus of their 'profiler' and the special features of the locality; this aspect is particularly stressed by those authors who have had experience of profiling (Drennan, 1990; Cernik and Wearne, 1991). For example, a poverty profile as outlined by Blackburn (1992) may be appropriate for practitioners working in deprived areas. Also, as data collection progresses, areas of relevance may emerge warranting more detailed information; thus, uniform operational terms are often not possible.

Those authors who offer guidance on the factors of the community profile also vary in specificity. The description by Hawtin et al. (1994), for example, involves the extensive collection of data relating to housing, environment, health and resources. They suggest that this information can be obtained by published sources such as Census material, interviews and questionnaires in the community, 'streetwork', or casual observation, thus combining quantitative with qualitative approaches. Guidance regarding the practical application and measurement of these factors is outlined.

The most comprehensive suggestions for the content of a community health profile appears to be offered by Luker and Orr (1992); although originally developed from a health visiting perspective, it is pertinent to all practitioners. Twelve topics are selected, ranging from organizations and power and leadership information to health status of the community and health action potential. The authors argue that they have drawn upon knowledge from sociology, psychology, epidemiology and social policy for this selection. They also suggest a range of local informal and formal sources of data (housing, social service and voluntary departments), and official sources, such as Census information. Despite the seemingly extensive range of components, specific guidance on how to operationalize the criteria is limited, highlighting the skill and organization involved in the practicalities of completing a profile. Other measures, such as the health profile (Twinn et al., 1990), a school health profile (RCN, 1992) and the practice profile (RCN, 1993), outline more abridged versions of the above, but with differing perspectives.

Several authors, such as Drennan (1990), focus on factors for specific practitioners. Drennan suggests that data from district nursing caseloads, in addition to demographic and social information about clients, should also include documenting aspects such as nursing dependency levels, discharges and admissions and reduction in nursing care over the past month. Drennan states that these criteria were established following an extensive literature search and 'brainstorming' sessions with a representative working group. Assessment tools for the identification of individual and family needs are again most extensively offered by authors such as Luker and Orr (1992), and also Bell (1993). A more specific and contemporary outline of data sources for a community profile from a health visiting perspective is offered by Cowley and Billings (1994a), used for the initial phase of the 'Family Health Needs' study. The aim of this study was to identify indicators of need to determine local health visiting specifications for contracting. Table 23.2 outlines the data sources and provides approaches to the type and method of data collection. For the study, the target population consisted of families with children under 18 years old. This study has been used to provide an illustration of the processes involved in profiling a practice population.

Collecting the data

For the collection of data, it must also be considered that some commercially-minded organizations, such as new Hospital Trusts, have become increasingly reluctant to part with information without reimbursement, identifying the costs associated with profiling (Cowley and Billings, 1994a). Problems can also be experienced in tracing key personnel within bureaucratic organizations, and considerable patience is needed. However, despite these difficulties, some data sources are relatively easy to access. These include local public health departments, where acquisition of the annual report can reduce time-consuming searches for health-related epidemiological statistics. Also, housing departments have alliances with most statutory and voluntary agencies in the community and either regularly fund, or know of local research projects or initiatives that are health related, so therefore are a valuable source of material. For the 'Family Health Needs' project, for example, local reports were available on issues such as the experiences of mental health patients in the community.

Most purchasing health authorities now have information departments which may supply reasonable amounts of health data free of charge. In addition, local health commissioners and representatives at the Family Health Services Authority are generally involved in accumulating data for needs assessment that may be of use to the profiler. Again, in the example described above, local research had been undertaken regarding accidents among the under fives and the work of specialist health visitors involved in child protection issues, and was made available for the 'Family Health Needs' project. Although many of the above sources will have used Census data, comprehensive and locally pertinent booklets of Census information are usually made available by the planning departments in local government offices at a small charge, or are accessible at

Table 23.2 Type and method of data collection per data source

Data source	Quantitative data	Qualitative data
OPCS: County Council, Planning	Census data: Small area statistics	–
Government departments: Home Office Department of Trade and Industry	National statistics: Crime Home/leisure accidents	–
Public health:	Epidemiological data: Mortality/Jarman scores	–
Trusts: Paediatric Family and Child Psychiatric Family Planning	Statistical health data: Special needs children Prevalence/referral studies Service provision	–
Health Commissioners: Family Health Services Authorities Locality Commissioners Area Health Authorities	Statistical health data: Locality statistics	–
Local statutory agencies: Housing Social Services Police Careers County Council Environmental Health	Statistical data: Strategic document Child protection figures Crime statistics Destination statistics Road traffic accidents, Unemployment statistics Local surveys, complaints	Informal interviews (health perceptions)
Local voluntary agencies: Shelter	Statistical data: Homelessness figures	Informal interviews (health perceptions)
Local projects: Trinity DDU Mental health Under 5s accidents Child protection	Statistical data:	Informal interviews (health perceptions)
Community Practitioners: School Nurses, CPNs Education Welfare Officers Health Visitors Specialist Nurses	–	Focus groups (health perceptions)
Health Visitors	Caseload analysis: 102 families	Informal interviews (health perceptions)
GP unit	Practice profile: Demographic/morbidity information	–

libraries. As well as providing national statistics, Census data are obtainable for electoral wards and enumeration (clusters of streets) districts, which can be valuable in identifying characteristics of small neighbourhoods.

Once again using the project identified earlier, the health visiting profile was collected using a columned schedule on A3 paper designed by the author, to examine the health situation per family unit. This enabled the extraction of a range of material from the documentation, such as social class, family structure, breastfeeding patterns, child health and family health issues. Information was documented on the schedule in numerical or, as with the child and family health issues, coded format. This allowed a simple analysis to take place highlighting the incidence of breastfeeding and accidents which could then be compared across caseloads. This information was supplemented by interviews with the health visitors responsible for the caseloads, where further material relating to aspects such as family social support networks were elaborated upon and other coping mechanisms. This data was also coded and entered on the schedule and provided an important 'positive health' perspective, rather than focusing upon problems within families, an aspect elaborated upon later.

The objective of the GP practice profile was to extract health information from the computer software about families with children under 18 and obtain broader baseline data concerning the population, such as mortality and morbidity figures and an age/sex breakdown. This aspect of the profile compilation proved to the most challenging, as there were numerous difficulties associated with data accessibility. With relatively new computer software having been installed in the practice, the degree to which health information about the population could be extracted, without recourse to lengthy documentary analysis, was limited due to the lack of input of such data at the time of the research.

As health information related to the practice population on an individual level, and details of family health were not available, the first step was to plot the geographical location of families on a large street map giving electoral ward boundaries. This allowed Census, some epidemiological data and deprivation scores to be applied to the populations in the differing wards. Plotting of families with pre-school age children was unproblematic, being extracted from health visiting caseloads. However, families with children aged 6–18 years required a list of all individuals between those ages from the computer, matching names and addresses (a complex process as families frequently had children with different surnames), and eliminating those who had pre-school siblings, as these were already plotted. The eventual list was also checked for accuracy by the reception staff, who have a wealth of knowledge about the families in their practice population. The difficulty highlights the importance of appropriate software using family units, which would overcome some of the difficulties experienced.

Having completed the first step, a range of more general morbidity information about the practice population was obtained by exploring the data banks. Once the access procedure had been identified, it became relatively easy to request information from the computer, such as numbers of people with hypertension, heart disease or attempted suicides. According to the practice manager, these data were approximately 80% accurate. It was decided to relate information to 'Health of the Nation' classifications (coronary heart disease and strokes, cancers, mental health, accidents and HIV virus and AIDS) to facilitate cross-comparison between GP caseloads, making the data more useful to both purchasers and providers of health care. Of interest was the fact that mortality data was not available at practice level, nor from other local sources such as the Family Health Services Authority, which would appear to be a fundamental omission. Wider epidemiological data, which is mostly concerned with death rates, could not therefore be used for comparison purposes in this project. Positive indicators of health were also obtained, such as the numbers attending for immunization and cervical screening. A 'snapshot' picture of all antenatal patients was also acquired, using hospital booking forms and a schedule upon which to collect the information.

However, it must be acknowledged that the reliability of this information should be treated with caution, with data only giving broad indications of the health status of the practice population. Also, accuracy of data between GPs within a practice varied considerably, making cross-comparison between populations largely invalid. However, with the increasing pressure placed upon fundholding GPs to produce accurate health information for contracting (NHSME, 1992), practitioners should find the situation improving.

As health information about the 6–18-year-old children was difficult to access, the inclusion of small focus groups of health care professionals in contact with this age group of children was necessary. The qualitative data obtained from these professionals, perceptions of the health status and social situation of children in the practice provided an illuminating overview of their health needs. It is appreciated that practitioners compiling profiles of their areas may find this data source impractical, being time consuming and difficult to arrange.

Data analysis

Having acquired a range of information from multiple sources, if the profile is to influence the direction of nursing services as suggested, practitioners must then interpret and aggregate the material into meaningful indicators of need, which will in turn guide nursing practice. There is very little, if any, clear guidance within the literature about this analysis, and would appear to be the Achilles' heel of profiling. For example, where profiling has been used to determine nursing strategy, there is little evidence within these studies to suggest an identifiable research approach to data collection and analysis in profiling, which makes the findings, conclusions and ultimately action difficult to interpret.

In an attempt to overcome these problems, Cowley and Billings (1994b) have applied the use of the case study design suggested by Yin (1989) to the data from the community profile. The unique strength of this design is to allow the researcher to manipulate a multiple range of data, both qualitative and quantitative, while still permitting an investigation to retain meaningful characteristics of life events. The design was of a single-embedded type, using the community profile itself as the unit of analysis and incorporating 10 of the data sources or 'sub-units' as outlined in Table 23.2, which is demonstrated in Figure 23.1.

This design is flexible and allowed for more sub-units to be added

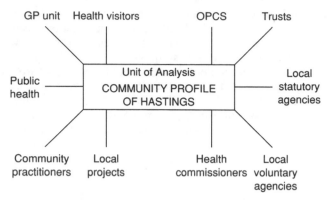

Figure 23.1 Single-embedded case study design, demonstrating unit of analysis and sub-units (OPCS, Office of Population, Census and Surveys)

as data collection progressed. The general analytical strategy was through the development of a case description by the tabulation and pattern-matching of themes identified within each sub-group. For example, a columned schedule was drawn up and, taking each data source in turn, the predominant themes were entered in columns. This process enabled sources to be cross-referenced for similarities and emerging patterns or trends and allowed the data to explain the health situation in the community and its personal impact on families. Mapping the data also facilitated visual interpretation of pattern-matching. At the same time, the practitioners used sources in the literature to match emergent themes to other health theories and research to help strengthen their position as potential indicators of need.

This method has been useful in making sense of multiple data sources and in the identification of broad indicators of need. It allowed for both quantitative and qualitative sub-units to be handled according to their methodological requirements and allowed integration of results in a meaningful way. Currently the project is collecting perceptions of health needs using semi-structured interviews. This qualitative data will be analysed and added as a sub-unit to the case study, to present an overall community health profile.

● Reliability and validity of empirical data sources

This final section of the chapter will focus on a critical review of three of the main empirical souces of data, namely Census information, indicators of social deprivation and epidemiological data. This is important in order to raise critical awareness of the more established and widely used forms of data.

Census data

Although the use of 1991 Census material in determining a range of population characteristics and circumstances is strongly recommended as a valuable source of information (Kennedy, 1992), authors have argued that Census variables such as age and ethnicity are not in themselves causes, nor necessarily indicators, of need (Stalker, 1993). Indeed, Robinson (1985) argues that such classifications may lend themselves to professional stereotyping in the process of needs assessment, rather than recognizing individual variation within the categories.

Census data also continues to request information using the head of the household on which to base social class. Despite differing economic activity between partners, this is still largely completed as that of the male partner in a household consisting of a couple (OPCS, 1992). McDowall (1983) highlights the shortcomings of this approach, particularly in relation to women. First, most women now work, with approximately $10\frac{1}{2}$ million women currently in employment in the UK (OPCS, 1992). Not classifying them individually by their own occupation may not only conceal health hazards, but also the earnings of working women may influence and improve the standard of living within the household. Difficulties with the unemployed, the elderly and children also arise, in that occupational class does not fully describe the circumstances in which they live (Whitehead, 1987). Thus the needs of large sections of the population may be hidden or over-estimated using this classification. Several alternatives have been put forward, such as the system of household class, based upon the occupation of the spouse who is economically dominant, as described by Arber (1987), or the child-centred Social Index (Osborn and Morris, 1979), a system which was intended to be more relevant to the home environment of the child rather than occupational class alone. Interestingly, the use of these systems has not yet been widely replicated and evaluated.

A further difficulty regarding Census data is its relevance to practitioners carrying out profiles in relation to the geographical distribution of results. The present availability of small area population statistics (electoral ward and enumeration district) has facilitated planners in identifying need, but it does not assist GP practices where populations may span a wide geographical area with three or four families per ward (Young and Haynes, 1993; Cowley and Billings, 1994a). This argument highlights the difficulties associated with 'goodness of fit' of the various data sources, which is a recurrent problem regarding meaningful profile compilation. Furthermore, the apparent under-representation of single people aged 16–44 in comparison to that of the 1981 Census has also caused speculation regarding the reliability of data in this group, particularly concerning potential poll tax evasion (OPCS, 1992). This has obvious implications concerning accuracy in identifying health needs. Also, assuming that the data was accurate in the first place, Census data becomes very rapidly out of date, a factor that creates difficulties for 'snapshot' population information (Stalker, 1993).

Indicators of social deprivation

As described earlier, although indicators of social inequality and deprivation are also important in estimating the health of a population (Whitehead, 1987; Stalker, 1993) there are problems attached to their measurement. For example, the scoring system developed by Jarman (1984) has been criticized for its bias towards using determination variables associated with the elderly (Thunhurst, 1985). Foy *et al.* (1987) and Chase and Davies (1991) have pointed out that the aggregated data may hide large variations between smaller groups such as the deprivation within a housing estate, that is situated in an area of relative affluence. However, enumeration data from the Census may now largely overcome this problem, by giving specific house number information. In addition, Whitehead (1987) points out that some indices combine direct indicators of deprivation such as overcrowding and unemployment with indirect measures of numbers of people 'at risk' of deprivation (i.e. single-parent families and ethnic minorities), where, as previously mentioned, not all people are deprived in these groups.

Townsend *et al.* (1988) have highlighted contradictions between scores when indices are monopolized by highly skewed variables such as ethnicity; for example, the indices developed by the Department of the Environment (DoE, 1983), and Jarman (1984) demonstrated that the most deprived local authority areas were in London, with none in the north. The indices used by Townsend *et al.* (1988) demonstrate the converse to be more the case. However, this problem may be overcome by choosing only indicators of material deprivation such as the proportion of households with no car, and unemployment (Townsend *et al.*, 1985), by employing more sophisticated statistical techniques (Wagstaff *et al.*, 1991), or by using 'grass root' surveys to check and extend the statistical results (Thunhurst, 1985).

Epidemiological data

The acquisition of epidemiological evidence has largely depended upon morbidity and mortality data. Stevens and Gabby (1991) argue that an epidemiologically sound assessment of needs is a vital inclusion to any profile and the ultimate development of the health service, focusing as it does on prevalence rates of death and disease. Although death rates are obviously a necessary concept for assessing disease, Patrick (1986) argues that these statistics have lost importance in assessing the health of a population. He adds that this is particularly so when death rates are low, with the majority of the population remaining alive but in varying states of health. Wilson (1981) adds that the increase in chronic conditions and development of medical treatment to prolong life, such as renal dialysis and insulin therapy, have contributed to the decreasing value of this data.

Thus information relating to the prevalence of disease would appear to have greater relevance to needs assessment (Mays, 1987). Stalker (1993), however, urges morbidity rates to be translated with caution, supporting critics of census and deprivation data stating that incidence must not be confused with actual need. Also, there are many inconsistencies in measurement, particularly in relation to mental health. McCollam (1992) discovered that the incidence of mental health problems is obtained in a variety of different ways and that differing methods used in one area produced different results of the prevalence of mental health needs. However, Bebbington and Davies (1980) acknowledge the difficulties in reaching consensus regarding criteria for measurement, and suggest that attempts to develop national indicators would meet with limited success.

Profiling: a health perspective

It cannot have escaped many readers that most data sources for profile compilation tend to focus upon disease, illness, social problems or other negative health states. There is a growing body of literature that acknowledges and criticizes the somewhat contradictory nature of an emphasis on disease as a way of assessing need to determine health.

Rijke (1993), for example, states that most medical research has been undertaken in academic settings or hospitals where a select group of the population with certain abnormalities and diseases are investigated. Rijke goes on to argue that focusing upon disease groups to estimate population needs is not profitable, as very little is known in medical science about the natural history of diseases in the general public (Lorber, 1980; Nelson and Ellenberg, 1982). Rijke (1993) states that there is an assumption that the occurrence of a disease is determined by a causal or 'risk' factor(s), and that the elimination of the disease is achieved by medical intervention or lifestyle changes. He argues that reducing certain factors does not necessarily lead to better health when applied to larger population groups, especially in relation to cardiovascular disease (Coronary Drug Project Research Group, 1980). Risk factors describe different patterns of health problems, but not the causes of different patterns, which are often connected to social inequalities (Niehoff and Schneider, 1993). Rijke (1993) therefore urges a scientific approach to research which studies health rather than disease.

To support his view, Rijke (1993) outlines research that has focused upon how people remain healthy. This points to factors such as autonomy, vitality and social support as being essential to the reduced frequency of physical complaints and illness, and maintenance of a sense of wellbeing (Rijke, 1985; Antonovsky, 1987; Rohe and Kahn, 1987). The importance of this perspective is increasingly being recognized and used in the field of nursing research. A study concerned with accident prevention in a Glasgow housing estate focused upon the 'near' accidents and the positive actions that mothers took to prevent recurrence (Roberts *et al.*, 1993). This provided valuable lay information that the authors felt would be more acceptable to other mothers.

Not only has this perspective considerable implications for the focus of current health education and promotion programmes, which work from a perspective of disease avoidance rather than health persistence, but it offers another dimension to the assessment of community and individual needs and service provision. Services such as health visiting, where practitioners have the necessary skills to assess these qualities, and potentially augment their deficiencies through facilitating empowerment and networking (Drennan, 1988), should be developed rather than eroded.

Profiling: the consumer perspective

The importance of including the consumer perspective when assessing needs cannot be overstated. Profiling has been accused of being restricted in providing a picture of health needs, limited as it is in many cases to the collection and collation of existing information from a service perspective (Peckham and Spanton, 1994). The latter is insufficient in explaining the experience of health at the interactive level (Stalker, 1993). Public consultation therefore is an aspect of profiling that is attracting considerable interest, offering a unique opportunity for the community to make their needs known and, theoretically, ensure that they are adequately addressed within plans (Clode, 1992). Criticism has been directed against health care professionals for setting the health agenda without consulting the public (Forrester, 1991).

Among both the general population (Richardson *et al.*, 1992) and health care professionals (Higgens, 1992) there appears to be increasing importance attached to the idea of consultation about health needs. The current wave of consumerism in health and social circles has, however, not occurred due to the sudden development of socially conscious managers. Phillips *et al.* (1994) state that the government's policy of controlling public expenditure and encouraging a mixed economy of care has introduced a strong element of enterprise culture into public service organizations. Central policy thus demands greater choice and independence for service users, demonstrated by their publications (DoH, 1990; NHSME, 1992).

Reviewing the various approaches to consultation, Bowling (1992) highlights numerous ways in which this can be achieved, namely consumer feedback via forums, public meetings, and consumer representation on user-groups. Local interview, postal or telephone surveys of views and satisfaction surveys have also been used (Roberts and Magowan, 1994). Bowling (1992) adds that observation techniques can also be applied in care settings where clients find difficulty in expressing views. The use of focus groups has also been advocated as a valuable method of exploring perceptions of need (Morgan, 1993). Indeed, the use of these groups has been enlightening, demonstrating consumer awareness of their contributive strengths and limitations in the needs assessment process (Cowley *et al.*, 1994).

Consultation is, however, not without its methodological difficulties. Focus groups, for example, are generally characterized by small numbers which raises questions regarding the ultimate reliability of the results, as demonstrated by Cowley *et al.* (1994). To overcome this problem, some studies have used a combination of techniques to obtain a more comprehensive picture of consumer need (Judge and Solomon, 1992). Also, the constraints of satisfaction surveys have long been recognized, relating particularly to the validity of current methods of operationalizing the concept of client satisfaction (Avis, 1994). A factor common to all approaches to consultation concerns reliability of sample selection. Rodgers (1994) and Bowling (1992) suggest that, where researchers do not strive to gain equity of response, there will be a tendency for the more articulate, less burdened consumers' voice to be heard loudest. Consultation therefore has the potential to reinforce inequalities in service provision, rather than address them.

However, obtaining the views of less articulate sections of the population has its constraints. In a community project based in Stirling, the needs of a sample of elderly people were obtained with the aid of a schedule (Hudson, 1992). Prior to the assessment, a 10-point question-naire was completed by the referrer, indicating the degree to which the elderly person was perceived to be 'in need'. Hudson (1992) documents the difficulties experienced by elderly people, who found expression of need not only arduous but also consistently linked need to availability of resources. This was in contrast to the referrers' perceptions, who generally identified multiple needs among the sample regardless of available service provision. Further complications were revealed in this study regarding the tension between carers' needs and those of the elderly person. Decisions regarding whose needs would drive the care plans thus became difficult. The study therefore highlights some important issues surrounding the complexities of needs assessment.

Once data from the consumer has been compiled by a chosen method, consideration must be given to its synthesis with broader health information into local policy. In an analysis of community plans, Richards (1991) noted that while most emphasized the importance of aggregation of data, few practical proposals for achieving it were made. This becomes increasing significant when considering the depth of information obtained by practitioners through individual needs assessment. Incorporating such information into meaningful policy statements can be complex and difficult. For example, unless the total population within an area can be targeted, bias may be an inevitable consequence and 'felt' need never be fully identified (Stalker, 1993). Conversely, converting the needs of individuals into meaningful components to guide policy may require a radical aggregation of felt need, so a true picture may never be demonstrated. However, focusing upon small groups within a loca-lity, such as carers or families of physically challenged children, may converge areas of need in a more meaningful way (Richards, 1991; Morris and Lindlow, 1993). Indeed, using a case study approach as advocated by Cowley and Billings (1994b) may also facilitate blending of data.

This latter argument highlights a concern regarding the ethical consequences of needs assessment that concerns not only the consumer perspective, but all methods of assessing need. Interestingly, the con-sideration of the ethical issues involved in obtaining information about a community both from statutory and informal sources appears to be largely absent from the literature (Cowley, 1993). This invasion of privacy becomes of increasing significance if a large percentage of the population from which data is being obtained will not benefit from any service provision. In addition, the often perceived unequal relationship between professionals and recipients of care (Becker, 1967; Dunnell and Dobbs, 1983) may mean that clients are placed in uncompromising situations in revealing personal details for the purposes of a profile. This is particularly evident when viewing the very personal components of the individual assessments, evidenced by questions relating to intimate physical and sexual needs (Bell, 1993). A balance must therefore be achieved between a desire to locate and provide for unexpressed needs and the right of citizens to maintain their privacy (Pinker, 1982).

Notwithstanding methodological and ethical issues, further contradictions to this approach to needs assessment are evident. For example, the financial costs are considerable (Richardson *et al.*, 1992), and the depth of information obtained will ultimately depend upon the methods employed. As there is no minimum standard to be achieved, cost restrictions may limit areas to obtaining superficial consumer data only, while still fulfilling government recommendations. Rodgers (1994) argues that the 'Citizen's Charter' is a case in point – with its 'vague promises and relaxed standards' it may leave the organization with a comfortable feeling that issues are being addressed.

Wistow *et al.* (1992) have argued that public consultation may be nothing more than tokenism in some areas. In their analysis of 22 English community care plans, it was discovered that, where consultation had been employed, methods differed considerably across regions. Importantly, the extent to which the results of the exercises had influenced the completed strategy documents and service specifications was far from clear, nor were there distinct evaluative accounts of how satisfactory the process had been. Respondents in the study by Cowley *et al.* (1994) were not uniformly convinced that their views were respected, either at an individual level or as part of a service planning exercise. Indeed, the findings by Richardson *et al.* (1992) support this powerlessness perspective and highlight the consumer's dilemma, by indicating that most respondents in their survey felt they were unable to influence decisions in health care, despite welcoming the opportunity. Studies are now emerging that document participants' frustration at the lack of feedback and positive action following consultation (Southampton and S. W. Hants. Health Commission, 1993).

However, it is within this context that the true paradox of community needs assessment occurs. Critics of the community care reforms have argued that without a substantial increase in resources, assessment of needs, however it is undertaken, becomes an almost meaningless exercise, since the services and support required by the population will not be available (Cornwell, 1992; Jack, 1992). The more comprehensive the assessment, the more inevitable the possibility that a plethora of social needs will be revealed that providers are unable to act upon, resulting in universal disillusionment. Cheetham (1991), while urging local authorities to use the results of assessment as a means of exposing unmet need and social ills, acknowledges the political risks involved if the shortfall between planned services, needs identified and resources available is demonstrated. Phillips *et al.* (1994) add that for care agencies to fully encompass the notion of consumerism is to make demands that both the public and professionals are unable to meet. It is therefore not surprising that superficial data collection and interpretation may become the preferred option.

In addition, the apparent mismatch between political aspirations and the realities appears to have created a certain amount of disillusion about the value and worth of needs assessment as a whole within professional opinion. Although policy appears to have largely pinned its hopes upon greater collaboration between community agencies and consumers, health care professionals are becoming increasingly unsure about their own organization's ability to realize this potential (Higgens, 1992). Indeed, Stalker (1993) points out that the changes required on the part of community agencies to undertake this task in terms of activity and skills are often underestimated and only fully realized once assessment is underway. For example, training staff is essential to facilitate their transition from assessor to assessed (Hudson, 1992), and in helping them to cope with the cultural shift of power to the consumer (Higgens, 1992), a change that cannot occur overnight.

Also, as the ultimate approach to needs assessment may depend upon the prevailing philosophy of a locality, variations between districts may make cross-comparison impossible. It therefore could be argued that an effective nationwide implementation of care in the community may be problematic to audit. Selecting the most suitable approach is only the first step. Indeed, Cheetham (1991) emphasizes the importance of careful consideration in this initial stage, as future community plans may hinge upon comprehensive and sound community needs assessments. But, as Stevens and Gabby (1991) point out, producing facts and figures to provide a comprehensive picture, coupled with staff training and development, are lengthy procedures, in contrast to the headlong rush to agree contracts. They continue by declaring the fear that needs assessment is being put to one side, with the consequence that the logical sequence of needs identification, service specification and contracts may be reversed.

● **Conclusion**
In conclusion, this chapter has attempted to debate definable methodological, ethical and contextual factors surrounding community needs assessment, highlighting the multi-dimensional difficulties surrounding the process. The issues raised have been discussed within the current political climate, and have recognized its influence in relation to community needs assessment. This arena served to highlight the inherent paradoxes and dilemmas within the needs assessment procedure. It has also attempted to demonstrate the potentially vital position of practitioners regarding data sources, which has yet to be fully recognized and taken advantage of.

In general, it must be stated that needs assessment literature tends to be characterized more by assumptions, predictions and, for the most part speculative rhetoric, rather than sound evaluative research, due possibly to its emergent nature. However, the difficulties associated with community needs assessment, coupled with its continued high political profile, dictate to a large extent the protracted but welcome appearance of needs assessment deliberation within health-related literature.

References
Antonovsky, A. (1987) The salutogenic perspective – towards a new view of health and disease. *Advances*, 4(3), 47–55

Arber, S. (1987) Gender and class inequalities in health: understanding the differentials. In *Inequalities in Health within Europe* (ed. A.J. Fox), Gower Press, Aldershot

Ashley, J. and McLachlan, G. (1985) *Mortal or Morbid? A Diagnosis of the Morbidity Factor*, Nuffield Provincial Hospitals Trust, London

Avis, M. (1994) Satisfying solutions: a review of issues in measuring patient satisfaction. Paper presented at the RCN Annual Research Conference, Hull.

Bebbington, A.C. and Davies, B. (1980) Territorial needs indicators: a new approach. *Journal of Social Policy*, **9**(2), 145–168

Becker, H. (1967) Whose side are we on? *Social Problems*, **14**, 241

Bell, I. (1993) Less impertinence, more partnership. *Health Visitor*, **66**(10), 370–372

Benson, J. (1976) The concept of community. In *Talking About Welfare* (eds N. Timms and D. Watson), Routledge and Kegan Paul, London

Billingham, K. (1991) *Community Profiles*, unpublished

Blackburn, C. (1992) *Improving Health and Welfare Work with Families in Poverty*, Open University Press, Milton Keynes

Blaxter, M. (1990) *Health and Lifestyles*, Routledge, London

Bowling, A. (1992) 'Local voices' in purchasing health care: an exploratory exercise in public consultation on priority setting. Needs Assessment Unit, St. Bartholomew's Hospital Medical College

Bradshaw, J. (1972) The concept of social need. *New Society*, **30**, 640–643

Bryan, S., Parkin, D. and Donaldson, C. (1991) Chiropody and the QALY: a case study in assigning categories of disability and stress to patients. *Health Policy*, **18**, 169–185

Buchan, H. and Gray, J.A. (1990) Needs assessment made simple. *Health Service Journal*, **100**, 240–241

Cernik, K. and Wearne, M. (1991) Going public. *Primary Health Care*, **1**(4), 26–27

Cernik, K. and Wearne, M. (1992) Using community health profiles to improve service provision. *Health Visitor*, **65**(10), 343–345

Chase, H.D. and Davies, P.R.T. (1991) Calculation of the underprivileged area score for a practice in inner London. *British Journal of General Practice*, February, 63–66

Cheetham, J. (1991) Community care: bridging the gap. *Community Care*, **870**, 24–25

Clode, D. (1992) Best laid plans. *Community Care*, **871**, 205–206

Colin-Thome, D. (1993) The public health nurse: a new model for health visiting? *Primary Care Management*, **3**(5), 4–6

Cornwell, N. (1992) Assessment and accountability in community care. *Critical Social Policy*, **36**, 42–52

Coronary Drug Project Research Group (1980) Influence of adherence to treatment and response of cholesterol in the coronary drug project. *New England Journal of Medicine*, **303**, 1038–1041

Cowley, S. (1993) Skill mix: value for whom? *Health Visitor*, **66**(5), 166–168, 171

Cowley, S., Bergen, A., Young, K. and Kavanagh, A. (1994) The challenging nature of needs assessment in primary health care. Paper presented at the Fourth Internation Primary Health Care Conference, London

Cowley, S. and Billings, J.R. (1994a) *Family Health Needs Project Report*, unpublished report, Primary Health Care Development Fund, King's College, London

Cowley, S. and Billings, J.R. (1994b) *A Community Profile of Hastings: Phase 1 of the Family Health Needs Project*, unpublished report, Primary Health Care Development Fund, King's College, London

Culyer, A.J. (1976) *Need and the National Health Service*, Martin Robertson, London

Day, L. (1992) Promoting the health visiting profession. *Health Visitor*, **65**(8), 270–272

Denny, E. (1989) The future of health visiting. *Health Visitor*, **62**(8), 250–251

DHSS (1988) *Public Health in England: The Report of the Committee of Enquiry into the Future Development of the Public Health Function*, HMSO, London

Dobby, J. (1986) *The Development of a Method for the Assessment of Health Visiting*, The Health Promotion Research Trust, London

DoE, (1983) *Urban Deprivation: Information Note No. 2 from the Inner Cities Directorate*, HMSO, London

DoH, (1989a) *Working For Patients*, HMSO, London

DoH (1989b) *Caring for People: Community Care in the Next Decade and Beyond*, HMSO, London

DoH (1989c) *The Role of the District Health Authority*, HMSO, London

DoH (1990) *Caring for People: Implementation Document – Assessment and Case Management*, HMSO, London

DoH (1992) *The Health of the Nation*, HMSO, London

DoH (1993) *Implementing Community Care: Population Needs Assessment, Good Practice Guide*, HMSO, London

Donaldson, C. and Mooney, G. (1991) Needs assessment, priority setting and contracts for health care: an economic view. *British Medical Journal*, **303**, 1529–1530

Donebedian, A. (1977) Some issues in evaluating the quality of nursing care. *American Journal of Public Health*, **5a**(10), 1833–1836

Drennan, V. (ed.) (1988) *Health Visitors and Groups: Politics and Practice*, Heinemann Nursing, Oxford

Drennan, V. (1990) Gathering information from the field. *Nursing Times*, **86**(39), 46–48

Dunnell, K. and Dobbs, J. (1983) *Nurses Working in the Community*, OPCS/HMSO, London

Forrester, P.H. (1991) Assessing health information needs. In *Promoting Choice: Consumer Health Information in the 1990s*, Consumer Health Information Consortium, Loughborough University

Foy, C., Hutchinson, A. and Smythe, J. (1987) Providing census data for general practice. *Journal of the Royal College of General Practice*, **37**, 451–454

Gooch, S. (1989) The health visitor's influence: imperatives for change. *Nursing Standard*, 25 October, 4–5

Goodwin, S. (1988) Whither health visiting? Keynote speech to the Health Visitor's Association Annual Study Conference, Health Visitors' Association, London

Goodwin, S. (1992) Community nursing and the new public health. *Health Visitor*, **65**(3), 78–80

Goodwin, S. (1994) Purchasing effective care for parents and young children. *Health Visitor*, **67**(4), 127–129

Harvey, J. (1994) Assessment of population health needs. Paper presented at the RCN Public Health Conference, London

Hawtin, M., Hughes, G. and Percy-Smith, J. (1994) *Community Profiling: Auditory Social Needs*, OUP, Buckingham

Higgens, R. (1992) Consumerism and participation. *Senior Nurse*, **12**(5), 3–4

Hubley, J. (1982) Making the community profile. *Journal of the Institute of Health Education*, **20**(1), 4–9

Hudson, H. (1992) Needs-led assessment: nice idea, shame about the reality? *Health and Social Care*, **1**, 115–118

Hugman, J. and McCready, S. (1993) Profiles make perfect practice. *Nursing Times*, **89**(27), 46–49

Hull, W. (1989) Measuring effectiveness in health visiting. *Health Visitor*, **62**(4), 113–115

Hunt, M. (1982) Caseload profiles – an alternative to the neighbourhood study. *Health Visitor*, **55**(11), 606–607

HVA (1994) *Professional Briefing: GP Fundholding*, Health Visitors' Association, London

Jack, R. (1992) Case management and social services: welfare or trade fare? *Journal of the British Society of Gerontology*, **2**, 4

Jackson, C. (1989) Wherefore to Oxfordshire? An interview with health visitors. *Health Visitor*, **62**(5), 159–160

Jarman, B. (1984) Underpriviledged areas: validation and distribution of scores. *British Medical Journal*, **289**, 1587–1592

Judge, K. and Solomon, M. (1992) Public opinion and the National Health Service: patterns and perspectives in consumer satisfaction. Paper presented to the Annual Conference of the Society for Social Medicine, University of Nottingham

Kennedy, A. (1992) The community health profile. *Community Outlook*, March, 16

Klein, L. and Thomlinson, P. (1987) Patchwork. *Nursing Times*, **83**(26), 39–40

Knight, B. and Hayes, R. (1981) *Self-Help in the Inner City*, Voluntary Services Council, London

Loomes, G. and McKenzie, L. (1989) The use of QALYS in health care decision-making. *Social Science and Medicine*, **28**, 299–308

Lorber, J. (1980) Is your brain really necessary? *Science*, **210**, 1232–1234

Luker, K. and Orr, J. (eds) (1985) *Health Visiting*, Blackwell Scientific Publications, Oxford

Luker, K. and Orr, J. (1992) *Health Visiting: Towards Community Health Nursing*, Blackwell Scientific Publications, Oxford

McCollam, A. (1992) *Community Care Planning for Mental Health in Scotland*, Scottish Association for Mental Health, Edinburgh

McDowell, D. (1983) Measuring women's occupational mortality. *Population Trends*, **34**, 25–29

Mays, N. (1987) Measuring morbidity for resource allocation. *British Medical Journal*, **295**, 703–706

Morgan, D. (ed.) (1993) *Successful Focus Groups*, Sage, Newbury Park, CA

Morris, J. and Lindlow, V. (1993) *User Participation in Community Care Services*, Community Care Support Force, Leeds

Nelson, K.B. and Ellenberg, J.H. (1982) Children who 'outgrew' cerebral palsy. *Pediatrics*, **69**, 529–536

NHSE (1994) *Health Visitor Marketing Project: Project Report July 1994*. National Health Service Executive, London

NHSME (1991) Assessing Health Care Needs: A DHA Project Discussion Document, National Health Service Management Executive, London

NHSME (1992) *Guidance on the extension of hospital and community health services elements of the GP fund-holding scheme from April 1993*, EL (92) 48, National Health Service Management Executive, London

Niehoff, J. and Schneider, F. (1993) Epidemiology and the criticism of the risk factor approach. In *Towards a New Science of Health* (eds R. Lafaille and S. Fulder) Routledge, London

OPCS (1992) *Census Newsletter: Coverage Check from the 1991 Census Validation Survey*, HMSO, London

Orr, J. (1992a) Health visiting and the community. In *Health Visiting*, 2nd edn (eds K. Luker and J. Orr), Blackwell Scientific Publications, Oxford

Orr, J. (1992b) Individual and family needs. In *Health Visiting*, 2nd edn (eds K. Luker and J. Orr), Blackwell Scientific Publications

Osborn, A. F. and Morris, A.C. (1979) The rationale for a composite index of social class and its evaluation. *British Journal of Sociology*, **30**(1), 39–60

Patrick, D.L. (1986) Measurement of health and quality of life. In *Sociology as Applied to Medicine* (eds D.L. Patrick and G. Scambler), Baillière Tindall, Eastbourne

Peckham, S. and Spanton, J. (1994) Community development approaches to health needs assessment. *Health Visitor*, **67**(4), 124–125

Phillimore, P., Beattie, A. and Townsend, P. (1994) Widening inequality of health in northern England, 1981–91. *British Medical Journal*, **308**, 1125–1128

Phillips, C., Palfrey, C. and Thomas, P. (1994) *Evaluating Health and Social Care*, Macmillan, Basingstoke

Pinker, R. (1982) An alternative view: appendix B. In *Social Workers: Their Role and Tasks*, National Institute for Social Work, Bedford Press, London

RCN (1992) *School Profiling*, Royal College of Nursing, London

RCN (1993) *The GP Practice Population Profile*, Royal College of Nursing, London

Richards, J. (1991) Consumer-oriented planning. In *Community Care Plans – the First Steps*, SSI Department of Health, London

Richardson, A., Charney, M. and Hanmer-Lloyd, S. (1992) Public opinion and purchasing. *British Medical Journal*, **304**, 680–682

Rijke, R. (1985) Cancer and the development of will. *Journal of Theoretical Medicine*, **6**, 133–142

Rijke, R. (1993) Health in medical science: from determinism towards autonomy. In *Towards a New Science of Health* (eds R. Lafaille and S. Fulder), Routledge, London

Roberts, H. and Magowan, R. (1994) Local sensitivities. *Health Service Journal*, 10 March, 30–31

Roberts, H., Smith, S. and Bryce, C. (1993) Prevention is better . . . *Sociology of Health and Illness*, **16**(4), 447–463

Robinson, J. (1985) Health visiting and health. In *Political Issues in Nursing* (ed. R. White), Wiley, London

Rodgers, J. (1994) Power to the people. *Health Service Journal*, 24 March, 28–29

Rodrigues, L. (1989) Whither health visiting: a PR exercise? *Health Visitor*, **62**(11), 335

Rohe, J.W. and Kahn, K.I. (1987) Human ageing: usual and successful. *Science* **237**, 143–149

Seedhouse, D. (1986) *Health: The Foundation for Achievement*, Wiley, Chichester

Southampton and S.W. Hants. Health Commission (1993) *Consumer and Public Health Commissioning: Learning from Experience*, Southampton and S.W. Hants Health Commission, Southampton

Stalker, K. (1993) The best laid plans . . . gang aft agley? Assessing population needs in Scotland. *Health and Social Care*, **2**, 1–9

Stevens, A. and Gabby, J. (1991) Needs assessment needs assessment. *Health Trends*, **23**(1), 20–23

Thayer, R. (1973) Measuring need in the social services. *Social and Economic Administration*, 7 May, 91–105

Thunhurst, C. (1985) The analysis of small area statistics and planning for health. *The Statistician*, **34**, 93–106

Townsend, P., Phillimore, P. and Beattie, A. (1988) *Health and Deprivation: Inequality in the North*, Routledge, London

Townsend, P., Simpson, D. and Tibbs, N. (1985) Inequalities in health in the city of Bristol: a preliminary view of statistical evidence. *International Journal of Health Service*, **15**(4), 637–663

Twinn, S. and Cowley, S. (1992) *The Principles of Health Visiting: A Re-examina-*

tion, Health Visitors' Association/United Kingdom Standing Conference, London

Twinn, S., Dauncey, J. and Carnell, J. (1990) *The Process of Health Profiling*, Health Visitors' Association, London

Wagstaff, S., Paci, P. and van Doorslaer, E. (1991) On the measurement of inequalities in health. *Social Science and Medicine*, **33**(5), 545–557

Whitehead, M. (1987) *The Health Divide*, Penguin, London

Williams, A. (1987) Health economics: the cheerful face of the dismal science? In *Health and Economics* (ed. A. Williams), Macmillan, London

Wilson, R. (1981) Do health indicators indicate health? *American Journal of Public Health*, **71**(5), 461–463

Wistow, G., Leedham, I. and Hardy, B. (1992) *A Preliminary Analysis of a Sample of Community Care Plans*, Department of Health, London

Yin, R.K. (1989) *Case Study Research: Design and Methods*, Sage Publications, Thousand Oaks, California

Yorkshire Health (1990) *Health Visiting: the Yorkshire Approach*, Yorkshire Regional Health Authority, York

Young, K. and Haynes, R. (1993) Assessing population needs in primary health care: the problem of GP attachment. *Journal of Interprofessional Care*, **7**(1), 15–27

24

Partnership in care

Sally Kendall

● **Introduction**

A number of reports and recent legislation have suggested directions for nursing practice largely determined by the concept of partnership in care. In order to make some sense of the plethora of literature which is available to practitioners in this field, it is appropriate to analyse this concept and its implications for community nursing practice from a critical research-based perspective. This chapter therefore aims to examine briefly the policy context of partnership, to review critically some of the literature which offers a conceptual analysis of partnership and to bring these perspectives together through an analysis of practice. Some conclusions about the ideology and the reality of partnership will be sought.

● **Partnership in the context of policy**

Among recent policies directed not only at a national level but also specifically at the nursing profession, there is evidence of an emerging ideology promoting the concept of partnership. Among these are The Children Act (DoH, 1990a), *The Health of the Nation* (DoH, 1992), *The Patient's Charter* (DoH, 1991), The Community Care Act (DoH, 1990b) and *Changing Childbirth* (DoH, 1993). While all these documents have been criticized for their rhetoric, there nevertheless appears to be some underlying principles which could potentially, at least, guide practice. The Children Act which sought to rationalize muddled and diverse legislation in relation to the care and protection of children, places far more emphasis on the needs of children and their perceptions of the world than those imposed on them by adults, as was evident in previous legislation. The rights of children are recognized, as is their right to consistency of care in order to reduce disruption and change and the right to be safe and protected from harm as well as the right to be respected as an individual. The implications for practice are profound since the Act is requiring both professionals and parents to re-examine their values and beliefs about children and their perceived needs and to accept that these may differ fundamentally from those held by the children. Indeed, working in partnership with parents, carers, other agencies and children themselves to protect children may require a new way of thinking for some practitioners.

The Health of the Nation is the response of the Department of Health (DoH, 1992) to the World Health Organisation (WHO) initiative for 'Health for All' (WHO, 1978). The DoH document sets out the agenda for health and the health service for the next decade in the form of five target areas for improving the health of the nation. These include reductions in coronary heart disease and strokes, cancers, accidents and improvements in mental health and sexual health. The document has been the subject of much criticism for its selection of targets which normal trends would achieve anyway and its total failure to address the effects of poverty on health (see, for example, the Public Health Alliance, 1992). Nevertheless, much of the potential of the policy rests on the ideology of partnership. This is seen in terms of individuals working in partnership with each other, of communities working in partnership with local services and of professional groups working in partnership with each other, a process summed up as 'healthy alliances'. The ideology stems from the WHO (1985) definition of health promotion which is described as 'a process of enabling people to increase control over and improve their health'. This theme is taken up in *The Patient's Charter* (DoH, 1991) where users of the health service are advised in the guide to primary health care that 'You will be treated as a partner in the care and attention you receive'. This implies partnership on a one-to-one basis with the doctor or the named nurse, whereas the notion of 'healthy alliances' and the essence of the Community Care Act 1990 is more directed towards partnership at a macro level where the individual is just one element of a system which operates at the social and political interface.

A range of issues are raised for the community nurse. What does partnership mean for the nurse and for the person or community? At what level should partnership happen? What effect will partnership have on health? The following sections will attempt to address these questions.

● **The meaning of partnership**

The concept of partnership has become a 'buzz word' in the nursing and health literature. It is necessary to explore the meaning behind the rhetoric and to examine its relevance to community nursing practice.

Most theories of nursing include a reference to partnership; the whole basis of primary nursing rests on the notion that nurse and patient will work together to achieve goals as the patient perceives them (Manthey, 1992). In addition, it is perceived as the basis for therapeutic care. For example, Meutzel (1988) describes a model for therapeutic nursing in which partnership is a key concept in the development of a therapeutic relationship. This is represented theoretically alongside concepts of intimacy and reciprocity, implying a relationship between the nurse and the patient which resembles that of mother and child or lovers. This representation of partnership requires the practitioner to have a great deal of self-awareness and reflexivity. Often, it appears as a taken-for-granted concept with little analysis of the skills and processes involved. Indeed, Salvage (1992) has warned against nurses taking the concept on board too lightly as she believes that, to be effective, nurses need a greater knowledge and understanding of psychotherapeutic theories and techniques. Salvage also argues that there are issues of power and control to be considered too. If nurses are perceived as those in possession of the expertise and knowledge in relation to health, the patient may prefer to accept a passive role (Parsons, 1951); equally, the nurse may find it difficult to relinquish the role of expert. Indeed, Waterworth and Luker (1990), found, in a small study of hospital in-patients, that some people were, in fact, reluctant collaborators in their care.

There is also a tendency in the literature to equate partnership with empowerment, as though the terms are interchangeable. Partnership can perhaps be seen as a surrogate term for empowerment, but it does not mean the same thing, neither does one automatically lead to the other. However, the author believes that in order to empower clients or communities, partnership is a necessary prerequisite. A partner has been defined by the *Oxford English Dictionary* as a sharer. As such, it could be argued that the community nurse should be able to share knowledge, expertise, skills, beliefs, values and decision-making with the client or family and to accept what they offer in these areas as both valid and respected, even when it differs fundamentally from her or his own views. As a partner, the practitioner should refrain from making judgements about the individual or family, but should be able to share perspectives on an equal footing. Ashworth *et al*. (1992) have addressed this issue in relation to patient participation and they suggest that

> *participation with others presupposes that each person is receptive to others' contributions, and that each is able to assume the receptiveness of the others.*

The social interaction that presumes partnership and participation also presumes to understand perceived roles and status as well as beliefs and attitudes underlying biases and prejudices of the other. These are dangerous assumptions in a health care system built on hierarchies, power and bureaucratic control.

Empowerment

In discussing the concept of partnership, issues of power and control arise and are inextricably linked to the notion that people or communities can be empowered through partnership. Tones (1991) has explored the concept of empowerment in relation to the psychology of control and health promotion. He suggests that

> *Empowerment refers to the process whereby an individual – or a community of individuals – acquires power, i.e. the capacity to*

control other people and resources. Self-empowerment focuses on the individual's capacity to control his or her own life.

Likewise, Kalnins *et al*. (1992) suggest that empowerment means

that people must feel that they have significant control over their health and the conditions that affect their health.

A third definition of empowerment suggested by Gibson (1991) is

a social process of recognising, promoting and enhancing people's abilities to meet their own needs, solve their own problems and mobilise the necessary resources in order to feel in control of their own lives.

These definitions seem to have developed from an understanding that lack of empowerment means that people perceive themselves as powerless and not in control of their own life or the conditions which determine health. Indeed, if it is accepted that the determinants of health extend beyond lifestyle and biomedical factors to environmental, social and political (as demonstrated, for example, by Blackburn, 1991, and Blaxter, 1990), then it can be argued that individuals may not be in control of their health and may need some help or support in the way previously described by Gibson (1991).

Lobstein (1992), in his work with the Food Commission, has commented, for example, on the need for poor families to provide 'comforting' foods in the form of crisps and hamburgers to their children, as this is more likely to be eaten and to fulfil the social and emotional aspects of eating rather than 'health' foods. If community health care nurses are to be involved in working in partnership with families and empowering children, it raises questions of the extent to which they have a role in enabling families to overcome the effects of poverty. This is a particularly interesting question when considered in the context of *The Health of the Nation* (DoH, 1992) which makes no reference to poverty as a determinant of ill health and therefore, presumably, implying that health professionals have no significant role in this field.

However, Tones (1992) has argued that community action initiatives may be useful in this respect, by empowering individuals to make up empowered communities. In turn, empowered communities may have some control over policy issues such as housing, planning of playgrounds and leisure centres, and the control of pollution. From this perspective, it can be argued that community health care nurses can do a great deal in terms of consciousness raising among children and their families to help them to develop the life skills needed to be pro-active. Much of this kind of work can be carried out at an individual and small group level, where the majority of community nursing is currently practised.

It may be possible for some practitioners to work at a community level using the Freire model of empowerment (Freire, 1972). Freire's approach stems from a Marxist ideology which advocates the emancipation of the working classes. In his native country, Freire believed that the most oppressed people in this impoverished South American society could be empowered through education. By working directly with communities and key workers, critical consciousness raising combined with education enables communities to recognize their own needs and start demanding for themselves the necessary changes. Drennan (1985) used some of the principles of Freire's work in a study in North Paddington of health visiting in a deprived London borough. She worked very closely with local communities, organizations and voluntary groups to enable needs to be identified and the communities themselves to begin to take health-related action.

Despite the encouraging work that has been done, Foster and Mayall (1990) found, in their longitudinal study of health education with families, that health visitors tended not to adopt this 'bottom up' approach to health education. However, generally the case for many practitioners working with the family, the client or the school will continue to be the major focus of their attention. It therefore seems logical to pursue the discussion within this context.

● Partnership in practice

An appropriate way to explore practising in partnership is through the presentation of the model case, as described by Walker and Avant (1983). A case study from health visiting practice is presented below, which attempts to demonstrate the issues of partnership, advocacy and empowerment and relationships in health promotion for the whole family:

Joanna and Richard Mead were expecting their second baby. Susannah was five years old and looking forward to the arrival of her new baby brother or sister. Their health visitor, Ann, had come to know the family well since the birth of Susannah and had seen Joanna regularly during her pregnancy as she had attended ante-natal classes. At the last of these classes, Joanna confided in Ann that she had not felt any fetal movements for over 24 hours. While not wanting to alarm Joanna unduly, Ann listened to her anxiety and suggested she went to the maternity unit that morning for fetal monitoring. When the baby boy was born the next day, Ann was immediately notified by the maternity unit as there were some manifest problems which were later to be diagnosed as Blackfan–Diamond syndrome. This meant that baby David had a cleft palate, no distinction between his chin and his neck, a poorly developed rib cage leading to respiratory problems and brain damage resulting from hypoxic seizures. He required an immediate tracheostomy, nasogastric feeding and oxygen therapy, as well as anti-epileptic therapy.

Ann visited Joanna and David in the maternity unit and it soon became obvious that, despite the immediacy of David's problems, Joanna had realized his poor prognosis and her one wish was to take him home to die with his family. Ann's first response was to resist Joanna's wishes. Ann felt that the family would have enough to cope with without the added responsibility of caring for a very sick baby. Through the trusting relationship she had developed with Joanna, she felt able to share this initial response. However, she then listened to Joanna's perspective on the problem and observed her lovingly handling David and managing his tubes like a veteran, using her additional knowledge and skill as a mother to anticipate his needs and care for him. Ann listened to what Joanna had to say about the need for the family to be together, for David to be in a home environment and for Susannah to know and care for her baby brother. Ann recognized that there were some important principles operating here of which the most paramount was the right of the child to be with his family and the rights of the family to lovingly care for their dying baby. Although David's health was extremely poor he had a right to a quality of life and the health of the rest of the family might be in jeopardy if they were forced to nurse him in hospital.

It soon became obvious, however, that the hospital personnel did not share this view and the opportunity to care for David at home was opposed by all concerned. The family needed to make a decision that was right for David and by enabling Joanna and Richard to weigh up all the possibilities, and communicate with hospital and community staff, Ann felt that the decision they had made to take David home had been arrived at through a process of participation. Ann found that through listening to Joanna, by observing and assessing her coping skills, by recognizing the importance of the baby's welfare, she was working in partnership with Joanna, and had become an advocate for David and his family.

Joanna and Richard spend the next few days convincing the hospital staff that they could manage David at home. Meanwhile, Ann investigated all possible support systems in the community. The Macmillan nurses were contacted, and the District Nursing Service and Community Service Volunteers. All were able to offer some help, albeit limited. The school nurse from Susannah's school was kept informed so that she was aware of the situation and its potential effects on the child. Finally, with the support of Ann's manager, David was allowed to come home. Joanna wanted life for him to be as normal as possible and to this end she took him out in the pram (with oxygen and suction!), allowed Susannah to hold and feed him and encouraged all who visited to have the courage to nurture David as they would a 'normal' baby. Ann learned a great deal about risk-taking, courage and love from this remarkable woman. She also learned about the importance of advocacy and partnership for promoting the health of the child in need. When David died a few weeks later, Ann was able to mourn for him with the rest of the family and the many other carers who had given support and practical help, in the knowledge that she had acted professionally by sharing perceptions, knowledge, skills and the decision-making process with the family.

This case study is a true story, although names have been changed to ensure confidentiality. While it could be seen as a rather extreme case, it serves to illustrate some important points about partnership and advocacy. First, where there is a perceived need, that need should be explored from the perspective of the person in need. In this case, the needs of David as a psychosocial being were paramount. It could be argued that a concentration on his biological need and the need to sustain life were more salient for the hospital staff, but this view does not take into account the health and needs of the whole family.

However, some research has shown that health visitors are not always able to share needs from the client's perspective. Indeed, for example, research by the author (Kendall, 1991a) found that health visitors used the interaction during a home visit to meet their own agenda and that perceptions of need differed between health visitors and their clients. Pearson (1991) also found that lay and professional perceptions of health may differ. Such studies indicate the need to reflect on professional values and develop skills in self-awareness and communication which will enable practitioners to put theory into practice.

Barker (1992), on the other hand, has demonstrated, in extensive research with health visitors, how working in partnership with families can have significantly beneficial effects. Perhaps one of the most interesting findings from his work has been that 'the most significant contribution to the changes in the children occurred as a result of changes in the mother's self-esteem'. These findings derived from an approach to practice which encouraged health visitors in the intervention group to 'work with families and as far as possible encourage them to find their own solutions to their problems'. There is a lack of qualitative evidence from Barker's studies of the process of partnership, perhaps demonstrating the need for a process-outcome approach to this area of research.

It is important to acknowledge that advocacy may be a traumatic and isolating experience for the professional concerned. In the case above, the health visitor found herself in conflict against hospital staff in support of this family, which without the support of her line manager could have been a destructive experience. At the same time, the community nurse must be accountable for her practice under the Professional Code of Conduct (UKCC, 1992). If promoting the health of the family and child within a framework of partnership was her aim, then she had to take on an advocacy role and be accountable for the risks which are inherent in this approach to care. Manthey (1992) has argued that risk-taking in the nursing professional is often associated with a punitive management style. According to her, nurses are unlikely to make risky decisions where they have to be accountable for their actions and may face retribution for 'mistakes'. This is especially the case when nurses are rarely conferred the authority to act in a way which is commensurate with the responsibilities they are expected to assume. From this perspective, partnership in its fullest sense is difficult to put into practice. The issue of participative decision-making is also raised here. Decision-making in a crisis can be particularly difficult for both the parents and the professionals (Bond and Kendall, 1990).

However, there is evidence to suggest that clients prefer to be involved in making decisions about their health (see, for example, Slimmer and Brown, 1985) and that children themselves can be involved in this process (Kaufman, 1985). It is important to reiterate that the process of participative decision-making does not just happen – it requires skill and insight on the part of the community nurses to be able to reflect on their own perceptions and to explore the perceptions of the client or family.

Finally, it is clear that by working in partnership with the family and other health professionals, by encouraging participative decision-making and acting as an advocate, the health visitor in the model case above helped to empower the family concerned by enabling them to take some control over the traumatic events in their lives. Through his parents and the support of the health visitor, David was empowered to enjoy the last few weeks in a family environment. From this perspective, through a partnership approach to care, the health of the whole family was promoted, although the cost to the health visitor in terms of self-confidence and stress may have been high.

It has been argued, then, that in order to work in partnership, community nurses may need to utilize the concept of empowerment if there is to be a meaningful outcome to practice. At the same time, a degree of doubt has been expressed at the extent to which practitioners are able to draw upon knowledge and skills which promote such an approach. For example, Kendall (1991a) carried out a detailed study of the health visitor–client interaction in which client participation was the phenomenon of interest. Findings from 62 transcribed interactions suggested that the health visitor largely controlled the encounter in terms of carrying through her own agenda, giving unsolicited advice, asking most of the questions and failing to elicit from clients their perceptions of the encounter or the health issue under discussion. The data demonstrated not only the lack of interpersonal skill but also no explicit recognition of the issues underpinning a partnership or empowering approach to enable the individual to have a greater sense of personal control over health-related matters. There may be several explanations for these findings, not least of which may be that touched on above, which is by maintaining control over the encounter the health visitor is less likely to generate any difficult decisions for which she or he will have to assume accountability.

Dennis (1987) identified three dimensions of client control using self-efficacy as a theoretical framework, in a study which aimed to identify activities which gave clients a sense of control during hospitalization. These dimensions were: knowing and fulfilling the patient role; being involved in decision-making; and directing interpersonal and environmental components. This study concluded that hospitalized patients wanted to have control over the people and events that had an impact on their wellbeing and quality of life. Extrapolating from the findings of this study, it seems appropriate that clients and families should be fully involved in understanding the role of the community nurse and their own roles as clients. This would involve making it explicit that the practitioner recognizes that the client has expertise rather than the practitioner taking on the role of expert. Also the community nurse could, within this theoretical framework, encourage client decision-making and enable individuals to take control over their environment and people around them.

Gibson (1991) identifies self-efficacy as one of the factors within the client domain of empowerment. However, such a role by the practitioner requires a knowledge of the concept of self-efficacy described by Bandura (1977) alongside considerable skill in eliciting perceived self-efficacy for which Bandura gives no guidance. This again implies that skills in communication are imperative and that the practitioner has the confidence to take responsibility for and be accountable for any decisions which are reached. For example, the practice nurse may advise a young girl about contraception on the basis that the girl's perceived self-efficacy in using contraception is high. In combination with a shared knowledge base and a collaborative approach, by understanding the risks of sexual encounters during the teenage years the practice nurse may be able to account fully for her actions and accept the risk that the young girl may become pregnant. The author has considered elsewhere the hypothetical application of self-efficacy theory to health visiting practice as a way to potentially empower parents (Kendall, 1991b). However, the theory needs to be empirically tested for its validity in a practice situation, in terms of its usefulness for identifying client needs, enhancing client participation and identifying client outcomes.

Research from other areas of community nursing also presents positive examples of nurses working in partnership. Ross (1988), for example, carried out a study from a district nursing perspective in which a drug guide for elderly people was evaluated. The drug guide itself was drawn up in consultation with other primary health care team members and was a response to the problem of compliance with drug therapy among elderly people in relation to principles of self-care and participation. Ross demonstrated that after using the guide with a sample of 90 people over 60 years in one practice population, an association was found with an improvement in patient knowledge of drugs, reduction in disagreement between doctors and nurses as well as between professionals and patients, and an improvement in the organization of medical records. The implications of this study are important in terms of working in partnership with colleagues and clients and the potential effect on the health outcomes for elderly people. Not only was their health promoted through an enhanced likelihood of the appropriate drugs being taken, but also their self-efficacy and sense of personal control was also potentially increased (in the studies by Ross this was not measured).

Methven (1989), in a study of midwifery practice, found that, compared to the traditional obstetric history-taking in the antenatal clinic, assessment interview using a nursing process approach produced information of much greater quality and quantity. This was achieved by recording interviews between midwives and pregnant women and repeating interviews using the nursing process. The research was limited by the fact that the researcher carried out the second interview herself. It nevertheless demonstrated the potential of using good interviewing skills and an approach to care grounded in the concept of partnership.

● **Conclusion**

In many respects, some of the issues and ideas presented above may not be recognized as 'mainstream' care as far as community nurses are concerned. However, the author believes that the issues of empowerment and partnership must be confronted for effective practice in caring and health promotion. Although the targets set in *The Health of the Nation* (DoH, 1992) do not address the main determinants of ill-health, such as poverty and inequality, practitioners have to find effective ways of meeting these targets. By utilizing the concepts embedded in documents such as The Children Act (DoH, 1990a), *The Patient's Charter* (DoH, 1991) and *The Health of the Nation* (DoH, 1992), practitioners can identify strategies to enable them to take an empowering approach in health promotion. Community nurses are at the helm of this initiative, as they are working directly with clients, families and communities and could be particularly influential in changing the health of the nation.

There are a range of issues which are important for education and research in community nursing to address. The concept of partnership is one which needs to take a more prominent place in curricula and the knowledge underpinning this concept should be developed, particularly that pertaining to issues of power, control and empowerment. It is imperative that practitioners try to understand more about the client's perspective in this field and how well-designed research studies are conducted by appropriately prepared community nurses, to test the effectiveness in terms of health outcomes of putting this knowledge into practice.

Communicating effectively with the client and the family has to be the central aim of any course leading to a qualification in community health care nursing. However, there has been ample evidence from the literature, such as that of health visiting and midwifery, to demonstrate that this has not always been the case in practice (Sefi, 1985; Kirkham, 1989; Kendall, 1991a). It is now imperative that the opportunity is taken by educationalists and practitioners to rectify this situation. Although there is some evidence that this is already happening, by reflecting on and developing skills and knowledge providing insights into the process of care as well as outcome, it may be possible to develop genuine and positive partnerships in care.

References

Ashworth, P., Longmate, M.A. and Morrison, P. (1992) Patient participation: its meaning and significance in the context of caring. *Journal of Advanced Nursing*, **17**, 1430–1439

Bandura, A. (1977) Self-efficacy: towards a unifying theory of behavioural change. *Psychological Review*, **84**(2), 191–215

Barker, W. (1992) Health visiting: action research in a controlled environment. *International Journal of Nursing Studies*, **29**(3), 251–259

Blackburn, C. (1991) *Poverty and Health: Working with Families*, Open University Press, Buckingham

Blaxter, M. (1990) *Health and Lifestyles*, Tavistock/Routledge, London

Bond, M. and Kendall, S. (1990) *Improve Your Decision Making*, Distance Learning Centre, South Bank Polytechnic, London

Dennis, K. (1987) Dimensions of client control. *Nursing Research*, **36**(3), 151–156

DoH (1990a) *The Care of Children*, HMSO, London

DoH (1990b) *The NHS and Community Care Act*, HMSO, London

DoH (1991) *The Patient's Charter*, HMSO, London

DoH (1992) *The Health of the Nation*, HMSO, London

DoH (1993) *Changing Childbirth*, HMSO, London

Drennan, V. (1985) *Working in a Different Way*, North Paddington Health Authority, London

Foster, M.-C. and Mayall, B. (1990) Health visitors as educators. *Journal of Advanced Nursing*, **15**(3), 286–292

Freire, P. (1972) *Pedagogy of the Oppressed*, Penguin, Harmondsworth

Gibson, C.H. (1991) A concept analysis of empowerment. *Journal of Advanced Nursing*, **16**, 354–361

Kalnins, I., McQueen, D.V., Badsett, K.C. *et al*. (1992) Children, empowerment and health promotion: some new directions in research and practice. *Health Promotion International*, **7**(1), 53–59

Kaufman, D. (1985) An interview guide for helping children make health care decisions. *Pediatric Nursing*, **11**(5), 365–367

Kendall, S. (1991a) An analysis of the health visitor client interaction. The effect of the health visiting process on client participation. Unpublished PhD thesis, King's College, London University

Kendall, S. (1991b) A home visit by a health visitor using Bandura's theory of self-efficacy. In *Caring for Children: Towards Partnership with Families* (ed. A. While), Edward Arnold, London

Kirkham, M. (1989) Midwives and information giving during labour. In *Midwives, Research and Childbirth*, Vol. 1 (eds S. Robinson and A.M. Thomson), Chapman and Hall, London

Lobstein, T. (1992) Commentary on eating among poor families. *Sunday Times*, 31 Oct.

Manthey, M. (1992) *The Practice of Primary Nursing*, Macmillan, London

Methven, R. (1989) Recording an obstetric history or relating to a pregnant woman? A study of the antenatal booking interview. In *Midwives, Research and Childbirth*, Vol. 1 (eds S. Robinson and A.M. Thomson), Chapman and Hall, London

Meutzel, P. (1988) Therapeutic nursing. In *Primary Nursing: Nursing in the Oxford and Burford Nursing Development Units* (ed. A. Pearson), Croom Helm, London

Parsons, T. (1951) *The Social System*, Routledge and Kegan Paul, London

Pearson, P. (1991) Clients' perceptions: the use of case studies in developing theory. *Journal of Advanced Nursing*, **16**(5), 521–528

Public Health Alliance (1992) *The Health of the Nation: Challenges for a New Government*, Public Health Alliance, Birmingham

Ross, F. (1988) Information sharing between patients, nurses and doctors: evaluation of a drug guide for old people in primary health care. In *Recent Advances in Nursing: Excellence in Nursing*, Vol. 21 (ed. R.A. Johnson), Churchill Livingstone, Edinburgh

Salvage, J. (1992) The new nursing: empowering patients or empowering nurses? In *Policy Issues in Nursing* (eds J. Robinson, A. Gray and R. Elkan), Open University Press, Buckingham

Sefi, S. (1985) The first visit: a study of health visitor–mother verbal interaction. Unpublished MA dissertation, University of Warwick

Slimmer, L. and Brown, R. (1985) Patients' decision making process in medication administration for control of hyperactivity. *Journal of School Health*, **55**(6), 221–225

Tones, K. (1991) Health promotion, empowerment and the psychology of control. *Journal of the Institute of Health Education*, **29**(1), 17–26

Tones, K. (1992) Theory of health promotion. Unpublished paper presented at Promoting Health – International Research Conference for Nursing, Queen Elizabeth Hall, London, September

UKCC (1992) *Code of Professional Conduct for the Nurse, Midwife and Health Visitor*, 3rd edn, UKCC, London

Walker, L. and Avant, K. (1983) *Strategies for Theory Construction in Nursing*, Appleton Century Crofts, Norwalk, Connecticut

Waterworth, S. and Luker, K. (1990) Reluctant collaborators: do patients want to be involved in decisions concerning care? *Journal of Advanced Nursing*, **15**, 971–976

WHO (1978) *Primary Health Care*, Report of the International Conference on Primary Health Care held at Alma-Ata, USSR, 6–12 September, World Health Organisation, Geneva

WHO (1985) *Health Promotion*. A WHO discussion document on the concept and principles. *Journal of the Institute of Health Education*, **23**(1), 431–435

25

The role of the clinical nurse specialist: an approach to care

Angela Williams

● Introduction

Although the idea that nurses should consult experts outside their immediate work group has been acknowledged in the UK since the 1980s, the concept has not been well developed (Everson, 1981; Barron, 1983). It is in response to the identified need for greater knowledge and clinical expertise in the domain of patient and client care that the position has been changing. Any nurse acting as a resource and providing support in the management of patient and client care is required to practise within a framework of theoretically-based knowledge and combine that knowledge with clinical expertise. This chapter considers how nurses might act as a resource and provide support to other nurses; the roles and skills required when acting as a resource and providing support in patient and client care; and models of liaison between a 'resource and support nurse' and other carers. The development of the nursing speciality of lymphoedema is used as an example.

Stages along the nursing continuum

A developmental continuum exists between novice nurses and nurses with clinical expertise. Although experience is one component that differentiates the various levels of nursing expertise, experience alone does not make an expert nurse. According to Benner (1984), the expert nurse uses analytical problem-solving and underpins practice with detailed knowledge. However, it is important to recognize that the attributes of the 'expert nurse' and those of the 'clinical nurse specialist' (CNS) are distinguishable. What differentiates the CNS from the expert nurse is the depth and breadth of knowledge; the advanced clinical judgement; and clinical expertise which is evident in the judgement and decisions about both clinical and non-clinical variables (Spross and Baggerly, 1989; Kitzman, 1989). Dirschel (1976) states that in order to meet the health needs of a community the nursing profession needs scholarly practitioners who can translate their advanced preparation into practice. Indeed, in America, the CNS has studied at a postgraduate level (masters or doctorate), this being a primary criterion before being considered a CNS.

In the UK, such criteria are not held – formal entry to a nursing speciality is located at a post-registration level, generally following syllabuses laid down by the National Boards for Nursing, Midwifery and Health Visiting which offer a theoretical and practice-based education in the chosen speciality (Cheay and Moon, 1993). In the new nursing speciality of lymphoedema until recently, there have only been study days and short courses offering training for a CNS in the subject. A diploma course is now available at one site in the UK.

In situations where nurses are not aware of the differences between the way in which the expert nurse and the CNS function, there could be role confusion (Castledine, 1986). Indeed, it is vital to recognize that specialization within an area of nursing practice does not mean that practitioners are necessarily CNSs. The different titles designated to the nurses infer the role and behaviour to be expected (Baker and Kramer, 1970).

The American Nurses' Association (ANA, 1980) describes specialization as 'a mark of the advancement of the nursing profession' and states it involves concentration on a selected part of the whole field of nursing. Societal and professional forces continue to shape the direction of nursing specialization. Societal forces that have contributed to the increase in specialization include growth in the amount and complexity of knowledge and technology and the focus of public attention on the need for specialization (Naisbitt, 1982). Professional forces include the presence within nursing of pioneers who test out new practices and obtain greater depth of understanding of a segment of nursing and nursing's desire to advance in a more clinical direction (Christman, 1965). The development of the CNS and the progress in lymphoedema treatment in the UK in the past decade are two responses to these forces. The American Nurses' Association (ANA, 1980) has identified five main factors that give rise to specialization, as shown in Table 25.1.

Obviously, within all levels of nursing a nurse can offer support and be a resource to colleagues. However, the degree of support and the amount of additional knowledge provided will in part be dependent on the nurses' knowledge of and interest in the particular topic. For patients and clients to benefit most effectively from the breadth of practical knowledge, a team of nurses needs to be aware of each other's interests and areas of advanced knowledge and be prepared to consult and advise each other as required. If a topic or appropriate depth of knowledge is

Table 25.1   Factors giving rise to specialization (From ANA, 1980, by permission)

1.	An increasing amount and complexity of knowledge and technology
2.	The need to obtain greater depth of understanding of a segment of nursing and to test new practices related to that segment of nursing
3.	The centring of public attention and funds on an area of nursing practice
4.	The complexity of services exceeding the prevailing knowledge and skills of general practitioners
5.	The expansion of part of a professional field

not available within the immediate team of nurses, specialized advice should be sought. In this way nurses can implement the widest and most current knowledge in patient and client care.

A CNS in lymphoedema care

An example of the implementation of patient and client care by professionals with differing levels of knowledge is illustrated in the UK by the Enfield Health Authority Lymphoedema Project (Williams, 1992; Williams, 1993a). The community-based lymphoedema service was initially set up in January 1992 supported by The Queen's Nursing Institute. A district nurse with an interest and basic knowledge of lymphoedema management was identified in each of the health authority's three localities. Overseeing the project was a nurse co-ordinator who was a CNS in lymphoedema, employed by another health authority. Prior to this development patients and clients with lymphoedema, as in the rest of the UK, were told they had to 'learn to live with it' or were offered a few sessions using a pneumatic compression pump (Badger, 1994).

The three district nurses, identified as the 'lymphoedema key workers', treated those lymphoedema patients and clients referred in their locality, in addition to the usual district nursing case load, and were supported and assisted by their primary health care colleagues. The co-ordinator was used as the key workers' resource and support in the management of those patients and clients with more complicated lymphoedema. All community nurses were encouraged to join visits and share in the care, and the general practitioners were regularly involved in discussions about the patients' and clients' progress. In this way there was informal learning about the condition. A multidisciplinary study session clarified the means of diagnosing lymphoedema and the use and value of the service. It was encouraging to note that there was a decrease in the number of inappropriate referrals and a steady referral rate, indicating greater awareness of lymphoedema and its inherent problems.

However, the number of patients and clients became too high to continue this system of lymphoedema care additional to the usual district nursing case load. It was therefore agreed that a community-based CNS in lymphoedema care was needed within this health authority to replace the non-clinical co-ordinator. This CNS would assist with the clinical practice as well as expand the educator and consultant roles. The CNS would act as the resource and support to the lymphoedema advisers in the district.

Using this model, the primary health care team, the lymphoedema advisers and the CNS all have an increasing knowledge of lymphoedema care. All levels of community nurses may be involved in the clinical practice, but refer to a colleague with greater depth of knowledge as their resource and support when required. In addition to improved patient and client care, each health care professional's position is maximized, encouraging personal development at all levels as well as improved patient and client care. By the end of the first year this model of care, involving a CNS acting as a resource to generic staff and care given by community nurses, appeared to have benefited both community nurses and the patients and clients. A similar finding was reported by Layzell and McCarthy (1993) with CNSs in HIV/AIDS in one regional health authority in England.

● **The CNS role**

Nurses as a resource and support

Acting as a resource and providing support encompasses many sub-roles related to direct and indirect patient and client care. The CNS who is expected to advance the nursing profession as a whole and to advance the speciality field is the definitive resource and support for patient and client care with expert clinical practice and advanced knowledge. Consideration of the sub-roles of the CNS will illustrate the roles and skills required in acting as a resource and providing support.

The CNS's task is complex, and many authors have described the various roles of the CNS (Sills, 1983; RCN, 1988; Barron, 1989). Hamric (1989) considered the CNS role from four perspectives:

● baseline or primary criteria before one can be considered a CNS
● four major sub-roles of the CNS which all must be practiced in some degree
● a set of skills or competencies the CNS uses in implementing the sub-roles
● variables significantly influencing the CNS role expression and implementation.

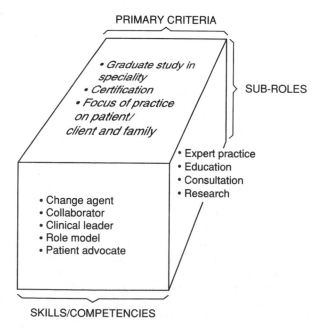

Figure 25.1 Core definition of the CNS (From Hamric, 1989, by permission)

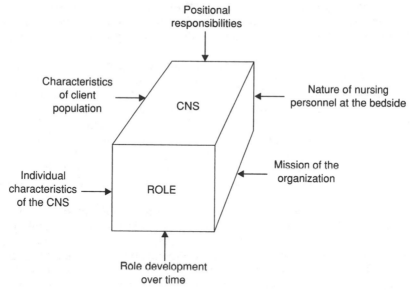

Figure 25.2 Variables influencing CNS role expression (From Hamric, 1989, by permission)

The first three sets of characteristics form the core definition of the CNS role (Figure 25.1); the fourth set, while not an inherent part of the definition, influences CNS role expression (Figure 25.2). Hamric considers that to fully implement the varied aspects of the practice a considerable period of role development is required. In addition, continued refinement of the role definition and expression of that role is essential. The remainder of the discussion in this section relates to the model developed for the CNS by Hamric (1989).

Expert practitioner

The role of the CNS has been implemented in a variety of ways but the direct care sub-role of the expert practitioner brings the expertise of advanced practitioners directly to the patient and client. This direct care sub-role may consist of two components. First, direct care that is regularly and systematically provided; secondly, episodic direct care provided to meet a specific need or solve a particular problem. The nature of practice will vary, enabling the CNS to assess specific patient and client concerns. The CNS can then act as a role model while working with the staff in providing care, demonstrating desirable practice behaviours for them to emulate (Metcalf *et al.*, 1984). Patient and client advocacy should also be evident in the CNS's work (see Chapter 28). This was identified in Fenton's study as a major function of the expert nurse in working with nursing staff, other professionals and the health care system (Fenton, 1985). The amount of time spent in clinical practice will vary, practising CNSs having stated that anywhere from 25% to 50% of a working week should be devoted to direct care (Welch-McCaffrey, 1986). Indirect activities have also been identified by Fenton (1985), among others, and include the development of standards of care and quality assurance activities.

There are a number of benefits the nursing profession can derive from CNS direct care, for example, collaboration with other disciplines enhancing the professional nursing profile. Collaboration which involves health care professionals functioning as colleagues and partners within a level hierarchy is one practice that the CNS will stimulate in this sub-role. Collaborative practice positively affects patients and clients and their families, the nurse, and allied health care professionals. It also results in improved job satisfaction, improved communication and understanding among health care professionals and professional growth and development.

However, Felder (1983) has outlined a number of situations that may be problematic for the CNS. These include nurses with feelings of resentment and territoriality, time pressures, lack of support, cost to the institution and role confusion. There are means by which the implementation of the expert practitioner sub-role can be managed more easily. For example, it is helpful to know the staff mix and each person's background experience and education to assist with determining the approach to care within the team. Administrative support for the sub-role is essential along with organizational/departmental resource support as required by the CNS to accomplish the clinical sub-role. In addition, working alongside other community health care nurses allows the CNS to integrate with the staff which avoids unnecessary friction. The sub-role requires clarification with the nursing staff, as illustrated in a survey of community nurses by Williams (1993b).

Educator

The traditional sub-role of educator is characterized as an indirect practice role. According to Priest (1989):

By definition the CNS is committed to furthering excellence in clinical practice and seeks innovative ways to share knowledge with other practitioners.

In comparison to most other nurse educators, the practice base for the CNS is patient and client care, thus facilitating more access to and control over the clinical environment. The CNS educator sub-role is almost unique because unlike with the majority of nurse educators, the educator role is not the sole function of her or his position, the remaining sub-roles having to be balanced with the educator role. The CNS participates in the education of staff, patients and clients and their families, and nursing students.

Participation in the education and professional development of all levels of staff is an appropriate function of the CNS. The clinical expertise and analytical skills of the CNS are fundamental assets to this role. Two established approaches to the sub-role are the participation in selected formal educational sessions and addressing individual learning and developmental needs of the staff. Welch-McCaffrey (1986) points out that the delivery of education must be in a variety of modalities and that the choice of method should be a purposeful one. However, this sub-role may suffer if staff are not readily available or motivated to learn, if there is a lack of institutional resources, or a lack of administrative support.

The CNS is in the ideal position and is equipped with the required skills and knowledge for patient and client and family education. This may be for the individual patient and client or group education. The CNS is not always the appropriate person to teach a patient and client who has identified with another health care professional as their key worker. In these cases the CNS can be used as a consultant to determine learning needs of the patient and client.

The CNS can facilitate learning in the practice setting by demonstrating her or his function and commitment to clinical practice. Knowledge can be gained not only by direct reading, but of equal importance are observation and participation. However, the success of the clinical experience depends upon the willingness of the CNS and student to discuss, describe and analyse the clinical practice issues as well as the amount of clinical practice time and support.

The educator sub-role extends to include staff, patient or client, family and student nurse education. The challenge for the CNS is to fulfil the sub-role, balancing it with that of expert practitioner, consultant and researcher.

Consultant

Consultation is an important aspect of the CNS role. According to Tarsitano et al. (1986), nurse administrators and CNSs regard the consultant sub-role as the function most valued by the nursing staff. The emphasis placed on the sub-role will vary over time with the expertise and needs of the staff, patients and clients, with the goals and priorities of the CNS fluctuating.

Caplan (1970) defined consultation as a process of communication between professionals which can be systematically taught, applied and analysed. The consultation process involves communication between the consultant, who is the specialist, and the consultee. The consultee acknowledges a problem and the need to seek specialized expertise, initiating a consultation. The consultant may offer education, clarification, diagnostic formulation and additional problem-solving strategies. The consultee accepts or rejects the recommendations from this collaborative relationship, the consultee remaining responsible for the patient and client care.

Caplan (1970) describes consultation as a complex process requiring an understanding of the theoretical frameworks relevant to nursing consultation; some examples include the consultation process, communications, change theory, nursing process, problem-solving and conflict resolution. The cognitive and interpersonal skills important in developing this sub-role include high degrees of self-awareness and interpersonal skill, effective time management, ability to assess the varying levels of needs and abilities, accepting the decision-making power of the consultee, and feeling comfortable with a significant degree of autonomy (Barron, 1989).

Establishing the consultant sub-role of the CNS involves generating positive working relationships, developing alliances, negotiating professional roles, clearly defining the sub-role to staff and inviting regular feedback on their perceptions of the sub-role. Indeed, the first step in promoting consultation involves educating staff about the consultative service available to them and the means to request consultation. It is the CNS–nurse relationship which is central to effective CNS consultation. However, as previously stated, since the idea of consultation with other nurses is not well developed in the UK, both CNS behaviours and staff responses might impair this relationship (Everson, 1981; Barron, 1983). The CNS can be viewed as a threat by staff for many reasons, including intimidation by the educational preparation of the CNS, envy of the autonomy of the CNS's position, implications of inadequacy by their presence, fear of takeover of their work and an extension of administration. To minimize these potential misconceptions, the CNS should remain visible and available, getting to know the staff to build trust and confidence. The CNS responding to a request for consultation should avoid an imposing entrance, avoid criticism which could enhance feelings of incompetence and should encourage support and give constructive feedback. One positive benefit of the consultative process is that not only does the CNS assist the staff with assessment, but also facilitates a holistic perspective by helping the staff examine their own perceptions, feelings and behaviours as well as those of patients and families (Fife and Lemler, 1983). The CNS consultant also liaises with physicians and other health care professionals. The overlap and interface of care in these situations will need to be negotiated, as it is inevitable that the role as consultant will at times complement, overlap or even contradict the opinions of others (Barron, 1983). The CNS must always focus on improving the quality of the nursing care for patients and clients.

Clinical leadership skills, including problem-solving, setting priorities, exercising authority by virtue of one's expert power base and providing emotional and situational support, are clearly required for the consultant sub-role's smooth implementation. Indeed, Spross and Donoghue (1984) suggest that 'clinical professional leadership is inherent in the CNS role – it is not optional'. Effective leadership skills are used to accomplish the goal of improving patient and client care directly and indirectly.

Researcher

Nurses with direct patient and client contact are encouraged to participate in research. Indeed, Schlotfeldt (1974) suggests that the commitment to inquiry should be possessed by all nurses (see Chapter 11). The sub-role of researcher is a required component of the CNS role; however, the interpretation of this sub-role ranges from the actual conduct of research to its application in clinical practice. Cronenwett (1986) reported that many CNSs felt unsuccessful in achieving the expectations of the research sub-role. McGuire and Harwood (1989) also suggest that it is naive and unfair to expect all CNSs to be interested and involved in research at the same level, describing the role in research at three separate levels:

- Level 1. To interpret, evaluate and communicate to nursing staff research findings pertinent to the specialization
- Level 2. To test and apply the findings of research produced by other researchers
- Level 3. To replicate the research of others, precepting students in research projects, generating original studies and collaborating with other nurses and physicians.

Storr (1988) suggests that implying that the interpretation of the research sub-role is synonymous with the discovery of knowledge is unrealistic and promotes a disservice to the CNS. McGuire and Harwood (1989) acknowledge that the level of activity would depend on several factors, emphasizing that the evaluation, communication and utilization of new knowledge should be the focus of the CNS's practice, the utilization of research in practice being the most important component of the research sub-role. As a clinical expert the CNS is aware of clinical problems which need to be addressed through research utilization. The application of research is a process through which research findings are critiqued, implemented, evaluated and disseminated. The CNS can act as a change agent, facilitating pro-active change to improve patient and client care. Through the utilization of research findings, the gap between knowledge generation through research and use of research findings in practice can be narrowed, a gap that according to Padilla (1979) '. . . has been difficult to bridge'. Participation at any level of research involvement will enable the CNS to contribute substantially to the continually expanding body of knowledge which underlies nursing practice, as well as fulfilling one of the components of the CNS role. Sills (1983) states:

Indeed, central to the position of the CNS is a set of ideas about change. Inherent in all that the CNS does is the fundamental notion of attempting to alter or change the course of some human experience.

● Working with a resource nurse

There is little written concerning nurses' utilization and communication system with the CNS. The method of communication and liaison between nurses and the CNS will specify the degree of utilization of the CNS and have differing degrees of impact on patient and client care, nurses' and CNS job satisfaction and development. Griffiths (1994) reported that specialists were needed in the community but not at the expense of training the community nurses themselves; and when a condition is less common, the generalist nurse has access to working with the specialist nurse. The following three models of care are proposed for applications in practice: parallel care, supported care and shared care.

Parallel care

In parallel care, as illustrated in Figure 25.3, the CNS and nurse practice their direct patient and client care independently. Both nurses will have been asked for their intervention from either the same or different sources, such as both from the General Practitioner or one from the patient or client's General Practitioner and the other from a hospital department. There is no case management discussion to agree and co-ordinate the care required. No readily identifiable 'key worker' may lead to the patient or client receiving too little support. As previously described, the patient or client receives direct care from the CNS and the nurse. For the CNS, direct care will boost job satisfaction but could easily encroach into time allocated for the other sub-roles. The skills of role model and clinical leader will be under-used with a danger of existing nursing expertise being overlooked. There could also be frustrations and overlap of care by the two nurses, created by different care and delivery systems being used. Territorial feelings may be fostered by the nurse in conjunction with role confusion. For the patient or client there may be conflict and confusion from the separate care inputs which will heighten any anxiety. The CNS's competencies of patient and client advocate and collaborator with other health care professionals are likely to be perceived as a threat by the nurse, thus straining working relationships further. Skilled education is received by the patient or client from the CNS, but the nurse is unable to learn from this if the liaison with the CNS is poor. Indeed, the patient or client is in danger of receiving conflicting advice from the two separate nurses and the CNS of under-utilizing the sub-roles of the specialist practitioner. The CNS is likely to encounter difficulties implementing research findings, since any change may be viewed as potentially threatening, which may result in the CNS having difficulty in acting as a change agent.

The parallel care model uses the sub-roles and skills and competencies of the CNS inadequately, as is illustrated by the example of a woman with lower limb lymphoedema following surgical treatment for cervical cancer. The hospital consultant may refer her to the lymphoedema CNS and, in addition, the ward staff would refer her to the district nurse on discharge. Since there is no discussion of cases between the CNS and the district nurse, the patient or client would go on receiving lymphoedema treatment from the specialist, the district nurse only learning about the treatment for lymphoedema from her observations when with the patient or client. All of the problems highlighted above could develop for the patient and client, district nurse and the CNS – a wasted opportunity for development and understanding for everybody.

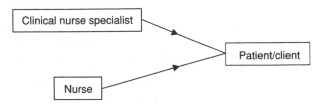

Figure 25.3 Parallel care

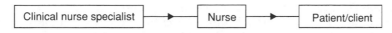

Figure 25.4   Supported care

Supported care

In supported care (Figure 25.4), the nurse delivers direct care, the CNS only offering indirect care via the case management discussions. The patient or client receives direct care from the nurse alone. The CNS loses any satisfaction from direct care, is unable to fulfil her functions as a role model and patient and client advocate in practice, and operates only from the periphery of the delivery system. The skill of clinical leader is lost in this model, in which the patient or client liaises with the one nurse and is probably unaware of the indirect input from the CNS. Any requirement for collaboration with other health care professionals should be accepted, the input being discussed when planning the patient and client care. The patient or client receives education from the nurse alone, possibly advised from the CNS, but no direct input.

The lack of clinical practice involvement limits the extent of the educator sub-role of the CNS and the extent of motivation by the nurse. The consultancy sub-role is accessible to the nurse, but may be potentially under-used due to the lack of contact in clinical practice. The support and advice will be offered, but limited according to the nurses' appreciation of the need for additional resources and advice.

The application of research findings is possible, but extension of the sub-role beyond this initial level is limited by minimal teamwork in the clinical setting. Even so, the CNS can pursue change in clinical practice in this situation.

Although the supported care model stimulates greater use of the sub-roles and skills of the CNS, further advancement is limited primarily by the lack of direct care in the clinical practice setting. Once again, the woman with lymphoedema secondary to cancer treatment provides an illustration. The district nurse would be giving the lymphoedema treatment knowing that if she perceived the need for additional advice the CNS was available. Without more direct care by the CNS there is the risk that additional measures could be taken in the management of the problem.

Shared care

In shared care (Figure 25.5), the CNS and the nurse deliver co-ordinated direct patient and client care as agreed in case management

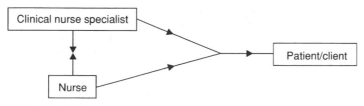

Figure 25.5   Shared care

discussions. The patient or client receives prearranged direct care from the CNS and nurse, giving job satisfaction for the CNS and allowing her time to pursue her other sub-roles. The CNS is able to implement her clinical leader and role model skills, enhancing patient and client care without threatening the position of the nurse. The relationship between the CNS and the nurse should be strong, there being a full understanding of each other's roles. The patient or client benefits from this co-ordinated shared approach, having both nurses in a position to be advocates. The close liaison between the two nurses augments the educational possibilities, at both a formal and informal level. The nurse is easily motivated and able to fully implement the educator sub-role of the CNS. The patient or client also receives direct and indirect learning as required from the CNS. The CNS's sub-role of consultant, using collaborative skills, is fully used in clinical practice and at case management meetings planning care. A developed relationship between the CNS and the nurse will encourage the nurse to comfortably use the CNS without feeling threatened in her role. Credibility will flourish easily for the two practitioners and their roles.

The shared care model enables the progression to more advanced levels of the research sub-role. The theory–practice divide, when it exists, can be acknowledged and narrowed without unnecessary threat to the nurse. In addition, change will be possible to advance nursing care. Indeed, this model of care is existing, using the sub-roles and skills and competencies of the CNS fully to the advantage of the patient or client, nurse and CNS. The author believes this model to be the one of choice for effective care in the community, the CNS being a resource as opposed to only a provider of specialist care, contributing significantly to raising standards of patient care. Returning to the case example, an initial joint meeting between the CNS and the district nurse to plan optimum care would ensure that the most appropriate nurse was giving care within a supportive structure. Additionally, the patient, district nurse and CNS would benefit from the structure of care.

Clearly, each of the three models utilizes the clinical nurse specialist sub-roles in varying degrees. Consideration of which model is most likely to be implemented in different practice settings relates to the role development of the practitioners.

● **Role development for the CNS**

Role development for the CNS occurs in sequential phases involving a process of skill acquisition and changing focus of practice (Holt, 1987). Baker (1987) developed model activities, clustered according to the number of years in the role. In this model, in years one and two the focus is on establishing role identity through direct care functions, years three and four are directed to change agent activities and years five and six focus upon the consultant sub-role. According to Baker's interpretation it would seem likely, using the model identified above, that parallel care would initially be established, moving through supported care to shared care as roles evolve.

Another approach to understanding role development focuses on the experience of the new CNS. Baker (1979) identified four phases of role development: orientation, frustration, implementation, and reassessment. Hamric (1989) conducted a study involving 100 practising CNSs, some with less than three years' experience as a CNS and others with over three years' experience. Seven definable phases were identified: orientation, frustration, implementation, integration, frozen, reorganization and complacent. The first three are analogous to the first three categories described by Baker (1979). Details of the phases experienced by CNSs in their first position were compared with those in their second. The first three phases were shorter for the latter group but not necessarily easier. It was identified from the study that the CNS's own sense of confidence and role clarity assists role development, but variables in the setting, especially the amount of support available, are important factors. The factors identified by respondents as facilitating and obstructing role development in the study of Hamric (1989) are listed in Table 25.2.

These studies by Baker (1979) and Hamric (1989) illustrate the different models representing the complex nature of CNS role development for which there has been little systematic investigation. Recker (1991) considered the perception of the CNS's responsibilities in the field of critical care. Staff members with less than two years' experience were more likely to identify the educator and clinical practice sub-roles. Staff with more than two years' experience usually identified all sub-roles. The difference between the two groups of staff may be related to the amount of time they have with the CNS and the context of the contact. Clearly, nurses are in a key position to influence aspects of the CNS role, including the pattern of liaison with the CNS. It is likely that a confident nurse who identifies the CNS's roles will establish shared care as opposed to the nurse who lacks confidence and is unable to liaise with a CNS.

The evolution of the CNS role is characterized by continued defining, refining and refocusing – demonstrating a dynamic process.

Table 25.2   Factors facilitating or obstructing CNS role development

Facilitating role development		Obstructing role development	
1.	Peer support	1.	Administrative problems
2.	Administrative support	2.	Lack of other's understanding the role
3.	Self-characteristics, e.g. self-confidence	3.	Intra-professional problems, e.g. staff resistance to change
4.	Role characteristics, e.g. independence	4.	Time pressures
5.	Mentor	5.	Self-characteristics, e.g. impatience, insecurity
6.	Experience	6.	Lack of peer support
7.	Colleagues from other disciplines	7.	Inter-professional problems, e.g. with physicians
8.	Other, e.g. flexibility, commitment	8.	Role characteristics, e.g. incompatibility with organizational goals

● **Conclusion**
Over the past two decades there have been striking changes and advances in nursing practice. The growth of the CNS provides an important example. There are an increasing number of specialities in nursing, some surging ahead of medical specialization, for example in lymphoedema. Lymphology is not a recognized medical speciality in the UK as it is in some countries and as such is an example of an area of expertise outside of medicine (McGee, 1993). Therefore, CNSs play a key role in influencing nursing practice with their focus in clinical practice as an expert practitioner. This, in conjunction with academic training and theory-based clinical practice, will guide clinical practice developments and be in a position to challenge the traditional perception of a nurse carrying out the physician's orders. For this to happen, academic training as well as clinical practice for the CNS needs to develop so that CNSs are the experts clinically, with advanced knowledge. In addition, an important issue is how to structure nursing care to maximize the benefits of specialized input and minimize the drawbacks. Establishing the shared care model, employing nurses with specialist knowledge and skills to act as a resource to existing staff as opposed to direct care specialist posts, is vital to this issue.

References
ANA (1980) *Nursing: A Social Policy Statement*, American Nurses' Association Kansas City, MO

Badger, C. (1994) Pause for thought: nurses use research – don't they? *European Journal of Cancer Care*, **3**, 63–66

Baker, C. and Kramer, M. (1970) To define or not define: the role of the clinical nurses specialist. *Nursing Forum*, **9**(1), 41–55

Baker, P. (1987) Model activities for clinical nurse specialists' role development. *Clinical Nurse Specialist*, **1**(3), 119–123

Baker, V. (1979) Retrospective explorations in role development. In *The Clinical Nurse Specialist and Improvement of Nursing Practice* (ed. G.V. Padilla), Nursing Resources, Wakefield

Barron, A. (1983) the CNS as consultant. In *The Clinical Nurse Specialist in Theory and Practice* (eds A.B. Hamric and J. Spross), Grune and Stratton, New York

Barron, A. (1989) The CNS as consultant. In *The Clinical Nurse Specialist in Theory and Practice* (eds A.B. Hamric and J. Spross), W.B. Saunders, Philadelphia

Benner, P. (1984) *From Novice to Expert: Excellence and Power in Clinical Nurse Practice*, Addison-Wesley, Menlo Park, CA

Caplan, G. (1970) *The Theory and Practice of Mental Health Consultation*, Basic Books, New York

Castledine, G. (1986) Clinical nurse specialists. *Nursing Practice*, **31**(4), 213–214

Cheay, Y.L. and Moon, G.M. (1993) Specialism in nursing: the case of nursing care for elderly people. *Journal of Advanced Nursing*, **18**, 1610–1616

Christman, L. (1965) The influence of specialisation on the nursing profession. *Nursing Science*, **3**, 446–453

Cronenwett, L.R. (1986) The research role of the clinical nurse specialist. *Journal of Nursing Administration*, **16**(4), 10–11

Dirschel, K.M. (1976) The conception, gestation, and delivery of the clinical nurse specialist. In *Quality Patient Care and the Role of the Clinical Nurse Specialist* (ed. R. Rotkovitch), Wiley, New York

Everson, S. (1981) Integration of the role of the clinical nurse specialist. *Journal of Continuing Education in Nursing*, **12**(2), 16–19

Felder, L. (1983) Direct patient care and independent practice. In *The Clinical Nurse Specialist in Theory and Practice* (eds A.B. Hamric and J. Spross), Grune and Stratton, New York

Fenton, M.V. (1985) Identifying competencies of clinical nurse specialists. *Journal of Nursing Administration*, **15**(12), 31–37

Fife, B. and Lemler, S. (1983) The psychiatric nurse specialist: a valuable asset in the general hospital. *Journal of Nursing Administration*, **13**(4), 14–17

Griffiths, J. (1994) Community nurse attitudes to the clinical nurse specialist. *Nursing Times*, **90**(17), 39–42

Hamric, A.B. (1989) Role development and functions. In *The Clinical Nurse Specialist in Theory and Practice* (eds A.B. Hamric and J. Spross), W.B. Saunders, Philadelphia

Holt, F.M. (1987) Executive practice role – editorial. *Clinical Nurse Specialist*, **1**(3), 116–118

Kitzman, H.J. (1989) The CNS and the nurse practitioner. In *The Clinical Nurse Specialist in Theory and Practice* (eds A.B. Hamric and J. Spross), W.B. Saunders, Philadelphia

Layzell, S. and McCarthy, M. (1993) Specialist or generic community nursing care for HIV/AIDS patients? *Journal of Advanced Nursing*, **18**, 531–537

McGee, P. (1993) Defining nursing practice. *British Journal of Nursing*, **2**(20), 1022–1026

McGuire, D.B. and Harwood, K.V. (1989) The CNS as researcher. In *The Clinical Nurse Specialist in Theory and Practice* (eds A.B. Hamric and J. Spross), W.B. Saunders, Philadelphia

Metcalf, J., Werner, M. and Richmond, T. (1984) The clinical nurse specialist in a clinical career ladder. *Nursing Administration Quarterly*, **9**(3), 9–19

Naisbitt, J. (1982) *Megatrends*, Warner Books, New York

Padilla, G.V. (1979) Incorporating research in a service setting. *Journal of Nursing Administration*, **9**(1), 44–49

Priest, A. (1989) The clinical nurse specialist as educator. In *The Clinical Nurse Specialist in Theory and Practice* (eds A.B. Hamric and J. Spross), W.B. Saunders, Philadelphia

RCN (1988) *Specialities in Nursing*, Royal College of Nursing, London

Recker, D. (1991) Staff nurse's view of the clinical nurse specialist. *Nursing Management*, April, 64L

Schlotfeldt, R.M. (1974) Cooperative nursing investigations: a role for everyone. *Nursing Research*, **23**(6), 452–456

Sills, G.M. (1983) The role and function of the clinical nurse specialist. In *The Nursing Profession: A Time to Speak* (ed. N.L. Chaska), McGraw-Hill, New York

Spross, J.A. and Baggerly, J. (1989) Models of advanced nursing practice. In *The Clinical Nurse Specialist in Theory and Practice* (eds A.B. Hamric and J. Spross), W.B. Saunders, Philadelphia

Spross, J.A. and Donoghue, M. (1984) The future of the oncology clinical nurse specialist. *Oncology Nursing Forum*, **11**(1), 74–78

Storr, G. (1988) The clinical nurse specialist: from the outside looking in. *Journal of Advanced Nursing*, **13**, 265–272

Tarsitano, B., Brophy, E. and Snyder, D. (1986) Demystification of the clinical nurse specialist role: perceptions of clinical nurse specialists and nurse administrators. *Journal of Nursing Education*, **25**, 4–9

Welch-McCaffrey, D. (1986) Role performance issues for oncology clinical nurse specialists. *Cancer Nursing*, **9**(6), 287–294

Williams, A.E. (1992) Management of lymphoedema: a community-based approach. *British Journal of Nursing*, **1**(8), 383–387

Williams, A.E. (1993a) Management of lymphoedema: a community-based approach. *British Journal of Nursing*, **2**(13), 678–681

Williams, A.E. (1993b) Steps to develop a working relationship. *Professional Nurse*, **8**(12), 806–812

26

Promoting positive and healthy lifestyles

Sarah Cowley

● Introduction

There are many positive approaches which community nurses can use to promote healthy lifestyles and a selection of illustrative examples will be included in this chapter. Most importantly, it will critically explore what is meant by the term 'lifestyle', drawing a sharp comparison between the holistic, contextual origins of the term, and the contemporary tendency to target isolated 'lifestyle factors' such as diet, smoking or alcohol-intake, in the name of health promotion.

There is no doubt that these factors are linked with poor health in a variety of ways. Although a clear, systematic approach can be extremely useful, very strictly focused programmes are likely to be counter-productive to the promotion of positive and healthy lifestyles. The reasons for this contention will be explained in more detail, after the term 'lifestyle' has been examined to explore its origins and recent usage.

● Lifestyle

Coreil *et al.* (1985) offer a theoretical discussion and selective literature review which traces the origins of the term 'lifestyle'. They suggest that it was first used to refer to the unity, goal-directedness and uniqueness of a person's actions, and explain that the way people live their lives tends to be both subjectively determined and heavily influenced by early childhood experience. Notions of integration, social and cultural context, and the linking of different aspects and styles into a unified whole, were considered important features in the early use of the term. In view of this, it was anticipated that growing use of the term indicated increasing awareness of a humanistic and holistic concept of mankind, and a corresponding rejection of mechanistic or deterministic views.

This broad interpretation seemed to underpin the way 'lifestyle' was used by the World Health Organisation (WHO), in their publication which proposed 38 targets aimed at achieving 'Health for All' by the year

2000 (WHO, 1987). These targets included five directed at promoting lifestyles conducive to health. The WHO define lifestyle in relation to collective and individual experiences and to conditions of life; the range of options open to an individual is confined to the area in which these different aspects overlap (Kickbusch, 1986). Accordingly, the five 'lifestyle targets' are widely focused. One concerns the development of healthy public policy; another focuses on the role of families and other community groups in developing social support systems. A third proposes improvements to educational programmes which enhance the knowledge, motivation and skills of people to acquire health.

The next two targets propose increases in positive health behaviour, such as balanced nutrition, non-smoking and appropriate stress management; and decreasing health-damaging behaviour, like over-use of alcohol, use of illicit drugs, dangerous driving and violent social behaviour. The idea was to encourage people to develop a positive view of health, to recognize the right of individuals to self-determination and to self-care and to emphasize health as a social, rather than medical concept (Kickbusch, 1989). However, these atomistic approaches have been picked up and used as a sole focus in many programmes which claim to be promoting health. In England, for example, specific targets relating to diet, smoking and use of alcohol have been incorporated in the government's strategy document, *The Health of the Nation* (DoH, 1992). General Practitioners were encouraged to establish clinics focusing on single aspects of health-related behaviour, by the use of bonus payments linked to numbers of patients seen in this way.

The importance attached to goal-directed programmes stems from a commercial management perspective, which holds that greater efficiency is achieved from purposeful, clearly measurable activities, than from those which appear unfocused or unclear to the workers undertaking them (Peters and Waterman, 1982). The 'Health of the Nation' strategy was proposed as part of a wider move to improve efficiency within the National Health Service. This helps to explain the determination, even within the government's consultative proposals (DoH, 1991), to identify specific, measurable targets. This targeting of isolated lifestyle factors follows a wide trend noted by Coreil *et al.* (1985). The majority of the recent articles they reviewed referred to 'lifestyle' in the sense of specific behaviours identified as risk factors for disease and accidental death. Typically, the underlying assumption was:

> *the notion that personal habits are discrete and independently modifiable, and that individuals can voluntarily choose to alter such behaviours. Little, if any, attention is given to altering the larger society in which individuals participate.*

Health promotion programmes which are based on such assumptions fail to deal adequately with the sociocultural context of behaviour – a major weakness in the lifestyle modification approach (Coreil *et al.*, 1985). The rest of this chapter will explore the reasons for this assertion. It will suggest strategies that community nurses can use which avoid the pitfalls associated with single focus programmes, yet still succeed in promoting positive and healthy lifestyles.

● Who defines the problem?

One reason for the apparent inability of single focus health promotion programmes to modify lifestyles may be that they target 'problems' which are professionally defined. Indeed, some professionals convey an impression of believing they have a moral right to decide what kind of behaviour is 'proper' and which is a 'problem', in the name of health promotion. However, the so-called problems may seem irrelevant to the difficulties faced by the client at the time; this mismatch can lead people to believe that professionals are unaware of the real health issues which concern them.

When, for example, a community action group was established to improve squalid housing conditions in a Glasgow housing estate, the local people explained that the doctors and community nurses had been prepared to write letters to the council, but not to become any further involved in the campaign (Seymour, 1991). The tenants presumed the professionals were 'too busy'. However, they also suspected that the doctors and nurses underestimated the impact of damp and mould on the physical and mental health of people living there, citing their tendency to talk about things like 'brown bread and jogging' as scornful evidence of this belief. There is a great deal of research to support the tenants' view that poor housing has a serious and adverse effect on health (see, for example, Martin *et al.*, 1987; Platt *et al.* 1989; Fisher and Collins, 1993; Ineichin, 1993).

Repeatedly, surveys of how people view their own health demonstrate differences between lay and professionals' views (Cornwell, 1984; Calnan, 1987; Blaxter, 1990). There is a tendency for health workers to underestimate both the extent and usefulness of lay knowledge and coping networks, and the difficulties which people have to overcome to achieve healthy lifestyles, particularly if they are living on a limited income (Mayall and Foster, 1989; Blackburn, 1991; Pearson *et al.*, 1993).

> ● Health-promoting strategies which are most likely to effect real changes in lifestyle are those which can harness, rather than undermine, these lay networks and knowledge.

In some circumstances, this may mean changing an approach to service provision, or making a special effort to ensure that it reaches people who need it. A health visitor working with elderly people in London, for example, realized that the local Asian population tended not to use the standard health service provision very readily, despite having higher rates of non-insulin-dependent diabetes and coronary heart disease than the indigenous population (Thompson, 1993).

The health visitor began by learning as much as she could about the Asian community, until they realized that her respect for their ways was genuine and based on a thorough knowledge. The real 'breakthrough' occurred when she was given permission to begin a 'look after yourself' course within a local day centre for elderly Asians (Redmond, quoted in Thompson, 1993). The course was popular, and future courses were modified as the participants explained, through an interpreter, what they wanted to hear about. Gradually, as the Asian population became more familiar with the health visitor and learned from her about the mainstream services which were available, they began to use them. Subsequently, the nearby hospital was persuaded to run a clinic especially geared to their needs.

Likewise, in a collaborative initiative between health and education workers, and the charity 'Save the Children', a project designed to improve uptake of services by travelling familes in the Midlands began by asking them what they wanted (Tyler, 1993). They asked for antenatal care, and for women's and children's clinics. The project workers developed client-held records for both children and adults, and established an accessible weekly clinic for them. By listening to the travelling families, they gained a deeper understanding of the difficulties faced in a community where illiteracy is common, and access to mainstream health and education services frequently denied because of prejudice and regulations which fail to acknowledge their particular needs (Reid, 1993). The workers were then far better placed to act as advocates on behalf of the families; for instance, explaining to accident and emergency staff that General Practitioners will often refuse to accept these families on their list – in such cases, the only way to access a medical opinion may be by 'inappropriately' attending the nearest hospital.

In addition, there has been considerable concern about how mental health services seem to be used least by those who might gain most, for example, people who use illicit drugs or drink excessive amounts of alcohol (Shanks, 1992). Often, those who are most in need of help fail to access it, sometimes because of concerns about the stigma associated with such services, because they feel professionals will not understand their predicament, or because they do not see themselves as having a problem. In Manchester, a community mental health service was planned, which aimed to overcome such difficulties by involving potential clients from the start (Newbigging *et al.*, 1989).

The Powell Street community mental health centre was established in a small terraced house, in a working class residential area. Local people and self-help groups were involved in planning the service from the start; the centre was available for them to use alongside professionals, such as community nurses and the community drugs team. The service planned to improve accessibility by emphasizing informality, an open referral system and involvement of the whole community from the start. Targeting a geographically defined population, rather than people who had been diagnosed as having a specific mental illness or problem, was intended to remove stigma and enable the service to engage in pro-active, preventive work, as well as responding to people who needed immediate help.

The centre adopted a social model of health, which values the views of those who would use it, encouraging their involvement at every stage; this helped to encourage integration of people with mental health problems into the community, rather than singling them out as 'different'. This focus on developing the role of communities and social support systems is consistent with the WHO view of promoting healthy lifestyles, as it can gradually influence the cultural beliefs which shape the way people live their lives.

Long-term gains

In comparison, programmes which focus on a clearly measurable aspect of behaviour can seem relatively rapid. However, evaluations tend to suggest that they lead to relatively few long-term health gains. This seems to be particularly the case if professionals decide both the topic and the target group to receive health education, without any consultation or collaboration. Rowland and Maynard (1993), for instance, examined a programme which targeted a sample of young people who had been identified by professionals as drinking excessive amounts of alcohol; the programme led to very limited changes among the adolescents, who had not considered that they had a problem. Similarly, few smoking cessation programmes seem to be sucessful in making an impact on the numbers of smokers (Graham, 1993a; Walsh and Redman, 1993).

Likewise, the majority of dieters tend to revert quite quickly to their former eating patterns and soon regain all, or more than, the weight they had lost (Ogden, 1992). Overall, the number of people regarded as overweight in the UK continues to rise, but the reasons for some people consuming more food than they need to meet their energy requirements are imperfectly understood (Barker and Cooke, 1992).

It is important to recognize that food intake is not only about nutrition. Patterns of eating are associated with deeply-held beliefs and cultural meanings, so changes may involve considerable upheaval. In a study which examines issues of responsibility and control in the feeding of families, for example, Charles and Kerr (1986) discovered that many women aimed to avoid conflict by only preparing food which their partner liked. In most instances, this would be a 'cooked dinner', usually with the pastry and fatty foods which were considered 'suitable' for men. Those who lived with domineering or abusive partners were particularly aware that offering food which did not accord with this cultural view of a 'proper meal' was to risk a violent outburst and family discord.

Also, while the extent of obesity remains a source of concern, the pattern of fat distribution may be a more significant predictor of health problems than a person's total weight (Ashwell, 1991). Little is known about what influences fat distribution throughout the body, but it seems to be more closely linked to genetic make-up than to dietary intake. Nevertheless, there is a considerable industry based on promulgating special dietary products and regimens. Many of them are of doubtful benefit, but some manufacturers direct their marketing strategies at community nurses, because of their role in offering nutritional advice. A popular selling point is the promise of rapid weight loss, and the view that even if this is not sustained, a brief improvement would be better than none at all. However, such changes may be harmful in themselves; there is growing evidence that the variability in body size caused by a pattern of intermittent dieting leads to greater health problems than remaining at a stable, if heavy, weight (Lissner *et al.*, 1991).

> • Health promotion strategies which show most promise in the long term are those that encourage sustained rather than sudden changes, and which specifically avoid the risk of replacing one harmful behaviour pattern with another.

A small terraced house in Cope Street, Nottingham has been used as a base from which young parents could work in partnership with professionals to identify practical and workable ways of overcoming difficulties they faced (Billingham, 1989). The health visitors who set up the scheme respected their clients' views, and learnt to work as group facilitators, and as a resource for the users of the house. At the start of each group, for example, those participating were asked to say what they wanted to gain from attendance; the programme was then jointly decided according to those wishes. One group established in this way aimed to help people make sense of claims being made on food labels (Billingham, 1990). This allowed the women to discuss the different influences on how they chose their family diet; they were empowered in deciding for themselves what kinds of food they wished to have, and how to introduce any changes.

This approach is quite difficult to evaluate in relation to specific dietary targets. However, a qualitative study of those attending showed that most people felt they had gained more control over their lives, improved their self-image and benefited in some tangible, often individual and personal, way from attending the centre (Mackeith *et al.* 1991). Thus, the approach is consistent with the WHO proposal that healthy lifestyles can be promoted by educational programmes which enhance the knowledge, motivation and skills of people to acquire health.

● A positive resource

An important belief which underpins the promotion of healthy lifestyles is that health is a positive resource for life, and not the reason for living (WHO, 1986; Seedhouse, 1986). Health education programmes which emphasize giving up preferred behaviours with little apparent reward may inadvertently imply the opposite; that is, that 'being healthy' requires one to adopt a miserable and negative way of living. Alternatively, 'healthy behaviour' may be adopted so obsessively as to create difficulties. The influence of crank diets, excessive exercise or overdosage with vitamin supplements provide examples.

> • Successful health promotion strategies are more likely to emphasize positive health gains than negative aspects of behaviour.

This positive idea was adopted by an occupational health nurse, who was aware of the unhealthy patterns of 'relaxation' adopted by men working on a building gang erecting tower blocks in a development area (Berns, 1991). The men were mainly living in temporary lodgings away from their families, and spent the evenings drinking heavily in the local pub. Although she did not question them about their drinking habits, the nurse was often asked to supply paracetamol as a hangover cure, and she became aware that, despite their 'macho' image, many of the men were isolated and lonely. They worked in small teams which had no reason to meet and mix with each other; apart from the drinking sessions, most had no other social outlet.

Hesitantly, the nurse started a social club, initially arranging group outings to the theatre and to restaurants. As the club began to flourish, so the number of requests for hangover cures reduced; the men started to take an interest in identifying alternative social events for themselves – the club became known as 'Alternatives'. A sense of community developed on the building site: heavy drinking sessions no longer seemed to be the only option; friendships and informal support systems were formed.

Similar positive spin-offs have been reported where elderly people have been involved in setting up and running social gatherings, rather than being expected to sit passively, listening to lectures about 'health' from professionals (Meade and Carter, 1990). The strategy emphasizes enjoyable aspects of adopting a healthy lifestyle, and develops informal social systems which enable positive, health-enhancing behaviour to be adopted more easily than health-harming ones.

Limits to individual choice

Just as concentrating on behaviour patterns overemphasizes physical health at the expense of mental health or social wellbeing, so focusing on individuals minimizes the structural and political causes of ill-health. There is no doubt that behaviours like smoking, lack of exercise and poor diet contribute substantially and significantly to health problems. However, there is growing evidence to show that the people who are most likely to adopt unhealthy behaviour patterns are those who live in poor economic circumstances, who are vulnerable or in frail mental health, or who lack supportive social networks; that is, the people whose mental health and social wellbeing is already poor (Blackburn, 1991; Whitehead, 1992; Graham, 1993b).

Graham (1984, 1993a) describes how women may smoke to help them cope with daily crises such as a constantly demanding child or crying baby. Smoking a cigarette affords a small period of personal time and space in which they can relax and recover from the stress. This enables them to achieve a sense of wellbeing, albeit at the long-term expense of their physical health. Women living in poverty, and those with heavy caring responsibilities, perhaps for disabled children or elderly dependants, seem particularly vulnerable to the use of smoking as a coping strategy (Graham, 1993a, 1993b; Blackburn, 1993).

Lack of money may deny them the choice of, perhaps, taking children out for the day, buying toys, paying for childminding or respite care; they may have no separate room to retreat to for a small break.

In such circumstances, even though they are usually well aware of the potential harm it may cause them, smoking can seem like the only 'luxury' in their lives. It may be the only aspect of their lives over which women feel they can exercise control, to help them cope with the many stresses imposed by their living situation.

These observations challenge the notion that an 'unhealthy' way of behaving is the primary cause of ill-health. It seems more reasonable to view negative behaviours as the *result* of poor mental or social health, stemming from a social and economic situation that is politically, rather than individually, determined.

> • Health promotion strategies need to take full account of the inseparable and interactive nature of social, mental and physical aspects of health. This means recognizing limits to individual choice, and any constraints arising from the socio-economic and cultural context in which people live.

Blackburn (1993) suggests that smoking cessation work should tackle the conditions which lead women to smoke in the first place, rather than the blaming approach of advising the smokers about how much they are harming their health, and that they should stop. Instead, she advocates improving the circumstances within which women live, perhaps by ensuring that they are receiving all the welfare benefits to which they are entitled, or by finding ways of reducing the social isolation of carers.

Social support is a crucial practical and emotional resource for women with heavy caring responsibilities; this highlights the importance of community nurses offering a continuing programme of one-to-one support. Health visitors are well placed to support mothers of young children in this way, while district nurses and community psychiatric nurses may be aware of stressed carers of the elderly or mentally ill. People who are vulnerable to smoking also seem particularly unlikely to seek assistance for their own needs, even if their general health is poor. For such people, an offer of non-judgemental, unconditional and ongoing support may be the most important first step in any smoking strategy (Blackburn, 1993).

Edwards and Popay (1994) demonstrated that social support is not generally recognized as a suitable role for health care professionals by their managers, so it may be necessary to explain the health promoting relevance of supportive activities to purchasers of community nursing. In addition, community nurses can work to influence local policy initiatives, by explaining the link between smoking and a lack of facilities that might help to relieve the burdens of care – such as good playgrounds, day nurseries and locally accessible health centres. The aim is to empower people to adopt healthy lifestyles because that is the easiest and best choice for them – rather than to blame them, and create guilt because their circumstances lead them to adopt unhealthy patterns of living.

● **Conclusion**

This chapter has explained that promoting positive and healthy lifestyles requires a more integrated and holistic approach than one which targets single aspects of behaviour alone. It has been argued that very strictly focused programmes may be counter-productive to the promotion of positive and healthy lifestyles. Such approaches tend to be ineffective in the long term, as the behaviours are defined as 'problematic' by professionals, rather than by the people that indulge in them. Also, such targets seem to present 'health' as something which is negative, rather than as a positive resource for life. Concentrating on individual behaviour patterns overemphasizes physical health, at the expense of mental health or social wellbeing. Focusing solely on individual behaviour emphasizes personal guilt and blame, and minimizes the structural and political causes of ill-health.

Health-promoting strategies which are most likely to effect lasting changes in lifestyle are those which harness, rather than undermine, lay networks and knowledge. They should encourage sustained, rather than sudden changes, and take steps to avoid the risk of replacing one harmful behaviour pattern with another. Successful strategies are more likely to emphasize positive health gains than negative aspects of behaviour. Projects need to take full account of the inseparable and interactive nature of social, mental and physical aspects of health, recognizing limits to individual choice, and constraints arising from the socio-economic and cultural context in which people live.

Some examples have been offered to illustrate how community nurses have used a variety of creative and locally sensitive health-promoting strategies, which avoid the potential pitfalls of single focus programmes. These examples have not always been explicitly intended to promote healthy lifestyles, but they accord with the philosophy of health promotion espoused by the World Health Organisation (WHO, 1984, 1985, 1986). They demonstrate the vast potential, for community nurses, for using the opportunities afforded by their work to promote truly positive and healthy lifestyles.

References

Ashwell, M. (1991) Obesity in middle-aged women. In *Nutrition, Social Status and Health: Special Needs of Children, Women and Elderly People* (ed. J. Butriss), National Dairy Council, London

Barker, R. and Cooke, B. (1992) Diet, obesity and being overweight: a qualitative research study. *Health Education Journal*, **51**(3), 117–121

Berns, J. (1991) Building in health. *Nursing Times*, **87**(49), 26–29

Billingham, K. (1989) 45 Cope Street – working in partnership with parents. *Health Visitor*, **62**, 156–157

Billingham, K. (1990) Learning together: a health resource pack for working in groups. Nottingham Community Unit, Nottingham

Blackburn, C. (1991) *Poverty and Health*, Open University Press, Milton Keynes

Blackburn, C. (1993) Gender, class and smoking cessation work. *Health Visitor*, **66**(3), 83–85

Blaxter, M. (1990) *Health and Lifestyles*, Routledge, London

Calnan, M. (1987) *Health and Illness: The Lay Perspective*, Tavistock, London

Charles, N. and Kerr, M. (1986) Issues of responsibility and control in the feeding of families. In *The Politics of Health Education* (eds S. Rodmell and A. Watt), Routledge, London

Coreil, J. Levin, J. and Jaco, E. (1985) Lifestyle – an emergent concept in the socio-medical sciences. *Culture, Medicine and Psychiatry*, **9**, 423–437

Cornwell, J. (1984) *Hard-earned Lives: Accounts of Health and Illness from East London*, Tavistock Publications, London

DoH (1991) *Health of the Nation: A Consultative Document for Health in England*, HMSO, London

DoH (1992) *The Health of the Nation: A Strategy for Health in England*, HMSO, London

Edwards, J. and Popay, J. (1994) Contradictions of support and self-help: views from providers of community health and social services to families with young children. *Health and Social Care in the Community*, **2**(1), 31–40

Fisher, K. and Collins, J. (1993) *Homelessness, Health Care and Welfare Provision*, Routledge, London

Graham, H. (1984) *Women, Health and the Family*, Wheatsheaf Books, Guildford

Graham, H. (1993a) Women's smoking: government targets and social trends. *Health Visitor*, **66**(3), 80–82

Graham, H. (1993b) *Hardship and Health in Women's Lives*, Harvester Wheatsheaf, Hemel Hempstead

Ineichin, B. (1993) *Homes and Health: How Housing and Health Interact*, Spon, London

Kickbusch, I. (1986) Lifestyles and health. *Social Science and Medicine*, **22**, 117–124

Kickbusch, I. (1989) Self-care in health promotion. *Social Science and Medicine* **29**(2), 125–130

Lissner, L., Odell, P., D'Agostino, R. *et al*. (1991) Variability of body weight and health outcomes in the Framingham population. *New England Journal of Medicine*, **324**, 1839–1844

Mackeith, P., Phillipson, R. and Rowe, A. (1991) 45 Cope Street: Young mothers learning through group work: an evaluation report. Nottingham Community Health, Nottingham

Martin, C., Platt, S. and Hunt, S. (1987) Housing conditions and health. *British Medical Journal*, **294**, 1125–1127

Mayall, B. and Foster, M.-C. (1989) *Child Health Care: Living with Children, Working for Children*, Heinemann Nursing, London

Meade, K. and Carter, T. (1990) Empowering older users: some starting points. In *Power to the People* (ed. E. Winn), King's Fund, London

Newbigging, K., Cadman, T. and Westley, J. (1989) 'Powell Street' Community Mental Health Centre. In *Changing Ideas in Health Care* (eds D. Seedhouse and A. Cribb), Wiley, Chichester

Ogden, J. (1992) *Fat Chance: The Myth of Dieting Explained*, Routledge, London

Pearson, M., Dawson, C. Moore, H. *et al*. (1993) Health on borrowed time? Prioritizing and meeting needs in low income households. *Health and Social Care in the Community*, **1**(1), 45–54

Peters, T. and Waterman, R. (1982) *In Search of Excellence*, Harper and Row, London

Platt, S., Martin, C., Hunt, S. *et al*. (1989) Damp housing, mould growth and symptomatic health state. *British Medical Journal*, **298**, 1673–1678

Reid, T. (1993) Partners in care. *Nursing Times*, **89**(33), 28–30

Rowland, N. and Maynard, A. (1993) Standardized alcohol education: a hit or miss affair? *Health Promotion International*, **8**(1), 5–12

Seedhouse, D. (1986) *Health: The Foundations for Achievement*, Wiley, Chichester

Seymour, J. (1991) Whose health is it anyway? *Nursing Times*, **87**(15), 16–18

Shanks, J. (1992) Where have all the clients gone? *Nursing Times*, **88**(18), 34–35

Thompson, J. (1993) Healthy relations. *Nursing Times*, **89**(44), 50–52

Tyler, C. (1993) Travellers' tales. *Nursing Times*, **89**(33), 26–27

Walsh, R. and Redman, S. (1993) Smoking cessation in pregnancy: do effective programmes exist? *Health Promotion International*, **8**(2), 111–128

Whitehead, M. (1992) *Inequalities in Health*, Penguin, Harmondsworth

WHO (1984) *Health Promotion: a WHO Discussion Document on the Concepts and Principles*, World Health Organisation, Copenhagen

WHO (1985) *Targets for Health for All: Targets in Support of the European Regional Strategy for Health for All*, Regional Office for Europe, World Health Organisation, Copenhagen

WHO (1986) *Ottawa Charter for Health Promotion*, An International Conference on Health Promotion 17–21 November, Ottawa, Canada, World Health Organisation

WHO (1987) *Nursing and the 38 European Regional Targets for Health for All: a discussion paper*, World Health Organization, Geneva

27

Policies affecting health care: the practitioner's role

Sarah Forester

● **Introduction**

The past decade has witnessed a major change in the relationship between nursing and politics. Many authors (e.g. Gott, 1985; Salvage, 1985; Clay, 1987; Mason, 1990) have argued that political awareness and the ability to influence change are now an essential part of nursing professionalism. Two major factors have contributed to this process.

The first is the evidence of the link between socio-economic factors affecting health and the continued inequalities in health status demonstrated in the Black Report (Townsend *et al.*, 1988), and *The Nation's Health* (Jacobson *et al.*, 1991), both of which have been instrumental in shaping a nursing view of the politics of health. Secondly, changes in the management of the health service embodied in the White Paper *Working for Patients* (DoH, 1989) and the focus on preventive health strategies as set out in *The Health of the Nation* (DoH, 1992) have highlighted the need for nurses in the UK to justify their approaches in terms of health outcomes.

Community health care nursing has developed an ideology and models of care which emphasize a holistic approach in terms of health promotion, partnership and clients, patient advocacy and empowerment. In order to demonstrate the value of this approach to patient and client care, it is important for practitioners to have an understanding of the politics of health, since not only do nurses need to able to articulate the political influences on their work, but they must also be able to use and drive those influences as part of practice. In their daily work, nurses in the community have always been at the interface of rhetoric and reality in recognizing and working with varying influences on their client's health. The consequences of inequalities in health have been known for a long time. This has highlighted the need to develop strategies and policies to address those inequalities which will have a real impact on health status. One of the key principles of health visiting identified by CETHV (1977) is to influence policies affecting health. It is not surprising that this was reaffirmed more recently as being 'vitally important and as relevant as ever to practice' (Twinn and Cowley, 1992). This function is now being extended to other community nurses in the UK as it becomes integral to the core skills of community health care nurses (UKCC, 1994).

This chapter therefore will explore how community health care nursing can influence policies affecting health. However, influencing the multiplicity of social, economic and political factors which affect clients' lives is not only challenging and complex, but can also be very demoralising and unempowering for the individual nurse. For this reason, health will be considered in terms of not just health status but also how clients experience the health and social care services. Townsend *et al.* (1988) demonstrated that inequalities in health are strongly linked with unequal use of health care provision, highlighting the importance of the contribution of every community health care nurse. This contribution may be at a number of different levels, for example:

- individual service delivery
- locality/district level
- national level.

Some of the factors influencing political competence and how this area of practice might be developed will be explored and provide a framework for this chapter.

● Individual service delivery

Primary health care is not only the first point of entry into the health care system, but for an increasing number of clients it is the sole provider of both preventive and rehabilitative care. Community nurses must recognize their part in this system and in particular their role in decision-making. Robinson (1992) suggests two particular issues of relevance here. First, that nurses are unable to see their work within a broad policy context and, secondly, the view that decisions about care priorities are based on a consensus view, despite a long history of nursing losing out to those professional groups with more powerful interests.

These views are borne out in the ways in which community nurses practice. Through the mechanism of health profiling, workload and caseload management, targeting, contracting and negotiating referrals with General Practitioners, community nurses can be very influential in deciding who receives care, how it is to be delivered, how often and by whom. Against a background knowledge of inequalities in health, these decisions can be crucial in affecting change in health outcomes. A recognition of the power of these decisions may be uncomfortable but needs to be articulated if progress is to be made. Nurses must consider their roles in the broad policy context, and reflecting on practice in this respect means analysing what is informing decisions in relation to the care that is given. Indeed, nurses need to question whether decisions about workload and effective interventions are being led by nursing knowledge or are being influenced by economic and political demands. By beginning to articulate these varying influences, nurses can develop political awareness and identify where their power lies and how it may best be used.

An interesting example of how this may operate is found in the work of Cameron *et al*. (1989) in Birmingham. They found that disabled and elderly black people were under-represented in district nurse caseloads. In addition, those who received district nursing services were disadvantaged in their interactions with nurses because of stereotyping, miscommunication and language barriers. One reason for their under-representation was found to be the gate-keeping role of GPs. While the authors suggest that this is an area which needs further investigation, there are implications for community health care nurses in practice. Nurses who are aware of this issue could review their workload and stimulate discussion with Primary Health Care Teams to analyse factors influencing the under-representation of this client group. Following this process, agreed goals can be developed and referral patterns monitored. Nurses may also need to review their own educational needs to improve the quality and effectiveness of care. This type of action is within the sphere of influence of an individual nurse and may prompt colleagues into similar action, thus increasing the possibilities of changing policy and practice.

Another issue of relevance at this level is the nurse's role of rationing health care. A primary concern for nurses is the maintenance of adequate staffing levels to ensure equitable standards of care. In the community setting, where demand is seemingly endless, this debate needs to be overtly addressed. Robinson (1992) suggests that this kind of issue is often kept off the formal policy agenda or disguised as nurses' inability to manage resources adequately. Nurses have been loath to refuse care for patients, of whom many are often among the most vulnerable groups in society. This is illustrated in a study of a survey of patients receiving terminal care (Jacoby, 1990).

District nurses interviewed in this study identified occasions where not only requests for home visits had been refused, but also more frequently where heavy workloads and staff shortages resulted in the quality of care being diminished which caused them distress. The explicit demonstration of this latter point could become a key tool for nurses when arguing for greater resources to meet client needs. Ong (1991) outlines some key features of consumer satisfaction with district nursing services. With the move towards consumer satisfaction being a key feature in demonstrating the quality of services, community health care nurses need to develop tools to record any substantial claims for greater resources.

The introduction of community waiting lists may also be a way forward (Cottingham, 1988). The political impact of hospital waiting lists has been immense. Along with this there is a need for a full and open debate on skill mix (see, for example, Cowley, 1993). Nurses should not entrench themselves into old roles, but work collaboratively with nursing colleagues to better meet identified needs. Naish and Twinn (1992) have argued that nurses working in the community have placed the emphasis on their roles rather than the practice outcomes of nursing intervention, which has got in the way of meeting current political challenges in care. It is only through addressing these issues that community health care nurses can begin to really influence the service that clients want and need.

● Locality/district level

There are perhaps wider opportunities for nurses to influence policy at the locality/district level. The purchaser/provider philosophy currently experienced in health care in the UK has emphasized the need for profiling and assessment of need in determining service provision. The introduction of case management by The NHS and Community Care Act (DoH, 1990), and the increasing role played by community nurses in this process, allows practitioners to gather evidence of problems in responding to client/patient needs such as gaps in service provision. Community nurses can be influential in two main ways:

● setting programmes of action in response to identified needs which includes influencing the agendas of purchasing authorities and general practitioners
● developing and demonstrating the value of different approaches in working in response to agendas set by others such as purchasing authorities.

The potential role of nurses in purchasing will be discussed as an example of practitioners influencing the policy agenda and, in addition, different approaches to the delivery of care, particularly those of community development and public health, are considered to highlight the need to examine policy implications for practice.

Nurses and purchasing

It is becoming clear that there are major opportunities for community nurses to influence the purchasing role of health authorities. However, as this role develops it is becoming more apparent that a pure epidemiological approach to assessing health needs is limited in actually achieving health outcomes. Data at district level frequently consists of relatively small numbers making interpretation of need difficult to assess. Therefore, although problems may be identified, there is little information available as to the appropriate strategies to achieve change. A report by the King's Fund College (1993) suggests that nurses are an ideal group to fill some of these gaps. In particular, it suggests a strong role for community nurses in 'contract specification and negotiation, information analysis and influencing fund holding General Practitioners' decisions', thereby explicitly demonstrating the political contribution required of community nurses in their practice.

There is a need to elaborate on the process of achieving health gain, in particular by practice becoming more user focused and practitioners considering intersectoral working. Goodwin (1992) highlights the problem of public health led needs assessment becoming remote from both users and care deliverers unless a more 'bottom up' approach is adopted, reaffirming the significance of a 'local voices' concept (King's

Fund College, 1993). This concept implies finding ways of communicating with and educating user groups to articulate their needs as well as finding ways of crossing the purchaser/provider divide. This highlights the need to tap into the informal knowledge of primary health care workers as well as that recorded in their records. In particular, community nurses hold a significant amount of knowledge about local networks as well as the influences which shape clients' health behaviour. Community nurses have contacts with formal and informal user groups and the communication skills to put all these together to develop strategies to influence health. It is this kind of sophisticated level of local knowledge that policy-makers require to respond to the health needs of local populations, once again highlighting the political role played by community nurses at district level.

Community nurses have a long history of compiling and interpreting local health data. Indeed, as suggested by Cernic and Wearne (1992), neighbourhood studies have gathered dust in desk drawers for years. If nurses are to be truly influential in health gain, they must begin to use this information to inform practice and to demonstate to purchasers of health care the most effective health strategies. Drennan (1990) describes how a comprehensive collection of information from fieldworkers can be used to identify trends and determine service development and resource allocation. Information collected from district nursing teams about, for example, clients who only require nursing intervention to meet their hygiene needs showed great variation in one area of the district to another. Evidence suggests that this raised questions about the provision of other services across the district. Since district nurses are becoming more involved in working with social service providers of social care and case management, there is the opportunity for them to become key players in identifying whether changes in service provision meet health needs as well as identifying gaps in that provision.

Nurses must also be able to identify the impact of nursing interventions, since purchasers of health care who are able to directly contract for nursing services need to be influenced as to the most appropriate nursing approach to meet the health outcomes they require. Barriball and Mackenzie (1993) suggest that more research is needed to find methods of outcome measurement. Campbell *et al.* (1995) have produced a framework to identify outcomes and effectiveness in the more complex, qualitative realms of community nursing practice. What is needed is the ability to use this information in the policy-making arena of purchasing. In order to achieve this outcome, nurses have to take on the responsibility of marketing their services, particularly their contribution to the assessment of need. The marketing of health visiting project (NHSE, 1994) has provided one model for this exercise and anecdotal evidence suggests that this is already being used by other community nurses such as Macmillan nurses.

Influencing the policy agenda

An important example of nurses influencing local policies can be seen in the work of community and homeless people: with access to the conditions of homeless families, community nurses have played a major role in articulating the needs of this vulnerable group. Cross (1988) describes how local action generated the establishment of specialist services and this has been repeated in other areas of the UK. Health visitors campaigning at local and then at national level have succeeded in contributing to major identification of needs for this group and in developing alternative ways of working (Conway, 1988). This energy has resulted in, for example, the funding of a full-time worker at a major professional organization (Health Visitors' Association) who continues to campaign for better services. This type of development removes the debate from the local level of providing better services to the crucial question of housing policy. Indeed, through the work of groups like SIGH (Special Interest Group for Homeless) at the Health Visitors' Association, health workers collectively have the power effectively to use the information they hold about health and homelessness to change policy. In particular, by working collaboratively with other housing groups they can provide evidence to campaign for good affordable housing for all, which is at the core of the problem.

Of the many examples of community nurses working with and on behalf of homeless people, there are common strategies which include:

- publicizing the identified needs – to managers, local campaigning groups, the media
- joining with other practitioners and other local workers to establish joint initiatives
- using experiences gained in the field to influence national policies.

This is a model of political action that can be applied to other client groups. A further example of this model is described by Hutchings and Gower (1993), in which a study of needs of clients referred to community mental health services highlighted employment status as having a major impact on their mental health. Having identified this need, community mental health nurses were instrumental in establishing a multi-agency project which provides both a service and campaigns on employment issues.

Community health development

In trying to develop policies to be more effective in meeting identified health needs, the growth of the 'community development' movement provides a useful model (see Chapter 31). This model, which involves lay participation, has been used effectively by some community nurses to develop health policy. However, Whitehead (1989), in reviewing the community development movement's contribution to the development of policy within the context of health promotion, highlights five areas of tension in this type of initiative which need to be addressed for progress to be made. These are:

- different priorities between the community and funding body
- threat to local health workers
- the need to achieve instant results

- unrealistic expectations of what can be achieved
- evaluation conflicts.

All these issues are relevant to community nurses and many will be familiar to practitioners who are trying to demonstrate effective practice in health promotion. In particular, the different priorities of clients and service providers need to be clearly articulated. An example is provided by *The Health of the Nation* (DoH, 1992) targets for smoking or childhood accidents which appear to make very complex health issues simple to achieve. By focusing on single, mostly physical problems, it ignores social and emotional influences such as poverty, social isolation and poor environments which are often more pressing concerns for client groups considered most at risk.

Currently, community nurses, in particular health visitors, continue to see their priorities as working with women and families since research has demonstrated their gatekeeping role in family health (Graham, 1990). In order to do this in an effective and sensitive way, there is a need to address the total concerns of those women, not the single health issue as suggested by some policy documents. Graham (1990) and Blackburn (1992) both clearly demonstrate how complex and difficult it can be caring for family health in poverty. They also highlight the effects this has on women's health, for example their smoking habits or inability to access preventive health services. It is clear that an individual casework approach, which has been the traditional approach of the health visitor, is inadequate in both meeting the needs of these clients and in addressing governmental targets. Edwards and Ramsey (1992), in describing the PATCH project, provide a good example of a community health development project by a health visitor to address the needs of isolated families in poor housing conditions. The philosophy of the programme is to start from the user perspective to create confidence in clients' parenting skills as well as enabling parents themselves to begin to tackle other problems such as housing. Key features in the success of this scheme seem to be the collaborative working with the voluntary sector in establishing the scheme and the long-term nature of the work. Indeed, to establish groups and effective working relationships requires patience and a long-term view. Consumer satisfaction is an important measure of success, and evaluation over time has demonstrated increased uptake of health and other local services. Projects like this must be assessed in an appropriate way – merely using medical measures are ineffective at every level. However, this approach to practice needs a change in philosophy as well as policy in those purchasing bodies who wish to see measurable health improvements. It is therefore important that practitioners demonstrate the effectiveness of these types of approaches to health care. They can provide community nurses with a powerful tool to influence the health policy of purchasers.

Another important issue to consider in community development work which has implications for policy is the changing relationship practitioners experience with patients and clients. A similar issue, but in a different context, has been experienced with the introduction of patient-held records. Holland *et al*. (1993) described how this approach to practice required practitioners to re-examine their whole relationship with clients, in particular to embrace a more equal power-sharing approach. Other community nurses face the same challenges as they increasingly work in partnership with carers (Ong, 1991). From these new approaches to practice, it is apparent that traditional practice in community nursing has always incorporated unequal power relationships. This has necessarily allied nurses with the prevailing health policies which has led to victim-blaming attitudes and rendered many nurses powerless to influence change. By demonstrating a variety of approaches to different health needs and client groups, community health care nurses do not become entrenched in traditional roles, thus becoming more able to influence change.

The power relationship between different nursing groups also needs to be examined in order to enable practitioners to work together to influence health policies. Sutcliffe (1991) reports on an interesting initiative where the concept of neighbourhood nursing team, combined with the process of profiling and the introduction of the World Health Organisation's 'Health for All' (WHO, 1991) principles, has led to many new nursing initiatives. A nurse-led community health clinic provides a range of easily accessible primary health care services, including health promotion activities, within the context of mental health. Nurses having established agreements of care with clients are in the process of involving consumers in the planning and delivery of care. This is a good example of how community development approaches can be adapted to mainstream health care provision. Indeed, the techniques and philosophy of community development do not have to be restricted to special projects and provide practitioners with the opportunity of developing health policy which meets the needs of patients and clients.

Developing new strategies for the delivery of care, particularly working with groups and communities, enables community nurses to demonstrate the worth of these different approaches. This can be used to influence purchasing teams in health authorities and perhaps more directly GP fundholders. Community health care nurses need to reflect on the power relationships surrounding their work and through that reflection be able to work for change, thereby demonstrating the significance of their political role to practice.

Public health alliances

The development of GPs contracting for community nursing services has focused the debate about the public health role of community health care nurses. There is a danger that public health and health promotion work will once again be split from each other in the working practices of community health care nurses. While it is not appropriate to enter into the full debate here, some of the ways community health care nurses can contribute to public health, in particular environmental issues, will be discussed since this is particularly relevant to policies affecting health. The previous discussion has highlighted how community health care nurses can influence the debate on working policy. However, the introduction of water metering in some areas in the UK and the ensuing health problems, especially among families living in poverty, has taken many community health care nurses back to the public health roots of community nursing. Potrykus (1993) illustrates this point with an example of community health care nurses joining with other workers and members of the public in campaigning against metering. Community nurses, again because of their access to a wide range of homes, play an important role in collecting data to support campaigns such as this. It is suggested that many water-borne infections are going unrecorded as well as the stress and mental health problems that worrying about water bills is having on families. Health visitors in this area have joined the Public Health Alliance, a national organization with local centres, which aims to campaign about, and monitor, public health issues and how policy affects them. By working intersectorally in this way, practitioners have the opportunity to directly influence policy.

Other examples of environmental health hazards taken up by community health care nurses are described by Seymour (1990). High concentrations of nitrates in water breaching pollution guidance and the link between radiation emissions and childhood cancer are issues taken up by community nurses, either by giving general advice, initiating campaigns or joining existing campaigns. It is important that community nurses do not let the drive of market forces of the purchaser policy of health care dilute or lose their public health role. The emphasis put on public health as a core skill in community health care nursing within the Report on Post Registration Education and Practice (UKCC, 1994), will ensure that public health policy remains an influential sphere of practice within community nursing.

The key to all these actions is for community health care nurses to use the information they hold in a political way. For the most part this means practitioners sharing that information, first with clients, since this encompasses the process of empowerment facilitating long-term change. This objective may seem unobtainable when faced with the multiple needs of some clients, but it is important that practitioners keep this fundamental philosophy at the forefront of their practice if interventions are to be effective in meeting health needs. However, it would be naive to think that this approach to work is all that is needed. Community health care nurses need also to work on behalf of those vulnerable groups with whom they have contact and to do this nurses need to share information with other practitioners and begin to develop a collective view and strategy for the health needs appropriate to their communities. Collective voices are more powerful in the political arena and also protect individuals from the fear of victimization, a fear which can be a real barrier to action when the employment situation is precarious and conditions of service are changing. Discussion of possible political strategies within nursing teams at neighbourhood or locality level also provides support for a nurse or nurses who may be involved in taking strategies forward. This highlights the need for a decision-making process which legitimates political networking as a key part of the team's function.

Finally, having developed a group view community nurses need to establish links with the key players in the policy-making process. Initially this will be with purchasing bodies: health authorities, public health directorates, local authorities and fundholding general practitioners. In addition, formal and informal networks need to be developed with a range of different organizations involved in collaborative projects not only with the health service but also with voluntary sector and community-based agencies. Although there is no blueprint for this process, analysing what has been effective in their own as well as others' practices, will enable nurses to develop their skills within this important aspect of practice.

● National level

At a national level, community health care nurses need to grasp the opportunity to be effective advocates for their clients. As a group of professionals who are in daily contact with people with overt health needs, as well as the homeless, children, elderly, and disabled people, and other particularly vulnerable groups, community nurses are well placed to observe the effects of health and social policies. The collective strength of nursing is important in articulating the needs of these groups, providing a clear ongoing critique of policies affecting health and demonstrating how effective policies and strategies may be delivered in practice.

In order to achieve this, nurses need a strong united voice across the different disciplines of nursing in the community. As new roles develop, such as those of practice nurses and nurse practitioners, instead of taking a defensive position or entrenching themselves in traditional roles, community health care nurses should work collaboratively with these groups of practitioners. Indeed, to influence the national agenda the breadth of community nursing practice and the contributions of different skills must be valued and demonstrated. Community nursing development units, such as that described by Gooch (1993), provide the opportunity of demonstrating the value of nursing innovation in meeting complex health needs.

As the implications of GPs directly purchasing nursing services begin to take effect, the management and delivery of the totality of community nursing services will need to be increasingly reviewed. Community health care nurses must be aware of the changes and be pro-active in arguing for nursing-led services that respond to local need. It is important that community health care nurses are represented at all levels of policy-making, particularly when there is an emphasis on the market forces within health care.

In order to promote innovation in practice and provide a collective voice on important practice issues, community nurses need to ensure they use the power provided by professional organizations and trades unions. This requires individual nurses to take responsibility not only to be active in these organizations, but also keeping up to date with the activities of these organizations on behalf of community health care nursing. Indeed, it is the responsibility of field workers to keep nursing leaders informed of practice activities and initiatives in order to promote a strong lobby for change.

In addition, national organizations can be influential in using the media to highlight issues in health care. This may be achieved by lobbying inside and outside government organizations and contributing to policy-making through activities such as participation in select committees. Active trades unions and professional bodies are also able to establish links with workers in other social care agencies in both the statutory and the voluntary sector. Greater collaboration between bodies representing health and social care workers becomes increasingly important as the move to community-focused care becomes a reality. By working intersectorally and associating with national campaigns and pressure groups, organizations representing community health care nursing can also exert an important political influence.

● Conclusion

To review the role of nurses in influencing policies affecting health, nurses need to reflect on their strengths and weaknesses as political operators, a process in which education plays a particularly significant role. Indeed, pre- and post-registration nurse education now includes the development of political awareness through social policy studies. However, it is essential that practitioners become part of the processes involved in influencing health policies. In order to do this, it is necessary to:

- recognize the political nature of community nursing roles
- continue to demonstrate the link between socio-economic factors and health, for example by poverty profiling
- use this information to change practice to influence purchasers and to keep these issues in the public domain
- act together across professional boundaries to empower nurses by support and increased collaboration in nursing teams, recognizing the importance of health outcomes rather than traditional roles
- develop collective strategies in primary health and social care teams and by making alliances with other statutory and voluntary agencies
- extend the scope of practice to include political action, recognizing responsibility and accountability in this respect.

Above all, nurses cannot afford to be complacent; a consensus view in health care is not relevant either to the health problems of the next decade or to the way health care is at present being delivered. It is important for practitioners to remember that the professional code of conduct (UKCC, 1992) requires nurses to

act always in such a manner as to promote and safeguard the interests and well being of patients with clients.

This cannot be achieved without trying to influence policies affecting health.

References

Barriball, K.L. and Mackenzie, A. (1993) Measuring the impact of nursing interventions in community: a selective review of the literature. *Journal of Advanced Nursing*, **18**, 401–407

Blackburn, C. (1992) *Improving Health and Welfare Work with Families in Poverty – Handbook*, Open University Press, Milton Keynes

Cameron, E., Badger, R. and Evers, H. (1989) District nursing – who are the black patients? *Journal of Advanced Nursing*, **14**(5), 376–382

Campbell, F., Cowley, S. and Buttigieg, M. (1995) *Weights and Measures; Outcomes and Evaluation in Health Visiting*, HVA, London

Cernic, K. and Wearne, M. (1992) Using community health profiles to improve service provision. *Health Visitor*, **65**(10), 343–345

CETHV (1977) *An Investigation into the Principles of Health Visiting*, Council for Education and Training of Health Visitors, London

Clay, T.(1987) *Nurse: Power and Politics*, Heinemann, London

Conway, J. (ed.) (1988) *Prescription for Poor Health – The Crisis for London Homeless Families*, LFC MA SHAC/SHELTER, London

Cottingham, M. (1988) Rationing community care. *Nursing Times*, **84**(11), 16–22

Cowley, S. (1993) Skill mix: value for whom? *Health Visitor*, **66**(5), 166–168

Cross, A. (1988) Improving health care for the homeless. *Health Visitors and Groups; Politics and Practice* (ed. V. Drennan), Heinemann Nursing, Oxford

DoH (1989) *Working for Patients*, HMSO, London

DoH (1990) *The National Health and Community Care Act*, HMSO, London

DoH (1992) *The Health of the Nation*, HMSO, London

Drennan, V. (1990) Gathering information from the field. *Nursing Times*, **86**(39), 46–48

Edwards, R. and Ramsey, S. (1992) Health visiting on a playbus: a community approach. *Health Visitor*, **65**(5), 169–771

Gooch, S. (1993) Healthy options. *Nursing Times*, **89**(8), 41–43

Goodwin, S. (1992) Nurses and purchasing. *Senior Nurse*, **12**(6), 7–11

Gott, M. (1985) Politics and professionalism: nursing. *Nurse Education Today*, **5**, 274–276

Graham, H. (1990) Behaving well: women's health behaviour in context. In *Women's Health Counts* (ed. H. Roberts), Routledge, London

Holland, S., Emms, E., McNaughton, A., Philips, J. and Whitney, G. (1993) Preparing for parent held child health records. *Health Visitor*, **66**(4) 139–140

Hutchings, J. and Gower, K. (1993) Unemployment and mental health. *Community Psychiatric Nursing Journal*, **13**(5) 17–21

Jacobson, B., Smith, A. and Whitehead, M. (1991) *The Nation's Health*, 2nd edn, King's Fund, London

Jacoby, A. (1990) More demand, less care. *Nursing Standard*, **5**(7), 54–55

King's Fund College (1993) *The Professional Nursing Contribution to Purchasing*, NHSME Nursing Directorate, London

Mason, D. (1990) Nursing and politics: a profession comes of age. *Orthopaedic Nursing*, **9**(5), 11–17

Naish, J. and Twinn, S. (1992) Excellence in the community. *Nursing Times*, **88**(23), 45–47

NHSE (1994) *Health Visiting Marketing Project: Project Report*, NHSE, Leeds

Ong, B.N. (1991) Researching needs in district nursing. *Journal of Advanced Nursing*, **16**, 638–647

Potrykus, C. (1993) Building an alliance against disconnection. *Health Visitor* **66**(5), 150

Robinson, J. (1992) Introduction: beginning the study of nursing policy. In *Policy Issues in Nursing* (eds J. Robinson, A. Gray and R. Elkan), Open University Press, Milton Keynes

Salvage, J. (1985) *The Politics of Nursing,* Heinemann Nursing, London

Seymour, J. (1990) Water water everywhere. *Nursing Times,* **86**(44), 60–61

Sutcliffe, P. (1991) Changing practice – practising change. *Nursing,* **4**(35), 19–21

Townsend, P., Davidson, N. and Whitehead, M. (1988) *Inequalities in Health: The Black Report and the Health Divide,* Penguin, Harmondsworth

Twinn, S. and Cowley, S. (1992) *The Principles of Health Visiting: A Re-examination,* HVA/UKSC, London

UKCC (1992) *The Scope of Professional Practice,* UKCC, London

UKCC (1994) *Post Registration Education and Practice: Final Report,* UKCC, London

Whitehead, M. (1989) *Swimming Upstream. Trends and Prospects in Education for Health,* King's Fund Institute, London

WHO (1991) *Health for All Targets: A Health Policy for Europe,* WHO, Copenhagen

28

Advocacy

David Sines

● Introduction

The British Government, in common with trends which can be identified in many areas of the Western world, has demonstrated a commitment to enhancing the powers that patients and clients have in respect of their negotiation rights to receive effective and efficient service responses from health service provider agencies.

In the UK, *The Patient's Charter* (DoH, 1991) had been the 'flagship' of this approach and requires Health Authorities to provide consumers with information and means of representation to inform their judgements and evaluation of public sector provision.

This chapter explores the concept of advocacy and considers the implications for practising nurses and colleagues as they aim to involve service users in all aspects of the health care delivery process.

● Advocacy

Advocacy may simply be defined as the process of acting for, or on behalf of, another person. Williams and Schoultz (1982) define advocacy as:

> *speaking or acting on behalf of oneself or another person or an issue, with self sacrificing vigour and vehemence.*

The nurse's role in exploring the concept of advocacy is well summarized by Murphy and Hunter (1984):

> *The goal of the nurse is not to receive gratification from other health professionals but rather to help the patient obtain the best care even if it means going against hospital administration and other health care professionals.*

The nurse needs to consider this quotation in relation to new working arrangements in NHS Trusts and within the purchaser/provider culture (see Chapter 8).

The advocacy role is therefore far from straightforward and demands that nurses should be prepared to undertake complex and, sometimes, controversial roles in support of the primacy of their patients' and clients' interests. In so doing, their role includes:

- to uphold the rights of persons without prejudice or discrimination
- to act always in the patient's best interests
- to act as an intermediary between the person and those providing or seeking to provide services for that person.

Fowler (1989) describes four models of advocacy:

- guardian of patient rights
- preservation of patient values
- champion of social justice in the provision of health care
- conservator of the patient's best interests.

Each of these functions is interdependent and requires the nurse to acquire and apply effective assertion and negotiation skills. A major component of the advocacy role is the extent to which the nurse succeeds in empowering her or his clients in order to enable them to take an active role in determining their own futures (which will include decisions about their health status and the provision of care). This may involve the development of self-advocacy skills which aim to enhance the person's ability to speak out and act on their own behalf.

Such schemes require active consideration and must commence with an acknowledgment that both the nurse and the client accept that their relationship must be based on equality, trust and mutual respect. The self-advocacy issue will be addressed later in this chapter, but serves as an important reminder that the primary goal of the advocacy role must be, at all times, to avoid patronizing clients by inflicting either personal or professional agendas.

Consequently, the interests of the advocate must never supersede those of the client, and Walsh (1985) warns nurses of the 'dangers of developing their own autonomy at the expense of those they wish to serve'. In this respect care must be taken to resolve power issues that might arise as a natural consequence of working as members of multi-professional teams, before engaging in representation issues for clients.

One other key issue to be addressed is the extent to which it might be said that nurses can, in fact, be true advocates for their patients and clients. Sutor (1993) argues that patient advocacy is an impossible goal until it is enshrined within a legal framework which protects both nurses and their clients from possible sanction from their employers. It is in this latter respect that nurses have learnt, sadly to their own cost, that there is a price to pay for speaking up for their clients.

● **Advocacy, accountability and ethical considerations**

The nurse's role as advocate is identified in the Code of Professional Conduct (UKCC, 1992b) and requires that nurses act always to uphold public interest. In a supplementary document *Exercising Accountability*, the UKCC (1989) advises that:

Advocacy is concerned with promoting and safeguarding the well-being and interests of clients. It is not concerned with conflict for its own sake.

The advice about conflict is an attempt to remove the presumption that advocating for others always involves some form of confrontation or adversarial quest. However, in the pursuit of this responsibility, nurses are also reminded that conflict may be unavoidable if it is considered that the patient's best interests are being compromised or if professional standards are reduced to an unacceptable level.

Examples involving conflict might include complaints about low staffing levels, inappropriate skill mix, the imposition of clinical treatments on persons who are unable to provide informed consent, or the premature discharge of a person from hospital care in the absence of acceptable home care arrangements.

Such situations involve negotiation with doctors, managers and other members of the inter-disciplinary team. Marshall (1991) notes that nurses often require the support and understanding of their professional colleagues. This may not always be achievable, particularly if other members of the multi-disciplinary team are unwilling to consult or collaborate with their nursing colleagues.

For example, some doctors have voiced their arguments against nurse advocacy by:

- presuming that it is their responsibility to give information and to discuss issues relating to diagnosis and prognosis
- suggesting that nurses are not adequately prepared for the responsibilities of advocacy
- relegating the nursing role to a subservient status, thus preserving the power base of the medical profession.

Nurses, of course, do not have to accept these unfounded arguments and are increasingly invited to mediate decisions between their medical colleagues and their patients and clients. They may be ideally placed to share information with clients and to assist in follow-up interviews to validate the extent to which clients have understood the rationale for their diagnosis, prognosis and treatment.

Management encounters may also compromise the nurse's role. Staff may find that they are occasionally confronted by ethical issues which urge them to report matters to their employers. As part of their employment contract, nurses are bound to maintain confidentiality and this includes a responsibility to clients and patients and to one's employers who act as guardians of case files and other formal documents.

In the introduction to the text *Secrets* (Bok, 1984), the key issues facing such questions of confidentiality are raised; conflicts are explored between the motives one has for either revealing or concealing the secrets conferred on us by others:

We are all, in a sense, experts on secrecy. From earliest childhood we feel its mystery and attraction. We know both the power it confers and the burden it imposes. We learn how it can delight, give breathing-space, and protect. But we come to understand its dangers, too: how it is used to oppress and exclude; what can befall those who come too close to secrets they were not meant to share; and the price of betrayal.

The study of ethics is primarily concerned with the question of how we should treat people and this must involve active deliberation of issues relating to truth-telling (veracity) and beneficence. The latter is one of the key principles that governs nursing practice and aims always to provide good and well-intentioned consequences for clients. However, while this might seem to be a valued ideal it may, in practice, conflict with the philosophy of care offered in the work setting.

Nurses will be judged in respect of the extent to which they conform to expectations of standard morality (virtue) and consequently uphold the rights of their clients. However, nurses may not always find it easy to behave accordingly and occasionally, when faced with moral dilemmas, are sometimes expected to act against the dictates of their conscience in order to execute their duties.

This leads us to consider the contemporary issue of whistle-blowing which places this dilemma into context. One of the reasons suggested for the failure of nurses to report either poor or unacceptable practice to their managers (or to the general public) has been the potential fear of reprisals from their managers. Employees are confronted by split loyalties to their clients, their profession, the general public, their employers and to themselves. Nurses are trained and inducted to obey rules and regulations which are primarily upheld in accordance with administrative protocol. As nurses become more aware of critical issues confronting standards of practice, so they reflect on the deficiencies in care delivery systems.

In the field of nursing, even the act of truth-telling can be fraught with difficulties. For example, to share a patient's concerns about her prognosis a nurse may find that she is unable to tell the truth due to medical advice to the contrary. Other situations might relate to low staffing levels and the effect these may have on a nurse's ability to provide an acceptable level of care for her clients. Repeated written reports to managers to improve the skill mix of the team might go unheard and eventually a crisis might confirm the nurse's worst fears that she was unable to provide a safe level of care to her clients. Not only might she face personal disciplinary action, but she may be faced with a moral dilemma of whether to produce evidence of her previous representations to her employers. The threat of losing one's job might well militate against disclosure and thus discourage the nurse to blow the whistle.

This, then, is the moral dilemma facing nursing, and the extent to which they can be said to be true advocates for their clients must always remain a question for critical evaluation. The American Nursing Association has already recognized that there should be an established mechanism for reporting and handling incompetent or unethical practice at work; this is undertaken within a system of reporting and representation without fear of reprisal for nurses (Muyskens, 1982).

The extent to which nurses may act as effective advocates for their patients and clients within the present professional and legal systems of the UK is somewhat limited. Despite major advances, the extent to which nursing has been afforded equal status with medicine remains questionable, and yet nurses are certainly encouraged to advocate on behalf of their clients and their new educational curricula address the advocacy issue both critically and responsively.

● **Developing consumer involvement**

The advocacy issue is not limited to the nursing profession and transcends the main agenda for the provision of health and social care. For example, The NHS and Community Care Act (DoH, 1990) recommends the involvement of consumers and their representative groups in all aspects of health care delivery and evaluation. The social care agenda also encourages partnership in care management and new complaints procedures have been published to advise consumers of their representation rights. Information leaflets have also been published to advise patients and clients of their expectations for accessing health and community services.

Nurses also have a specific role to play in representing the needs of consumers through involvement in the statementing process with children with special needs (DoH, 1981). Similarly, The Disabled Persons (Consultation, Representation and Services) Act (DoH, 1986) focuses attention on the needs to involve consumers at all stages of the assessment and care delivery process through the involvement of appointees and advocates. The Children Act (DoH, 1989) also emphasizes consultation and representation and its enactment will demand the acquisition of advocacy skills among nursing staff.

The government states that the purpose of public involvement is 'to ensure that the values and preferences of the public influence local plans and strategies' (Welsh Office, 1992). The key aims of this process are to match service responses to local needs and to assist in the determination of the style and quality of service provision.

Involving the public in this way is one strategic attempt to ensure that public agencies remain accountable to the electorate for the achievement of health gain. The development of a people-centred service requires:

● identification of the main consumers of present and future services
● eliciting fully and accurately the values and preferences of the community and its component groups
● communicating the information received, and at all times to inform the planning process of health care delivery
● acknowledgement of the importance of ensuring that plans respond to actual consumer demands and preferences.

Listening to consumers requires the active involvement of front-line workers in this process. These will often be nurses who have the opportunity of working closely with consumers at the coal-face of service delivery. There are many ways of capturing the views of the public, to assist them to identify the things that are important to them and to their health care status. Personal communication and mutual respect would appear to be the most effective means of gaining insight into such issues.

Community health care nurses can facilitate access to the representative views of individuals, groups and communities through the application of both research and epidemiological techniques. The techniques that might be applied are:

- in-depth interviews with clients and their families
- focused discussion groups with selected members
- patient associations and discussion groups
- holding opportunistic discussion groups
- surveys: questionnaires, structured and semi-structured interviews
- analysis of statistical records
- consultation with voluntary groups
- holding public meetings
- analysis of complaints and suggestion schemes.

● Impaired autonomy and advocacy

Nurses will often find themselves working with people who have impaired autonomy. People with learning disabilities, mental health needs and elderly persons with advanced dementia are examples of groups of people for whom autonomous decision-making may be impaired.

In such situations nurses must extend opportunities for consumer involvement, and one method of facilitating the achievement of this objective is the establishment of self-advocacy groups. In so doing it should be noted that primary consumers are not the only consumers who have an interest in the provision of care services. Secondary consumers such as parents, partners and other carers also have views and these must be heard. However, care should be taken to make a clear distinction between the wants, needs and views of both groups (which may occasionally be in conflict with each other).

Established services for such clients may have introduced a series of mechanisms for determining the needs of clients. Individual planning process, care management and shared action planning (Brechin and Swain, 1987) are all examples of mechanisms or processes whereby professional staff have engaged in active dialogue with clients to assess needs and to plan services in active partnership in a formal way. The individual planning process works in partnership with individuals, their families, representatives and carers to identify, assess and find ways of meeting their needs. To be meaningful, great care must be taken to ensure that consumers are engaged in all stages of the care process. It is vital, therefore, that they understand and feel valued and comfortable in the process. Their views should be respected and plans should be shared collaboratively with other agencies who may be involved or influential in meeting specified goals and targets.

The important role of voluntary organizations should also be remembered and their ability to represent consumer interests has been well acknowledged by all government departments.

Putting the person first would appear to be an appropriate description of the primary aim of the advocacy process. Services must always focus first on the individual and should attempt to respond to the needs, wishes and preferences of the person as a whole. In order for this to be accomplished, individuals need to have the self-confidence and verbal ability to make their needs and views known. This is particularly important in formal meetings and with groups of people they do not know well – membership of self-advocacy groups or the use of a citizen advocate (a person who agrees to represent the interests of a client without legal sanction or remuneration).

● Self-advocacy

Self-advocacy may be defined as enabling individuals to make choices, to make their own decisions and to assume control over their lives. It is often described as 'speaking up for yourself', but when taken seriously this has far greater significance.

People make decisions every day about what they want to wear or eat and choose where they want to go and with whom to share their time. These decisions are often taken for granted, but for a person with impaired autonomy (such as a person with a learning disability or mental illness) others often assume control over their lives. They may not have the opportunity, the self-confidence or the encouragement to make these decisions.

A key to ensuring that people do speak for themselves lies in the extent to which they are empowered to express their views both individually and collectively. The self-advocacy movement assists people to meet together and to speak with a united voice, thus enabling them to express their views. The result may be to assist people in achieving local and national changes in policy on issues that affect all individuals with similar needs.

● Citizen advocacy

Not all individuals wish to or are able to express themselves. Many individuals have the capacity for participating in the decision-making process, but need time to think and to articulate their position and to make up their minds. It can also take time to explain the options available and reasons for certain courses of action.

In these circumstances, the presence of a person who knows the individual well, has spent time getting to know them, and explaining the options in advance in a relaxed and non-threatening manner, may be able to interpret responses provided at a meeting for clients. The independence of citizen advocates is essential in order to avoid the possibility of conflicting interests.

Citizen advocates are a valuable support to people with impaired autonomy and should be encouraged to support people who, for one reason or another, are unable to represent themselves in public. They require training and support themselves and access to information about important decisions that might affect the lives of their partners.

● Practical implications

It is of little use to anyone if the principles outlined in this chapter are ignored. People need to be encouraged to speak for themselves and to be represented when they so wish. It is essential if the government's strategy of client involvement is to work, to ensure that health care professionals examine their own agendas for self-fulfilment and personal advancement.

A partnership between client and professional carer is quite acceptable as long as both partners in the process are aware of the potential conflicts of interests that might occur in the relationship.

One of these refers to the calculation of risk and the endorsement of action chosen by clients themselves, which may not be supported by professional carers. Take for example a person with a learning disability who expresses a desire to marry. Who makes the final decision? Advice, counselling and support will be needed, but at the end of the day as long as the client understands the implications of the marital contract, there is no legal sanction to prohibit the marriage. True, there are issues to address such as child-bearing and potential abuse, but these must be addressed objectively and the risks should be assessed and calculated within the context of a shared action plan with the client and other relevant professionals.

There is no simple solution to such matters, but each must be judged in accordance with its individual merit. Risk-taking implies both moral and professional judgement and this forms the central core of the advocacy issue.

● Conclusion

Nurses are ideally placed to represent the views and wishes of their clients. However, they must acknowledge their professional position in this relationship and apply both moral and professional judgements.

Conflict must be handled carefully and judiciously in accordance with the UKCC (1992b) *Code of Professional Conduct* (with specific reference to issues relating to accountability) and the UKCC (1992a) document *The Scope of Professional Practice*. Taking a stand on behalf of clients requires a strong personal belief in the moral rightness of what one is doing.

The role of nurse advocate is an integral part of the nurse's duty to represent the primacy of interest of each client and patient whenever their autonomy is impaired. In accepting this responsibility, nurses must recognize their personal training needs, covert prejudices and personal obligations. They must inform their clients and empower them to share in all aspects care planning, delivery and measurement of its effectiveness.

References

Bok, S. (1986) *Secrets – The Ethics of Concealment and Revelation*, Oxford University Press, Oxford

Brechin, A. and Swain, J. (1987) *Changing Relationships – Shared Action Planning for People with Mental Handicaps*, Harper and Row, London

DoH (1981) *The Education Act*, HMSO, London

DoH (1986) *The Disabled Persons (Consultation, Representation and Services) Act*, HMSO, London

DoH (1989) *The Children Act*, HMSO, London

DoH (1990) *The NHS and Community Care Act*, HMSO, London

DoH (1991) *The Patient's Charter*, HMSO, London

Fowler, D.M. (1989) Social advocacy. *Heart and Lung*, **1**, 18

Marshall, M. (1991) Advocacy within the multi-disciplinary team. *Nursing Standard*, **27**(6), 28–31

Murphy, C. and Hunter, H. (1984) *Ethical Problems in the Nurse–Patient Relationship*, Allwin and Bacon, Boston

Muyskens, J.L. (1982) *Moral Problems in Nursing*, Rowman and Littlefield, Totowa, N.J.

Sutor, J (1993) Can nurses be effective advocates? *Nursing Standard*, **7**(22), 30–33

UKCC (1989) *Exercising Accountability*, UKCC, London

UKCC (1992a) *The Scope of Professional Practice*, UKCC, London

UKCC (1992b) *Code of Professional Conduct for Nurses, Midwives and Health Visitors*, UKCC, London

Walsh, P. (1985) Speaking up for the patient. *Nursing Times*, **81**(18), 24–27

Welsh Office (1992) Local strategies for health – developing public involvement. Guidance Notes, NHS Directorate, Cardiff

Williams, P. and Schoultz, B. (1982) *We Can Speak for Ourselves*, Condor Books, London

29

Initiating and managing change

Annabel Broome

● **Introduction**

Change is all around us and is here to stay, and is affecting community care in the NHS at least as much as in other organizations. This chapter is concerned with different types of change and the choices of approach that community health care nurses might need to make when they are trying to help others change, or are struggling to come to terms with changes others have imposed on them.

It focuses on the leadership styles which different changes need and the steps community health care nurses as team players and leaders can make to plan and implement the changes they want. It will also address some ways of diagnosing a healthy organization. Unless an organization has a fitness for change, and a healthy culture, the necessary changes may not be possible. This chapter is also about the way changes are made. It draws heavily on the author's experience of organizational changes in many settings, which have value in trying to understand the community care setting. So, it is about designing both what to change as well as how to make the changes.

In any change it is necessary to be clear about the culture that is to be created, so the way the changes are made demonstrate the new culture, rather than the old (Atkinson, 1990). For instance, in a hierarchical organization, change can be undertaken less sensitively (and in the short term, quite effectively) by using a hard 'tell' style. Individuals with power at the top of the organization design and implement the change and tell everyone else what to do. People lower down the organization will have little idea of the overall purpose of the change and will feel less involved and committed than those at the top. As a result they may be reluctant to contribute all their energy to the new culture.

Success in creating long-lasting change commences with leaders being clear about what they are trying to do and bringing people alongside them, building commitment and being seen to lead (Tichy and Devanna, 1986).

The author has noted in her work with a wide variety of organizations that leaders often have to work hard to become the kind of leader that others can believe in and follow. In addition to being convincing, they often have to struggle to find a way of convincing themselves that the changes are good. Until the leaders are convinced, they cannot be convincing. Each leader has to find a personal vision to be able to lead well. Lack of leadership commitment and vision results in ineffective change, and leaders who lack these necessary attributes may need to consider their own position in the organization.

Many staff in the NHS and in primary health care have been struggling with the new ideas which they feel have been imposed in them. In the new contract environment, many primary health care staff have felt ambivalent about driving the changes through. Some have not liked the values or the new practices the changes represent. Although this way of imposing change is painful, it is nevertheless a perfectly legitimate way to do it, and it works. However, each person has to find a way, individually, to work with the new culture and drive the changes forward. One Family Health Services Authority (FHSA) manager told the author that she was unsure of whether the reforms would actually improve the services she managed. She was struggling to find some good in the new design, so she could become convincing. After lengthy discussions she said: 'Well, I suppose it has made us more concerned about how limited money is spent, we have had to prioritise more, and it has meant I question more how my staff spend their time, and whether it is on the most worthwhile tasks.' She was beginning to find her own reasons for being convinced, and so she could start to build commitment in others.

This development was important for the manager because she wanted to make substantial changes that would last. For this, she needed to demonstrate visionary leadership to give a clear direction in order that commitment was built with people becoming so involved that they too wanted the changes to last. The rest of the chapter is about such changes.

● Critical success factors for change

The modern NHS operates on the principles of the internal market. To understand change within the new NHS it is helpful to examine other organizations which operate market principles. Kanter (1984) looked at organizations that are flexible, and change and shift as the market changes. She found two characteristics:

- strong horizontal relationships between professionals
- weaker vertical or hierarchical relationships.

Innovative organizations in the 1990s use flexible, cross-professional teamworking. Many Primary Health Care Teams work well, whereas others have a high level of inter-professional wrangling and territorial posturing. This is common in many organizations with highly developed professional identities and skills. As is the case in all organizations, a Primary Health Care Team which encourages a climate of role and skill-flexibility will be more innovative and use scarce resources to greater advantage than in a similar team where rigid role boundaries exit (Rosen, 1989). In order to achieve this teams need to:

- be able to tolerate uncertainty and manage conflict
- have a high level of personal security
- have a capacity to see both the detail and the 'wide angle' picture or strategic view at the same time
- have good communication skills
- have a wish to share success
- have a clear and open motivation for the changes
- be tenacious about new plans, and flexible enough to deviate from them when necessary
- be visionaries.

So it is apparent that good leaders should be able to facilitate flexible teamworking. To do this they require a range of leadership skills (Hersey and Blanchard, 1976) which are focused flexibly to match different situations, depending on whether the emphasis is on getting the task done or developing the people. These activities are discussed more fully in the later section on 'Leadership'.

Shifting the focus to change, Hutchinson (1989) sought to test attitudes to change among senior managers from 70 leading UK companies. Two questions about making changes were asked of senior managers in both the public and private sectors:

1.   What aspects do you give most attention when making changes?
2.   What aspects do you think are the most important to give attention to during the change?

The results show that, though managers readily recognized and understood the need to focus on certain aspects essential to change, such as vision, they did not necessarily spend time on those aspects which they considered the most important. First, they gave more attention to:

- maintaining existing performance while effecting change
- top management defining the desired future
- changing the organizational structure
- relying on top management diagnosis
- assigning responsibility for transition
- diagnosing the current situation.

However, they considered that the following features of change are the most important aspects of the process to focus on:

- having clear change goals
- agreeing key issues with all people affected by the change
- encouraging the learning of new behaviours
- senior management setting new example
- keeping staff informed during transition
- involving people in future visions.

From this study it is possible to learn that even if managers know the issues and the theory of successful change, it is easy to get 'blown off course' by the immediate demands of managing an organization or a team in the 'here and now'. The general lessons for community health care nurses is the same as for other professionals: be clear about the changes that are needed, make sure senior people model the changes and involve people right from the start in the design of the changes, and do not depend only on the most senior people to drive the process.

When considering the major roles that any all-round manager needs to perform, Mintzberg (1973) divides them into three major components:

- interpersonal roles of figurehead/leader/liaison
- informational roles of monitor/disseminator/spokesperson
- decisional roles of entrepreneur/disturbance handler/resource allocator/negotiator.

From these components it is possible to see that the decisional roles are particularly important as the key to successful change. However, the constraints or realms of authority are different for each job. Stewart (1976) has written about the need for clarity about the freedoms of action of the leader or manager in making changes. Community health care nurses in wanting to change things or influence their team members will need to be clear about the boundaries of their role. The following scenario provides one example:

A primary health care team was trying to decide a strategy for the future based on the health needs of the local population. They started by listing all the things they did now, and then all the things they wanted to do. In this way each team member from each profession made a huge 'wish list' of all the services they had always wanted to deliver. A plan was then formulated and forwarded to the FHSA. The FHSA sent the list back and said: 'Thank you, but can you now send us a plan that is an agreed list (agreed with all the primary health care team), with agreed priorities, that is built up from the health needs of your local population?'

In order to do this, each profession had to come together to make their corporate vision, values and time-frame more explicit. They had to spend time listening to each other, and, because of the different data and perspectives they all had, they had to deal with the conflicts that this open discussion generated, as they decided what their practice population needed. Held together by their common goals and discovering a shared set of values, they then had to pull the ideas together and set priorities for change. Individual team members became more assertive and challenging of the 'titular' leaders – the General Practitioners. Resistance was noticed in some team members who felt comfortable with the status quo and saw no benefit in changing things. In managing this change process, the vision was all important because, without some general agreement about what everybody was working towards, there could be no successful future. But by redesigning the future themselves, even the most resistant staff became more questioning of the present. This is illustrated by the following comment: 'So if all the Community Nurses were on site and had an office here, we could

co-ordinate with the doctors better, we would know what was going
on quicker with the whole family, we would avoid conflicting
advice, and we could use the comfy rooms for child clinics and I
would have a place to take a lunch break.'

The team was beginning to work the issues, and conflict was beginning to
come out in the open, and leaders were emerging. In this example,
finding a way of working more closely together in a geographical sense
was the first step to agreeing, as a team, where to start with the changes.

● **Where to start in the implementation of change**

Planning change

First, in any change it is important for people to understand where
they are aiming for with the change (*vision*). A vision should be stated in
very general terms – it is not a blueprint or a detailed floor plan (this
comes later in planning tactics, or the next steps to achieving change).
Secondly, it is important to diagnose where things are *now*, and what is
going well and badly with the current way of doing things. Lastly, it is

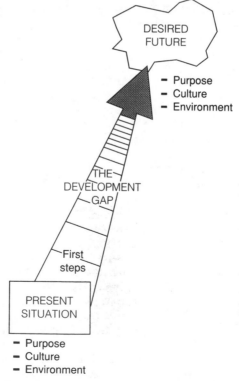

Figure 29.1 The change process

necessary to plan the steps to achieve the change. Figure 29.1 illustrates the stages in the process of planning change.

Several times in this chapter the importance of shaping vision has been discussed. In deciding the shape of the vision, any leader needs to keep in mind an image of a healthy team or organization. A definition of a healthy organization is one which learns, changes, renews and develops according to changing circumstances (Beckhard and Harris, 1987; Broome, 1990). This requires the organization to:

- have a strategic view
- energize others lower in the system
- create a structure that follows function
- make decisions at a level 'where the information is held'
- reward what is known as well as what is done
- have a relatively open communication system
- reward collaboration
- manage conflict (do not suppress it)
- relate well to people around
- value individuals and individuality
- actively learn through feedback.

Steps in designing the future

Once the ideal future team or organization is planned, the structure needs checking with the attributes identified above. Then the 'key' people (members of the team and others who will be affected by the changes) need to 'come on board' so that the vision can be built with them.

So the third stage is to build up a shared vision throughout the organization. One problem the author has experienced in the community nursing service is that each different professional group builds their own vision which they find difficult to share or indeed find any common ground among the whole team. So the services to the patients come second to the professional needs. An example is provided from an interesting discussion between members of a PHCT:

> The Practice Manager was suggesting that her practice vision which was to become the biggest, best and most profitable practice in 'M' was not shared by the rest of the team. Indeed, though they all wanted to provide better services, there was hesitation about getting bigger. There was particular hesitancy about growing through marketing and building competitive advantage for their practice. It was clear that unless she found some sound common ground, she would have trouble building her own vision into one that was shared.

One of the key success factors at this early stage in team change is the need for strong leadership, and the ability to be explicit about what the group vision is. The second is building total commitment for the changes. Both of these depend on the leader's ability to build up a vision, and to encourage people to support it.

Blocks to getting to the vision

After identifying the vision, it is helpful to identify factors blocking its achievement. These factors might be people, policies, practices, attitudes or behaviours which will prevent the vision from becoming reality. Some of the blocking will be by people who want to remain the same, and resist the vision. A decision will be needed as to whether these people are essential to the changes, or whether it is possible to ignore them.

It may be necessary to build a vision with the key people that is so compelling that they cannot resist it. An alternative is to expose any dissatisfaction with present practice which allows an exploration of the strengths of future plans.

Sensitive leaders take into account the stage of development of the team or unit. In the 1960s, Tuckman (1965) was proposing a development process for groups which went through four phases: forming, storming, norming and performing. But some teams never develop, and some GP practices have become fixed in their ways. A kind of uneasy equilibrium has been reached, and some have a hesitancy to begin the 'storming' phase, to avoid conflict or differences. It is often the job of the newcomer to get some leverage into the system, and to help the others see more rewarding possibilities (the vision) and also to recognize or emphasize the dissatisfactions with the current ways of doing things, and move the group on. However, it is important to acknowledge that this can be very uncomfortable or even a painful experience for the newcomer.

Dealing with resistance

Whether practitioners initiate changes themselves because of their own ideas or beliefs, or whether they are trying to cope with other people's imposed changes, resistance is a common reaction. One way of understanding resistance is to unravel the three parts of the process of change that have just been identified. This approach is based on the expectation that resistance will be high if the cost of change is also high.

There are three lever points to change:

- the prospect of a better (more exciting, profitable, fulfilling) future, than the present
- a real dissatisfaction with how things are now (uncomfortable, stressful, unrewarding)
- some ideas of how to change things.

The change equation outlines these three elements. All three dimensions are necessary for effective change:

$$\text{Vision} \times \text{Dissatisfaction} \times \text{First steps} > \text{Cost of change}$$

But when these three dimensions exist:

- a wish to do things differently (a shared vision)
- increasing unhappiness with the current situation (dissatisfaction)
- a shared understanding of what to do next (first steps)

there is a chance that the very natural tendency to resist will be overcome, and the change will look more attractive.

Building vision

People with strong leadership skills more often build strong visions and energize people around them. Often this is described as good managerial skills, but it may be suggested that there are good managers who are not leaders, and these will have more difficulty using visioning to lead significant changes.

An example from primary health care is that of a good practice manager or team leader who is good at facilitating the members of the PHCT systematically through difficult times, but may see change in the short term as a series of tasks. However, when visioning is called for, they may have difficulty inspiring and building commitment in the team, to a longer term future. Leadership is what is wanted here. Indeed, not all leaders are good managers, and good managers are not necessarily good leaders. It is the two together that will deliver excellence.

First steps

A good leader is one who will communicate a clear vision and build commitment for it. If the level of dissatisfaction is sufficient, then some first steps need planning. People need to know what to do. This can follow a sequence reached through a series of questions:

- Do we need more data, before we can make plans?
- How well will the current structure/human resources/information and decision systems and reward systems help us deliver the vision?
- Who, among the key people, are ready for this change?
- Which people are capable of making it happen?
- Who will be doing what in the change tasks?

Addressing these questions in a systematic way allows a transition plan to be formed. This is time consuming and needs resources to be allocated specifically to the change effort. Some change experts such as Beckhard and Harris (1987) describe the transition state as a rather different state, and recommend addressing it as such. However, a different view is that successful organizations need to build a fitness for change, and have a readiness and responsiveness for change. A fit organization is one which is constantly learning (Pedler *et al.*, 1991) and can move quickly and flexibly in response to new conditions.

A further example from community nursing follows:

One Locality Manager said: 'I want to swing things round, I want the service to become more preventive, and more efficient, but the problem is lack of systems. I do not really know precisely what activity we are up to, I do not know what it costs, and I do not know if it is effective.' This manager simply has not got the systems to give him the data he needs, in order to start making a diagnosis for change.

It is particularly difficult to take on change if there are few additional resources to find out what is going on, to develop the change plans and implement them, and, later on, to assess whether changes have been effective. Yet, this is what is asked of community health care nurses and their managers. Setting up such systems takes resources such as time, people and information technology. And making major change also needs extra resources to maintain services alongside the new work (Beckhard and Harris, 1987). The Locality Manager above needed to consider realistic changes – first, to develop the means of managing information, then to consider the more radical changes he wanted. At times this need is recognized, for instance with the additional resources that have been allocated to Fundholding General Practitioners, to help with the additional work during the transition to setting up new information and financial systems.

● **Leadership**

The concept of leadership and the ways in which leaders drive change has already been considered: it motivates and gives enthusiasm, sets direction and builds commitment. Leadership is essential when difficult changes are required. Not all nurses like the recent NHS reforms, but if they choose to stay and work in the new system, and help the changes through, then they have to find some way of becoming committed and be a champion of the 'new' ideas. To make significant changes to the way things are done in an organization, resistance needs to be overcome, and people need to be given a clear picture of the future the leaders are aiming at. Then they will be encouraged to 'buy into' the change and begin to drive it themselves.

Many managers now talk of cultural design (Pettigrew, 1979) and developing quality (Atkinson, 1990) and empowerment (Belasco, 1990), enabling the workforce to take responsibility for their part in the process, and use of influence (not power), and the need to bring the workforce with them, without the need to use positional power. All this puts greater demands on managers' and team leaders' skills in building a clear joint purpose.

Sometimes the changes people have to make challenge top peoples' values. So they are struggling with their own ambivalence, while trying to give a high profile lead, and to 'sell' a new vision to staff, who need to be energised to put their energy behind all these changes. Unless they can be convincing, they will have trouble leading others. An example is provided by one Senior Manager in the NHS who said: 'I had to go for the job, I had no option, my kids are young and I have known nothing else but the NHS. But now I find I am having to sell ideas to my colleagues that they do not like, and I do not believe in.'

However, this problem is not unique to health care or even to nursing. The process of change is equally disruptive to other professions. Indeed, a high street bank manager said: 'I did not come into the bank to sell insurance, or become a shop keeper. I miss the old bank, I knew where I was, I was respected in the town community. Now people see me as a sharp businessman, charging for everything, and I am not sure I want to be part of it.'

So what is leadership?
Burns (1978) shows that research identifies characteristics of leaders. They are:

- communicate a clear vision of the future
- develop a culture of change
- dynamically manage their boundaries (keep in touch and influence the boundaries to their part of the organization)
- develop the people in the organization, by creating a learning community.

They also need to be skilled in assessing the forces:

- in themselves
- in others
- in each situation

and have a flexibility of approach to deliver the behaviour that best fits all three. Good leaders need a range of different behaviours for different situations if they are to manage change effectively. The skill is in selecting the appropriate behaviour for themselves and the people they are trying to influence, to meet the demands of the particular situation.

Other authors suggest that the competence of the follower or subordinate is important (Hersey and Blanchard, 1976). If they are competent, then the leader can use a style which will give others responsibility. Different people have skills in some areas and not others, so the style needs to shift accordingly. For example, a new member of the team will be good at some things and not others. For the tasks with less competence, the leader will need to coach on the job and build up the skill, but if they have the necessary skill, then the leader will need to give them responsibility. But some leaders are more comfortable with one style than another, and fail to shift style when their team member shows unexpected skill in one area. They keep on coaching, failing to recognize when it is not necessary for all tasks, creating frustration for both of them. At other times, particularly in a critical situation, the most important thing is to get the task done quickly and well. The style of leadership then should be directive and decisive. At a different time, it may be more appropriate for the leader to listen to the team member and shape their behaviour, rather than being directive. So, the good manager assesses each situation, the other person's skill, the demands of the situation, and adapts their style accordingly.

At times the task focus is crucial (when the follower or team member is less mature or unskilled) and there is a need to direct or coach the team members depending on their skill. But at other times (when the skill is high and they are well motivated), managing the person is most important and in this situation support or delegation is essential.

The following list shows the range of different behaviours a manager needs to be able to deliver, to meet different tasks, with people of differing commitment and competence (Hersey and Blanchard, 1976):

Directing. Leader provides specific instruction for follower, and closely supervises the task accomplishment.

Coaching. Leader explains problems and decisions, sets boundaries, gets suggestions from follower, but directs task accomplishment.

Supporting. Leader makes decisions together with the follower, and supports efforts to the task accomplishment.

Delegating. Leader turns over decisions and responsibility for implementation to follower.

So, this raises the question of whether leaders are just good managers. Authors such as Burns (1978) and Turrell (1986) state that the most effective leaders:

- motivate and inspire
- have and communicate a long-term, strategic vision
- use influence not positional power
- build common commitment
- simplify
- relate emotionally
- challenge and support
- empower others.

However, they suggest that managers:

- are task-centred
- use formal channels and methods
- have a short/medium term focus
- make decisions
- solve problems.

Tichy and Devanna (1986) have differentiated two styles of leadership: the transformational and the transactional. The transformational leader demonstrates more of the emotional, encouraging strategic, visionary style, and the transactional manager fulfils more of the steady, operational logical manager's role. In this way some differentiation is made between managers and leaders, the leader falling more into the transformational category and the manager into the transactional. This is illustrated by Table 29.1.

Table 29.1 The features of managers and leaders

Transformational leadership	Transactional management
Empowers	Bargains
Inspires by vision, ideals	Task-centred
Mixes home and work	Separates home and work
Long-term focus	Medium/short term focus
Challenges	Coaches
Rewards informally, personally	Rewards formally
Is emotional, turbulent	Is orderly
Simplifies	Complicates

Different styles of leadership need to be appropriate to the development of the organization. It is the transformational style that is more important in the early stages of development. For example, when a team or unit is in the formative stage there is emphasis on innovation, energizing by visioning and building new skills and commitment. For instance, a new company or team at the *pioneer phase* needs strong entrepreneurship, while a team or organization which has been established longer and is reaching the *differentiation phase* needs a steadier style, where roles and relationships become more complex and differentiated and more management and production systems need to be developed to help manage the tasks and monitor what it is doing.

Many readers will have encountered the experience of new practices setting up, and the team is enthusiastic and flexible. If anything needs doing, anyone will do it. However, as the team gets more established, and the practice develops policies and standard ways of doing things, so the flexibility reduces, and the professional staff may become more territorial and systems driven. As primary health care gets more of the slice of resources, so the teams will have to struggle with this problem, and be aware that renewing and flexible working needs to be balanced against the need for systems and structures.

● **People in change**

Earlier, the situation was described of resistance being particularly common when changes are imposed. Resistance is demonstrated by the way people behave. Frequently they will:

● procrastinate
● deny (the importance or significance)
● distort messages and meanings
● reject ideas out of hand.

If these behaviours are experienced within the team it is important to check whether there is some resistance. It is really important to work with the resisters, particularly if their help is required.

An estimate of an individual's commitment to change, and their readiness and capability of following it through, will depend on their level of security. For instance, someone who is low in security may reject or distort the messages they are being given by the leaders. Alternatively, those at a reasonable level of security will behave differently, and begin to:

- listen
- explore
- build on new ideas
- problem solve with the team.

Once people are at this stage, planning can start.

● **Conclusion**

The NHS is going through major, imposed changes, which are meeting a level of resistance. Using a simple tool (the change equation), the chapter has outlined some of the processes that need addressing. It also draws on examples of change in community care in the NHS and also of some market place companies. The experiences are different, but the conclusions are similar. In community care, many changes involve different professional groups with their different visions and ideas. The skilled change agent will help team-mates build a common vision of the future, enthuse others and build a way of working together, which transcends professional boundaries.

A culture of change and renewal needs to be modelled and encouraged. There is a wealth of skill in interpersonal communications at all levels in these community teams, but these need to be mobilized to more corporate goals. All staff will need to understand and be skilled in managing the uncomfortable process of taking people through their resistance. In addition, sufficient resources need to be devoted to any transition process, so current services can be maintained, while clear change goals are set and met.

References

Atkinson, P.E. (1990) *Creating Culture Change: The Key to Successful Total Quality Management*, IFS Publications, UK

Beckhard, D. and Harris, T. (1987) *Organisational Transitions; Managing Complex Change*, 2nd edn, Addison Wesley, USA

Belasco, J.A. (1990) *Teaching the Elephant to Dance*, Century Business, UK

Broome, A.K. (1990) *Managing Change*, Macmillan, London

Burns, J.M. (1978) *Leadership*, Harper and Row, New York

Hersey, P. and Blanchard, K. (1976) *Situational Leadership*, Centre for Creative Leadership, Greenboro, NC, USA

Hutchinson, C. (1989) *Managing Change; A Survey*, Sheppard Moscow, Chislehurst, UK

Kanter, R.M. (1984) *The Change Masters*, Allen and Unwin, London

Mintzberg, H. (1973) *The Nature of Managerial Work*, Harper and Row, New York

Pedler, M. Burgoyne, J. and Boydell, T. (1991) *The Learning Company*, McGraw-Hill, New York

Pettigrew, A.M. (1979) On studying organisational cultures. *Administrative Science Quarterly*, **24**, 570–587

Rosen, N. (1989) *Teamwork and the Bottom Line*, Erlbaum Associates, New Jersey, USA

Stewart, R. (1976) *Contrasts in Management: A Study of Different Types of Managers' Jobs, their Demands and Choices*, McGraw-Hill, New York

Tichy, N.M. and Devanna, M.A. (1986) *The Transformational Leader*, Wiley, Chichester

Tuckman, B.W. (1965) Developmental sequence in small groups. *Psychological Bulletin*, **63**, 384–399

Turrell, E.A. (1986) *Change and Innovation. A Challenge for the NHS*, Institute of Health Services Management, London

30

Case management

Ann Bergen

● **Introduction**

Since the mid-1980s the term case management has become very much part of the community care language within the new economy of health care which includes the contract culture and consumerism. In common with many new approaches to the delivery of health care, case management can remain dangerously ill-defined, ill-executed and based on ill-researched evidence if taken at no more than surface value. It is the aim of this chapter to explore a little below the surface in order not only to shed conceptual clarity on the term, but also to evaluate the current state of research in the area. More importantly, perhaps, it aims to draw out the implications and issues relevant to community nursing based on current evidence related to community nursing practices.

● **Definitions and models**

It is probably no exaggeration to suggest that there are as many definitions of case management as there are case management projects extant. Indeed, commentators have seen the very substance of an ideology within this diversity, the creed of which is based on developing approaches to care reflective of local needs (Beardshaw, 1991; Knapp *et al.*, 1992). However, a number of commonalities may be identified wherever case management is seen to operate, and these may be broadly encapsulated in the definition offered by Onyett (1992):

> *Case management is a way of tailoring help to meet individual need through placing responsibility for assessment and service co-ordination with one individual worker or team.*

This generic description is derived from the North American origin of case management, with its stress on co-ordination as a counter to service fragmentation and spiralling health costs (Beardshaw and Towell, 1990). Nevertheless, within this broad brush statement it is possible to identify the ideals and operational procedures which could be said to characterize case management, as the summation of many of the themes already highlighted in this and previous chapters, and therefore relevant to contemporary Britain. While the overt 'managerial' (including resource management) function implicit in the title is emphasized by some (Cambridge, 1990), the case manager–client interface, with its individualized focus, has served as the vehicle for the promotion of ideals of client advocacy (Thornicroft, 1991) (see Chapter 28), partnership with clients and other agencies (DoH, 1989) (see Chapter 24) and education for empowerment (Richardson and Higgins, 1991; Repper and Peacham, 1991). Further, client groups selected for case management span the range of contextual settings, as well as the age ranges and health status considered in earlier chapters. Finally, operational guidelines for the implementation of case management have often conceived of it in terms of five core functions or stages (DoH, 1989; Richardson and Higgins, 1991), at least some of which have already been a focus of discussion:

- selecting specific individuals for attention (case finding or targeting)
- seeking to understand their needs (assessment)
- working out a plan of action to meet these needs (individual programme planning – IPP)
- putting the plan into effect (service delivery)
- keeping in touch to see how the plan is working and making changes as appropriate (monitoring/review/evaluation).

The varying emphases given by different projects to these functions and values is dependent upon their context and, the cynic might say, on the overriding political and managerial imperatives. These variations can be illustrated in the three-model framework used for classifying case management, as identified by Beardshaw and Towell (1990), which are those of 'brokerage', social entrepreneurship and co-ordination.

For instance, advocacy is a prominent feature of the 'brokerage' model, where the case manager acts as an independent 'go-between' for a client and links services to needs. This is an approach which has occasionally been adopted in British case management for people with physical disabilities (Hunter, 1988; Pilling, 1992) or learning disabilities (Archer and Robertson, 1990; Richardson and Higgins, 1990, 1991). However, its derivation from North American practices, where case managers are commonly agents independent of service provision, has meant it has less relevance to Britain where case managers tend to be service based or linked (Beardshaw and Towell, 1990).

Resource and budgetary control are central to the social entrepreneurship model (Beardshaw and Towell, 1990), where the case manager holds a devolved budget for the purchase of an individual's care from within and outside statutory agencies. Devolved financial accountability is ideologically conducive to the provision of individualized, needs-led care packages and was a feature of the pioneering Kent Community Care Scheme and its derivatives (Challis and Davies, 1986) upon which much post-Griffiths thinking in the UK was predicated (DHSS, 1988).

Beardshaw and Towell's third model of case management focuses on the co-ordination dimension of case management and entails the assumption by members of multidisciplinary teams of responsibility for arranging and monitoring care for specific clients in addition to their professional roles with regard to other clients. The case manager is thus an extension of the keyworker role, which is a term derived from the prime workers with elderly people in residential accommodation and, therefore, inclusive of the case manager's involvement in service provision (Beardshaw and Towell, 1990). The model has been described in practice by Dant *et al.* (1989) in case management for elderly people and, while it clearly has the advantage of being less disruptive in terms of role change for practitioners, it opposes the government's concept of separating assessment from service provision.

As a postscript to the issue of definitions and models it may be pertinent to allude to the lack of semantic consensus as to which term best comprehends the ideals and processes described above. While the term case management, as used in the UK, became enshrined in the public consciousness following its endorsement in the White Paper *Caring for People* (DoH, 1989), it became superseded by the apparently more politically correct phrase care management in subsequent, post-consultation policy guidance. This was on the grounds that ' "case" was regarded as demeaning to the individual and misleading in that (it) is the care, and not the person, that is being managed' (DoH, 1991a). The implication that the two terms are interchangeable, and that their usage is really only a matter of sensitivity and preference, has meant that a number of authorities, such as the King's Fund have followed suit (Beardshaw, 1991). However, Onyett (1992) argues that

> although the word 'case' has unfortunate medical overtones and users have stressed that they are not cases to be managed, the phrase does emphasize the individual focus of case management that is perhaps its only wholly unequivocal characteristic.

Furthermore, because case management 'involves assessing and meeting users' needs rather than managing service provision ("care") *per se*', it is more appropriate than the alternative care management which 'obscures the central features of this approach, a focus on the needs and strengths of individual users'. Other commentators (Hunter, 1988; Ryan *et al.*, 1991) also argue for a recognition of two levels of describing this modality of care delivery and it is of interest to note that many of the more recent project evaluations (Richardson and Higgins, 1991; Knapp *et al.*, 1992; Pilling, 1992; Ford *et al.*, 1993) continue to use the term 'case', an indication, perhaps, of where the focus should be angled in the evaluation of the new community care. This is also the term which will continue to be used in this chapter both because of the intended individual focus and because of the supranational currency the term already enjoys both in general and as applied to nursing.

● **The literature – research and practice**

The link between research, policy and practice cannot automatically be assumed to operate in a linear fashion, as any nurse aware of the research–practice gap will testify (Hunt, 1981). The UK experience of the development of case management as a central component of the 'Care in the Community' initiative provides a useful example. While, for example, the Kent, Darlington and Gateshead models of case management (Challis and Davies, 1986; Challis *et al*., 1989, 1990) were highly influential in post-Griffiths thinking and explicitly mentioned in the subsequent White Paper itself (DoH, 1989), the degree of congruency between the initial Implementation and Guidance Documents (DoH, 1990, 1991a, 1991b) and actual service practices must currently be subject to some doubt. Official policy relating to, for instance, the clear position of social services as lead agencies, the separation of assessment and service provision and the stress on devolved budgetary management cannot necessarily be said to effect a logical link between these specially funded, time-limited projects and the operationalization of case management as part of mainstream care delivery. Indeed, the few instances where initiatives have been set up with a view to long-term continuation have demonstrated the greatest problems in realizing noble ideals in the real world of limited resources (Richardson and Higgins, 1991). This will necessarily limit the degree to which either research findings or policy statements can inform health and social care (including nursing) practice.

That said, health care professionals have, hopefully, come some way since the climate of the early 1980s when the debate on community care was described as 'often based on tangentially relevant research and seemingly dominated by anecdote' (Knapp *et al*., 1993). Pilling (1992) gives an indication of just how far, in terms of quantity of published research, in her comprehensive review of the growing body of literature. However, this predates the recent important work of authors such as Knapp *et al*. (1992) and Ford *et al*. (1993), and it is, therefore, worth summarizing the state of the art on the subject.

The literature on case management spans its target client groups as envisaged by the government, that is, the dependent elderly (Challis and Davies, 1986; Dant *et al*., 1989), people with learning disabilities (Archer and Robertson, 1990; Richardson and Higgins, 1991), those with mental health problems (Onyett, 1992) and with physical disability (Pilling, 1992). In addition to single project evaluations, programmes set up and funded by the Department of Health (Knapp *et al*., 1992), the King's Fund (Hunter, 1988; Beardshaw, 1991) and Research and Development for Psychiatry (RDP) (Ryan *et al*., 1991; Ford *et al*., 1993) have more recently been comprehensively documented. Some, notably in England, such as the Department of Health 'Care in the Community' programme (Knapp *et al*., 1992) and projects for clients with learning disabilities and mental health problems, are specifically geared to resettlement in the community following de-institutionalization. Others, especially those concerned with older people (Challis and Davies, 1986) are focused more on maintaining the independence of people already in the community and preventing hospital admission.

In addition, there is a significant social service orientation in the majority of projects, which is perhaps reflective of governmental policy in the UK, although the development of multidisciplinary case management teams is a feature of some, particularly those with a mental health focus. It is within this multidisciplinary framework that community nurses receive most attention. For instance, in Gateshead's Social and Health

Care Scheme a senior nurse worked with a social worker, registrar in community medicine and physiotherapist within a social entrepreneurship model with an emphasis on assessment and decentralized budgeting, but not service delivery (Challis *et al.*, 1990). A district nurse participated in the Andover project by acting as case manager for one of her existing clients (Archer and Robertson, 1990). Seventeen mental health nurses were involved in the case management teams evaluated by RDP – now the Sainsbury Centre) (Ford *et al.*, 1992).

This apparent marginalization of nurses is, perhaps, disappointing in view of the government's suggestion that, where an individual's health needs predominate, 'they [nurses] may be the most appropriate practitioners to assume the responsibilities for care management' (DoH, 1991a). Even more disappointing, perhaps, is the lack of published work with a nursing focus, especially by nurse researchers. More project analyses like that of the Blaydon project are needed for the light they shed on the realities of case management practices for community nurses (Peck, 1991).

However, even given this recent plethora of general research, its quality needs careful assessment before it can appropriately guide practice. Ryan *et al.* (1991) rehearse some of the pitfalls in the evidence for case management in terms of poor descriptions of the processes involved, thereby making comparisons difficult, as well as failure to adequately define the expectations of such projects, leading to an abundance of no change outcomes.

There remain, however, problems inherent in researching case management where internal and external validity are central to the design. Establishing cause-and-effect relationships are always notoriously difficult where the multiple intervening variables of any care setting are present and so-called control groups difficult to identify. Similarly, generalizing from a limited number of the multiplicity of case management models must obviously be handled cautiously, especially when the models themselves are embodied in specially funded projects, and therefore not necessarily representative of the reality to come.

Weaknesses and difficulties notwithstanding, it is possible to draw some conclusions from the body of research on British case management. The comprehensive review carried out by Knapp *et al.* (1992) of the 28 DoH 'Care in the Community' projects, which covered a variety of client groups and using multiple methods of evaluation, concluded:

> *Case management can be used as an instrument for identifying client needs and abilities, involving service users in decision-making, translating broad care principles into practice, planning and co-ordinating service packages for matching resources to needs, monitoring achievements, carrying out reassessments and introducing relevant financial information into comparatively routine community care processes.*

However authors such as Ford *et al.* (1993), in their similarly favourable review, also warn of problems inherent in, and limits to, case management and caution that it should not, therefore, be seen as an automatic panacea.

● Implications for community nursing

While it would be imprudent to claim to predict future practices with any degree of accuracy from research findings alone, some extrapolation here is justified in order to comment on the possible role of community nurses within the case management remit. Bergen (1992) highlights three key questions as a starting point for this debate and these will be addressed below, drawing on recent literature, research in progress and both health policy and professional agendas (Bergen, 1993, 1994).

The first question pertains to the suitability of nurses for the case management role. The encouragement given to community nurses in the White Paper *Caring for People* (DoH, 1989), combined with general reasoning, might suggest they were an ideal group to assume this new role. They have, after all, frequent contact with the client groups singled out as most appropriate for case management (those older people who are mentally and/or physically frail, those with mental health problems and learning disabilities) and have demonstrated a *de facto* assumption of the role in anecdotal reporting in the British nursing press (Henderson, 1990). Indeed, the ideals of case management, as enumerated above, seem eminently compatible with those of nursing (Morrison, 1991).

Hunter (1988), however, cautions against overenthusiasm here, despite the acknowledged supporting evidence. He argues that, because nurses are usually service providers, they may experience difficulty in remaining sufficiently independent to perform an advocacy role and overplay the importance of nursing care to the possible exclusion of other necessary support. Moreover, while health visitors often demonstrate a reluctance to focus their efforts on the priority groups mentioned, district nurses have traditionally been found to be slow in acquiring the new skills which would be necessary (Bowling, 1981). For both groups, the notion of teamwork within primary health care is often more rhetoric than reality.

Although Hunter's doubts were voiced before the current moves within nursing to redefine the Scope of Professional Practice (UKCC, 1992b), this ambivalence in the literature of the immediate post-Griffiths era is perhaps not misplaced. Even on the eve of community care implementation, commentators such as Thomas (1992) seemed to be unclear as to the role of nursing, whereas others were inclined to divergent views, varying from announcing practitioners' self-proclaimed enthusiasm, on the one hand (Brittian, 1992), to ignorance on the other (Mason, 1992). This reflects the enormous variation in practice noted in preliminary research (Bergen, 1993, 1994) and supported by the findings of the Audit Commission (1992).

The second question relates to the issues which must be addressed by nurses, which include whether they should assume the case management role and which model should be adopted. It seems likely on current evidence that many nurse case managers will adopt the third of the models proposed by Beardshaw and Towell (1990), combining the role with keyworking within the multidisciplinary team. Case management by teamwork is particularly favoured by community psychiatric nurses

(CPNs) (Drozd and Gabell, 1991) and community nurses for people with learning disabilities (Ovretveit, 1992). Although this means overriding the UK government's preferred option of concentrating the core functions within one individual, the sharing of tasks is compatible with the definition used in this chapter (Onyett, 1992). In particular, it appears that CPNs wish to retain a care delivery function both as a hedge against the potential for de-skilling (Trotter, 1992) and because keyworking also sits comfortably with the care programme approach (Ryan *et al.*, 1991). Authors such as Squire (1993) and Rodrigues (1992) occasionally argue that nurses have been placed firmly on the commissioning side of the purchaser–provider divide, though this is perhaps more accurately perceived as occurring at the care management level, as described above.

It follows from the adoption of the multidisciplinary team extension model that many nurses will be acting concurrently as case managers for targeted clients within their caseload, while continuing their conventional professional role with respect to the remaining clients in their case load. Squire (1993) suggests that this has led to role overload and, therefore, caseload numbers may need monitoring. In addition, most nurses will be service linked, which gives them extra influence in negotiating for services. However, it may risk compromising a disinterested advocacy role, which is the strength of the independent model. While most nurses will probably operate within a health agency, there appears to be a growing trend for secondment to social services in order to utilize nursing skills (Korczak, 1993; Squire, 1993). This brings with it the attendant problem of diffused accountability and nurses must be aware of responsibility towards the profession and their patients as described in the *Code of Professional Conduct* (UKCC, 1992a). In addition, there are issues about their responsibilities to line and professional managers.

One of the inevitable issues which will need to be addressed by nurses, irrespective of the model of case management, is that of inter-agency relations. Almost without exception, accounts of case management projects mention the difficulties of redefining roles within a broader inter-professional framework. This has led, on occasions, to acrimonious debate or demarcation issues, particularly between nursing and social work and with staff working in more traditional ways (Lieberman, 1990; Rodrigues, 1992; Squire, 1993; Brunnen and Korczak, 1993). Adequate multidisciplinary preparation and training in the lead-in period to such projects would seem to be essential if such problems are to be minimized. However, evidence suggests this preparation to be currently lacking (George, 1993). Also lacking, but equally important, is the provision of professional supervision in light of the stressful aspects of case management work noted by some nurses (Squire, 1993; George, 1993).

There is little doubt that ethical issues will continue to loom large in the real world of case management. The potential conflict between service aims (for example, hospital closure) and client choice (for instance, to remain in hospital) noted in the Wakefield project (Richardson and Higgins, 1990) is not the only issue over which compromise may be necessary. Lieberman (1990), in describing the EPIC project in

Stirling, highlighted the impossible question of what happens to clients when a project's budget ceiling is reached. The UKCC (1989, 1992a) emphasizes nurses' prime responsibility towards clients and it is, indeed, encouraging to note that the health visitor on the case management team of this particular project was very clear about her own professional accountability. However, this ideal is not always easy to effect. Indeed, where rationing and compromises are inevitable, it may well place nurses in an invidious position.

Two final areas of concern for nurses involved in case management initiatives are those of administrative burdens and coping with change. The extra paperwork generated through the new assessment procedures in particular has been noted (Carlisle, 1992; Squire, 1993). Another issue is the pace with which the necessary change has been introduced (Carlisle, 1992; Fry, 1992). All these issues appear to be emerging across a wide range of nurse-related projects on the evidence of current research (Bergen, 1994).

But, lest it be thought that the prospect for community nurses in case management is seen to be a wholly negative experience, the outcomes resulting from those initiatives already evaluated are encouraging. Whether in terms of enabling dependent clients to remain at home, the increasing focus on consumer evaluation or some other measure, the evidence appears to be that case management can be a positive practice happening for nurses and their patients in the community (Steward, 1990; Drozd and Gabell, 1991; Brunnen and Korczak, 1993; Squire, 1993).

● **Conclusion**

There is, however, much still to be done in the area of nursing research into case management, the third key area for debate highlighted above. The more substantial general research has, perhaps, led the way here at least methodologically, if not in focus. The danger, without such research, is that positive outcomes will fail to be linked, within the multi-agency input, to particular nursing dimensions. The challenge for practice in the 1990s is for nurses to demonstrate their potential in the area, without diluting the professionalism which is uniquely theirs.

References

Archer, R. and Robertson, G. (1990) *Andover case management project: services for people with a mental handicap*. First Year Report, Hampshire Social Services, Winchester

Audit Commission (1992) *Community Care: Managing the Cascade of Change*, HMSO, London

Beardshaw, V. (1991) *Implementing assessment and care management: learning from local experience 1990–1991*. King's Fund College Paper 3, King's Fund, London

Beardshaw, V. and Towell, D. (1990) *Assessment and case management: implications for the implementation of 'Caring for People'*. King's Fund Briefing Paper 10, King's Fund, London

Bergen, A. (1992) Case management in community care: concepts, practices and implications for nursing. *Journal of Advanced Nursing*, **17**, 1106–1113

Bergen, A. (1993) Towards community care: methodological and sampling issues in obtaining a preliminary overview of current nursing practice. *Journal of Health and Social Care in the Community*, **1**, 307–318

Bergen, A. (1994) Case management in community care: identifying a role for nursing. *Journal of Clinical Nursing*, **3**, 251–257

Bowling, A. (1981) *Delegation in General Practice: A Study of Doctors and Nurses*, Tavistock, London

Brittian, O. (1992) Community nurses' views on care management. *Health Visitor*, **65**(10), 365–367

Brunnen, V. and Korczak, E. (1993) Making teamwork work. *Primary Health Care*, **3**(3), 6–8

Cambridge, P. (1990) Ways forward. *Community Care*, **837**, 25–28

Carlisle, D. (1992) All change. *Nursing Times*, **88**(22), 28–30

Challis, D., Chessum, R., Chesterman, J., Luckett, R. and Traske, K. (1990) *Case Management in Social and Health Care: The Gateshead Community Care Scheme*, PSSRU, University of Kent, Canterbury

Challis, D., Darton, R., Johnson, L., Stone, M., Traske, K. and Wall, B. (1989) *Supporting Frail Elderly People at Home: The Darlington Community Care Project*, PSSRU, University of Kent, Canterbury

Challis, D. and Davies, B. (1986) *Case Management in Community Care: An Evaluated Experiment in the Care of the Elderly*, PSSRU/Gower, Aldershot

Dant, T., Gearing, B., Carley, M. and Johnson, M. (1989) *Keyworkers for elderly people in the community: case managers and care co-ordinaters*. Open University/Department of Health and Social Welfare/Policy Studies Institute, Project Paper 1, Milton Keynes

DHSS (1988) *Community Care: Agenda for Action* (the Griffiths Report), HMSO, London

DoH (1989) *Caring for People*, White Paper, HMSO, London

DoH (1990) *Caring for People – Implementation documents. Draft guidance: assessment and case management*, HMSO, London

DoH – Social Services Inspectorate (1991a) *Care Management and Assessment: Practitioners' Guide*, HMSO, London

DoH – Social Services Inspectorate (1991b) *Care Management and Assessment: Managers' Guide*, HMSO, London

Drozd, E. and Gabell, M. (1991) Working together. *Senior Nurse*, **11**(2), 36–40

Ford, R., Cooke, A. and Repper, J. (1992) Making a point of contact. *Nursing Times*, **4**(88), 40–42

Ford, R., Repper, J., Cook, A., Norton, P., Beadsmoore, A. and Clark, C. (1993) *Implementing Case Management*, Research and Development for Psychiatry, London

Fry, A. (1992) Caring for the community. *Nursing Times*, **11**(88), 16–17

George, M. (1993) The good, the bad and the ugly. *Nursing Standard*, **7**(28), 22–23

Henderson, A. (1990) The monitoring of psychiatric patients. *Nursing Standard*, **4**(3), 28–31

Hunt, J. (1981) Indicators for nursing practice: the use of research findings. *Journal of Advanced Nursing*, **6**, 189–194

Hunter, D.J. (1988) *Bridging the Gap: Case Management and Advocacy for People with Physical Handicap*, King Edward's Hospital Fund, London

Knapp, M., Cambridge, P., Thomason, C., Beecham, J., Allen, C. and Darton, R. (1992) *Care in the Community: Challenge and Demonstration*, PSSRU, University of Kent at Canterbury/Ashgate

Korczak, E. (1993) Preparing for joint assessment. *Primary Health Care*, **3**(2), 6–8

Lieberman, S. (1990) It can be done. *Community Care*, **843**, 26–28

Mason, P. (1992) Gathering momentum. *Nursing Times*, **88**(22), 26–28

Morrison, A. (1991) The nurse's role in relation to advocacy. *Nursing Standard*, **5**(41), 37–40

Onyett, S. (1992) *Case Management in Mental Health*, Chapman and Hall, London

Ovretveit, J. (1992) Fulfilling the need for a co-ordinated approach. Case management and community nursing. *Professional Nurse*, **7**, 264–269

Peck, E. (1991) *From genesis to revelation: an evaluation of the creation and operation of the Blaydon assessment and care management pilot project*. HMSU Occasional Paper No. 11, University of Newcastle upon Tyne

Pilling, D. (1992) *Approaches to Case Management for People with Disabilities*, Disability and Rehabilitation Series No. 1. Jessica Kingsley, London

Repper, J. and Peacham, W. (1991) A suitable case for management? *Journal for Psychiatric Nurses (Nursing Times)*, **87**(12), 62–65

Richardson, A. and Higgins, R. (1990) *Case management: reflections on the Wakefield case management project*. Working Paper No. 1, Nuffield Institute/ University of Leeds, Leeds

Richardson, A. and Higgins, R. (1991) *Doing case management: learning from the Wakefield case management project*. Working Paper No. 4, Nuffield Institute/ University of Leeds, Leeds

Rodrigues, L. (1992) A bright future for community nursing. *Health Visitor*, **65**(10), 363–364

Ryan, P., Ford, R. and Clifford, P. (1991) *Case Management and Community Care*, Research and Development for Psychiatry, London

Squire, C. (1993) Health visiting and the case manager role. *Health Visitor*, **66**(4), 127–129

Steward, H. (1990) Help from home. *Health Service Journal*, **100**(5182), 24–25

Thomas, J. (1992) Package deals. *Nursing Times*, **88**(29), 48–49

Thornicroft, G. (1991) The concept of case management for long term mental illness. *International Review of Psychiatry*, **3**, 125–132

Trotter, B. (1992) Team spirit. *Nursing Times*, **88**(28), 33–35

UKCC (1989) *Exercising Accountability*, UKCC, London

UKCC (1992a) *Code of Professional Conduct for Nurses, Midwives and Health Visitors*, 3rd edn, UKCC, London

UKCC (1992b) *The Scope of Professional Practice*, UKCC, London

31

Community development: innovation in practice

Fedelmia O'Gorman

● **Introduction**

In the past 20 years or so, a growing community health movement has arisen in the UK with its origins based on the successes learnt from the economic and social regeneration programmes in the developing world. Indeed, community participation is now on government agendas, particularly since the World Health Organisation Alma Ata Declaration (WHO, 1978) and the 38 targets for 'Health for All by the Year 2000'. Subsequent work in the Ottawa Charter (WHO, 1986) and 'Healthy Cities' projects (Ashton and Seymour, 1988) have challenged statutory sectors to adopt strategies to combat inequalities in health through reorientation towards primary health care, community participation and intersectoral co-operation.

Community development is the term most frequently used to describe an approach which aims to maximize community participation in the planning and implementation of health-enhancing activities. The Alma Ata Declaration stated the case for community development.

The community development process prioritises work with disadvantaged and deprived groups in society, often around issues related to inequalities in health. To address these inequalities the communities must be empowered to take their place in an equal partnership at all levels of decision making related to their health.

This statement encompasses all the key ingredients of the community development movement. Put more simply, community development is a process by which a community defines its own needs and acts to make them known to service providers. The purpose of this chapter is therefore to explain, clarify and relate the concepts of community development to community health care nursing practice. The first stage of the process is to define the terms making up the concept of community development.

● **Community**

The word community has a multiplicity of meanings and uses. It has international connotations such as 'the European Community', while at a national level 'the whole community' often refers to either the population in general or to localities. It is used to describe occupational roles in public services, especially in the Health Services, with terms such as community nurses and dietitians commonly used. Community is frequently thought of as either a geographical locality, a neighbourhood, or a set of relationships. Williams (1976) described it as a 'warmly persuasive word', whereas other authors have described it in terms of a social structure or social activity (Luker and Orr, 1992), evoking notions of people caring for each other, or solidarity, security and sense of belonging (Clarke, 1973).

Communities may be hard environments to live in, however. Noisy or disruptive neighbours, petty crime and assaults – or the fear of these – can mar the lives of vulnerable people in particular. There may be partisan loyalties based on cultural or religious differences, for example between Catholics and Protestants in certain areas of Northern Ireland, or racial tension in inner city areas in Britain. Weiner (1975) describes the factional effects of a hierarchical structure based on extended family networks in a local community in Belfast.

Mayo (1994) argues that communities' own concepts of themselves are dynamic and changing rather than constant and static. This may be because of gradual processes of social changes, but may also be as a result of an event or crisis which acts as a catalyst. An illustration is provided by the 1984–85 mining strike: in communities where strike action was solid, community solidarity was strengthened, but in other villages where some miners worked on, old conflicts were exacerbated (Waddington *et al*. 1991). Another example is that of the Ancoats community in Manchester which mounted collective action when the local accident and emergency wing was threatened with closure, and thus avoided closure (Sutcliff, 1994).

In other communities, activity is initiated as a result of raised awareness of a long-standing problem. An example is provided by the Blackstaff Community Project, where during a meeting of the local community centre management committee, made up of a representative of user groups, the issue of Belfast's centenary celebrations arose. Local people noted that some housing in the area had hardly improved in those hundred years. A community profile developed which included not only poor housing but also health status, health services and the general environment (Blackstaff Community Health Profile, 1991).

● **Meanings of health and lay perceptions of health**

In addition to the plethora of evidence about structural inequalities in health, there is now a substantial amount of literature about people's perceptions of their health, and maintenance of health and disease. Definitions of health have been debated before and since the famous WHO (1946) declaration of health as not just the 'absence of disease', but instead a holistic concept involving a complete sense of 'well being'. Health has also been identified as a function or an experience. Among functional explanations is that of Parsons (1951), who viewed health as the capacity to create wealth (Calnan, 1987). Experiential explanations include health as a 'capacity for human development' (Kelman, 1975). Anderson (1984) defined health as a:

- product or outcome
- capacity or potential to achieve goals or perform functions
- dynamics process, or
- as an attribute.

A useful review of definitions of health is provided by Seedhouse (1986). Lay perceptions of health reflect these explanations of health (Blaxter and Paterson, 1982). Williams (1983) and Pill and Stott (1982), in separate studies, found that health was perceived mainly as absence of disease and the ability to work, therefore, a functional capacity. Cornwall (1984) argues that lay health beliefs may be broadly divided into two different types: public and private. Public accounts include moralistic ideas of worth, justice or fairness. People see bad health as a punishment or a lottery. The ultimate responsibility for health loss or maintenance is with the individual. Private accounts are much more to do with context such as gender, personality and social class. The first explanation fits with traditional medical ideology and current government policy, which emphasizes individual responsibility. The latter accords with the WHO, Alma Ata and the Ottawa Charter, which acknowledge social determinants of health.

Blaxter and Paterson (1982) describe pragmatic attitudes towards health among working class women which reflect the realities of their lives. First, there were lower expectations of normal health and, secondly, women in the study tended to redefine ill-health as normal. Ability to work and 'no time' to be ill were shown to be important coping factors which fit with lower expectations and experience of life. A more recent study by Popay (1992) supports this view.

Responsibility for health maintenance is also the subject of continuing debate. Issues include whether health policies should reflect needs perceived by the people or whether they should be directed by government policy. This raises questions as to whether health policies should have an individualist or collective orientation. Graham (1979) argues that current health policies place too much responsibility for health on individuals, particularly as socio-economic disadvantages in themselves may be sufficient to impede behaviour change (Graham, 1984).

Pill and Stott (1982), in their research in South Wales, found that attitudes towards responsibility for health differed in ways which have important implications for health promotion activities. People in the study divided into three groups:

- lifestylists – those who stressed the importance of making appropriate choices in lifestyle to improve health, such as not smoking
- moralists – those who believed that individuals should not 'give in' to ill health
- rejecters – those who refuted the notion that the individual was responsible for his own health.

In a later study, Calnan (1987) found that middle class women were more likely to favour individual responsibility for health than working class women. In addition, middle class women were more likely to believe in the preventability of major diseases such as cancer and heart disease. Calnan explains the scepticism of working class women in terms of their relative deprivation and lack of control of major factors which influence their quality of life.

Indeed, these views of working class respondents in studies on lay perceptions of health reflect the 'culture of poverty' described by Lewis (1968), a culture characterized by marginality, helplessness and dependence. Working towards behavioural changes by individuals may be an extremely difficult task if these socio-economic and cultural factors are not taken into account. Blaxter and Paterson (1982) suggest that behavioural changes for health require an orientation by the individual towards the future, which may be impossible for individuals burdened by poverty or other disadvantages.

Lay health workers

Along with contextual factors inherent in lay perceptions of health is the relationship between health professionals and clients which is characterized by a mismatch of language usage, knowledge base and values. A study by Rogers and Shoemaker (1971) looked at the conditions necessary for behavioural change through the work of opinion leaders. More effective communication is possible where both the person giving and the person receiving the message share the same culture and values.

The underlying theory known as innovation diffusion has shown successful outcomes, most notably in the North Karelia Project in Finland (Puska, 1995). There, opinion leaders were recruited to assist in a comprehensive community-based programme to reduce the high rates of cardiovascular disease in the region. After four years, cardiovascular disease was reduced significantly compared to the rest of Finland. In addition, there was a 28% decrease in smoking as well as changes in dietary and exercise habits.

In some programmes, lay health workers are employed to act as change agents, by helping the community to develop awareness of the factors causing ill-health through education, and assisting them to change such factors. Underpinning this concept and the ethos of community development in general is the work of Friere (1973). He believed that through the education process, when both teacher and learner gain from each other's experience, the community can achieve 'critical awareness' and so be empowered to act. Lay health workers have been employed in north and west Belfast to assist the health visiting and district nursing teams in the first instance. They have been accepted by clients and patients often because of the fact that they were not professional. Indeed, their success has been attributed to the fact that 'she wasn't a professional and she wasn't family' (Lay Health Workers' Project, 1990).

In developing or poor countries, lay workers have also been used to fill a gap in the absence of other health professionals. With the advent of skill mix, this role is occurring in the UK also. The work of village health workers or community health workers will be determined by local needs, mainly for health education and basic health care procedures such as immunizations. This is known as a service extension role, which has been described as extra hands to do the work (Walt, 1990).

Lay health workers in Belfast have straddled both service extension and change agent roles by developing work with local communities, particularly women's groups. Peer education programmes have been used as an effective way of getting health messages about drugs and sexual health to young people. In communities with non-English-speaking members, Asian lay workers have been used to provide health promotion. Newman and Ramaiah (1990) describe a scheme for a mainly Muslim population in Middlesbrough. In Nottingham, an Asian community Mothers' scheme provides support for mothers in that community (Jackson, 1992).

Therefore, following the definitions of the major concepts making up community development, the main features of the community development process (adapted from Gulbenkian Foundation, 1968; Bryant, 1972; Hubley, 1979) can be described as:

- holistic, in that it recognizes the relationship between the individual and the environment – it does not compartmentalize problems into health, housing, environment or education
- it is area based as it does not target individuals' behaviour or target groups within a community
- it encourages the community to identify their own needs rather than impose professionally determined priorities
- it assumes the need to confront discrimination or racism and to involve marginalized groups
- it acknowledges that outcomes are often unpredictable which has implications for the type of evaluation used
- it provides resources for health information and support for self-help groups.

In addition, implicit with the process, is collaboration and co-operation between statutory and voluntary agencies and the community. The overall aim is to work together to reduce inequalities in health and in access to health care.

● The history of community development

As stated earlier, community development has it origins in economic and social regeneration programmes in developing countries. The success of programmes led health planners to use this approach to tackle health inequalities in emerging countries and later in developed countries (Walt, 1990). Indeed, the impetus for countries to adopt community development methods arose from:

- the rediscovery of inequalities in health, in particular the links with poverty, and the fact that affluence did not 'trickle down' to improve the lives of the poor

- the disillusionment with medical models of care and 'high tech' medicine in the prevention and treatment of many of the major health problems of communities, such as malnutrition
- an association with the shift to primary health care and adoption of preventive and health promotion strategies (Rifken, 1985).

In Britain, lessons learnt from the developing world and the American 'War on Poverty' in the 1960s resulted in a Community Development Project launched by the Home Office in 1969. The projects in 12 local authority areas were considered by the Home Office to be part of 'a radical experiment' involving central and local government, voluntary agencies and the universities in a 'concerted search' for solutions to deprivation (Lee and Smith, 1975).

The Gulbenkian Report *Community Work and Social Change* (Gulbenkian Foundation, 1968) led to the establishment of community development posts within social work and community education sectors. In the following years the number of such posts and projects has multiplied, tackling social, economic and environmental problems as well as health issues. In addition, welfare and self-help groups, the feminist movement and black and ethnic minority movements campaigned and pressurized to increase awareness of and demand action against institutionalized racism and sexism as well as health issues (Mayo, 1994).

The consequence of this activity was the establishment of alternative approaches to health care and social support such as Well Women's centres, child care, Women's Aid and Rape and Incest lines. All of these approaches are examples of the radical shift in women's expectations and autonomy, and their contribution to the growth of the community development movement.

Another contributory factor to community development was the publication of the Black Report (Black, 1980) on socio-economic inequalities in health. Although not welcomed by the government, it showed that there were large differences in mortality and morbidity which favoured higher socio-economic groups. These inequalities were not being redressed by existing health and social services. The report, which became a model for similar work in other countries, also highlighted what is called the 'inverse care law', namely that those most in need are least likely to receive health care (Hart, 1971). In the 1990s, even with new methods of analysing data, such as 'years of potential life lost', there is a widening differential between the best and the least well off in society. Indeed, an analysis by Smith *et al.* (1990) indicates that 10 years after the Black Report there are:

- widening social class differences in mortality
- widening social class differences in health and illness
- trends in distribution of income which suggest that further widening of mortality differentials may be expected
- health inequalities, which have been shown in all countries which collect similar data.

It is factors such as these which have led to the growth of community development as a means of providing alternative health care to overcome the health problems.

● **The process of community development**

This is the development of dialogue between the professional worker and community, with the aim of working in an equal partnership. It demands the sharing of knowledge, skills and experience which for those professionals concerned means acknowledging that people know what their needs are. It means being non-directive even when the perceived needs of the community differ from those of the professional (Batten, 1967).

However, as discussed in Chapter 28, members of the community may not have the confidence or the skills to articulate their needs, nor indeed is there consensus between individuals within groups about their needs. The aim of the community development approach is to build trust, and develop skills and confidence in the group as a whole and in individual members. To facilitate the process the worker must be skilled at listening and communicating. This requires workers to be non-judgemental and honest when there are issues which are beyond their capabilities. The emphasis must be on the identification of needs, prioritizing them and facilitation of activities to address them. Indeed, in community development the process is considered as important as the outcomes of a project. The underpinning aim is empowerment, so that the community are no longer 'passive recipients' of health care and professional expertise, but 'active doers', who are autonomous and self-reliant. The worker aims to be an enabler in this process and not a provider. This process is outlined in Table 31.1.

The important element in the community development approach is co-operation, not only between professional workers and the community but also between these and local representatives of statutory and

Table 31.1 Process of community development (After Youd and Jayne, 1986)

1   Get to know community:
        use local statistics
        develop a community profile
2   Contact informal leaders:
        listen to their perceived needs
3   Jointly decide on priorities for action:
        if possible, plan short-, medium- and long-term objectives
        decide on what to tackle first
4   Decide jointly on details of what is to be done:
        who will do it
        when and how they will do it
5   Identify resource needs:
        sources of funding
6   Decide on evaluation
7   After an activity, such as health fair or course on health issues,
        analyse evaluation and identify unforeseen problems
8   Plan future action
9   Share with a wider audience:
        report
        publicity or exhibition

voluntary agencies. By working co-operatively, community mistrust and long-standing barriers will slowly lessen. Implicit within this process is the essential role of community participation.

● **Community participation**
The WHO Alma Ata Declaration (WHO, 1978) states that

People have the right and duty to participate individually and collectively in the planning and implementation of their health care.

The UKCC Code of Professional Conduct (UKCC, 1992) states that nurses, midwives and health visitors should work in a co-operative way with patients and clients, foster independence, and recognize lay involvement in the planning and delivery of care. However, participation is a word which has many shades of meaning, ranging from real power on decision-making to mere token consultation (Hubley, 1979).

Token consultation or involvement may be a means of achieving community compliance with local health promotion priorities determined by the statutory organization. To illustrate this concept, the example of a Community Health Trust, required to work towards 'Health of the Nation' targets for a purchasing Health Authority or Board, is considered. Although a smoking cessation course may be started in a local community centre with permission from the centre user committee, whether it is successful or not is a variable which is not within the control of even the most energetic health professional. Participants need to feel that they share control in deciding course content; indeed, one of the recognized truths of the community development movement is that a sense of ownership is a vital ingredient to the success of any community health project (McCloskey and O'Gorman, 1991).

This type of community involvement is a commonly used method of working with community groups in the planning and implementation of health activities. However, a more participative approach will establish the felt needs of the community as a starting point for action. An additional advantage of this approach is that needs such as high numbers of child accidents may highlight environmental problems such as poor housing, busy through-traffic or dangerous play areas, which can then be addressed by an intersectoral approach to health care.

Many models of community participation are used in the variety of current community health care projects in the UK. The degree or level of participation depends largely on where the project was initiated, and

Table 31.2 Community participation models (After Rose and Watt, unpubl., by permission)

Model	Knowledge bases	Who sets goal
Involvement	Medical science	Health professionals
Partnership	Medical science and experience	Health professionals and community
Grassroots/community	Experience	Community

whether by a professional worker and/or the community. The main types of models are summarized in Table 31.2. The following discussion gives practical example of each of the models.

Models of community participation

Involvement
This is the approach of most preventive strategies in the health service whether at a primary, secondary or tertiary level. It is professionally led, and encourages compliance by the consumers of health services in achievement of health gain through the prevention or early detection of disease and the promotion of healthy life styles.

> The Strelley Nursing Development Unit in Nottingham has explored new ways of targeting need and working in partnership with clients and the community. Twenty-one wide-ranging projects have been undertaken on topics such as community profiling, women's health and domestic violence, food and child accident prevention (Brummell, 1993).
>
> Reduction in teenage pregnancies in the South Kent Community Healthcare Trust area is an initiative by a school team based on research on the perceived needs of local young people. Clinic sessions are held to provide information, counselling and practical help for the under-19 age group. In the first year the conception rate dropped by 16% or 85 fewer conceptions (DoH, 1993).

Partnership
Regardless of how the project is initiated, in this model all participants share in the development of the work. The resulting sense of ownership brings positive outcomes which go beyond achieving narrow definitions of health gain. The term partnership is now embedded in most mission statements in every part of the NHS, presenting challenges and opportunities for all practitioners in the community.

> The 45 Cope Street Health Project is an example of multi-disciplinary work initiated by health visitors and midwives. Its aims are to work in partnership with young pregnant women and parents to help them to improve their health by building self-confidence and self-esteem (Billingham, 1989; McKeith *et al.*, 1991).
>
> The Pilton Community Health Project was originally founded by a health visitor in the early 1980s. It has developed a wide range of programmes in the Pilton area of Edinburgh with a high level of

participation by local people. Activities include working with groups through all age ranges and stages of life on projects such as a food co-operative, a Mental Health Forum and Tranquillizer campaign, conferences and events on women and food (Wynn-Williams, 1986).

Grassroots- or community-led initiatives

This is probably the most common model of community participation, with a history which predates professional involvement. It was the success of the community at finding solutions to local environmental, housing and social problems which attracted policy-makers to alternative ways of tackling health problems. Community groups who organize themselves often utilize the services of various professionals to share information.

The Women's Information Group is an umbrella group for women's groups in Belfast. For 14 years, monthly information days have been organized to provide a forum for education on a wide range of topics such as benefits, housing, health and child care. Two hundred women attend the information days from all parts of Belfast, with transport and crèche provided.

● Evaluation of community development programmes

Evaluation is an integral part of community development projects primarily because funders usually require progress reports to justify the financial support provided. In addition, project workers are also accountable to their employers, to the community and to their professional body. One definition of evaluation is the use of information to assess the effectiveness of the programme as well as to establish whether aims have been achieved (CAPT, 1993). In a comprehensive study of evaluation in community projects, Feuerstein (1986) states that evaluation 'simply means to assess the value of something'.

In most nursing and health promotion activities, outcomes are used to evaluate delivery of service and change in lifestyles, respectively. A quantitative approach such as this is not appropriate in community development where, as previously discussed, process is equally important. Qualitative methods will therefore produce more meaningful information to enable a project to develop.

In an account of process evaluation in 45 Cope Street, Rowe and McKeith (1991) describe how individuals, groups and workers provide feedback on their feelings about the content and progress of the project work, which includes courses, group sessions and the processes used.

Feuerstein (1986) recommends this type of participatory evaluation as a way of making methods suit the people and their situation.

The success of the community development approach and therefore factors to be evaluated include:

- raised self-esteem, knowledge and skills among all who participate
- provision of a model which can be replicated
- generation of discussion within the neighbourhood and organizations involved
- ongoing assessment of the impact, achievements and problems which can inform future planning.

Evaluation also highlights factors which need to be considered at the project planning stage. The major ones are as follows (adapted from Youd and Jayne, 1986 and Feuerstein, 1986):

- Identification of the expectations and values of the planning group.
- The aims and objectives of the programme. These need to be broken down into manageable strategies by asking: What needs to be done? How is it going to be achieved? What is the timescale? Most community development work will include:
  - (a) short-term projects, such as planning a series of meetings or an information day
  - (b) medium-term projects, such as building a neighbourhood profile
  - (c) long-term projects such as securing core funding.

All of these require interim goal-setting:

- The development of a recording system and decisions as to who is going to collate the information and to whom the information is aimed.
- Funding organizations will require as much 'hard' data as possible. Examples of recording methods include questionnaires, interviews, attendance sheets, and notes on meetings. Decide on the best time to collect information.
- An analysis of information and the best method to present the results. Several methods may be necessary to disseminate information about a particular piece of work, including:
  - (a) a detailed report for funders/employers of statutory agencies
  - (b) a summary report for the local community, press releases or articles for local media, public launch, making a video.
- On the basis of new information consider if aims and objectives have been met, and decide on strategies for future development.

Evaluation linked to other research can be used to inform purchasers or commissioners of service about areas of need and the value or potential of innovative practice. In the absence of measurable outcomes, it can be used to audit core values such as equity and user satisfaction, which commissioners are responsive to (Goodwin, 1995).

● **Barriers to community participation**

Professionalism

Community health care nurses have a high level of expertise in primary, secondary and tertiary prevention of ill-health. This knowledge base and their professional status have traditionally given them the authority to decide what clients need rather than what the client wants (Goode, 1966). These elements in the professional role of nursing provide a major barrier to an equal partnership between nurses and their clients, whatever the care setting. Indeed, although nurses see themselves as advocates for clients, professionalism can in itself mitigate against this because of the unequal share of power and knowledge (Porter, 1988). Therefore, meaningful participation requires nurses to re-orientate their attitudes towards patients, clients and communities. This involves an acceptance of the rights of individuals to be involved in planning and policy-making and abilities of people to make their own health choices. However, it is important to acknowledge that community health care nurses may also have limited input into policy-making within the provider unit and even less into purchaser policy-making. 'Health of the Nation' targets determine the direction of much health promotion work which may make it difficult to engage in community development work with an open agenda.

In addition, hostile or negative attitudes towards community development work on the part of other colleagues and managers may be a problem. These may take the form of ambivalence or ignorance of the work or a lack of recognition of its validity, particularly if a proposed project is not explicit in purchaser/provider contracting. The community development process may also pose difficulties for demonstrating measurable outcomes, particularly within the short term. GP fundholders may wish to purchase only activities related to their practice population. Therefore, resources for the work may be difficult to find, with project nurses having to spend a considerable amount of time and energy identifying funders. All these issues highlight the fact that the methods used in a participative approach to practice require skills which may demand additional training for practitioners.

Barriers within the community

The community may also have difficulties in participating in community development projects due to the lack of confidence in working with professionals. They may lack the necessary organizational skills, as well as feeling hostile and helpless. In addition, there may be no clear consensus on specific issues within groups about what needs to be done or how it will be tackled. The community may also feel that the professionals concerned have a hidden agenda, particularly where previous interventions, such as housing or health surveys, have left them feeling that they were used for information gathering, especially if they were not informed of outcomes. Other examples include the decline of activities generated from outside or achieving little due to lack of resources or because the worker moved to another job. In addition, they may be unsure of the commitment which will be required of them.

Limits of participation

There are also major issues about which a local community has little opportunity to change collectively. Government policies determining unemployment rates, social benefit levels, NHS provision, food prices all provide examples. Indeed, however effective in generating local action on certain issues, a community development approach will have limited power in effecting major change on needs such as the cost of living. Community groups can, however, lobby local statutory authorities to make their needs known. By networking with other community organizations, community action is much more likely to be effective. Project reports circulated widely, and local media interest, can raise the profile of community activities. Inter-agency co-operation in community development work also increases the likelihood of statutory response. A range of actions may result from successful community activity, and possible examples are as follows:

- implementation of traffic-calming measures in an area where child accident rates are high
- repair of pavements, street lighting, poor housing, or other environmental improvements
- new bus routes
- keeping a local hospital or accident and emergency department open
- obtaining premises from housing authorities for a Women's Centre, environmental groups, playgroups or food co-operatives
- obtaining funds from Voluntary Trusts or Inner City schemes
- forming interest groups for women or elderly people, local health forums and tenants' groups
- networking with other community groups.

Practitioners need to accept that not all initiatives will be successful. However, despite setbacks it is essential to keep to the principles of a participative process which demands honesty as well as positive attitudes. One way of achieving this is to identify targets or aims which can be divided into short, medium or long term. There are usually many issues which need action, so that even if the project has setbacks in achieving some aims, others can progress. By adopting this approach many projects can become successful.

● Issues for community health care nursing

Community profiles

An important component of community development is identifying the health needs of a locality. Profiling, as described in Chapter 23, is one way of achieving this. Obviously, from a community development approach it is most successful when there is active participation by the community. This will need to include communication with key people within the community, both formal and informal leaders, and listening carefully to what they have to say. The use of surveys has the potential to provide information about the perceptions of the community; however, the community should be involved in deciding issues to be included within the questionnaires. Indeed, with some training local people can conduct the interviews and participate in formulating recommendations once the results have been analysed. The Moyard Health Profile (Ginnety, 1985) and the Blackstaff Community Health Profile (1991) provide details of the process of working with communities on developing local profiles.

Health of the nation

The 'Health of the Nation' strategic framework for health targets in England, as well as the parallel strategies in Scotland, Wales and Northern Ireland, have become core objectives for the NHS. At a local level, provider units are required to work towards achieving the stated goals within the key areas. This presents challenges for practitioners attempting to work towards an empowering partnership within communities, where priorities may not be those of the key targets of the 'Health of the Nation' document (DoH, 1992). However, developing a dialogue with the community will allow information about the key targets to spread, which will allow possible methods of combining local needs with health service contracting obligations to emerge. Examples in practice include community action on accident prevention, healthy eating groups and food co-operatives as ways in which 'Health of the Nation' targets have been tackled.

Other examples of community development approaches within the 'Health of the Nation' framework can be found in the NHSME (1993) publication. This includes health visitors in Gateshead who have incorporated both the targets of 'Health of the Nation' and a community development philosophy in five localities. Activities include profiling, working with existing groups, 'drop-in' centres, multi-agency co-operation, networking between groups and safety loan schemes, as well as events such as community festivals, a safety pantomime and a road show. Indeed, although the 'Health of the Nation' is targeted at individual behaviours, it assigns responsibility for action on health across all sections of society. This presents exciting opportunities for collaborative work between health services and other agencies, which in turn presents a major challenge for practitioners in the community.

● Conclusion

The concepts of consultation, participation and partnership have been explicitly stated in all government White Papers since *Working for Patients* (DoH, 1989). Most health authorities support the underlying principles of community development and resource innovative projects, though misunderstandings about the meaning of community development continue. Therefore, this is a time more than ever before, of exciting opportunity and challenge for practitioners to work alongside communities in order to identify health needs and find ways to make an impact on inequalities in health.

References

Anderson, R. (1984) Health promotion: an overview. *European Monographs in Health Education Research*, **6**, 5

Ashton, J. and Seymour, H. (1988) *The New Public Health*, Open University Press, Milton Keynes

Batten, T. (1967) *The Non-directive Approach in Group and Community Work*, Oxford University Press, London

Billingham, K. (1989) 45 Cope Street: working in partnership with parents. *Health Visitor* **64**, 156–157

Black, Sir Douglas (Chair) (1980) *Inequalities in Health. Report of a Research Working Group*, DHSS, London

Blackstaff Community Health Profile (1991). EHSSB, Belfast

Blaxter, M. and Paterson, E. (1982) *Mothers and Daughters. A Three Generational Study of Health Attitudes and Behaviour*, Heinemann, London

Brummell, K. (1993) The public health role at Strelly. In HVA Community Development Interest Group Newsletter, London

Bryant, R. (1972) Community action *British Journal of Social Work*, **2**(2), 205

Calnan, M. (1987) *Health and Illness, The Lay Perspective*. Tavistock Publishers, London

CAPT (1993) *Approaches to Local Child Accident Prevention*, The ALCAP Pack, Child Accident Prevention Trust, London

Clarke, J. (1973) *A Family Visitor*, Royal College of Nursing, London

Cornwall, J. (1984) *Hard Earned Lives*, Social Science Paperbacks, Tavistock Publishers, London

DoH (1989) *Working for Patients*, HMSO, London

DoH (1992) *Health of the Nation. A Strategy for England*, HMSO, London

DoH (1993) *Health of the Nation. Targeting Practice, The Contribution of Nurses, Midwives and Health Visitors*, Department of Health, London

Feuerstein, M.T. (1986) *Partners in Evaluation: Evaluating Community Development and Community Programmes with Participants*, Macmillan, London

Friere, P. (1973) *Education for Critical Consciousness*, Sheed and Ward, London

Ginnety, P. (1985) *Moyard Health Profile*, EHSSB, Belfast

Goode, W.J. (1966). Professions and non-professions. In *Professionalization* (eds H.M. Vollmer and D.L. Mills), Prentice-Hall. Englewood Cliffs, N.J.

Goodwin, S. (1995) Commissioning for health. *Health Visitor*, **68**(1), 16–18

Graham, H. (1979) Prevention and health: every mother's business, sociology of the family, a comment on child health policies in the 1970s. In Harris R. (ed.). *A Sociology of the Family: New Directions for Britain*, Sociological Review Monograph 28, University of Keele

Graham, H. (1984) *Women, Health and the Family*, Wheatsheaf, Sussex

Gulbenkian Foundation (1968) *Community Work and Social Change*, Longman, London

Hart, J.T. (1971) The inverse care law. *Lancet*, **1**, 405–412

Hubley, J. (1979) *Community development and health education*. Discussion paper prepared for the Working Party on Behavioural Research Priorities of the Chief Scientist's Office, Scottish Home and Health Department

Jackson, C. (1992) Community mothers: trick or treat? *Health Visitor*, **65**(6), 199–201

Kelman, S. (1975) The social nature of the definition problem in health. *International Journal of Health Services*, **5**, 625–642

Lay Health Workers' Project (1990) *An Evaluation*, Eastern Health and Social Services Board, Belfast

Lee, S. and Smith, G (1975) *Action-Research in Community Development*, Routledge and Kegan Paul, London

Lewis, O. (1968) *La Vida*, Panther Books, London

Luker, K. and Orr, J. (1992) *Health Visiting: Towards Community Health Nursing*, 2nd edn, Blackwell, Oxford

McCloskey M. and O'Gorman, F. (1991) Blackstaff Community Health Project, *Blackstaff: a community's response to poor housing and ill health*. Paper presented at Housing and Health Conference, Society of Environment Health Officers

McKeith, P., Phillipson, R. and Rowe, A. (1991) *45 Cope Street: young mothers learning through group work*. An evaluation report. Nottingham Community Health, Nottingham

Mayo, M. (1994) *Community and Caring*, St Martin's Press, New York

Newman, A. and Ramaiah, S. (1990) Fit for life in the mosque in South Tees. *Health Visitor*, **63**(9), 310–311

NHSME (1993) *Targeting Practice: The Contribution of Nurses, Midwives and Health Visitors*, Department of Health, London

Parsons, T. (ed.) (1951) *Towards a General Theory of Action*, Harvard University Press, Cambridge, Mass.

Pill, R. and Stott, N. (1982) Concepts of illness causation and responsibility: some preliminary data from a sample of working class mothers. *Social Sciences and Medicine*, **16**, 13–51

Popay, J. (1992) My health is alright, but I'm just tired all the time. In *Women's Health Matters* (ed. H. Roberts), Routledge, London

Porter, S. (1988) Siding with the system. *Nursing Times*, **84**(41), 30–31

Puska, P. (1995) Communication with the population: the North Karelia project. *Journal of Human Hypertension*, **9**(1), 63–66

Rifken, S. (1985) *Health Planning and Community Participation*, Croom Helm, Kent

Rogers, E. and Shoemaker, F. (1971) *Communication of Innovations, a Cross-cultural Approach*, The Free Press, New York

Rose, H. and Watt, A. (unpubl.) *The Background to Community Development in Health*, Bradford University

Rowe, A. and MacKeith, P. (1991) Is 'evaluation' a dirty word? *Health Visitor*, **64**(9), 292–293

Smith, G.D., Bartley, M. and Blane, D. (1990) The Black Report on socio-economic inequalities in health 10 years on. *British Medical Journal*, **301**, 373–377

Sutcliff, P. (1994) Ancoats. Community health in Action. *Health Visitor*, **67**, 1–30

UKCC (1992) *Code of Professional Conduct*, 3rd edn, UKCC, London

Waddington, D., Wykes, M. and Critcher, C. (1991) *Split at the Seams? Community, Continuity and Changes after the 1984-5 Coal Dispute*, Open University Press, Buckingham

Walt, S. (ed.) (1990) *Background to Community Health, The Evolution of a Concept*, Open University Press, Buckingham

Weiner, R. (1975). The rape and plunder of the Shankill. In *Community Action: The Belfast Experience*, Norman Press, Belfast

Whitehead, M. (1988) *The Health Divide*. In *Inequalities in Health*, Penguin, London

WHO (1946) *Constitution*, World Health Organisation, Geneva

WHO (1978) *Alma Ata, Global Strategy for Health For All by the Year 2000*, World Health Organisation, Geneva

WHO (1986) *Ottawa Charter for Health Promotion*, World Health Organisation, Copenhagen

Williams, R. (1976). *Keywords*, Croom Helm, London

Williams, R. (1983) Concepts of health: an analysis of lay logic. *Sociology*, **17**, 185–204

Wynn-Williams, C. (1986) Personal communication. Granton Community Health Project, Edinburgh

Youd, L. and Jayne, L. (1986) *Salford Community Health Project: The First Three Years*, Higher Broughton Health Centre, Salford

Index